◆

# CHILD
# MALTREATMENT

## A CLINICAL
## GUIDE AND REFERENCE

SECOND EDITION

**G. W. Medical Publishing, Inc.**

St. Louis

TO PATTY, PATRICK, LISA,
GABRIEL AND DACEY

◆

# CHILD
# MALTREATMENT

## A CLINICAL
## GUIDE AND REFERENCE

SECOND EDITION

## JAMES A. MONTELEONE, M.D.

Professor of Pediatrics and Gynecology
Saint Louis University School of Medicine
Director of the Division of Child Protection
Cardinal Glennon Children's Hospital
St. Louis, Missouri

## ARMAND E. BRODEUR, M.D., M.RD., L.L.D., F.A.C.R., F.A.A.P.

Professor Emeritus of Radiology and Pediatrics
Saint Louis University School of Medicine
Emeritus Director of Pediatric Radiology
Cardinal Glennon Children's Hospital
Director of Radiology
Shriners Hospital for Crippled Children—St. Louis Unit
St. Louis, Missouri

## G. W. Medical Publishing, Inc.
St. Louis

Publisher: Glenn E. Whaley

Design Director: Glenn E. Whaley

Editor: Elaine Steinborn

Production Manager: Charles J. Seibel III

–Book Design/Page Layout: Christine Bauer, Sue E. White
–Print/Production Coordinator: Charles J. Seibel III
–Cover Design: G.W. Graphics
–Production: Christine Bauer, Sue E. White

Indexer: Linda Caravelli

Publisher:

G. W. Medical Publishing, Inc.
2601 Metro Blvd., St. Louis, Missouri 63043 U.S.A.
ph (314) 298-0330 fax (314) 298-2820
http://www.gwmedical.com

Library of Congress Cataloging in Publication Data
    Child maltreatment / [edited by] James A. Monteleone. -- 2nd ed.
        p.    cm.
    Includes bibliographical references and index.
    Contents: [v. 1]. A clinical guide and reference -- [v. 2]. A comprehensive photographic reference identifying potential child abuse.
    ISBN 1-878060-22-8 (casebound : v. 1 : alk. paper). -- ISBN 1-878060-23-6 (casebound : v. 2 : alk. paper)
    1. Child abuse--Diagnosis. 2. Battered child syndrome--Atlases. 3. Battered child syndrome--Diagnosis. 4. Child abuse--Reporting. I. Monteleone, James A.
    [DNLM: 1. Child Abuse. 2. Child Abuse--atlases. 3. Wounds and Injuries--in infancy & childhood--atlases. WA 320 C53483 1997]
RA1122.5.C49 1998
618.92'858223--dc21
DNLM/DLC
for Library of Congress                97-41395
                          CIP

# CONTRIBUTORS

**Pasquale J. Accardo, M.D.**
Professor of Pediatrics
New York Medical College
Director of Pediatrics
Westchester Institute for Human Development
Valhalla, New York

**Richard C. Barry, M.D.**
Professor of Pediatrics
Saint Louis University School of Medicine
Director of Emergency Care Services
Cardinal Glennon Children's Hospital
St. Louis, Missouri

**Karen M. Bly, R.N., B.S.N., M.A., M.Ed.**
Nurse/Counselor
Child Protection Unit
Cardinal Glennon Children's Hospital
St. Louis, Missouri

**John R. Brewer, M.D.**
Associate Clinical Professor of Pediatrics
Saint Louis University School of Medicine
Medical Director of Grace Hill Neighborhood Health Clinics
St. Louis, Missouri

**Armand E. Brodeur, M.D., M.Rd., L.L.D., F.A.C.R., F.A.A.P.**
Professor Emeritus of Radiology and Pediatrics
Saint Louis University School of Medicine
Emeritus Director of Pediatric Radiology
Cardinal Glennon Children's Hospital
Director of Radiology
Shriners Hospital for Crippled Children
St. Louis Unit
St. Louis, Missouri

**Mary E. S. Case, M.D.**
Associate Professor of Pathology
Saint Louis University Health Sciences Center
Chief Medical Examiner
St. Louis, St. Charles, Jefferson and
Franklin Counties, Missouri

**Kevin Coulter, M.D.**
Associate Clinical Professor
Department of Pediatrics
University of California, San Francisco
Medical Director
Center for Child Protection
San Francisco General Hospital
San Francisco, California

**Oscar A. Cruz, M.D.**
Associate Professor of Ophthalmology
Saint Louis University School of Medicine
Director of Pediatric Ophthalmology
Cardinal Glennon Children's Hospital
St. Louis, Missouri

**Bradley V. Davitt, M.D.**
Assistant Professor of Ophthalmology
Cardinal Glennon Children's Hospital
Saint Louis University School of Medicine
St. Louis, Missouri

**Cassandra K. Dolgin, B.A., J.D.**
Member of the Missouri Bar
Assistant Attorney General
Office of the Missouri Attorney General
Jefferson City, Missouri

**Richard P. Easter**
Chief Investigator
State Technical Assistance Team (STAT)
State of Missouri

**Timothy J. Fete, M.D.**
Associate Professor of Pediatrics
Saint Louis University School of Medicine
Director of the Division of General Academic Pediatrics
Cardinal Glennon Children's Hospital
St. Louis, Missouri

**Allan D. Friedman, M.D., M.P.H.**
Associate Professor, Department of Pediatrics
Case-Western Reserve University
Director, Department of Pediatrics
St. Joseph Mercy Hospital–Oakland
Pontiac, Michigan
Senior Medical Staff
Henry Ford Health System
Detroit, Michigan

**Sheilah Glaze, M.S.W., L.C.S.W.**
Medical Social Worker
Cardinal Glennon Children's Hospital
St. Louis, Missouri

**Jesse A. Goldner, M.A., J.D.**
Professor of Law
Director of the Center for Health Law Studies
Saint Louis University School of Law
Professor of Pediatrics
Professor of Law in Psychiatry
Saint Louis University School of Medicine
St. Louis, Missouri

**Michael Graham, M.D.**
Professor of Pathology
Co-director, Division of Forensic & Environmental Pathology
Saint Louis University School of Medicine
Chief Medical Examiner,
City of St. Louis, Missouri
Deputy Medical Examiner,
St. Louis and Jefferson Counties, Missouri

**E. Richard Graviss, M.D.**
Professor of Pediatrics and Radiology
Saint Louis University School of Medicine
Director, Diagnostic Imaging
Cardinal Glennon Children's Hospital
St. Louis, Missouri

**Stuart L. Kaplan, M.D.**
Professor of Psychiatry
Saint Louis University School of Medicine
Director, Division of Child and Adolescent Psychiatry
Chief, Child Psychiatry
Cardinal Glennon Children's Hospital
St. Louis, Missouri

**Donna M. (Prenger) Kolilis, B.S., Business Administration**
Director of Administration
Missouri Public Service Commission
Past Administrator
State Technical Assistance Team (STAT) and
Child Fatality Review Program
Missouri Department of Social Services

**Gus H. Kolilis, B.S., Education**
Chief, Missouri Capitol Police
Missouri Police Chiefs Association
International Police Chiefs Association
Past Director
State Technical Assistance Team (STAT) and
Child Fatality Review Program
Missouri Department of Social Services

**Gregory D. Launius, M.D.**
Instructor, Department of Radiology
Saint Louis University School of Medicine
St. Louis, Missouri

**Atchawee Luisiri, M.D.**
Associate Professor of Radiology
Saint Louis University School of Medicine
St. Louis, Missouri

**Sandra H. Manske, R.N., M.A., J.D.**
Member of the Missouri Bar
St. Louis, Missouri

**Vicki McNeese, M.S.**
Staff Psychologist
Cardinal Glennon Children's Hospital
Adjunct Instructor of Psychology
Saint Louis University
St. Louis, Missouri

**James A. Monteleone, M.D.**
Professor of Pediatrics and Gynecology
Saint Louis University School of Medicine
Director of the Division of Child Protection
Cardinal Glennon Children's Hospital
St. Louis, Missouri

**Lynn Douglas Mouden, D.D.S., M.P.H., F.I.C.D., F.A.C.D.**
Associate Chief, Bureau of Dental Health,
Missouri Department of Health
Jefferson City, Missouri

**Wayne I. Munkel, M.S.W., L.C.S.W.**
Supervisor of Social Services
Cardinal Glennon Children's Hospital
Lecturer, School of Social Work
University of Missouri–St. Louis
St. Louis, Missouri

**Peggy S. Pearl, Ed.D.**
Professor, Department of Consumer and Family Studies
Southwest Missouri State University
Springfield, Missouri

**Colette M. Rickert, LPCC, A.T.R.-BC**
American Art Therapy Association
American Counseling Association

**Anthony J. Scalzo, M.D., F.A.A.P., A.C.M.T.**
Professor of Pediatrics
Division of Emergency Medicine
Medical Toxicologist and Director, Division of Toxicology
Saint Louis University School of Medicine
Medical Director, Missouri Regional Poison Center at
Cardinal Glennon Children's Hospital
St. Louis, Missouri

**Michael J. Silberstein, M.D.**
Professor of Radiology and Pediatrics
Saint Louis University School of Medicine
St. Louis, Missouri

**Patricia M. Sullivan, Ph.D.**
Professor, Department of Otolaryngology and
Human Communication
Creighton University School of Medicine
Director, Center for Abused Children with Disabilities
Boys Town National Research Hospital
Omaha, Nebraska

**Thomas R. Weber, M.D.**
Professor of Surgery
Saint Louis University School of Medicine
Director of Pediatric Surgery
Cardinal Glennon Children's Hospital
St. Louis, Missouri

**Thomas F. Weeston, M.D.**
Resident of Child Psychiatry
Saint Louis University School of Medicine
Cardinal Glennon Children's Hospital
St. Louis, Missouri

**Barbara Y. Whitman, Ph.D.**
Associate Professor of Pediatrics
Saint Louis University School of Medicine
Director, Family Services and Family Studies
Knights of Columbus Developmental Center
Cardinal Glennon Children's Hospital
St. Louis, Missouri

**James J. Williams, M.D.**
Staff Pediatrician
The Permanente Medical Group
Redwood City, California
Attending Pediatrician
San Francisco General Hospital
San Francisco, California

## THE G.W. MEDICAL PUBLISHING MISSION

*To become the world leader in publishing and information services*

*on child abuse, maltreatment and diseases, and domestic violence.*

*We seek to heighten awareness of these issues and provide relevant*

*information to professionals and consumers.*

A portion of our profits is contributed to non-profit
organizations dedicated to the prevention of child abuse
and the care of victims of abuse and other children
and family charities.

## FOREWORD TO THE SECOND EDITION

We live in a society beset by escalating endangerment of children. At least 1,011,628 children under 19 years of age were victims of abuse and neglect in 1994 and more than 1,000 of these were known to have died as a result. (National Center for Health Statistics, United States, 1996-1997 and Injury Chartbook. Hyattsville, MD: 1997). However, the true number of victims is surely far greater than reported, and the deleterious effects on those children who survive these cruel acts persist for a lifetime.

Dr. Monteleone and his collaborators provide a compelling litany of information to assist in realistically confronting the problem. They underscore risk factors that contribute to abuse, and national statistics show that many of these are dramatically increasing. For example, there has been a doubling of single parent households over the past 25 years, from 4 million to 8 million. Over the same period, the proportion of births out of wedlock has increased from about 11% to 32%.

The authors further illustrate a frequent dilemma—protecting the child while assuring that caregivers are not unjustly accused. All too often this task can seem impossible, the effort and personal emotional risks too great, and the frustrations inevitable.

The importance of strong commitments to accuracy and action goes beyond merely providing a child the opportunity for survival to adulthood. The long-term consequences of such inattention have been made abundantly clear: the abused later become the abusers, and, if unchecked, the whole process will be repeated and amplified in future generations. All who are committed to child health, social improvement, and legal protection must educate themselves carefully about these difficult issues. We must accept our responsibility as advocates for all children at risk. Without this help, they can neither run nor hide from the perpetrators of their misery.

C. George Ray, M.D.
Professor and Chairman
Department of Pediatrics
Saint Louis University
School of Medicine
St. Louis, Missouri

# PREFACE TO THE SECOND EDITION

The first edition of *Child Maltreatment: A Clinical Guide and Reference* was well received by the practitioners dealing with abused children, and serves as the solid foundation on which this revision is based. The expansion represented by this second edition reflects areas that have come to be recognized as important by those dealing with child abuse, as well as more in-depth treatment of topics discussed in the first edition. Seven chapters have been added, covering a range of topics. In addition, more than 40 new illustrations have been included, many in the new Art Therapy chapter.

To further our understanding of the child who is at risk for abuse, a chapter on Developmental Influences has been added. The stages of development that children pass through are described and factors that influence child abuse explained.

The multidisciplinary team approach to caring for children who are abused is emphasized in chapters on Art Therapy, Psychopathology and the Role of the Child Psychiatrist, Developmental Influences, Oral Injuries, Forensic Findings, and Child Fatality Review Teams. Specialists in each of these areas offer insights regarding approaches to managing child maltreatment, including procedures for evaluation and practical guidelines for handling cases.

Another new chapter, Failure to Thrive, helps the reader to understand how to differentiate neglected and abused children from those with organic failure to thrive. This distinction is important in the evaluation of many cases of child maltreatment.

The material in chapters from the first edition has also been updated. There is additional information and illustrations regarding fetal abuse and the use of dolls in disclosures of abuse, an expanded understanding of the credibility of children, and a completely revised printing of the Missouri Child Fatality Teams protocols.

The companion volume to this book, *Child Maltreatment: A Comprehensive Photographic Reference Identifying Potential Child Abuse,* has also been expanded, with the addition of over 180 new photographs. Two new chapters — Art Therapy and The Medical Examiner — have been added, with extensive descriptions of the cases being illustrated. Together these two references present a comprehensive source of information covering all areas of Child Maltreatment.

It is hoped that with the addition of these new chapters and the expansion of existing material, the practitioner who deals with any area of child maltreatment will be fully equipped to assess any situation appropriately and determine the best course of action. The focus of all our work is the children — and we offer this volume as a powerful tool to use in creating a better future for them.

James A. Monteleone, M.D.

# REVIEWS OF THE FIRST EDITION

*"I've been in this business for over 20 years, and this is the first time I can honestly say a reference work has surpassed our expectations.* **Child Maltreatment** *is an invaluable tool to make accurate assessments of child abuse."*

Lloyd Malone, Administrator
El Paso County
Department of Social Services
Colorado Springs, CO

*"The photographic atlas is extremely helpful in evaluation of suspected child abuse injuries. We are not doctors, but we must recognize retinal hemorrhages and long bone and other skeletal injuries caused by abuse." "It's the most comprehensive child abuse reference we've ever seen."*

Deborah Gelb
Manhattan District Attorney
Child Abuse Bureau
New York, NY

*"The picture atlas provides valuable photos." "We only have one two-volume set and we guard it with our lives, it's that valuable. It's a great training aid for our new people. Great resource!"*

Phil Setter
Child Protection Supervisor
Colorado Springs, CO

*"This two-volume set of comprehensive and very valuable material on Child Maltreatment and Abuse is a welcome and timely addition to our understanding of this global problem. Every chapter is an excellent reference for all health care professionals, social services, law enforcement, hospitals, attorneys and anyone who cares for victims of child abuse."*

Ranjit N. Ratnaike, M.D.,
F.R.A.C.P., F.A.F.P.H.M. Director,
International Health Programs,
Department of Medicine,
Queen Elizabeth Hospital
South Australia

*"The books are a state-of-the-art comprehensive text that clearly explains the multiple aspects of child maltreatment. It should serve as an excellent reference source."*

Allan D. Friedman, M.D.
Department of Pediatrics
Saint Louis University School of Medicine
St. Louis, MO

*"I feel that these two books will soon be the pre-eminent references on the issues of child abuse and neglect; and they should be required reading for all health care professionals who work with children and families."*

Lynn Douglas Mouden, DDS, MPH
Associate Chief
Bureau of Dental Health
State of Missouri

*"This two-part book* **(Child Maltreatment)** *provides a comprehensive understanding of the issues raised in child maltreatment cases. It is critical reading for all professionals in the child protection field–attorneys, social workers, law enforcement officers and health care professionals."*

Clire Sandt
American Bar Association
Center on Children and the Law
Washington, D.C.

*"Most comprehensive set of books available on child abuse." "Excellent resource for physicians who care for victims of child abuse. An excellent reference for hospital emergency rooms, physicians, medical students and residents in training!"*

Mark Bugnitz, M.D.
LeBonheur Hospital
Division of Pediatric Critical Care
University of Tennessee
Memphis, TN

*"The Atlas provides the type of high quality detailed photographs of abuse-related injuries that front-line professionals need to understand the complexities of child abuse. We have found this two-volume set particularly valuable to the non-medical professionals to gain a better understanding of injuries children have received and the implications of any related medical diagnoses. The quality of the publication is outstanding."*

Charles Wilson, MSSW
Executive Director
National Children's Advocacy Center
Huntsville, Alabama

*". . . This product is a most valuable reference work for all persons who are involved in the care of children. I have strongly recommended it to concerned colleagues, students, residents and nurses." "You have provided an important service to child advocacy with these books!"*

C. George Ray, M.D.
Professor and Chairman of Pediatrics
Saint Louis University
Health Sciences Center
St. Louis, MO

*". . . these two texts are an absolute necessity for the library of every emergency room, police department, school administration training office and child welfare agency!"* ★★★★★ *"A must-have reference for...any officials who must confront and deal with this issue!"*

Wayne Hill, Sr., BCFE, FACFE
Book Review
Forensic Examiner / Mar-Apr '96

*"There are helpful sample documents, including excellent forms for telephone referrals in cases of child abuse and telephone screening for possible abuse. The book (volume one) also presents sample questions for use in interviewing parents and children about sexual abuse . . . the book's accessibility and relevance make it a fine reference for clinical personnel dealing with child abuse. . . The book's style makes it accessible to nonmedical providers . . . The book of photographs*

*(volume two) addresses an important need in the field of pediatrics . . . The text accompanying the photographs repeatedly emphasizes important issues, including the need to question the proferred history and the need for a developmental assessment of the child in every case of possible abuse . . . The presentation of radiologic differential diagnosis is clear . . . the discussion of the physical examination of sexually abused children is a gem, with a table of the genital findings in abused girls, as well as unusual findings in nonabused children. This section alone makes the book worthwhile . . . Another valuable section, perhaps the most valuable of all, concerns the sexual abuse interview. The authors present a developmentally appropriate approach to interviewing children of various ages . . . these are worthwhile books. Busy clinicians will find the book of photographs especially useful."*

The New England Journal of Medicine
April 6, 1995, Vol. 332, No. 14

*". . . a wonderful addition to the core reference shelf of professionals who work with children . . . The collective expertise represented by the authors is a solid foundation of authority for this work . . . an impressive range of quality photographic records of children's injuries, both abusive and accidental . . . The writing styles are coherent and readable . . . several chapters do an excellent job of laying the ground work for a deeper understanding of violence within families and against children . . . This book also does an excellent job of describing the ambiguities of actual clinical situations. Many cases are described, followed by the examination details and thought process that led to a determination of abuse or of accidental injury . . . Overall, this is a very valuable addition to the reference shelf . . . very readable and accessible, while presenting a complete review of the broad range of abuse . . . This very comprehensive work will meet most needs for both the new learner and the experienced professional."*

Archives of Family Medicine
American Medical Association
Vol. 4, October 1995

# FOREWORD TO THE FIRST EDITION

The abuse and misuse of children are not unique to any time or location. Indeed, infanticide, the ultimate outcome of violence against children, has, throughout various times in history, been an accepted procedure to rid society of deformed and sickly newborns as well as children who were felt to impose an economic hardship to a family unit or community.

In America, the medical profession's role in identifying child abuse was noted in 1946 when Dr. Caffey, a radiologist, described the specific association between healed fractures, subdural hematomas, and child abuse. It was not until 1962, however, when Dr. C. Henry Kempe and his associates published their sentinel paper in the *Journal of the American Medical Association*, that medical professionals recognized the battered child syndrome. Over the next three decades, researchers and practitioners gathered data and advanced the body of scientific knowledge concerning the various etiologies of abuse (psychological, social learning, sociological, cultural, and others), tools/methods to facilitate victim-sensitive interviews (anatomically detailed dolls, puppets, drawings, computer programs, videotaping, etc.), the techniques to enhance the identification of abuse (colposcopy, serologic and immunologic analyses, diagnostic imaging, etc.), and subsequently modalities which address post-assessment interventions (play therapy, art therapy, formal psychological testing, court testimony, etc.).

The various disciplines dealing with abused children represent an interactive and dynamic community of professional groups, including social service, medical, judicial, law enforcement, mental health, and government systems. Each discipline has a specific role both in responding to the violence and interacting with other members of the community — it is the availability and coordination of these independent systems in responding to victims that define the nature and the parameters of the overall response. This lesson is aptly portrayed in this book. Drs. Monteleone and Brodeur and their co-authors have integrated more than 30 years of experience as members of the Cardinal Glennon Child Protection Team with the training and skills they acquired as active participants in the closely knit St. Louis Interagency Task Force.

Many recent books dealing with child abuse and neglect focused on a single aspect of child abuse. Others, in their efforts to reach a broad audience, have omitted crucial information. Drs. Monteleone and Brodeur are to be congratulated. These two physicians and their co-authors have successfully written an exhaustive two-volume reference book to meet the needs of the various disciplines. This text will guide the reader on his or her journey from the initial chapters on the identification and reporting of child abuse, through the more technically complex sections on the medical aspects of diagnosis, to the final chapters focusing on court testimony and the prevention of child abuse.

This comprehensive resource is published as a two-volume set complete with colored illustrations and diagrams. The information is provided in a manner which should hold the interest of both the dilettante and the seasoned professional. In summary, the single criticism noted by this reader is that the authors should have written their very valuable textbook sooner. This text should be considered recommended reading for each of the various disciplines involved in the field of child abuse and neglect regardless of whether the learner is entry level or emeritus.

Howard B. Levy, M.D.
Department of Pediatrics
Grant Hospital of Chicago

# PREFACE TO THE FIRST EDITION

This reference was created to help physicians diagnose child maltreatment, recognize those children at high risk for abuse and neglect, and realize strategies for prevention and intervention in abuse cases. Although the text is approached from a medical point of view, the information contained will also be beneficial to other health care professionals, social service workers, attorneys, law enforcement workers, state agencies, and others who might be involved with abused children. Information concerning physical and psychological abuse, neglect, and sexual abuse, as well as their legal aspects, is collected here in a single volume.

In the mid-1980's the St. Louis Child Abuse Network was involved in a project to review deaths and catastrophic injuries in children that resulted from abuse. The results of that study were released to the media and presented at several medical conferences but were not published. This study was unique in that it collected data not only on severely abused children and their families but also on control groups of mildly abused and nonabused children and their families. Along with other studies at the time, it showed the value of reviewing not only the circumstances of the deaths of abused children, but also the circumstances of suspicious deaths. In 1992 the State of Missouri enacted legislation providing for the establishment of death review teams throughout the state. We share the information about how to set up a death review mechanism in this text.

In the past, books focused on the social aspects of child abuse. But many practitioners believe that the social aspects of child abuse should be the domain of social agencies. Most clinicians want to be able to recognize abuse and to know what to do after they decide they have reason to suspect abuse. While the "why" and the "who" are important, the "how" and the "what" are foremost in their minds and must be addressed.

Recent books written on sexual abuse in children give only passing mention of the importance of the child's disclosure and interview, focusing rather on the physical examination and the physician's role in the process. We believe that the most important aspect of evaluating the sexually abused child in particular is her or his disclosure, because all of the other elements depend on what the child says. The physical examination should not stand alone; it has been proven inadequate because 60% to 70% of the children who have been sexually abused have no physical findings of abuse. In addition, an effective interview determines the "credibility" of the child's statement. Current texts on abuse lack information concerning this vital component.

The contributors to this reference are experts in their fields. Since we felt strongly that no one person could effectively address all aspects of child abuse, we sought specific expertise in each area. These individuals have been involved in child protection activities for significant periods of time and are acknowledged as extremely competent by both their peers and the legal system.

Our laws allow parents broad freedom with regard to child rearing, and this book is not challenging parental rights. We must, however, in our schools, through the media, and in our churches teach parenting skills, proper forms of discipline, normal child behavior, proper toilet training techniques, and effective communication methods. The primary caregiver must have these skills. Clinicians must know when to step in and instruct families in these skills with the goal of preventing child abuse. It is hoped that this book will prove valuable in these endeavors.

James A. Monteleone
Armand E. Brodeur

# TABLE OF CONTENTS

## CHAPTER 13: MULTIPLE PERSONALITY DISORDER . . . . . . 269

## CHAPTER 14: PSYCHOPATHOLOGY AND THE ROLE OF THE CHILD PSYCHIATRIST . . . . . . 281

## CHAPTER 15: SEXUALLY TRANSMITTED DISEASES IN ABUSED CHILDREN . . . . . . 301

## CHAPTER 19: FAILURE TO THRIVE: A RECONCEPTUALIZATION

## CHAPTER 20: PSYCHOLOGICAL ABUSE

♦

# CHILD MALTREATMENT

## A CLINICAL
## GUIDE AND REFERENCE

SECOND EDITION

# Chapter 1

# Identifying, Interpreting, and Reporting Injuries

James A. Monteleone, M.D.
Armand E. Brodeur, M.D.

*A 3-year-old girl was taken to the emergency room after she had fallen down the stairs. She was unconscious and unresponsive. On physical examination, she was found to have ecchymotic areas on her face, chest, abdomen, back, and thighs. All of the injuries were acute and of the same age. CT scan of the head revealed a massive occipital subdural hematoma, and an abdominal CT revealed a laceration of the liver. A social service consult was requested, and the incident was reported to the hotline.*

*The mother was 19 years old and single. She was living with a paramour. The Division of Family Services stated that the child had a similar episode 6 months earlier when the case was opened. The previous incident had been substantiated as abuse, and the child was returned home with the understanding that the paramour would move out of the home. In describing the current incident, the mother said that she and the paramour had gotten "stoned" and the child was thrown against the wall, kicked, and slapped. The child survived, but she was permanently mentally incapacitated. She is presently living in a vegetative state in a chronic rehabilitative state hospital.*

*The mother and paramour were found guilty of child abuse and sentenced to prison.*

Child abuse involves every segment of society and crosses all social, ethnic, religious, and professional lines. The definition of child abuse can range from a narrow focus, limited to intentional inflicted injury, to a broad scope, covering any act that impairs the developmental potential of a child. Included in the definition are neglect (acts of omission) and physical, psychological, or sexual injury (acts of commission) by a parent or caretaker. Intent is not considered in reporting abuse; protection of the child is paramount.

According to the United States Department of Health and Human Services report (1980), the national incidence of countable child maltreatment was 9.8 children per 1,000 population. This totaled about 625,100 children. In 1988 this agency reported that 16.3 children per 1,000 population, or 1,025,900 children, were maltreated. Whether these data reflect an increase in the occurrence of child maltreatment or an increase in the ability of professionals to recognize and report cases is arguable.

We live in a violent society. Children are often the targets of that violence. The violence is most apt to occur in the home and be perpetrated by a family member. Some studies suggest that people who were abused as children are more apt as adults to become perpetrators of abuse than are those who were not abused as children. Social factors—poverty, unemployment, and isolation—are major factors increasing the risk of child abuse (Gelles, 1982).

The diagnosis of the classic battered child who presents with multiple injuries in differing stages of healing is easy for the experienced physician. Determining, with certainty, whether a single injury is accidental or intended is difficult. Inflicted injury is diagnosed when the physician is certain that a single injury in a child could not have been the result of the circumstance described by the caretaker. This decision is based on the physician's clinical experience and reliance on studies in the literature.

Effective strategies to deal with and prevent abuse must involve many disciplines. No one individual, whether pediatrician, radiologist, psychiatrist, nurse, social worker, or juvenile officer, can have all of the answers and consistently make correct decisions without the input from other professionals on the team.

Previously, references dealing with child abuse have concentrated on the social factors—the *who* and the *why* of child abuse. This reference, while not ignoring the who and the why, emphasizes the *what* and the *how*: *what* is abuse, *what* to do when one suspects abuse, and *how* to do it.

## ◆ IDENTIFYING CHILD ABUSE

### NORMAL CHILD DEVELOPMENT AND BEHAVIOR

In evaluating injuries, the age of the child is crucial. Infants who are basically immobile and who are receiving good care rarely suffer injury. When they reach the mobile stage and are learning to walk or crawl, single bruises are generally found as a result of their many falls. Multiple bruises, involving multiple body areas, require multiple impacts, and the history should reflect multiple incidents.

With some exceptions, a child cannot roll over until at least 4 months of age, often not until about 6 months of age. A child will not crawl until about 10 months or walk until about a year old. He will not run well until age 2 and cannot ride a tricycle until about 3. It is also about this time that the child climbs the stairs alternating feet *(see Denver Developmental Screening Test, p. 24).*

Accidental injuries require specific motor skills on the part of a child. A fall from a bed is not possible before the child can roll over; a fall down the stairs is not plausible until the child can crawl. The ability to turn a circular-motion hot water knob and turn on the tap is not possible until approximately 2 years of age. Therefore a 2-month-old infant cannot roll over, let alone crawl, to a radiator to sustain a burn or get into a toxin, and a 2-year-old who has severe buttock burns could not have ridden a tricycle into a space heater.

Occasionally an injury is blamed on a sibling. This explanation is feasible, since children often are abusive to their siblings. However, the evaluator must determine if the injury could have occurred as described and if the sibling is developmentally mature enough to have initiated the injury. It may be necessary to test the child or sibling to see if the action attributed to him or her is possible.

Explanations of injuries must be evaluated using common sense or a sound knowledge of the consequences of routine accidents in the home. For example, a 17-month-old cannot burn his buttocks by climbing onto a space heater and sitting on the top without burning his hands and legs in the climb—assuming he can climb. Similarly, a 5-month-old cannot spontaneously sustain a severe rectal tear and dilated anus, nor can he suffer multiple skull fractures and internal abdominal injuries in a fall from the couch. Finally, a fractured femur does not generally occur when a 5-month-old tangles his leg in a blanket while rolling over.

## CONDITIONS THAT HAVE BEEN CONFUSED WITH ABUSE

A number of conditions over the years have been mistaken for child abuse and have been reported to state protective agencies. It is important that mandated reporters know these conditions and make an effort to identify them. Although it is tragic to miss recognizing a child who has been abused, it is equally tragic to falsely accuse a caretaker of abuse, especially when the child is ill and the allegations add to the caretaker's concerns for the child. A number of systems can be involved: the skin, involving easy bruisability and burns; the skeletal system, with fractures and other bony changes; the eye; and the central nervous system. A list of those conditions that have been reported or that the authors have encountered is given in **Table 1-1**.

Many of the conditions listed in Table 1-1 are one-time occurrences. However, the potential for many more such mistakes is enormous. These unfortunate mistakes can usually be avoided by taking a careful personal and family history and conducting a thorough physical examination. Although a differential diagnosis is not usually needed in abuse, it is needed to avoid these errors.

### Table 1-1. Conditions That Have Been Mistaken for Abuse

| Condition | Presentation | Reference |
| --- | --- | --- |
| Mongolian spots | Apparent bruising to back and buttocks | Asnes, Dungy, Oates, Wheeler and Hobbs, Wickes and Zaidi |
| Postmortem lividity | Bluish discoloration to dependent areas (buttocks, back, ankles) after death | Kirschner and Stein |
| *Folk Medicine* | | |
| Vietnamese | | |
| Coining, Cao gio | Bruises along bony prominences of rib cage, back, and chest | Anh, Du, Golden and Duster Leung, Saulsbury, and Hayden, Silfen and Wyre, Yeatman et al |
| Chinese | | |
| Spoon rubbing | Can include hematuria | Bryan, Rosenblat and Hong |
| Moxibustion | Small circular incense burns at therapeutic points | Feldman, Lee, Reinhart, and Ruhs |

**Table 1-1. Conditions That Have Been Mistaken for Abuse–*Continued***

| Condition | Presentation | Reference |
|---|---|---|
| Russian Cupping | Circular ecchymotic areas to the back | Asnes and Wisotsky |
| Latin American Cupping (ventosos) | Circular first-degree burns to back, abdomen, or chest | Sandler and Haynes |
| Arabs and Jews Maquas | Small deep burns at the site of disease | Rosenberg |
| Mexican Caida de mollera (fallen fontanelle) | Shaken infant syndrome, closed head injury | Guarnaschelli et al |
| Phytophotodermatitis psoralens in plants (limes, parsnips, figs, etc.) | Linear streaking of the dermis to face, hands, chest, and lower legs; may blister. Hand prints may form where the adult touched child | Coffman et al |
| *Easy Bruisability* | | |
| Hemophilia | Ecchymotic areas in various parts of the body at various stages of healing | O'Hara and Eden, Schwer et al, Wheeler and Hobbs |
| Vitamin K deficiency | Cutaneous or internal hemorrhages | Carpentieri et al, Kaplan, Wheeler and Hobbs |
| Leukemia | Ecchymotic areas, contusions, death | McClain et al |
| Henoch-Schonlein purpura | Purpuric lesions on various areas of the body—face, eyes, arms, legs, etc. | Brown and Melinkovich |
| Disseminated intravascular coagulation, meningitis | Multiple bruises, death | Kirschner and Stein |
| Erythema multiforme | Bruises and purpura on various areas of the body | Adler and Kane-Nussen |
| Ehlers-Danlos syndrome | Bruises, scars, open wounds on the head, knees, elbows, or chin | Owen and Durst, Roberts et al, Saulsbury and Hayden |
| *Burns and Burn-like Lesions* | | |
| Epidermolysis bullosa | Blisters to pressure areas | Colver et al, Winship and Winship |
| Impetigo | Blisters resembling cigarette burns | Kaplan, Oates, Wheeler and Hobbs |
| Car seat burn | Blisters, first- and second-degree burns to back, neck, and/or extremities | Schmitt et al |
| Frostbite | Linear burns at moisture points, such as the cheeks, chin, lips, glove and sock lines | Monteleone |
| Wringer injury | Burns to axilla | Monteleone |

**Table 1-1. Conditions That Have Been Mistaken for Abuse–*Continued***

| Condition | Presentation | Reference |
| --- | --- | --- |
| Congenital indifference to pain | Numerous old and recent cuts, scars, bruises, burns | Spencer and Grieve |
| Brain tumor or brain aneurysm | Shaken infant syndrome | Kaplan, McLellan et al |
| Osteogenesis imperfecta | Multiple unexplained fractures | Gahagan and Rimza, Paterson and McAllion |
| Hypogammaglobulinemia or cystic fibrosis | Failure to thrive | Carpentieri et al, Copeland, Wheeler and Hobbs |
| Hair tourniquet | Swelling, erythema of toe or penis | Oates |
| *Genetic Disorders* | | |
|    Mitochondrial disorder, congenital adrenal hyperplasia in a male, diabetes insipidus | Multiple SIDS, severe dehydration, failure to thrive | Monteleone |
|    Methylmalonic acidemia | Poisoning | |
| Congenital syphilis | Periosteal reaction, fractures | Fiser et al, Horodniceanu et al, Kaplan |
| Copper deficiency | Multiple bony abnormalities | Bays |
| Vitamin C or D deficiency | Fracture, metaphyseal and epiphyseal changes | Kaplan |
| Caffey's disease | Swelling of lower extremities | Wheeler and Hobbs |
| Toddler's fracture | Spiral fracture of lower one-third of tibia in toddlers | Kaplan |
| Fractures from passive exercise | Stress fractures to long bones seen in cerebral palsy patients who are receiving physical therapy | Bays |
| *Self-inflicted Injuries* | | |
|    Cornelia de Lange syndrome Lesch-Nyhan syndrome Head-bangers | Variety of cutaneous injuries, bites, burns, and bruises | Bays |

## FOLK MEDICINE

Physicians should become familiar with folk medicine practices in their community and work with organizations that sponsor immigrants in order to educate these individuals concerning acceptable medical care. Among the practices that have been found are the following:

*Cao Gio* is a form of folk medicine practiced by Southeast Asians. The healers follow traditional folk medicine when they rub a coin or a spoon heated in oil on an ill child's neck, spine, and ribs. The practice can cause a burn or abrasion (Gellis & Feingold, 1976) (**Figure 1-1 a,b**).

*Cupping (ventosos)* is practiced by some Latin American and Russian cultures. A vacuum is created under a cup or glass by placing a small amount of material under the vessel on the skin and burning the material. First- or second-degree burns of the area can result.

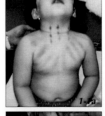
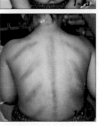

*Figure 1-1 a,b. This is a 4-year-old South Asian girl with severe asthma. Note the typical lesions of coining along the rib cage, back and front. The neck injuries are not typical, but are also coining lesions.*

*Moxibustion,* practiced by Southeast Asians, is a form of acupuncture in which lighted sticks of incense or other material from the herb artemisia are used to make small circular burns on the skin at therapeutic points.

Bedoins, Arabs, and Jews use a treatment called *maquas,* in which hot metal spits or coals are applied to areas near the site of the disease or on a traditional "draining point." Small burns are produced at the site.

*Caida de Mollera* (fallen fontanelle), which is practiced by Hispanics, is an attempt to elevate the fontanelle in children dehydrated from diarrhea and vomiting by holding the child upside down (Guarnaschelli et al., 1972). Retinal hemorrhages may result.

All of these forms of folk medicine are abusive practices done out of ignorance. Every effort should be made to prevent their continuance.

Some states have legislation declaring that it is acceptable to treat an ill child with prayer instead of medical care, provided the religious treatment is in accord with the tenets and practices of a recognized religion, such as Christian Science. However, certain states have removed the faith-healing exemptions from child endangering and neglect statutes, and other states may follow.

## ACCIDENTAL VERSUS INFLICTED INJURIES

Differentiating accidental injuries from inflicted injuries is important in the management of injured children. Errors in diagnosis are both catastrophic and costly for the child and the family. If inflicted injury is not recognized, the child is left in the care of persons who may injure him again. If the diagnosis of inflicted injury is incorrect, parents are wrongfully accused and investigated, and the child and parents may be separated.

**A caretaker rarely reports to an emergency room or physician's office stating that he has abused his child. He will try to convince the staff that the injury resulted from an accident initiated by the child. In order to diagnose abuse one must first believe that abuse is a possibility and effectively eliminate the potential of an accident having produced the presenting injury(ies).**

Children are forward moving and frontal explorers; therefore most accidental injuries involve only one plane of the body, the frontal plane. Specific frontal locations affected are the forehead, nose, chin, palms, elbows, and shins—areas where the bone is close to skin.

Palmar hand injuries can be accidental, occurring when breaking a fall or when exploring a dangerous object, such as a hot iron or a piece of machinery. However, both the palms and the backs of the hands are common areas where punishment is inflicted, and the physician should be alert to the possibility of abuse when there are injuries in these areas, especially when the injuries are symmetrical.

Injuries to the buttocks, genitalia, abdomen, back, and lateral areas of the body, especially the sides of the face, are frequently indicative of abuse. Abdominal bruising is unusual even with blunt trauma. Genital and perianal bruising is usually intentional.

**The evaluator must determine if the injury could have occurred as described. Then it must be determined if this particular child is developmentally mature enough to have caused the injury.** If the parents state that the child sustained the injury by doing something that he is not developmentally able to do or if the injury is too severe to be caused by the incident described, then the history given is incorrect and the evaluator must conclude that the injury was nonaccidental.

*Why does an abusive injury or situation go unrecognized? Several reasons may be cited:*

1. The mandated reporter may not be able to accept that a parent could abuse a child.

2. The examiner may not want to get involved or interfere in what he believes is, rightfully, a family situation.

3. If the examiner lacks proper training in observation, abuse may be overlooked.

4. In general, people tend to believe what they are told and base decisions on that belief.

5. Finally, perhaps most often, when the severely injured child presents to the emergency room, medical staff members concentrate on the problem at hand—respiratory arrest, cardiac arrest, shock, or convulsions—and miss the larger question of overall etiology.

## ♦ INTERPRETING ABUSE INJURIES

### CUTANEOUS INJURIES

Skin injuries are the most common and easily recognized manifestations of maltreatment of children. Human bites are strong indicators of abuse. Bruises can vary from superficial injuries, such as first-degree burns and abrasions, to deeper injuries, ranging from lacerations to second- and third-degree burns. Patterns and locations of these injuries are clues to suspecting child abuse.

### HUMAN BITES

Human bites are intentional and are common injuries in abuse. Trube-Becker (1977) reported 48 autopsied child abuse cases and noted that 11 of the 48 showed human bite marks. He found evidence of bites on the limbs, abdomen, and cheeks. Recognizing human bite marks is particularly important in child abuse cases because forensic dentists can study them and help determine the perpetrator of these injuries (Levine, 1984). Sims et al. (1973) reported three cases of human bite marks occurring in child abuse that were used to identify the perpetrator.

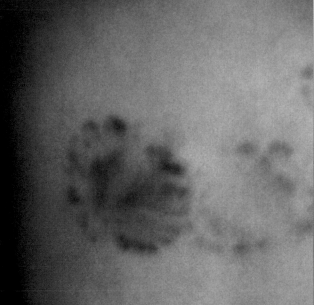

**Figure 1-2.** *Bite injury showing three components.*

Human bite marks can be easily overlooked if one is unaware of their characteristics. The location of bite marks on infants tends to differ from the location on older children. Bite marks around the genitalia or buttocks are usually seen in infants and are inflicted as punishment. Older children have bites associated with assault or sexual abuse; they are generally multiple, random, and well-defined and may be associated with a sucking mark. The sucking mark may be the only indicator noted if sexual abuse has occurred.

There are three components of a human bite to look for: the bite mark, the suck mark, and the thrust mark (**Figure 1-2**). Bite marks are ovoid areas with tooth imprints, and shape and size are significant. The suck mark is caused by a pulling of the skin into the mouth, creating a negative pressure. The thrust mark is caused by the tongue as it pushes against the skin, which is trapped behind the teeth. The inner portion of the bite mark may show no abnormality or may contain the suck or thrust mark. These two marks are similar in appearance in that each resembles a contusion in the center of the mark. To accurately identify a bite mark, each component must be recognized.

The anterior teeth give the human bite mark its configuration, which is the shape of the dental arch. Generally, no one tooth stands out (in contradistinction to the canines in animal bites), and the marks are irregular in size, shape, and position.

The incisor teeth leave narrow rectangles, the canines leave triangular shapes, and the premolars make circular marks. The canines are more likely to be recognizable in bites from adults than in bites from children.

Early recognition of a human bite mark is critical to preserve valuable information. The body should not be washed or an autopsy begun before the marks have been photographed. A measuring device, such as a ruler, should be placed in the field to be photographed and thereby document the size of the mark. A child's bite can be distinguished from an adult's bite by measuring arch and tooth widths. Moorees (1959) found that the difference between a 5-year-old child's arch width and an adult's is approximately 4.4 mm for the maxilla and 2.5 mm for the mandible. The cumulative widths of the six upper teeth of the child were 10 mm smaller than those of the adult. In the lower arch, the differences were approximately 7 mm. If puncture marks from the canines are visible in the bite, it is possible to distinguish bites of permanent teeth (older than age 8) from primary teeth bites because the distance of separation is greater than 30 mm.

## BRUISES

The skin can be a window to deeper injuries. Hemorrhage into deep subcutaneous tissues, such as muscle, will work its way to the surface. The accumulation of blood under the skin will be evident for a number of days, changing color as it ages. A fresh injury is red to blue, with the blue color caused by blood outside the vessels and the red component due to vasodilation with arterial blood visible in vessels; in 1 to 3 days it becomes deep black or purple; in 3 to 6 days the color changes to green and gradually brown; in 6 to 15 days it passes from green to tan to yellow to faded; and finally it disappears. The younger the child, the quicker the color resolves (Wilson, 1977).

Multiple bruises or bruises in inaccessible places are indications that the child has been abused (**Figure 1-3**). In addition, babies who are not mobile do not usually have bruising. The toddler who is learning to walk typically has frontal bruising, as stated earlier. Severe bruising is unlikely. In the older child (age 2 to 5), some parts of the body, such as the knees, shins, forehead, and elbows, are bruised often because these portions of the body are contact points.

Bruises, ecchymoses, and hematomas are the result of abuse when they occur in areas of the body that are unlikely to be injured accidentally. Multiple bruises and bruises of the buttocks or the genital area are usually not accidental. Bruises in different stages of healing are the result of repeated trauma and indicate abuse when the parents give a history describing a single accident. **A significant discrepancy between the physical findings and the history is the cardinal sign of abuse.**

Bruises that take the shape of a recognizable object are generally not accidental. Loop marks are caused by a flexible object, such as a belt, electric cord, or clothesline, folded on itself and used to beat the child (**Figure 1-4**). Multiple curvilinear loop marks on the child are pathognomonic of abuse. These bruises are usually ecchymotic but can be lacerations or abrasions. A hand imprint on a child's face after a slap and finger and thumb marks on an arm or leg where the child was grabbed or squeezed are inflicted injuries. Belt buckles and other synthetic objects used to inflict punishment leave recognizable imprints on the child's skin. Rope burns, bruises, or scars around the arms, ankles, neck, or waist are evidence that the child was tied (**Figure 1-5**). Many of these injuries leave long-lasting scars. There have been incidences when the penis is tied to prevent bed-wetting or pinched as

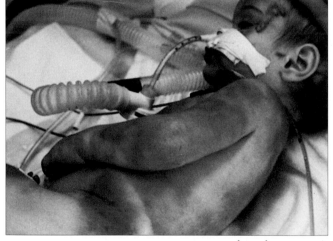

*Figure 1-3*. Child with multiple bruises involving multiple surfaces, on inaccessible places, and in various stages of healing.

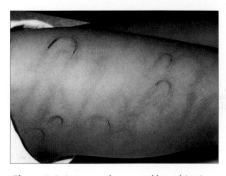

*Figure 1-4*. Loop marks caused by whipping with extension cord.

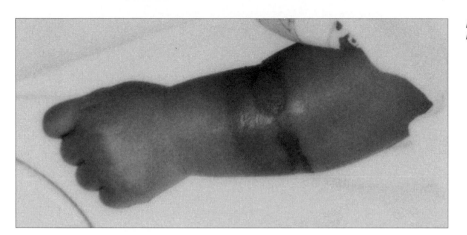

*Figure 1-5*. Circular bruising of wrist caused by restraints.

punishment for soiling (**Figure 1-6**). At autopsy, ligatures around the neck may be identified as a series of small hemorrhages seen in the trachea.

Parents can claim that a child suspected of being abused bruises easily. Coagulation studies, including platelet count, prothrombin time, and partial thromboplastin time, should be ordered in an abuse workup when the child has bruises. Bleeding time is a good screening test in some patients with platelet dysfunction. For completeness, coagulation studies should be ordered for all children presenting with marked bruising. Bleeding disorders, such as hemophilia, are usually diagnosed at an early age, but occasionally a mild form does not manifest until the child is older. The usual age for a bleeding disorder to become evident is when the child begins to walk and cruise, or with the eruption of the first tooth. This, coincidentally, is also the age when child abuse occurs frequently. It is important to note that hemophilia is a stress-producing disease, and hemophiliac children are at increased risk for being abused. Their tendency for easy bruising can mask an intentional injury.

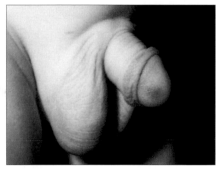

*Figure 1-6*. Ecchymosis of glans penis caused by pinching. Child was disciplined for soiling himself.

## HAIR LOSS

Hair loss (alopecia) can be a manifestation of child maltreatment. Traumatic alopecia occurs when parents pull their child's hair, frequently using the hair as a handle to grab the child and jerk or drag him. Pulling can cause hemorrhage under the galea aponeurotica, which has a rich supply of blood vessels. This accumulation of blood can be an important clue in differentiating between abusive and nonabusive loss of hair. Alopecia can also be a sign of latent syphilis.

*Traumatic alopecia* is defined as the forceful pulling of hair or the breaking of hair shafts by friction, traction, or other physical trauma. The usual causes of traumatic alopecia are trichotillomania or extreme cosmetic practices. Trichotillomania is conscious or subconscious self-induced alopecia caused by plucking, pulling, breaking, or cutting of the hair. The scalp is the most common site of involvement, but the eyebrows and eyelashes may also be affected. The patient plucks, twirls, or rubs hair-bearing areas, resulting in the loss or breakage of hair shafts. Most affected individuals are under varying degrees of emotional stress. Some have severe psychological problems.

Extreme cosmetic practices that can cause this condition are tight braiding or ponytails; the use of tight rollers, barrettes, head bands, or rubber bands; hair straightening practices such as teasing or pulling, or frequent brushing with nylon bristles; and the use of hot combs and petrolatum. Other common causes of traumatic alopecia include pressure, as is seen on the occiput of infants who lie on their backs or are in the habit of "head-banging"; prolonged bed rest in one position, as in chronically ill persons or neglected children; thermal or electric burns; repeated vigorous massage; a severe blow to the scalp; and avulsions, such as may occur after abusive hair-pulling.

*Alopecia areata* is a common disorder characterized by the sudden appearance of sharply defined round or oval patches of hair loss. Recent evidence suggests that an autoimmune process may cause this disorder. Another possible cause of bald patches is fungal infections, for example, ringworm. The diagnosis of alopecia areata is based on its clinical presentation—a sudden appearance and the circumscribed, nonscarring pattern of hair loss. One or more round or oval well-circumscribed and clearly defined patches are usual. Occasionally the initial patches may be atypical, lacking a regular outline or demonstrating scattered long hairs within the bald areas. This will usually distinguish it from other forms of alopecia (Hurwitz, 1981).

## FALLS

In most cases, a trivial injury occurs when a child has a routine fall in the home, such as out of bed, from a sofa, off a chair, or down the stairs. There is usually no object, such as a tricycle or stroller, involved; leverage created by such objects and their weight can influence the fall. On some occasions, a single skull fracture, most often parietal, is sustained. None of these fractures is bilateral, diastatic, or greater than 1 mm in width. Intracranial pressure is not increased.

A child, reported to have had a routine fall, may present with a skull fracture, cerebral edema, retinal hemorrhages, subdural hematoma, or epidural hemorrhage. These severe injuries are incongruous with a routine fall, and the inconsistency indicates child abuse. The physician should suspect child abuse whenever the child presents with serious head injury, with or without skull fracture, as a result of a reported fall from a bed, sofa, or crib.

A fall down the stairs, especially when the stairs are not padded, will cause a series of bruises the size and shape of the stair edge. The bruises are usually on multiple body surfaces. Joffe and Ludwig (1988) studied 363 children who fell down stairs and reported that the falls resulted in bony injuries in 7%, head and neck injuries in 73%, extremity injuries in 28%, and truncal injuries in 2%; injury to more than one body part occurred in 2.7%. **No patients had life-threatening injuries and none required admission to an intensive care unit.**

Injuries caused by a fall from a car generally include abrasions. The wounds are usually dirty and contain particulate matter from the road surface and shoulder. The injuries can involve multiple body surfaces because, depending on the speed of the vehicle, the child will roll when he strikes the ground. His clothes should show evidence of the experience. Vehicular accidents are usually reported to the police. In suspicious cases, if the police are unaware of the existence of such an accident, further investigation is warranted.

### STUDIES OF FALLS

*Falls were the subject of several studies, which are summarized here:*

**Hall et al. (1989)**—Reviewed records from a Medical Examiner's Office and found 18 cases in which a fall of 3 feet or less was associated with fatal head injury. The study was performed as a critique of therapies and practices necessary to prevent fatal outcomes. The authors were not primarily interested in the differentiation between accidental and inflicted injuries. Unfortunately the histories given to explain the falls were not challenged when the children were admitted to the hospital, so explanations for the severe injuries were accepted and the diagnosis of child abuse was not entertained. No other study has concluded that falls of this distance, 3 feet or less, are fatal in children.

**Helfer et al. (1977)**—Studied 246 children under 5 years of age who fell out of bed, documenting the degree and severity of cerebral injuries. Results from the review of these incidents revealed 85 reports of children who fell to the floor from heights of approximately 90 cm (about 36 inches).

*The 85 incidents resulted in the following injuries:*

57—no apparent injury; 17—small cuts, scratches, and/or bloody noses; 20—bump and/or bruise; 1— fracture of the skull with no serious sequelae (the child fell off an emergency room cart and had no signs of soft tissue injuries over the site of the fracture). Of the 85 incidents documented, two children had bumps on the forehead, one with a bruise on the back and one without injury. X-ray films taken following these incidents did not identify any fractures other than the one noted.

**Nimityongskul and Anderson (1987)**—Using a similar study, concluded that children are not seriously injured in short falls.

**Smith et al. (1975)**—Studied long falls of children from buildings and found that the shortest falls that resulted in death were from the four-story level (about 30 feet).

**Snyder et al. (1977)**—Studied 100 falls of children and adults and concluded that life-threatening injury required at least a 15-foot fall. They found just one child death after a presumed 10-foot fall.

**Williams (1991)**—Reported on 106 infants and children whose injuries resulted from falls that were witnessed by a second person. Only one death occurred, resulting from a 70-foot fall. There were falls of up to 15 feet with no injury, and minor injury or simple fractures were found in 77 patients.

**Chadwick et al. (1991)**—Examined fatal outcome of injury in 317 infants and children who were seen at a children's trauma center with injuries and a history of a fall. Caretakers of 7 of 100 children who died gave a history of a fall of less than 4 feet. No deaths occurred in 65 children who fell from 5 to 9 feet, and one death occurred in 118 children who fell from 10 to 45 feet. The fall that produced the single death in the long fall group, 10 to 45 feet, was not observed nor was a report of a scene investigation found for the case. Head injuries were the cause of death in all of the children in this study. The head injuries were subdural hematoma, cerebral contusion with brain swelling, or both. All seven patients had fresh subdural bleeding and cerebral edema and one had a skull fracture. The child who presumably fell from the second story had a markedly depressed parietal skull fracture with underlying bleeding. The child survived the head injury but died 6 weeks later from sepsis. Five of the seven fatal cases with short fall histories, less than 4 feet, had evidence of other injuries, including old fractures, bruising on the trunk and extremities, genital injury, or more than one impact site on the head.

If the histories of short falls are accepted as explaining the deaths, the conclusion could be reached that the risk of death is greater for children who fall from a distance of less than 4 feet than for those who fall from 5 to 9 feet or from 10 to 45 feet. Chadwick et al. (1991) concluded that the histories given to explain the injuries of the seven fatal falls noted in his study were falsified and emphasized the importance of early reporting to initiate an investigation at the scene. Vital information about the sites is best obtained by trained investigators who examine the alleged fall scenes and interview witnesses as soon as possible.

## EXTERNAL HEAD, FACIAL, AND ORAL INJURIES

The head is a common area of injury; approximately 50% of physical abuse patients have head or facial injuries. The reported incidence of intraoral injuries is low, most likely because the mouth is often not examined. Detailed dental examinations were performed on 170 physically and sexually abused children who were presented to a pediatric emergency department over a 4-month period. Approximately 25% of the physically abused children and 15% of the sexually abused children demonstrated injuries in and around the mouth. The injury patterns differed between the two groups of children (Bernat, 1992). Further information on injuries to oral structures is found in Chapter 3.

**Figure 1-7**. *Face injury caused by blow to the side of the face. Linear marks are caused by fingers.*

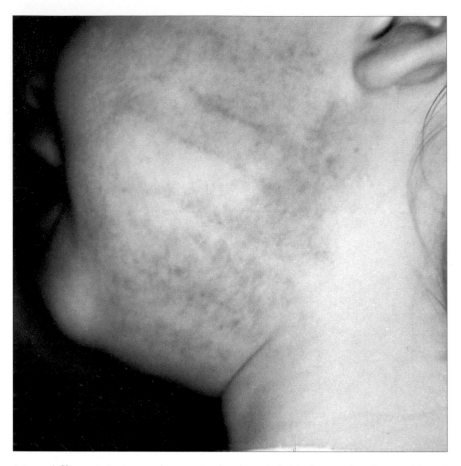

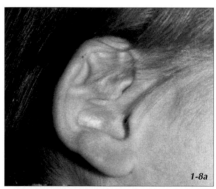

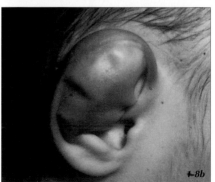

**Figure 1-8**. *Injuries to ear, **a,** old, and **b,** recent, caused by a blow to the side of the face. When the injury heals without medical intervention it leaves a distortion of the ear cartilage often called "cauliflower" ear.*

Many different injuries can be seen in the abused child. As stated earlier, accidental injuries to the face are usually frontal, involving the forehead, nose, chin, and incisor teeth. However, not all frontal injuries are accidental, and a careful history is needed to evaluate the reported accident's plausibility and consistency with the physical injuries.

Lateral injuries to the face, which are found on the ears, cheeks, and temporal and parietal areas (not including single parietal fractures), are highly suspicious for abuse (**Figure 1-7**). Hemorrhages around the ear and ear lobe or inside the ear canal are also important indicators of abuse.

Lacerations, hemorrhage, redness of the soft tissue membranes lining the external auditory canal, or swelling of its cartilage may be evidence of a severe blow to the ear (**Figure 1-8 a,b**). Such a blow may cause rupture of the tympanic membrane, with resultant hearing loss or infection secondary to opening of the middle ear chamber. The examiner must look for evidence of a lacerated drum when the membrane has not been perforated by infection or fistula.

The tin ear syndrome results from a slap or other blunt force to the ear (Hanigan et al., 1987). It is identified by bruising and hemorrhage in the helix and antitragus. If sufficient force is generated by the blow, unilateral hemorrhagic retinopathy, cerebral edema, and ipsilateral subdural hematoma may result. The cerebral damage results from the rotational acceleration of the head stretching and tearing the cortical veins. The findings in tin ear syndrome are similar to those with whiplash or shaken infants (Caffey, 1972).

If a black eye is present, the history must detail an appropriate injury to that side. It is difficult to break the tissues around the eye without damaging the nose as well, unless the black eye results from a direct blow, as from a fist. It is unlikely that a child will sustain two black eyes as the result of a fall unless the nose is broken also. If the child falls on the center of the face, injury to the nose will occur. This position of contact protects one or both eyes, and they should not be blackened (**Figure 1-9**). Bilateral suborbital bruising can occur secondary to blood seepage into loose tissue areas in cases where there has been a blow to the forehead, possibly from a swing or the corner of a table.

Hemorrhage in the upper eyelid often results when blood seeps down into periorbital tissues after an injury to the forehead or a subgaleal hematoma. Hemorrhage around the entire eye concentrically positioned as the result of a forehead injury is unlikely. Practitioners should be aware of the spontaneous black eye that occurs with malignant neuroblastoma, which may be associated with bony abnormalities palpable on the forehead. There are also rare occurrences of black eye(s) in blood dyscrasia.

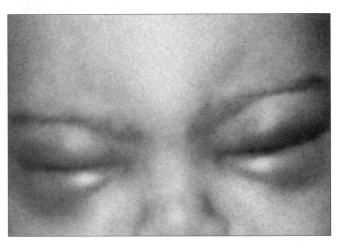

**Figure 1-9**. *Bilateral black eyes, when there is no broken nose, must be caused by at least two blows and cannot be explained by a single incident.*

## CLOSED HEAD INJURY— SHAKEN INFANT SYNDROME

In 1946 Caffey's initial report of the association of multiple fractures with chronic subdural hematomas in infants initiated the recognition of shaken infant syndrome. This syndrome is responsible for at least 50% of the deaths of children caused by nonaccidental trauma and also yields the most severe sequelae of abuse.

In the early 1970s Guthkelch (1971) and Caffey (1972) concluded that subdural hematoma, interhemispheric subarachnoid hemorrhage, and cerebral contusions in abused children were the result of a whiplash injury to the brain. Early studies were done before the availability of CT scans and therefore emphasized the most severe cases, those who were examined at autopsy. This form of abuse is comparable to those injuries seen in car accidents that result from acceleration-deceleration phenomena. The shaking produces a differential motion between the skull and intracranial structures as the head rotates on the neck. The differential motion causes stretching and tearing of the bridging vessels and the possibility of cerebral contusion or laceration as the brain moves within the skull.

Impact injury probably plays a major role in many closed head injuries. Scalp and subgaleal hemorrhages are often found in children who have died of abusive head trauma, and skull fractures, usually linear, are also common. Hahn et al. (1983) reported findings on 77 children, seen over a 10-year period, who suffered abusive injuries ranging from concussion to irreversible injury and death. Eight percent were believed to have been caused by shaking, 48% were caused by direct trauma to the face and head, and 35% resulted from dropping, throwing, or falling. The remaining children suffered impact trauma that was not directed at the head. Fifty percent had skull fractures, mostly parietal linear fractures. The intracranial injuries noted were 30 subdural hematomas, of which 22 were bilateral; 23 cerebral contusions; and 7 concussions.

The low incidence of shaking as an etiology in this group and the frequent finding of concealed impact injury in fatal cases of abuse raise questions about the biomechanics of inflicted head injury. Holbourn (1943) provided the first basis for analyzing head injuries secondary to impact phenomena of the head, but he did not evaluate the effects of acceleration-deceleration forces. Ommaya et al. (1968) noted that rotational injury without direct impact to the head could cause significant injury to the brain and followed a distribution suggested by Holbourn that corresponded to the regions of injury seen in abused infants diagnosed with the shaken infant syndrome. The degree of acceleration needed to cause a given injury is related to the duration of impact. Short duration impacts produce effects dependent on velocity change, not accelerational change alone.

Duhaime et al. (1987) reviewed 48 cases of shaken infants, seen over 8 years, for evidence of impact injury. Sixty-three percent of the patients had physical evidence of blunt impact to the head, as well as findings of retinal hemorrhage, subdural hematoma, subarachnoid hemorrhage, interhemispheric blood, or bilateral chronic subdural effusions. Thirteen percent had blunt extracranial trauma accompanying their intracranial findings, and 24% showed no physical evidence of a blow. Reliable histories were obtained for 40 of the cases and revealed that only one was apparently caused by shaking unassociated with other trauma. Analysis of the 13 fatal cases showed that all had evidence of blunt cranial trauma, but autopsy was necessary to demonstrate this finding in 7 of the 13 cases.

Duhaime et al. (1987) constructed mechanical models approximating the size, weight, and density of a 1-month-old infant. Three varieties of necks were devised and tested, and accelerometers were implanted in the head. Each model was tested at least 20 times, with vigorous shaking, by male and female adults. The occiput of each model was impacted against a metal bar or padded surface. The results showed that both the tangential and the angular accelerations were much higher with impact than with shaking. The authors concluded that, despite significant differences between the neck models, shaking did not generate accelerations great enough to produce concussion, subdural hematoma, or diffuse axonal injury. They determined the accelerations necessary based on estimates derived from the conversion equation proposed by Ommaya et al. (1968). (It should be noted that this conversion equation has not been verified for infants but has been verified in other nonhuman primates. Verification for adult humans has been provided from studies of motor vehicle accidents.)

Impact against a yielding surface will not alter the force delivered to the brain but can minimize the damage to external soft tissues. A boxer may be knocked unconscious, with injury to the brain, after impact from a gloved and cushioned hand yet suffer no facial bruising. In like manner, a child thrown against a soft crib mattress, bed, or carpeted floor can sustain severe brain injuries with no evidence of external damage.

**Shaking alone may produce the injuries seen in the shaken infant syndrome. When making this diagnosis, one should emphasize that an impact may have been involved in the injury even though no external evidence of injury is observed (Alexander et al., 1990).**

Table 1-2 lists the features in an infant that play an important role in creating shaken infant syndrome. Children under 2 years of age are prone to brain injury during severe shaking and severe shaking with impact because of the disproportionate size of the head compared to the body, the weakness of the cervical muscles, poor head and neck control, the higher water content of the infant brain, and poorer myelination of the brain, large subarachnoid space, and open fontanelles and sutures characteristic of this age.

What makes the shaken infant syndrome more difficult to recognize and diagnose than other forms of infant trauma is the usual absence of external evidence of trauma. In addition, the history given by the caretaker is usually deliberately

---

**Table 1-2. Mechanism of Shaken Infant Syndrome**

**Unique Features of Child Less Than 2 Years of Age**
Size of head relative to body
Weakness of cervical musculature
Poor control of head and neck
Anatomy of upper cervical spine and foramen magnum
Higher water content of brain
Minor degree of myelination
Large subarachnoid space

**Acceleration-Deceleration Phenomena**
Rotation of head on neck
Differential motion between skull and intracranial structures
Stretching and tearing of bridging vessels
Cerebral contusion and laceration

**Impact**

---

**Table 1-3. Presenting Signs and Symptoms of Shaken Infant Syndrome**

Altered level of consciousness
Somnolent yet irritable
Coma
Convulsions
Opisthotonic posturing
Respiratory problems
　Arrest
　Hypoventilation
　Cheyne-Stokes
Dead

---

misleading. The underlying pathophysiology is cerebral anoxia, ischemia, diffuse axonal injury, or a combination of all. **Table 1-3** lists the presenting signs and symptoms in an infant suspected to have shaken infant syndrome. The three essential components of the shaken infant syndrome are (1) closed head injury evidenced by altered level of consciousness, coma, convulsions, or death; (2) central nervous system (CNS) injury as evidenced by CNS hemorrhaging, laceration, contusion, or concussion; and (3) retinal hemorrhages. CNS injury can be documented with a CT scan or, if needed to clarify an injury, magnetic resonance imaging (MRI). It should be noted that approximately 40% of these infants have metaphyseal chip fractures of the long bones secondary to traction or shearing (Caffey, 1972). Therefore a skeletal survey should be included in the workup. This should also detect any vertebral injuries (Swischuk, 1969).

One should also look for evidence of impact, frequently indicated by bruises. In addition, routine skull films will help identify fractures, which may be missed by the CT scan if the fracture lies in the same plane as the CT slice. A radionuclide scan can help detect fresh fractures not visible on the routine radiograph.

As in any medical problem, a good history is paramount. It should be remembered that, as in other forms of child abuse, the history in these cases is apt to be misleading, false, or not available. An infant or toddler with a history of, or physical evidence of, altered level of consciousness must be suspected to have head trauma until proven otherwise. If a minor fall is given to explain the injury, child abuse, with closed head injury, should be suspected. As discussed earlier in this chapter, infants under 1 year of age rarely sustain devastating accidental head injury, and accidental severe head injury, as seen in an automobile accident, is usually witnessed.

While giving the CNS symptoms adequate attention, the examiner must also be aware that abdominal and/or chest trauma is often present and should be evaluated and treated. The workup of the child includes CT scans of both the head and the abdomen and chest (**Tables 1-4 and 1-5**).

Physical examination of the nude baby is essential to establish the presence of any signs of external trauma such as bruising and should include careful evaluation of hidden places such as the scalp, back, and buttocks. The physician must palpate the various areas of the skin and scalp for soft tissue swelling and the fontanelle for fullness or tension. The examination should also include the genital area. **It must be remembered that the absence of external injury does not rule out a diagnosis of shaken infant syndrome.**

Hypoventilation or Cheyne-Stokes breathing can alert the examiner to CNS injury. The neck should be examined for nuchal rigidity. **Most important, the examination must include evaluation of the optic fundi for retinal hemorrhage, which denotes severe trauma and is a necessary component in making the diagnosis of shaken infant syndrome.** Retinal hemorrhages in an infant without a history of severe accidental trauma constitute child abuse until proven otherwise.

As will be discussed in the chapter on the death review process, catastrophic injuries to children are costly in terms of survivor outcome. One third of these children die; one third, although they survive, are mentally and/or physically disabled and often require a lifetime of custodial care; and one third will have a good recovery. As we look at the three outcomes, the third, good recovery, is likely to be the most costly. The survivors often have severe emotional problems and develop into predators, becoming abusive and ending up in prison (Magid & McKelvey, 1987). Prevention through the early recognition of potential abusers is essential. These children, the apparent survivors, should receive extensive counseling.

| **Table 1-4. Suggested Diagnostic Studies for Shaken Infant Syndrome** |
| --- |
| History |
| Optic fundus exam for retinal hemorrhages |
| CT scan (head and abdomen) |
| MRI in selected cases |
| Lumbar puncture with precautions |
| Skeletal survey |
| Nuclear scan |
| Drug screen |
| Routine blood samples |
| Liver and pancreatic enzymes |

| **Table 1-5. Physical Findings in Shaken Infant Syndrome** |
| --- |
| Retinal hemorrhages |
| CNS (closed head) injury |
|   Bleeding (subdural, epidural, subarachnoid, subgaleal) |
|   Laceration |
|   Contusion |
|   Concussion |
|   Diffuse axonal injury |
| Bruises–facial, scalp, arms, abdomen, back |
| Soft tissue swelling |
| Skull fracture(s) |
| Other fracture(s) (long bones, ribs, metaphyseal) |
| Abdominal injuries |
| Chest injuries |
| Hypotension |
| Tense fontanelle |

## DROWNING

Drowning resulting from child abuse is difficult to distinguish from accidental immersion or from sudden and unexpected natural causes. Accidental drownings usually involve toddlers or older children in public areas—swimming pools, drainage ditches, lakes, and rivers—especially in rural areas. In cities, bathtubs are the major sites of accidental childhood drownings. Homicidal drownings usually occur in the home; the victims are young, either infants or toddlers. The pathologic findings of postimmersion syndrome suggest the cause of death. Foreign material in the lungs and injuries of the face are positive correlating factors indicating abuse. However, it is hypothesized that deliberate drowning is underreported and underdiagnosed because of the sparsity of physical evidence and clear criteria on which to base a diagnosis of abuse.

*Nixon and Pearn (also as Pearn & Nixon) in 1977 (a,b,c) described several features that serve to differentiate accidental from nonaccidental drowning:*

1. Accidental drowning occurs during the usual bath time when more than one child is present in the tub, and generally the older child(ren) left the youngest. The household routine is usually upset, resulting in a lapse of supervision.

2. Nonaccidental drownings or near-drownings occur in the bathtub at an unusual time of day with the drowned child alone in the bath.

3. The parents fit the sociopathologic profile of abusing caretakers, and a precipitating crisis, often a domestic problem, is present.

4. The abused children are older, usually between 15 and 30 months of age, compared with the usual age of 9 to 15 months for accidental drowning.

5. The depth of the bath water ranges from 5 to 35 cm (2 to 14 inches), and those children immersed 5 minutes or more die. Nixon and Pearn found that in cases of deliberate immersion, the child is held under the water until unconsciousness ensues.

6. There is often a history of previous abusive behavior by the parent or guardian or a history of alcohol and drug abuse.

7. There is a delay between the event and calling for help or finding the child, as evidenced by cerebral edema.

8. Postmortem pulmonary features of the postimmersion syndrome, characterized by widespread intraalveolar polymorphonuclear leukocyte infiltrates and edema of hyaline membranes, may be present.

In deaths that occur in the bathtub, the presence of foreign material in the lungs should be noted because it confirms the cause of death as drowning and the location of the drowning. The water from the reported immersion site should be analyzed and matched to that in the lung.

Griest and Zumwalt (1989) reviewed a series of accidental drownings of children between birth and 12 years of age. Irrigation ditch drownings prevailed among the toddler group, whereas lakes, rivers, and swimming pools were the prime location among older children. In bathtub drownings of older children there was a major contributing factor—cerebral palsy and epilepsy. In bathtub drownings of younger children the child was left alone in the tub by the parent or older sibling for a short period of time. In bucket deaths, the child was a toddler who was tall enough to tip himself into the pail, but not large enough to knock it over. The water in the bucket was heavy enough to weigh it down and deep enough to cover the child's nose and mouth.

## FETAL ABUSE

Fetal abuse involves a range of behaviors in pregnant women, or their partners, characterized by the nonaccidental performance of acts that can be detrimental to the fetus. These acts include a direct physical assault on the fetus, through the abdominal wall or via the vagina, or a failure to protect the fetus from an indirect assault, as with alcohol, nicotine, or drugs.

The cost of fetal abuse to society is considerable. It has been estimated that the risks to the fetus from maternal alcohol and nicotine abuse outweigh the risks of other medical conditions such as diabetes, toxemia, or Rh incompatibility (Sokol, 1981). No one knows what significance in utero physical assault has on abortion, prematurity, stillbirth, deformity, or mental retardation.

Condon (1985, 1986), in defining fetal abuse, differentiated behaviors directed at the pregnant state, that is, therapeutic or self-induced abortion, from behaviors aimed at the fetus itself. The former behaviors usually occur in early pregnancy, while the latter behaviors more often occur in late pregnancy. These studies showed that parents' attitudes toward "being pregnant" often bear little relationship to those toward the fetus itself, and the dichotomy "wanted" versus "unwanted" pregnancy is not clear-cut, with degrees of ambivalence prevailing. Even a "wanted" fetus may become the victim of abuse.

Although the incidence of fetal abuse is unknown, as with other forms of child abuse, fetal abuse is most likely underreported. Estimates of the incidence of fetal abuse due to alcohol or nicotine have been reported (Kwok et al., 1983; Streissguth et al., 1983). The fetal alcohol syndrome is the third most common known cause of mental retardation in the United States, possibly affecting 1 in 750 live births (Abel & Sokol, 1986). Between one half and two thirds of pregnant women consume some alcohol, and between 2% and 13% of all pregnant women acknowledge heavy consumption (Sokol, 1981; Kwok et al., 1983). A strong association exists between alcohol and cigarette use during pregnancy, with studies revealing that 25% to 35% of pregnant women smoke during pregnancy (Kwok et al., 1983; Streissguth et al., 1983), and 25% of these women smoke more than 20 cigarettes per day.

Until Condon (1985, 1986) reported several cases, no case of physical assault on the fetus through the anterior abdominal wall by the mother had been considered by experienced professionals. Condon noted that, if specific inquiry was made, the impulse to harm the fetus was not uncommon in pregnant women. The women involved did not satisfy the criteria for any psychiatric diagnosis, but their behaviors did resemble those of women who subsequently killed their babies shortly after delivery (Condon, 1986). Although spouse abuse of pregnant women has been reported, only Gelles (1975) speculated that sometimes the fetus was the target in spouse abuse of pregnant women. **Figure 1-10, a to d** are ultrasound images of a newborn who was severely injured in utero. His mother was beaten and kicked by her boyfriend, the child's father.

As stated, the risk of assaultive behavior is greatest in late pregnancy because of the stresses of the third trimester and because of progressive disenchantment, in both partners, with the pregnancy state in the final 2 to 3 months (Condon, 1985). Fetal abuse may be triggered by a woman's perception of rejection by her spouse, family, or doctor, because attention is directed to the fetus and not her. The perceived rejection may be responded to with a physical attack on her "rival," or a more passive neglect or failure to protect. This scenario of neglect can be likened to failure to thrive in the older child wherein poor weight gain and stunted development result.

The initial reactions of the medical community to reports of fetal abuse were that they were isolated, rare phenomena. Condon (1987) presents data, though preliminary, that dispute the rarity of the phenomenon, finding that, after interviewing 112 couples, 8% of pregnant women and 4% of expectant fathers acknowledged that they occasionally experienced an urge to hurt or punish their

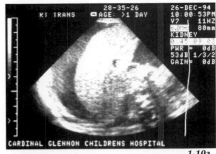
*1-10a*

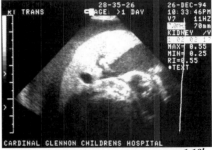
*1-10b*

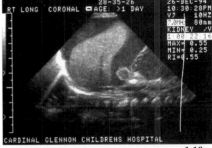
*1-10c*

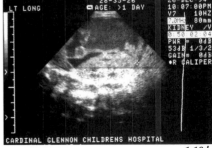
*1-10d*

**Figure 1-10.** *These are diagnostic ultrasound images of the abdomen of a newborn. **a** and **b** are transverse views of the liver and show extensive amounts of echogenic free fluid, which may represent blood-stained debris or meconium. **c** is a longitudinal view of the liver showing the organ floating in fluid. **d** is a longitudinal view of the left kidney showing the presence of an anterior collection of free fluid. At surgery the newborn was found to have a lacerated liver and pancreas; the fluid was blood. The lacerations cannot be seen clearly on ultrasound.*

unborn baby. The male partner was aware of the woman's urge to assault the fetus; 9% of fathers reported that they believed their female partner had experienced an urge to hurt or punish the fetus. When questioned about future child abuse, 8% of the women and 5% of the men acknowledged that they frequently had worries that they might lose their temper after the baby was born and harm the baby. The incidence estimates are probably conservative because the tendency to conceal this urge, based on shame, may result in underreporting. Condon warned that the data are preliminary and must be interpreted with caution. The worth in reporting them derived from the fact that they represent the only systematic attempt to explore expectant parents' feelings of aggression toward their unborn child; they suggest that an urge to hurt or punish the unborn child can be elicited in a significant number of expectant parents, suggesting that the phenomenon is not a clinical rarity.

## FETAL ABUSE AND SUBSEQUENT CHILD ABUSE

Is fetal abuse a precursor to later child abuse? In two of Condon's five cases, the abuse continued postnatally. Examining the characteristic low birth weight of abused children, it would seem that a correlation may exist. Smith and Hanson (1974), in a controlled study of abused children, found a fourfold increase in low birth weight, independent of social class. Klaus hypothesized that early maternal-infant separation, forced by a low birth weight, leads to subsequent dysfunctional bonding, predisposing to child abuse. This hypothesis has been challenged (Smith & Hanson, 1974; Herbert et al., 1982; Lamb, 1982). Alternatively, if alcohol abuse during pregnancy constitutes fetal abuse and leads to low birth weight and child abuse occurs frequently among low birth weight children, it could be surmised that alcohol abuse is a precursor of child abuse. The use of nicotine during pregnancy may also cause low birth weight and constitute fetal abuse.

Alcohol and nicotine clearly produce effects on the fetus. The possible effects of external physical trauma are speculative at present. The fetus is cushioned by the amniotic fluid, and it is unlikely that damage would be caused by external trauma. Abdominal trauma may precipitate labor with resultant prematurity and low birth weight. There is a need for further research in physical fetal abuse.

## FETAL ABUSE AND NEONATICIDE

Neonaticide is defined as murder of the baby during the first 24 hours of life. After reviewing the literature, Resnick (1970) concluded that hundreds and possibly thousands of neonaticides occur in the United States each year. Resnick noted that, unlike women who kill their older children, mothers who commit neonaticide are rarely psychotic. Neonaticide is usually committed because the child is not wanted. He went on to say that "passivity" is the most important personality characteristic differentiating women who commit neonaticide from those who obtain abortions. In fetal abuse, it is likely that passive acceptance, or denial, of an unwanted pregnancy is common and consequently elective abortion is not sought. Mothers who commit neonaticide suppress the reality of their pregnancy and make no preparations. They murder the infant when the reality of birth breaks through their defenses.

## SUFFOCATION

The number of young children suffocated by their parents is unknown, but smothering is being increasingly reported. The involved families generally have a high incidence of sudden death of other siblings; investigation determines that some of the siblings were also suffocated.

Meadow (1990) reviewed the cases of 27 young children from 27 different families who were suffocated by their mothers. Twenty-four reported previous episodes of apnea, cyanosis, or seizure, and 11 had 10 or more episodes. The episodes began between the ages of 1 and 3 months and continued until discovery or the child died, 6 to 12 months later. The 27 children had 18 older siblings who had died suddenly and unexpectedly in early life. Thirteen of the dead siblings had recurrent apnea, cyanosis, or seizures. Most of them at death were diagnosed as having sudden infant death syndrome (SIDS). Suffocation can also be confused with recurrent apnea, although suffocation has clinical features that may facilitate making the appropriate diagnosis before brain damage or death occurs.

Since many of the dead children and their siblings had an initial diagnosis of SIDS, the features of suffocation must be compared with those of SIDS. The classic features of SIDS are young age, previous good health of the child, lack of previous apnea or other illness, and rarity of a positive family history, together with a thorough, complete autopsy, including metabolic studies, which fails to find another cause of death. In suffocation cases, it is common to find a child more than 6 months old with previous apneic episodes, previous unexplained disorders, and a dead sibling.

Metabolic problems that may present as apparent SIDS include medium chain acyldehydrogenase deficiency (MCAD), type I glycogen storage disease, and carnitine deficiency. Urine chromatography may be difficult if the bladder is empty; other studies can be done on vitreous humor, blood, liver, or other frozen tissue.

There are families who have increased risk for multiple SIDS; therefore this possibility must be explored. Recurrent SIDS is probably more an environmental problem than a genetic one; there is no increased risk in first cousins or in monozygotic compared with dizygotic twins. Guntheroth et al. (1990) studied 251,124 live births by linked birth and death certificates from Oregon for a 10-year period to determine the risk of recurrence of SIDS. They found 5 recurrences among 385 subsequent siblings, for a rate of 13/1,000 live births.

In most of Meadow's cases, suffocation was suspected when no cause for the apnea was found. Recurrent apnea in a previously healthy child having no viral infection or cardiac, respiratory, metabolic, or neurologic abnormality is rare, and this factor combined with the unexplained death of a sibling led to the diagnosis. It is difficult to diagnose suffocation when it occurs for the first time and when it is a single act rather than repeated.

Suffocation may cause petechial hemorrhages, but it can result in brain damage and death without other findings. Therefore some deaths classified as SIDS may have been caused by the parents, as careful clinical, pathologic, and psychosocial studies of families have disclosed.

As in the Munchausen Syndrome by Proxy, there are few reports of suffocation of children by men; most acts of suffocation are committed by the natural mother. For more information on the Munchausen Syndrome by Proxy, *see Chapter 17.*

## NEGLECT

While not an injury, neglect is a presenting feature in many abuse cases. The symptoms of neglect reflect a lack of both physical and medical care. An unclean baby can be a strong factor in determining neglect, although the ability to accumulate dirt in skin creases and other unreachable places is a natural characteristic of infants and children. There are degrees of uncleanliness. Most babies get dirty during normal play and a bath removes the dirt. The degree of dirtiness that suggests neglect requires several baths to begin to remove it and is accompanied by an offensive odor. Feces and dirt in the skin folds and under the nails may be evidence of failure to provide for the child's basic needs. Diaper rash can be a key to the attentiveness and care attitudes of the parents. The skin of some babies is extremely sensitive, and some irritation and excoriation occur. But the diaper rash in these cases shows evidence of being cared for and seldom reaches the point where the skin is denuded, cracked, and bleeding. A baby with a constantly dirty perineum who is left in wet diapers sufficiently long for ammonia burns to occur is not being cared for adequately.

Multiple cat or dog bites and scratches indicate the child may be left unattended for long periods, another factor in neglect. If a parent fails to bring a child to a physician when the child has an infection of the skin and there is evidence that the illness has been present for some time, or if the child's condition is not improving with the treatment prescribed, assuming the diagnosis and treatment are correct, the parents are probably noncompliant, which constitutes medical neglect.

## ◆ REPORTING SUSPECTED ABUSE

Mandated reporters include physicians, dentists, podiatrists, nurses, psychologists, speech pathologists, coroners, medical examiners, child day care center employees, children's services workers, social workers, and schoolteachers. The physician reporter should be prepared and willing to express an opinion about the cause of the injuries, their seriousness, and the potential danger to the child; he must also be available to the court when needed *(see Chapter 27)*. Although other mandated reporters may be asked to testify, they are less likely to be called than the physician.

### QUESTIONING THE HISTORY

**The evaluator must remember that an explanation for an injury should not change when it is questioned or challenged.** If the history differs from parent to parent, with different history takers, or when challenged, it is very likely fabricated. Team members must communicate and share information. If the explanations offered differ significantly, further investigation is warranted. For example, a young father told a triage nurse that he found his son unconscious in the back yard at the bottom of the steps. He told the admitting physician the child was convulsing on the floor of the bedroom. The two did not check each other's notes, and the parent was sent home with two other children. Abuse was not diagnosed until 24 hours later when a skeletal survey revealed multiple old and new fractures.

Some parent advocacy groups do not consider any punishment of a child under the guise of discipline as child abuse. These groups consider the intent of the parent when the child was injured. Parents usually believe they are doing what is best for the child. Unfortunately, the injured child is not aware of the good intentions of the parent. As stated earlier, when deciding to report an injury, the mandated reporter concerned about a child's well-being should not be influenced by caretaker intent. The courts, law enforcement, and social services will decide what is best for the child and what influence intent will have.

### FALSE ALLEGATIONS

False reports of child sexual abuse are uncommon and represent only a small proportion of cases (Thoennes & Pearson, 1988). There is concern that many of the reports of sexual abuse determined to be unsubstantiated may be false. Even if false reports are uncommon, they should be a serious concern, not only because of the potential legal consequences of a false accusation, but also because of the distress caused the family and the child.

Alleged abuse of children, physical and sexual, is more common in divorce and separation situations than in stable families. An allegation of abuse is difficult to deal with when made between separated parents and must be carefully evaluated by the professionals involved. It can be a powerful weapon one parent uses against the other or become a ploy to use against each other, calling the authorities at each return of the child, who is trapped in a compromising situation. It can also be a true allegation of abuse and the child and family in need of help.

Hlady and Gunter (1990) reviewed the records of 370 children, of which 41 (11%) were involved in custody disputes; 31 children were female, 10 male; and 34 were alleged to be sexually abused, 7 physically abused. More than half were under 4 years of age. Of the 7 physical abuse children, 5 had corroborative evidence; 3 cases alleged neglect in addition. In a population of 110 children not involved in a custody situation, 48 (43.6%) demonstrated physical evidence of abuse. In the 34 children allegedly victims of sexual abuse, 6 (17%) had corroborative physical evidence of abuse. In a custodial group of 219 children reported as victims of sexual abuse, 33 (15%) had corroborative physical evidence.

Sexual abuse is usually secretive, involving two witnesses, abused and abuser. For good reasons, both parties may forget, or want to forget, the experience. Without a confession of guilt, one of those witnesses is lying. Jones (1986) suggested that the system may need to move away from true and false labeling and attempt an assessment based on degrees of probability. He studied 576 cases of sexual abuse reported to the Denver Department of Social Services and found 54% of the reports to be reliable. Nearly 22% were unable to be explored any further because of insufficient evidence. Nearly 17% of the reports were made by adults who were appropriately concerned and were not falsely creating an allegation. These cases were distinct from the fictitious accounts.

The fictitious reports were made by adults and/or their children and were broken down into two groups: 6.25% of the total number of reports were fictitiously made by an adult, and 1.56% by a child, for a total of 7.81% fictitious reports. *Jones made the following conclusions:*

> Female teenagers, between 12 and 17 years of age, suffering from post-traumatic stress disorder as a result of documented earlier sexual victimization, made the child generate fictitious allegations.

> Two adults involved suffered from major psychoses. Several of the adults were involved in custody disputes.

> Adults behind false allegations commonly were victims of sexual abuse when they were children and suffered from psychological aftereffects of the experience.

*Jones' study concluded:*

1. Fictitious accounts of child sexual abuse, although not common, do occur and involve children of all ages and sexes.
2. To diagnose these cases the evaluator must first accept the possibility that fictitious cases can occur.
3. The diagnosis depends on careful interviews of the child and parents as well as careful search for an explanation for the fictitious report, looking at the family situation and dynamics, and the presence or absence of the post-traumatic stress disorder in the children and parents. It should be noted that in many reliable accounts some of these features also existed.
4. Absence of emotion, threats, or coercion in the child's statement proved helpful in determining when the account was fictitious.
5. A symbiotic mother/child relationship was present in mixed or fused accounts. Fused accounts were made in custody disputes.
6. Those making fictitious accounts require psychological help.
7. Child developmental specialists should be involved in the initial investigation conducted by local social services to help detect fictitious accounts.

Many of the conclusions made by Jones in this study can also be applied to false allegations of abuse other than sexual.

## WHAT TO REPORT

Children's hospitals must have a Child Protection Team and must establish guidelines for recognizing and reporting child abuse. No numerical system or lab test is currently available to objectively evaluate abuse. While it may be relatively easy to determine some indicators, assigning a value to each is difficult. What is clearly abuse, what is probably abuse, and what is possibly abuse cannot be easily separated by a numerical system. The human factor remains in the equation, affecting what is reported and what is not. Knowing what and when to report requires a sound knowledge of what child abuse is, a familiarity with child development and behavior, an acquaintance with the child protection system, a knowledge of adult behavior, common sense, and a smattering of physics and biomechanics.

Various common abuse and neglect indicators can be rated on a relative value scale. The tables in this section rate as many of these situations as possible and assign a relative importance to each. It should be noted that these are guidelines only; no list is perfect. If one is to err, we recommend that the reader err on the side of the child. Errors that do not protect the child can be fatal. It is advisable that these lists be made available to clinic and emergency room personnel as reminders of what injuries and situations are suspicious for abuse. A protocol including these lists can be helpful as well as periodic in-service conferences to remind experienced and new personnel of the importance of recognizing abuse (**Tables 1-6, 1-7, and 1-8**).

---

**Table 1-6. Situations that are Possibly Child Abuse and Dictate a Report to the Authorities**

**Death of an Infant with Unknown Cause and Poor or Questionable History**

**Evidence of Emotional Abuse**
  Hair loss
  Suicide, runaway
  Drug use
  Child perpetrator
  Child has flat affect, is passive, demonstrates
    failure to thrive

**Neglect**
  Medical treatment delayed (depends on seriousness
    of condition)
  Failure to thrive with no medical condition
    to explain it
  First drug or toxin ingestion with suspicious history
  Repeated drug or toxin ingestion
  Small child(ren) supervised by child under 12 years
    of age
  Severe dehydration, underweight with no medical
    condition to explain it

**Head Injury**
  Subdural hematoma without appropriate history
  Fracture of the skull with suspicious or no history

**Thermal Injuries**
  Burns that involve neglect
  Burns with poor or no history

**Skeletal Injuries**
  Fractured long bone with no appropriate history

**Bruises**
  Multiple bruises
  Injuries that suggest the use of an instrument
  Injuries resulting from discipline in a child over
    1 year of age

**Intrauterine Abuse**
  Fetal neglect, no prenatal checkups, suspicion of
    drug or alcohol abuse, poor nutrition
  Psychotic mother who gives reason to suspect
    fetus is in danger
  Battered mother

**Sexual Abuse**
  Genital injuries
  Child prostitution

## Table 1-7. Situations that are Child Abuse and Dictate a Report to the Authorities

**Severe Neglect**
  Abandonment
  Long periods with no supervision; children from infancy to 8 years old left unattended
  Long delay in obtaining medical help for a serious injury
  Maternal deprivation

**Head Injury**
  Evidence of shaken infant syndrome
    —Altered level of consciousness
    —Closed head injury
    —CNS hemorrhaging
    —Retinal hemorrhages
  Catastrophic injury explained by routine fall

**Deliberate Thermal Injuries**
  Multiple cigarette burns in varying stages of healing
  Glove-and-sock pattern liquid burn
  Iron burns (shows iron pattern) on back, back of hand, or buttocks or curling iron burns in same areas
  Diaper area burns and doughnut-shaped burns
  Burns to the back of the hand
  Bilateral burns or injuries to hands

**Skeletal Injuries**
  Rupture of the costovertebral junction
  Posterior rib fractures

  Metaphyseal avulsion fracture
  Two or more fractures in different stages of healing
  Multiple skull fractures
  Long bone fracture in a nonambulating child

**Bruises**
  Bilateral black eyes without broken nose
  Skin bruises and lacerations in recognizable shapes, such as whip, belt, stick, fist, fingers, buckle, rope, or teeth
  Circumferential injuries (burns, bruises, lacerations, or scars) of the wrists, arms, ankles, legs, and neck
  Multiple bruises in inaccessible places, in different stages of healing
  An injury resulting from discipline in a child less than 1 year of age

**Trauma**
  Blunt trauma to abdomen or chest with inappropriate or no history
  Intrauterine abuse
  Crack baby or newborn or other child of drug-dependent mother
  Evidence of fetal injury or self-injury

**Sexual Abuse**
  Category IV of sexual molestation *(see Chapter 9)*
  Credible disclosure of abuse by child

## Table 1-8. Caretaker Indicators

**Strong Indicators**
  Explanation of injury not believable
  Explanations are inconsistent/changing story
  Paramour in the home
  Previously suspected of abuse
  Caretaker(s) understates the seriousness of child's condition
  Caretaker(s) projects blame to third party
  Caretaker(s) has delayed bringing child to hospital
  Caretaker(s) cannot be located
  History of substance abuse
  Caretaker(s) unable to function
  Child is not up-to-date on immunizations
  Child has severe diaper rash, is poorly kept, dirty
  Caretaker(s) is psychotic

**Nonspecific Indicators**
  Caretaker(s) is hostile and aggressive
  Caretaker(s) is compulsive, inflexible, unreasonable, and cold
  Caretaker(s) is passive and dependent
  Father is unemployed
  History of unwanted baby
  Caretaker(s) has unrealistic expectations of child
  Caretaker(s) is hospital shopper
  Frequent visits to the pediatrician without a medical reason
  Caregiver(s) overreacts to child's misbehavior

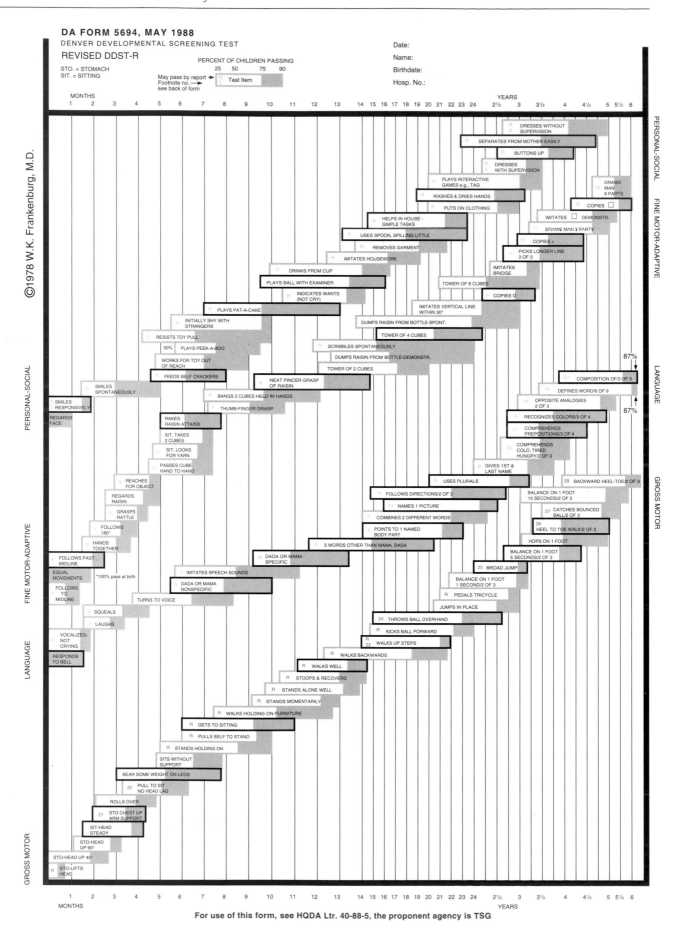

## ◆ BIBLIOGRAPHY

Abel, EL, and Sokol, RH: Fetal alcohol syndrome is now leading cause of mental retardation, *Lancet* 8517:1222, 1986.

Adler, R, and Kane-Nussen, B: Erythema multiforme: Confusion with child battering syndrome, *Pediatrics* 72:718, 1983.

Alexander, R, et al: Incidence of impact trauma, with cranial injuries ascribed to shaking, *Am J Dis Child* 144(6):724-726, 1990.

Anh, NT: "Pseudo-battered child" syndrome, *JAMA* 236:2288, 1976.

Asnes, RS: Buttock bruises–Mongolian spot, *Pediatrics* 74:321, 1984.

Asnes, RS, and Wisotsky, DH: Cupping lesions simulating child abuse, *J Pediatr* 99:267, 1981.

Barlow, B, Neiminska, M, Gandli, RP, et al: Ten years of experience with falls from a height in children, *J Pediatr Surg* 18:509-511, 1983.

Bays, J: *Conditions mistaken for child abuse,* The San Diego Conference on Responding to Child Maltreatment, San Diego, CA, 1993.

Bernat, JE: Dental trauma and bite mark evaluation. In S Ludwig and A Kornberg, eds: *Child Abuse*, Churchill Livingstone, New York, 1992, pp. 175-190.

Brown, J, and Mclinkovich, P: Schonlein-Henoch purpura misdiagnosed as suspected child abuse, *JAMA* 256:617, 1986.

Bryan, CS: Vietnamese coin rubbing, *Ann Emerg Med* 16:602, 1987.

Caffey, J: Multiple fractures in the long bones of infants suffering from chronic subdural hematoma, *AJR* 56:163-173, 1946.

Caffey, J: On the theory and practice: Its potential residual effects of permanent brain damage and mental retardation, *Am J Dis Child* 124:161, 1972.

Caffey, J: The whiplash-shaken-infant syndrome: Mutual shaking by the extremities with whiplash-induced intracranial intraocular bleedings, linked with residual permanent brain damage and mental retardation, *Pediatrics* 54:396-493, 1974.

Carpentieri, U, Gustavson, LP, and Haggard, ME: Misdiagnosis of neglect in a child with bleeding disorder and cystic fibrosis, *South Med J* 71:854, 1978.

Chadwick, DL, Chin, S, Salerno, C, Landsverk, J, and Kitchen, L: Deaths from falls in children: How far is fatal? *J Trauma* 31:1353-1355, 1991.

Coffman, K, Boyce, WT, and Hansen, RC: Phytodermatitis simulating child abuse, *Am J Dis Child* 139:239, 1985.

Colver, GB, Harris, DWS, and Tidman, MJ: Skin disease that may mimic child abuse, *Br J Dermatol* 123:129, 1990.

Condon, JT: The parental-fetal relationship: A comparison of male and female expectant parents, *J Psychosom Obstet Gynecol* 4:271-284, 1985.

Condon, JT: The spectrum of fetal abuse in pregnant women, *J Nerv Ment Dis* 174:509-516, 1986.

Condon, JT: The battered fetus syndrome, *J Nerv Ment Dis* 175:722-725, 1987.

Copeland, AR: A case of panhypogammaglobulinemia masquerading as child abuse, *J Forensic Sci* 33:1493, 1988.

Du, JNH: Pseudobattered child abuse syndrome in Vietnamese immigrant children, *Can Med Assoc J* 122:394, 1980.

Duhaime, AC, Gennarelli, TK, Thibault, LE, et al: The shaken baby syndrome: A clinical, pathological and biomechanical study, *J Neurosurg* 66:409, 1987.

Dungy, CI: Mongolian spots, day care centers and child abuse, *Pediatrics* 69:672, 1982.

Feldman, KW: Pseudoabusive burns in Asian refugees, *Am J Dis Child* 138:768, 1984.

Fiser, RH, Kaplan, JM, and Holder, JC: Congenital syphilis mimicking the battered child abuse syndrome: How does one tell them apart? *Clin Pediatr* 11:305, 1972.

Gahagan, S, and Rimza, ME: Child abuse or osteogenesis imperfecta: How can we tell? *Pediatrics* 88:987, 1991.

Ganaway, G: Historical truth versus narrative truth: Clarifying the role of exogenous trauma in the etiology of multiple personality disorder and its variants, *Dissociation* 2:205-220, 1989.

Gelles, RJ: Violence and pregnancy: A note on the extent of the problem and needed services, *Fam Coordinator* 24:81-86, 1975.

Gelles, RJ: The social context of child abuse. In EH Newberger, ed: *Child Abuse*, Little, Brown & Co, Boston, 1982, pp. 25-41.

Gellis, S, and Feingold, M: Cao Gio: Pseudobattering in Vietnamese children, *Am J Dis Child* 130:857-858, 1976.

Gennarelli, TK: Clinical and experimental head injury. In B Aldman and A Chapon, eds: *The Biomechanics of Impact Trauma*, Elsevier Science Publishers, Amsterdam, 1984, p. 103.

Golden, SM, and Duster, MC: Hazards of misdiagnosis due to Vietnamese folk medicine, *Clin Pediatr* 16:949, 1977.

Griest, KJ, and Zumwalt, RE: Child abuse by drowning, *Pediatrics* 83:41-46, 1989.

Guarnaschelli, J, Lee, J, and Pitts, FW: "Fallen fontanelle" (Caida de Mollera): A variant of the battered child syndrome, *JAMA* 222:1545, 1972.

Guntheroth, WG, Lohmann, R, and Spiers, PS: Risk of sudden infant death syndrome in subsequent siblings, *J Pediatr* 116:520-524, 1990.

Guthkelch, AN: Infantile subdural hematoma and its relationship to whiplash injuries, *Br Med J* 2:430, 1971.

Hahn, YS, Raimondi, AJ, McLone, DG, et al: Traumatic mechanisms of head injury in child abuse, *Childs Brain* 10:229, 1983.

Hall, JR, Reyes, HM, Horvat, M, Meller, JL, and Stein, R: The mortality of childhood falls, *J Trauma* 29:1273-1275, 1989.

Hanigan, WC, Peterson, RA, and Njus, G: Tin ear syndrome: Rotational acceleration in pediatric head injury, *Pediatrics* 80:618, 1987.

Helfer, RE, Slovis, TL, and Black, M: Injuries resulting when small children fall out of bed, *Pediatrics* 60:533-535, 1977.

Herbert, TM, Sluckin, W, and Sluckin, A: Mother-to-infant bonding, *J Child Psychol Psychiatry* 23:205-221, 1982.

Hlady, LJ, and Gunter, EJ: Alleged child abuse in custody access disputes, *Child Abuse Negl* 14:591-593, 1990.

Holbourn, AHS: Mechanics of head injuries, *Lancet* 2:438, 1943.

Horodniceanu, C, Grunebaum, M, Vkolovitz, B, and Nitzan, M: Unusual bone involvement in congenital syphilis mimicking the battered child syndrome, *Pediatr Radiol* 7:232, 1978.

Hurwitz, A, and Castells, S: Misdiagnosed child abuse and metabolic disorders, *Pediatr Nurs* 13:33-36, 1987.

Hurwitz, S: Disorders of hair and nails. In *Clinical Pediatric Dermatology*, WB Saunders Co, Philadelphia, 1981, pp. 361-383.

Joffe, M, and Ludwig, S: Stairway injuries in children, *Pediatrics* 82:457-461, 1988.

Jones, DPH: Reliable and fictitious accounts of sexual abuse in children, *J Interpersonal Violence* Vol. 1: June, 1986.

Junker, F, and Jonker-Bakker, P: Experiences with ritualistic child sexual abuse: A case study from the Netherlands, *Child Abuse Negl* 15:191-196, 1991.

Kaplan, JM: Pseudoabuse—the misdiagnosis of child abuse, *J Forensic Sci* 31:1420, 1986.

Kirschner, RH, and Stein RJ: Mistaken diagnosis of child abuse, *Am J Dis Child* 139:873, 1985.

Kravitz, H, Dricssen, G, Gomberg, R, et al: Accidental falls from elevated surfaces in infants from birth to one year of age, *Pediatrics* 44:869-876, 1969.

Kwok, P, Correy, JF, Newman, NM, and Curran, JT: Smoking and alcohol consumption during pregnancy, *Med J Aust* 1:220-223, 1983.

Lamb, M: The bonding phenomenon: Misinterpretations and their implications, *J Pediatr* 101:555-557, 1982.

Lanning, KV: Ritual abuse: A law enforcement view or perspective, *Child Abuse Negl* 15:171-173, 1991.

Lee, STS: Anterior stenosis from joss stick burns, *J Laryngol Otol* 104:497, 1990.

Leung, AKC: Ecchymoses from spoon scratching simulating child abuse, *Clin Pediatr* 25:98, 1986.

Levine, LJ: Bite marks in child abuse. In RG Sanger and DC Bloss, eds: *Management of Child Abuse and Neglect: A Guide for the Dental Professional*, Quintessence Publishing, Inc., Chicago, 1984.

Magid, K, and McKelvey, CA: *High Risk: Children Without a Conscience*, Bantam Books, New York, 1987.

McClain, JL, Clark, MA, and Sandusky, GE: Undiagnosed, untreated acute lymphoblastic leukemia presenting as suspected child abuse, *J Forensic Sci* 35:735, 1990.

McLellan, NJ, Prasad, R, and Punt, J: Spontaneous subhyaloid and retinal hemorrhages in an infant, *Arch Dis Child* 61:1130, 1986.

Meadow, R: Suffocation, recurrent apnea, and sudden infant death, *J Pediatr* 117:351-356, 1990.

Monteleone, JA: Unpublished observations, 1996.

Moorees, CFA: *The Dentition of the Growing Child*, Harvard University Press, 1959.

Nimityongskul, P, and Anderson, L: The likelihood of injuries when children fall out of bed, *J Pediatr Orthop* 7:184, 1987.

Nixon, J, and Pearn, J: Non-accidental immersion in bathwater: Another aspect of child abuse, *Br Med J* 271-272, 1977(a).

Oates, RK: Overturning the diagnosis of child abuse, *Arch Dis Child* 59:665-667, 1984.

O'Hara, AE, and Eden, OB: Bleeding disorders and non-accidental injury, *Arch Dis Child* 59:860, 1984.

Ommaya, AK: The head: Kinematics and brain injury mechanisms. In B Aldman and A Chapon, eds: *The Biomechanics of Impact Trauma*, Elsevier Science Publishers, Amsterdam, 1984, p. 117.

Ommaya, AK, Faas, F, and Yarnell, P: Whiplash injury and brain damage: An experimental study, *JAMA* 204:285, 1968.

Owen, SM, and Durst, RD: Ehlers-Danlos syndrome simulating child abuse, *Arch Dermatol* 120:97, 1984.

Paterson, CR: Osteogenesis imperfecta and other bone disorders in the differential diagnosis of unexplained fractures, *J Roy Soc Med* 83:72, 1990.

Paterson, CR, and McAllion, SJ: Child abuse and osteogenesis imperfecta, *Br Med J* 295:1561, 1987.

Pearn, J, and Nixon, J: Bathtub immersion accidents involving children, *Med J Aust* 211-213, 1977(b).

Pearn, J, and Nixon, J: Prevention of childhood drowning accidents, *Med J Aust* 616-618, 1977(c).

Putman, FW: The satanic ritual abuse controversy, *Child Abuse Negl* 15:175-179, 1991.

Putnam, N, and Stein, M: Self-inflicted injuries in childhood: A review and diagnostic approach, *Clin Pediatr* 24:514-518, 1985.

Reinhart, MA, and Ruhs, H: Moxibustion: Another traumatic folk remedy, *Clin Pediatr* 24:58, 1985.

Resnick, P: Murder of the newborn: A psychiatric review of neonaticide, *Am J Psychiatry* 126:1414-1420, 1970.

Roberts, DLL, Pope, FM, Nicholls, AC, and Narcis, P: Ehlers-Danlos syndrome type IV mimicking non-accidental injury in a child, *Br J Dermatol* 111:341, 1984.

Rosenberg, L, Amiram, S, Stahl, N, Greber, B, and Ben-Meir, P: Maqua (therapeutic burn) as an indicator of underlying disease, *Plast Reconstr Surg* 82:277, 1988.

Rosenblat, H, and Hong, P: Coin rolling misdiagnosed as child abuse, *Can Med Assoc J* 140:417, 1989.

Sandler, AP, and Haynes, V: Nonaccidental trauma and medical folk belief: A case of cupping, *Pediatrics* 61:921, 1978.

Saulsbury, FT, and Hayden, GF: Skin conditions simulating child abuse, *Pediatr Emerg Care* 1:147, 1985.

Schmitt, BD, Gray, JD, and Britton, HL: Car seat burns in infants; avoiding confusion with induced burns, *Pediatrics* 62:607, 1978.

Schwer, W, Brueschke, EE, and Dent, T: Family practice grand rounds: Hemophilia, *J Fam Pract* 14:661, 1982.

Silfen, E, and Wyre, HW: Factitial dermatitis-Cao gio, *Cutis* 28:399, 1981.

Sims, BG, Grant, JH, and Cameron, JM: Bite marks in the "battered baby syndrome," *Med Sci Law* 13:207, 1973.

Smialek, JE: Significance of Mongolian spots, *J Pediatr* 97:504, 1980.

Smith, MD, Burrington, JD, and Woolf, AD: Injuries in children sustained in free falls: An analysis of 66 cases, *J Trauma* 15:987-991, 1975.

Smith, S, and Hanson, R: 134 battered children: A medical and psychological study, *Br Med J* 3:666-670, 1974.

Snyder, RG, Foust, DR, and Bowman, BM: Study of impact tolerance through free-fall investigation. Prepared for Insurance Institute for Highway Safety by the University of Michigan Highway Safety Research Institute, Final Report 1977.

Sokol, R: Alcohol and abnormal outcomes of pregnancy, *Can Med Assoc J* 125:143-148, 1981.

Spencer, JA, and Grieve, DK: Congenital indifference to pain mistaken for non-accidental injury, *Br J Radiol* 63:308, 1990.

Streissguth, A, Darby, BL, Barr, HM, and Smith, JR: Comparison of drinking and smoking patterns during pregnancy over a six year interval, *Am J Obstet Gynecol* 145:716-724, 1983.

Swischuk, LE: Spine and spinal cord trauma in the battered child syndrome, *Radiology* 92:733, 1969.

Thoennes, N, and Pearson, J: Summary of findings from the sexual abuse allegations project. In EB Nicholson, ed: *Sexual Abuse Allegations in Custody and Visitation Cases*, American Bar Association, 1988.

Trube-Becker, F: Bite marks on battered children, *Z Rechtsmed* 79:73, 1977.

Wheeler, DM, and Hobbs, CJ: Mistakes in diagnosing non-accidental injury: 10 years' experience, *Br Med J* 296:1233-1236, 1988.

Wickes, IG, and Zaidi, ZH: Battered or pigmented? *Br Med J* 2:404, 1972.

Williams, RA: Injuries in infants and small children resulting from witnessed and corroborated free falls, *J Trauma* 31(10):1350-1352, 1991.

Wilson, EF: Estimation of the age of cutaneous contusions in child abuse, *Pediatrics* 60:751-752, 1977.

Winship, IM, and Winship, WS: Epidermolysis bullosa misdiagnosed as child abuse, *South Afr Med J* 73:369, 1988.

Yeatman, GW, Shaw, C, Barlow, MJ, and Bartlett, G: Pseudobattering in Vietnamese children, *Pediatrics* 58:616, 1976.

Young, WC, Sachs, RG, Braun, BG, and Watkins, RT: Patients reporting ritual abuse in childhood: A clinical syndrome, *Child Abuse Negl* 15:181-189, 1991.

# RADIOLOGY OF CHILD ABUSE

GREGORY D. LAUNIUS, M.D.
MICHAEL J. SILBERSTEIN, M.D.
ATCHAWEE LUISIRI, M.D.
E. RICHARD GRAVISS, M.D.

The role of radiology in child abuse is threefold: (1) identifying traumatic injury; (2) recognizing abusive origin; and (3) employing the optimal imaging modality to document findings. The radiologist's strength lies in identifying the type, extent, and age of the child's injury, as well as in distinguishing between accidental injury and inflicted abuse. This distinction is important, as the recognition of nonaccidental injury opens the door to intervention, thereby breaking the cycle of abuse.

The pediatric radiologist encounters a wide range of injuries resulting from child abuse. The most obvious are the physical injuries from intentionally inflicted trauma. Injury related to child neglect is equally important, since it is more common and harder to detect.

By being aware of the possibility of abuse and alert to its indications, the radiologist is able to identify the traumatic focus. Plain films are most effective in evaluating physical changes to bony structures. However, with the advent of additional modalities, less obvious but significant internal injuries can now be imaged when suspicion is high.

The radiologist plays a key role in the treatment team where he identifies, documents, reports, and testifies in cases of child abuse. In recognizing physical abuse, the radiologist must possess an awareness of the likely mechanism of injury. To this he adds his knowledge of the specificity of radiologic findings and the demographics of child abuse (Cameron, 1978; Merten, 1983).

Often it is the lack of correlation between the type of injury observed, the known mechanism required for its production, and the purported mechanism of injury that allows for the diagnosis of abuse (Swischuk, 1992). Maintaining a high index of suspicion for abuse in his differential diagnosis allows the radiologist to be among the first to note discrepancies between history and radiographic findings. He then selects the appropriate imaging modality to provide the optimal examination to confirm or deny the possibility of nonaccidental injury.

Included in the role of the radiologist is the responsibility to report suspected child abuse to the proper authorities and to work with them to prevent further injury (English & Grossman, 1989). One of the greatest benefits in diagnosing child abuse is the prevention of recurrence. For this reason, meticulous attention to technique and interpretation is essential, and statistically valid, high-quality images must be obtained so that confident testimony can be given (Leonidas, 1983).

It also falls within the radiologist's realm to consider the risk-to-benefit ratio for all examinations. The issue of cost versus diagnostic benefit is subjective and difficult to evaluate, given the implicit ethical considerations. Potential risks from ionizing radiation and complications of contrast or sedation must be weighed against the benefit of preventing further abuse.

In summary, the pediatric radiologist plays a strategic role in the diagnosis of abuse. His awareness of the mechanisms of injury, the optimal imaging modality, and the specificity of findings make him a key member in the team of caregivers of the abused or neglected child (**Table 2-1**).

---

**Table 2-1. Key Plain Film Findings of Abuse**

The pathognomonic metaphyseal-epiphyseal fracture, occurring at the ends of long bones, the acromial process of the scapula, and the clavicular ends.

Rib fractures in infants, multiple rib fractures, or posterior location correlate strongly with child abuse. (Rib fractures are uncommon sequelae of delivery or CPR.)

Fractures in multiple stages of healing.

Oblique long bone fractures in children under 18 months are suspicious for nonaccidental injury.

Vertebral fractures in infants are suspicious for abuse and require neurologic and skeletal follow-up.

Infantile subdural hematomas are best assumed to be indicative of nonaccidental injury in the absence of appropriate history and external signs.

Skull fractures that are depressed, cross the midline, or are occipital are suggestive of abuse.

---

## ◆ MODALITIES

The radiologist has at his disposal multiple methods of evaluating bony and soft tissue structures, including X-ray films, nuclear medicine, computerized tomography, magnetic resonance imaging, and ultrasound.

### X-RAY FILMS

Plain films provide the foundation for imaging nonaccidental injury in children. The radiographic skeletal survey has its highest yield in children under 2 years of age. After age 2, a more directed approach can be used, and after age 5, complete screening is usually unnecessary. Bone abnormalities themselves rarely result in long-term handicapping conditions. In performing radiologic studies for bone injuries the greatest benefit may be derived from documenting and dating abuse in the hope of preventing recurrence.

The skeletal survey should include a two-view chest with bone technique, a two-view skull, lateral lumbar spine, anteroposterior (AP) pelvis and AP views of the upper and lower extremities, including AP feet and posteroanterior (PA) hands (Kleinman, 1987). While the number of radiographs will vary with the size of the patient, the use of a single image, formerly called a "babygram," is no longer acceptable (Merten & Carpenter, 1990).

It is of great importance to maintain high technical standards in obtaining films in child abuse. One of the most frequent causes of missed or overdiagnosed cases of child abuse relates to poor quality films.

### NUCLEAR MEDICINE

Radiopharmaceuticals can be tagged and delivered to specific organs. Long scan times are required during imaging by the gamma camera. In children, sedation is frequently required. Radiation doses must be specific to each child to minimize exposure (Harcke, 1978). In addition, potassium perchlorate administration is useful to decrease the thyroid dose in technetium studies (Harcke, 1978).

In child abuse, bone imaging is the most commonly requested nuclear study to demonstrate osseous injuries not identified on standard X-rays (Merten & Carpenter, 1990). Bone scanning demonstrates abnormalities within hours of osseous injury and can show lesions missed on plain films (Harcke, 1978). These occult injuries may be nondisplaced traumatic fractures, stress fractures, and periosteal reaction. Injuries in regions difficult to evaluate on plain film, such as spine and ribs, can also be well seen (Harcke, 1978; Merten & Carpenter, 1990).

The high sensitivity of bone scintigraphy is offset by its low specificity. In addition, lesions adjacent to the growth plate can be missed entirely unless asymmetry is noted with the contralateral growth plate (Harcke, 1978). A high degree of technical precision is required, as even asymmetric positioning can cause abnormal activity on images.

The bone scan delivers a greater radiation dose than plain films, is less readily available, and costs more (Kleinman, 1987; Merten & Carpenter, 1990). Most nuclear medicine departments are not experienced in imaging children, and long scan times make patient motion a significant problem. Liver/spleen nuclear scanning is useful in evaluating splenic trauma, but the low specificity decreases its value for hepatic injury (Reece & Grodin, 1985).

## COMPUTED TOMOGRAPHY

Computed tomography has proven to be cost-effective and useful for evaluation of intracranial and intra-abdominal abnormalities (Merten & Carpenter, 1990). In the acute setting, CT is superior to MRI for the relative ease with which imaging can be performed in the unstable patient. In addition, CT is faster, less expensive, and not affected by rib and vertebral artifact, as is ultrasound (Kirks, 1983). CT is the examination of choice for children with suspected abdominal trauma (Kirks, 1983; Tolia et al., 1990). Specifically, CT facilitates the identification of splenic and hepatic injury in children without significant clinical complaint following blunt trauma.

A head CT is needed for evaluation of any child with a positive skeletal survey (Merten & Carpenter, 1990). It allows specific and sensitive detection of abnormalities such as extra-axial fluid collections, intraparenchymal and intraventricular hemorrhage, and cerebral edema (Reece & Grodin, 1985). CT is the method of choice for acute assessment of intracranial abnormalities and provides rapid, easy follow-up examination (McClelland et al., 1980).

There are, however, some limitations in intracranial CT evaluation. Small hemorrhages can be missed due to volume averaging. Subdural hematomas and fractures that lie in the plane of section can be missed entirely (Ball, 1989). Also, CT is relatively insensitive for the evaluation of small posterior fossa subdural hematomas, due to extensive artifact, unless coronal or thin sections are used (Zimmerman et al., 1978; Kleinman, 1987).

## MAGNETIC RESONANCE IMAGING

MR imaging, with its greater anatomic detail, is more sensitive than CT in detecting certain intracranial abnormalities, such as subdural hematomas, parenchymal contusions, and bleeding (Sato et al., 1989; Merten & Carpenter, 1990). MRI has the advantage of multiplanar imaging without ionizing radiation. Coronal planes and absent bone artifact improve sensitivity to posterior fossa hemorrhage and subdural hematoma (Alexander et al., 1986) (**Figure 2-1**).

Long MRI scan times frequently require sedation, as the technique is very sensitive to motion artifact. In the acute setting, it is even more

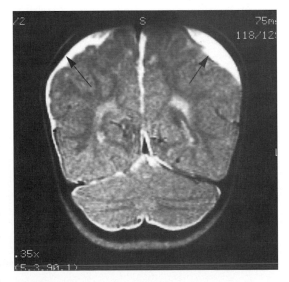

*Figure 2-1*. Coronal T2-weighted image demonstrating bright signal in bilateral subdural hematomas along parietal convexities (arrows).

difficult to obtain quality MRI examinations. Consequently, CT remains the modality of choice for intracranial assessment because of its availability and rapidity in the unstable patient.

MR imaging also allows the relative dating of subdural hemorrhage. This makes it useful in differentiating chronic subdural hematoma with ventricular enlargement from atrophy (Ball, 1989; Merten & Carpenter, 1990). MRI is of greater use in the subacute and chronic phases of central nervous system (CNS) evaluation of child abuse. Overall, MRI remains of limited value in nonaccidental injury.

## ULTRASOUND

Ultrasound allows the imaging of soft tissues without radiation exposure and is a safe and inexpensive means of examination. Ultrasound examinations are performed rapidly, with sedation rarely needed. In children under 2 years of age, ultrasound can be used to detect intracranial abnormalities, such as ventricular enlargement, cerebral edema, and intracranial hemorrhage. Large extra-axial fluid collections are visible, but smaller collections may be missed.

Ultrasound is often used as a screening tool in suspected nonaccidental abdominal injury, and the examination can be tailored to evaluate specific organs, such as the liver, spleen, pancreas, or kidneys. Evaluation via ultrasound is of particular use in identifying the sequelae of abuse, such as pseudocysts and pancreatitis (Merten & Carpenter, 1990). Free fluid or hemorrhage within the abdomen can be readily appreciated using ultrasound, as can retroperitoneal hematoma (Silverman & Kuhn, 1992).

A potential limitation for ultrasound examination is the technical variability that results from the different skill levels of sonographers. In addition, organs can be obscured by ribs, bone, and air artifact (Kleinman, 1987).

## ♦ DATING SKELETAL INJURY

The capacity to determine the age of a skeletal injury is critical to the radiologic diagnosis of child abuse (Merten & Carpenter, 1990). The differentiation between accidental and inflicted injuries depends as much on the ability to determine *when* as *how* the injury occurred. Dating injuries illuminates discrepancies between the radiographic findings and the history provided. Any incongruity can warn of possible abuse. Radiologic studies are also extremely useful in distinguishing old or healing bone injuries from new ones (McNeese & Hebeler, 1977). The presence of old *and* new fractures, suggesting that abuse took place over a period of time, is a strong indicator of nonaccidental injury in children.

The ability to determine the time of occurrence relies on the accepted radiologic and pathologic correlation for osseous injury. Following bone injury, hemorrhage occurs around the fracture, lifting the periosteum. An acute inflammatory change is initiated within hours and lasts approximately 3 days (Perper & Wecht, 1980).

In the first 4 days, histologic studies show that osteogenic granulation tissue has initiated the proliferative phase without radiographically appreciable healing. In this stage, soft tissue edema or a fracture line may be the only radiographic evidence of injury (Perper & Wecht, 1980). It is at this time that the radionuclide bone scan can detect subperiosteal change not yet evident radiographically.

A minimum of 5 days is required to see visible radiologic changes. In 5 to 14 days, a thin layer of subperiosteal new bone will be formed (Kleinman, 1987). By 10 days, the cellular collar, which includes osteogenic cells, is noted (Perper & Wecht, 1980). Within a week, woven bone is being formed for the temporary repair, which will correspond to the callus, the body's "splint" for the fracture. This callus calcifies 10 to 15 days after injury and can be difficult to appreciate initially (Swischuk, 1992).

It is not unusual for fracture sites in infants and young children to appear normal 6 months after injury. This healing process applies to the fracture of a long bone as well as to metaphyseal injury and rib fractures. However, fractures of the skull are an exception in that no significant healing reaction will occur for a minimum of 4 to 6 weeks (Cameron, 1978).

In summary, the dating of a fracture involves the recognition of soft tissue changes, fracture line visibility, calcification of callus, and ossification of new periosteal bone (Swischuk, 1992). The radiologist is able to correlate the physical and radiologic findings, keeping in mind the age of the injury and the mechanism of production.

## ♦ MULTIPLE FRACTURES

A maxim in the evaluation of plain films by the radiologist is that multiple fractures at multiple stages of healing are pathognomonic for child abuse (Swischuk, 1992). The concept of multiple fractures includes both injuries of a number of different bones as well as more than one site of trauma within the same bone (**Figure 2-2**). It is important for the radiologist to remember that although multiplicity of injury is a characteristic finding in nonaccidental injury in childhood, severe accidental trauma is another plausible explanation. Also, certain bone diseases can produce radiologic changes consistent with the multiple fractures of child abuse. Careful history and clinical correlation are essential.

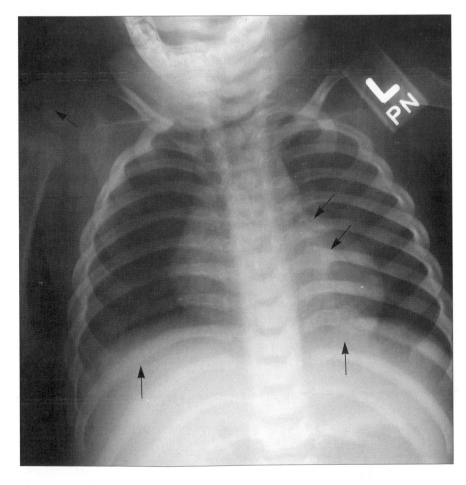

*Figure 2-2. AP chest radiograph demonstrates multiple fractures at varying stages of healing. A new right humeral fracture and multiple bilateral healing rib fractures are present.*

## ◆ EXTREMITIES

Skeletal injuries, in contrast to intracranial and abdominal injuries, are rarely life-threatening, can cause long-term deformity, and have higher specificity for abuse. The entire axial and appendicular skeleton can be a target for abuse, with the extremities being the most common focus.

The skeletal survey is the primary examination for musculoskeletal trauma. A standard skeletal survey consists of AP views of the extremities, including the hands and feet, AP and lateral skull views, AP chest and abdomen films, and a lateral thoracolumbar spine view. The risk-to-benefit ratio regarding radiation exposure favors the continued use of the skeletal survey (Ellerstein & Norris, 1984).

Physical signs suggesting skeletal injuries in abuse include tenderness, swelling, reduced range of motion, pseudoparalysis, and limb deformity. In the abuse setting these symptoms indicate the need for skeletal survey. Neurological changes should also initiate a skeletal survey, as 70% of abuse-related intracranial injuries have associated fractures (McNeese & Hebeler, 1977; Merten & Carpenter, 1990).

The skeletal survey is most beneficial in younger patients and children with extensive soft tissue injury. This relates to the observation that the younger the child, the greater the chance the fracture is from nonaccidental injury (Elliot, 1979).

Neonatal abuse requires special consideration. In utero conditions such as infection and rickets can cause osseous abnormalities. Injuries related to birth trauma and congenital skeletal dysplasia in the newborn may also present with bones in various stages of repair (Radkowski, 1983).

Fractures are found in slightly over one third of all physically abused children and represent over 80% of the total abuse-related injuries seen by radiology. Dislocations are uncommon in nonaccidental injury. Joint malalignment relates most often to metaphyseal-epiphyseal injury. True dislocations are usually associated with severe trauma. Relative weakness of the metaphyseal-epiphyseal region with resultant propensity for fracture spares the joint space ligaments from dislocating force (Kleinman, 1987; Merten & Carpenter, 1990).

### TYPES OF FRACTURES/MECHANISMS OF INJURY

In child abuse, skeletal fractures can be subdivided into those involving the metaphyseal-epiphyseal region and those involving the diaphysis. The metaphyseal-epiphyseal fractures include the classically described corner fracture, bucket-handle fracture, and metaphyseal lucency. Recent research has shown that these fractures represent varying appearances of the same injury (**Figure 2-3a,b,c**). They are pathognomonic for abuse because the force required for this type of injury is greater than that of a simple fall or accident (Silverman & Kuhn, 1992). They can occur in any bone adjacent to a growth plate, such as the clavicle or acromial process of the scapula.

Historically, metaphyseal-epiphyseal fractures were thought to represent avulsion of peripheral metaphyseal fragments at a site of fixed periosteal attachment. It is now known that shaking and jerking with attendant accelerating/decelerating forces produce a shearing effect resulting in transverse fractures in the weak, immature primary spongiosum layer. These transverse fractures along with the varying degrees of ossification in the fracture fragments and the projection of the radiograph combine to produce the multiple appearances of the same injury (Kleinman, 1987).

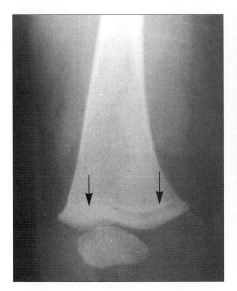

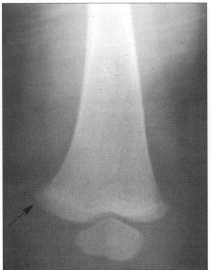

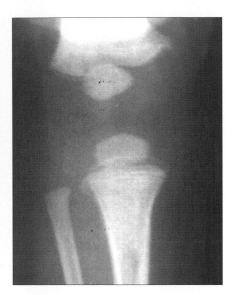

***Figure 2-3a***. *Fracture through the distal femoral metaphysis presents as abnormal lucency (arrows).*

***Figure 2-3b***. *Metaphyseal fracture presents as corner avulsion due to projection and thickness of ossified segments involved (arrow).*

***Figure 2-3c***. *Fracture across the entire metaphysis combined with nontangential projection produces characteristic "bucket-handle" fracture of child abuse.*

Fractures of the diaphysis are less specific for abuse than metaphyseal-epiphyseal fractures, but occur four times more often in abused children. Diaphyseal fractures are either oblique (spiral) or transverse. A single long bone fracture, coinciding with either the pathognomonic metaphyseal or multiple rib fracture injury patterns, should be considered nonaccidental without plausible history. Oblique fractures are caused by rotational or torsional forces applied to the limb, and transverse fractures result from a direct blow or a bending force. Torsional forces that produce the spiral fracture can be either accidental or intentionally inflicted. Without appropriate history, lower extremity spiral fractures in children who are not yet ambulatory imply abuse (**Figure 2-4**).

Subperiosteal hematoma is a common diaphyseal injury in child abuse. The loosely attached, highly vascularized periosteum of the diaphysis is easily lifted off the bone by hemorrhage from injury. Initial images show an intact cortex, but may reveal soft tissue edema related to the hemorrhage. Between 5 and 14 days after injury, an unbroken line of calcification reflecting periosteal new bone formation can be seen. Further healing will result in cortical thickening. Researchers have found that in cases of cortical thickening, there is often evidence to suggest rough handling or shaking (Tufts et al., 1982; Kleinman, 1987; Merten & Carpenter, 1990) (**Figure 2-5**).

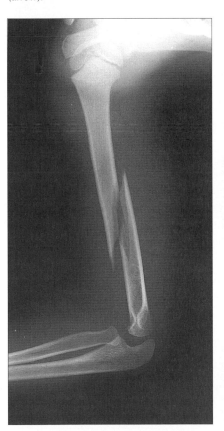

***Figure 2-4.*** *Single bony injury in a 4 1/2-year-old with Crouzon's disease. Films demonstrate oblique diaphyseal fracture with rotational component.*

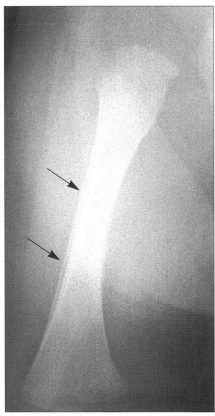

***Figure 2-5.*** *Examination demonstrates diaphyseal periosteal reaction (arrows) consistent with healing subperiosteal hemorrhage.*

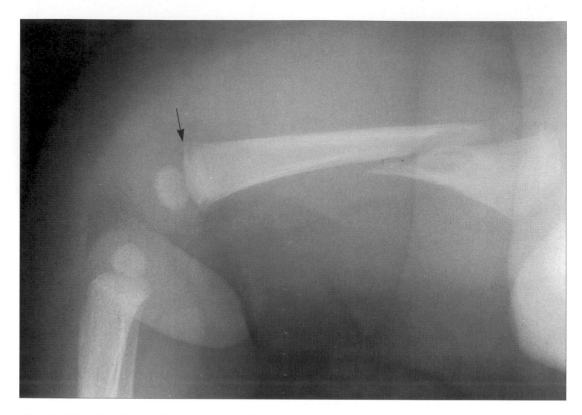

**Figure 2-6.** *Lateral radiograph demonstrating an oblique fracture of the right femoral diaphysis. Other metaphyseal fractures with varied stages of healing were present. Bucket-handle fracture is seen distally (arrow).*

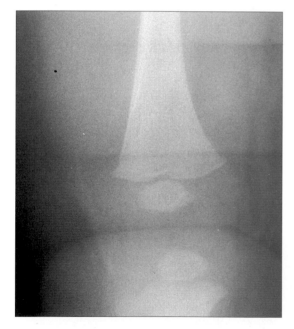

**Figure 2-7.** *Distal femoral metaphyseal-epiphyseal fracture presenting as a bucket-handle fracture in 4-month-old male.*

## ♦ REGIONAL SKELETAL INJURIES

### FEMUR

The femur is one of the most frequently fractured long bones in nonaccidental injury. Two peaks in incidence for femoral fracture occur, one at 6 months and the next at 3 years of age (Kleinman, 1987). Femoral shaft fractures are more common than metaphyseal-epiphyseal fractures, but are of lower specificity for abuse (Leonidas, 1983). As age increases, specificity decreases. The rotational mechanism of injury for an oblique fracture is highly suspicious for abuse in nonwalking children (Kleinman, 1987). These fractures require correlation with the history, presence of healing, and other injuries before being diagnosed as nonaccidental (**Figure 2-6**).

The distal metaphyseal-epiphyseal complex is fractured more often than the proximal (Kleinman, 1987), with lesions often bilateral due to flailing motion associated with severe shaking (**Figure 2-7**). The multiple growth plates in the proximal femur, with initial nonossification, make fractures in this region difficult to evaluate. Radiographic changes might show only subtle findings of soft tissue injury or abnormal alignment of the shaft relative to the pelvis. Arthrography or bone scintigraphy can aid in evaluating this region. Identification of proximal fractures is important, since proximal growth plate fractures have greater long-term sequelae than their more common distal counterparts.

### TIBIA AND FIBULA

Tibial shaft fractures are less common than metaphyseal fractures. In contrast to the femur, metaphyseal-epiphyseal fractures usually involve the proximal tibia

(Kleinman, 1987). Bilateral metaphyseal fractures of the proximal tibia are not uncommon and result from acceleration/deceleration forces produced by shaking (**Figure 2-8**).

The tibial diaphysis is a common location for subperiosteal hemorrhage and subperiosteal reaction. Fracture lines in shaft fractures are not always seen (Kleinman, 1987), and healing reaction can be the only indication of their presence. Rotational stress in a newly walking child is not unusual, is unintentional, and produces the so-called toddler's fracture, which usually occurs between the ages of 9 months and 3 years and should not be confused with abusive injury (Kirks, 1984; Kleinman, 1987) (**Figure 2-9**).

Fibular fractures are rare. Shaft fractures are often found in conjunction with tibial shaft fractures as a result of a direct blow. Distal and proximal fibular metaphyseal fractures are possible but rare (**Figure 2-10**).

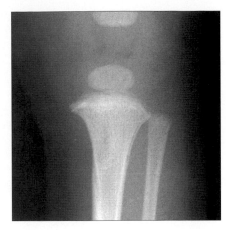

**Figure 2-8**. *The typical location for tibial metaphyseal-epiphyseal fractures is seen in this 3 1/2-month-old female with a bucket-handle fracture.*

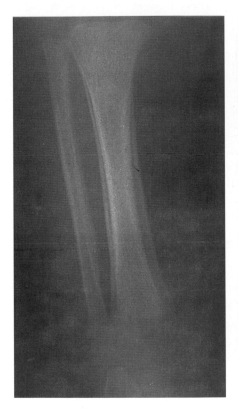

**Figure 2-9**. *Extensive tibial periosteal reaction with no fracture ever appreciated in this 7-week-old child with right parietal fracture and subgaleal hematoma.*

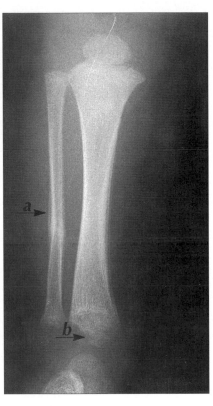

**Figure 2-10**. *AP view of the right tibia and fibula demonstrates healing reaction at a fibular fracture site (arrow a). Mild tibial periosteal reaction is also present, suggesting evolving subperiosteal hemorrhage. Also noted is a bucket-handle tibial metaphyseal fracture (arrow b).*

## FOOT FRACTURES

Foot fractures are not common, but their specificity for abuse is high. They more often involve older children. Of the multiple foot bones, the metatarsal is the most likely site of injury. For this reason, detailed foot views are helpful in the skeletal survey (Kleinman, 1987; Merten & Carpenter, 1990).

## HUMERAL SHAFT FRACTURES

Humeral shaft fractures tend to be oblique fractures arising from indirect torsion, such as grabbing the upper extremity distally and pulling or twisting. The less common transverse fracture is usually the result of a direct blow (**Figure 2-11**).

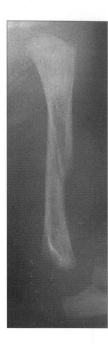

*Figure 2-11. An oblique fracture of the left humerus with rotational component is demonstrated in this 2-month-old female with multiple fractures.*

Other mechanisms of injury, such as shaking the child by the forearms or pulling the child up, are more often involved in injury to the metaphyseal-epiphyseal complexes. Injuries to the proximal growth plates, as in the femur, are difficult to evaluate because of their nonossified components. Subtle radiographic signs such as metaphyseal lucency or healing reaction may be the first plain film indication of trauma.

Another radiographic finding in metaphyseal-epiphyseal fractures is the displacement of the humerus away from the glenoid cavity (Kleinman, 1987). This occurs with greater frequency in association with severe trauma. An arthrogram can help confirm this finding.

Distinction between fracture separation and elbow dislocation is complicated by the nonossified nature of the distal humeral epiphysis. Statistically, fracture/separation is more common than dislocation. Prior to ossification, the olecranon lies medial to its expected location overlying the distal humerus in epiphyseal separation. After ossification of the capitellum at 3 to 4 months, the capitellar-radial relationship can be used to distinguish dislocation from metaphyseal-epiphyseal complex injury (Silverman & Kuhn, 1992) (**Figure 2-12**).

Supracondylar fractures are typical of accidental injury and are nonspecific for child abuse (Kleinman, 1987). They require correlation with other factors, such as history and degree of healing.

The literature reveals that forearm fractures represent 10% to 20% of all skeletal injuries from child abuse (Kleinman, 1987). This reflects the tendency to grab the upper extremities when shaking and pulling the child. Metaphyseal-epiphyseal injuries are much more common distally than proximally. The bucket-handle appearance is rarely seen, with most injuries presenting as metaphyseal lucencies or corner fractures (Merten & Carpenter, 1990).

Diaphyseal fractures of the radius and ulna occur in child abuse and are most often transverse. In these cases, blocking blows with the forearm corresponds to the known mechanism of injury for transverse fractures—that is, direct impact. Periosteal bone formation also presents in the forearm diaphyses as the manifestation of subperiosteal hemorrhage from direct blow or twisting injury (Kleinman, 1987).

## HANDS

It is suspected that hand fractures, like foot fractures, occur more frequently than the literature might indicate. This may reflect the failure to obtain quality hand radiographs (Kleinman, 1987). Fractures of the metacarpals can involve both the shafts and the metaphyseal-epiphyseal regions. Fractures or dislocations of the phalanges have been described in child abuse, possibly related to corporal punishment from direct blows.

## ♦ SPINE INJURIES

Fractures of the spine are infrequently associated with abuse. Those related to nonaccidental injury are often only a part of major trauma and may involve more than one site and level. The area of the spine most often involved is the thoracolumbar region. Abusive spine injuries are usually noted in infants and young children, with half occurring in children younger than 1 year. Most of these fractures are related to hyperflexion-hyperextension, either from shaking or direct blows (Cameron, 1978; Leonidas, 1983; Kleinman, 1987; Merten & Carpenter, 1990). Trauma to the spinal cord may occur without apparent bony injury. Swelling of the adjacent soft tissues may be the only plain film indication of spinal cord injury.

Most abusive injuries to the spine involve the vertebral body, and hyperflexion is the common mechanism of injury. Radiographic findings vary from subtle to severe anterior vertebral compression fractures. This often appears as a loss of bone

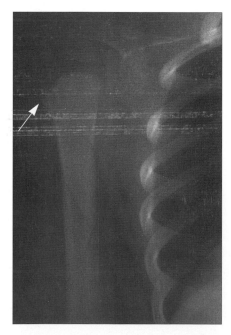

*Figure 2-12. Proximal metaphyseal avulsion of the humerus (arrow) is less common than distal metaphyseal involvement in abuse.*

on the anterosuperior and, less frequently, the anteroinferior margin of the vertebral body. With healing, sclerosis will be evident at the fracture site. Vertebral fractures are typically in the thoracolumbar spine, and a lateral view of this region in the standard skeletal survey provides optimal visualization (**Figure 2-13**).

Spinal trauma can cause anterior disk herniation with narrowing of the intervertebral disk space. Disturbance of the ring apophysis from disk herniation can alter vertebral body development with long-lasting debilitating effect. Disk space narrowing caused by abuse is less marked than that from infectious diskitis. The anterior corner notching is typically larger in abuse than in diskitis/osteomyelitis. When radiographic findings provide insufficient distinction from abuse, clinical and laboratory findings can help differentiate these entities (Kleinman, 1987).

Fractures of the posterior elements have been described by Kleinman as a result of hyperflexion-hyperextension injuries from shaking. Most often they present as spinous process avulsions at the interspinous ligament attachment. With time these show progressive calcification and ossification. These avulsion injuries of the posterior elements are stable. Only in rare instances has the unstable "hangman's fracture" been described. This may present as a subtle vertical lucency posterior to the body of C2 (Kleinman, 1987).

Subluxation of one vertebral body in relation to another may also occur in child abuse. Most subluxations are anterior or posterior and are effectively demonstrated on the lateral radiograph. Rare lateral subluxations have been described and would be seen on the AP view of the abdomen-pelvis. Cervical involvement is rare. Cervical pseudosubluxation at C2 is a common variant readily distinguished by means of alignments of the posterior elements. The method developed by Dr. Swischuk for this differentiation is readily available in Keats' *Atlas of Roentgenographic Measurement*. Pseudosubluxation is more common than true subluxation (Keats, 1985).

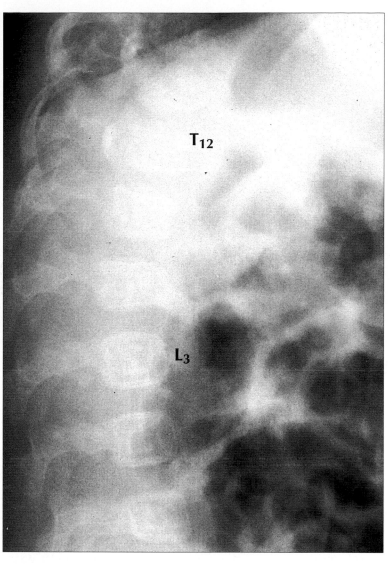

**Figure 2-13**. *Lateral thoracolumbar spine with compression fractures presenting as loss of height of the anterior L1 and L2 vertebral bodies in a child with intracranial injuries and skull fracture.*

Bone scintigraphy has been helpful in evaluation of posterior elements and transverse processes but is relatively insensitive for vertebral body fractures (Merten & Carpenter, 1990). Therefore the modality of choice remains plain films of the skeletal survey (Kleinman, 1987). Identification of spinal fractures requires careful examination of the thoracolumbar spine on the lateral view. Any vertebral fracture in an infant must raise the possibility of inflicted injury with resultant follow-up for abuse both clinically and radiographically.

## CHEST

Injury to the bony thorax occurs less frequently than extremity fractures in child abuse. Thoracic injury is of greater diagnostic specificity than extremity fractures

(Merten & Carpenter, 1990). Most chest injuries involve rib fractures and resultant complications. Accidental fracture of the rib cage is rare in infants and young children, as the rib cage is relatively compliant and resistant to injury from falls and accidental childhood trauma. The typical accidental injury occurs in children older than 2 years; a reversal of this age distribution is seen in abuse, with almost 90% occurring in children under age 2 years. Most rib fractures in abuse are multiple and located posteriorly, next to the costovertebral junction. The next most common fracture site is the lateral rib, with anterior costochondral separations occurring rarely. These last two sites are more often associated with extremely violent trauma.

Excessive squeezing of the chest can cause fractures at points of maximal stress. Ribs articulate with the spine at the costovertebral junction. As the ribs extend posterolaterally away from the spine, they overlie the transverse process. When squeezed, the ribs are bent over the transverse process, and injury can damage the periosteum or produce a fracture. As greater stress is applied, the force is transferred to the lateral and then the anterior ribs. This mechanism accounts for the location and equal age of multiple fractures in a single rib (Kleinman, 1987).

Although squeezing is the most often described mechanism of injury, direct blows to the chest can also cause rib fractures. The fracture occurs at the site of impact, often with an accompanying bruise (Alexander et al., 1990). Rib fractures are often initially invisible. The healing phase can cause asymmetric appearance of the posterior ribs from bone widening and sclerosis in posterior rib fractures. Lateral oblique films can help image lateral fractures. Callus formation may actually reveal the fracture line within the area of rib widening. The difficulty in imaging acute rib fractures has made the high sensitivity of the bone scan of great use in the difficult clinical situation requiring additional documentation of physical abuse.

Rib fractures related to delivery are rare, and incidental rib fractures in a patient with normal bones are highly suspicious for child abuse. The only mitigating factor would be a reasonable history of severe direct trauma to the chest. It should also be noted that although cardiopulmonary resuscitation (CPR) has been associated with rib fractures in adults, CPR in children rarely, if ever, causes fracture. Children have been known to present to emergency rooms with a supposed history of resuscitation and resultant fractures, and these explanations are often accepted without question (Feldman & Brewer, 1984). In light of this common misconception, unexplained rib fractures, specifically the posterior, are virtually pathognomonic for child abuse.

Underlying intrathoracic injury can result from severe squeezing. While pneumothoraces and subcutaneous emphysema can result from rib trauma, they are an uncommon occurrence. Pneumothoraces are best seen on the upright or decubitus chest radiographs. The decubitus films also reveal pleural fluid collections that may or may not relate to rib fracture. Pleural effusions may be a sign of associated pancreatitis, or they may actually represent a chylothorax. This can be the result of a severe compression injury that disrupts the thoracic lymphatic duct. Chylothoraces in the chest are located on the right, owing to thoracic duct anatomy.

The occurrence of pulmonary contusion as it relates to child abuse has not been well described in the literature, but given the incidence of rib fractures in child abuse, a higher frequency would not be surprising. Pulmonary infiltrates have been reported from both forced aspiration and as a result of infection related to neglect.

## CLAVICLE

The majority of clavicular fractures in abuse are in the mid shaft and are indistinguishable from those of accidental injury. Fractures of the medial one third of the clavicle shaft have a greater specificity for abuse. Avulsion fractures of either the medial or lateral clavicular apophyses are of greater diagnostic specificity for abuse. It is convenient to think of these as metaphyseal-epiphyseal lesions. Clavicle avulsion injuries often result from sudden traction of the associated arm. It is not surprising that they are frequently associated with proximal humeral injury.

Since scapular fractures rarely occur by accident, they are highly suspicious for child abuse. The most frequent site is the acromial apophysis. The next most fractured area is the coracoid process; glenoid fractures are uncommon (Merten & Carpenter, 1990). The rare fracture to the body of the scapula occurs as the result of a direct blow, whereas other scapular injuries are the result of indirect forces. Scapular fractures are difficult to evaluate radiographically, due to the scapula's location behind ribs and its anatomically complex shape. Bone scans can be helpful in the assessment of this difficult region.

### STERNUM

Sternal injuries are rare. This may relate to the multiple joints and resultant greater mobility, allowing dispersion of forces. Radiographically, they can present as sternomanubrial joint displacement or as defects along the cartilaginous edge of a sternal ossification center (Kleinman, 1987).

### PELVIS

Pelvic fractures are not commonly described in conjunction with nonaccidental injury in children. Occasional literature reports have noted periosteal reaction as subtle evidence of abuse. Kleinman suggests that, given the incidence of femoral fractures, fractures involving the adjacent pelvis should be more common, and careful attention to pelvic films may confirm this observation.

In summary, unexplained rib fractures are specific for abuse, as fractures to the ribs are uncommon in children under 2 years. Clavicular fractures involving the medial and lateral ends have a specificity for abuse equal to metaphyseal-epiphyseal lesions in the long bones. Scapular injuries are rare but highly specific for nonaccidental injury (see Table 2-1).

## ◆ CRANIOFACIAL INJURIES

Intracranial sequelae are the most serious and significant findings in child abuse. The incidence varies from 10% to 44%, depending on the study, on the children studied, and on the modality used (Sato et al., 1989). CNS injury may be the only manifestation of abuse; however, 70% have associated skeletal injuries.

The majority of fatalities in child abuse involve head injury. Morbidity and mortality are most significant in children less than 2 years old (90%). Residual changes can be seen in nearly 80% of those surviving intracranial injury. It is suspected that many cases of mental retardation can be ascribed to child abuse (Merten & Osborne, 1983; Reece & Grodin, 1985; Ball, 1989; Sato et al., 1989).

Important in CNS injury are the ramifications of shaking. As a mechanism of injury, shaking accounts for the presence of intracranial injury in children without apparent external trauma to the head. Acceleration/deceleration and rotational forces result in shearing injury to the intracranial contents. These shearing forces separate structures that have varying degrees of fixation/mobility and can result in retinal hemorrhage, extra-axial fluid collections, hemorrhage/contusion at the gray/white matter junctions, and cerebral edema (McClelland et al., 1980; Merten & Osborne, 1983; Ball, 1989; Merten & Carpenter, 1990). Direct blows to the brain can produce the same findings as shaking, with calvarial and extracranial injury. This is because both direct and indirect (shaking) trauma can produce the same rotation/shearing forces that cause intracranial injury. In many instances, shaking and direct blows occur together.

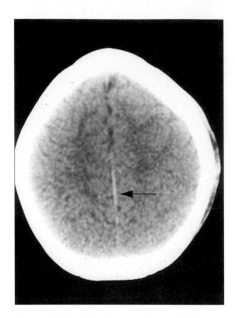

***Figure 2-14.*** *High density adjacent to the falx represents a subtle falcine subdural hematoma. Although it is common, the falcine subdural hematoma is easily missed.*

Several unique anatomic characteristics of the infant cranium make it susceptible to specific types of injuries. These include the increased elasticity from calvarial flexibility and sutural patency, as well as the increased plasticity from immature myelinization. Also, the child's brain floats in a relatively larger cerebrospinal fluid space than that of the adult. This renders the bridging veins vulnerable to tearing, with resultant subdural hematomas (Merten & Osborne, 1983; Alexander et al., 1990). The higher metabolic rate in children and infants, along with a higher vasoreactivity, makes children more susceptible to cerebral edema after intracranial injury (Merten & Osborne, 1983). The large head size of the child, combined with the relatively lax musculature of the neck, accentuates the acceleration/deceleration forces in injuries caused by shaking.

The brain is also injured secondarily through trauma to circulation and respiration. Direct trauma to the blood vessels supplying the brain and subsequent cerebral swelling may compromise brain vascularization. Strangulation with resultant asphyxia is another well-described means of producing cerebral edema (Merten & Osborne, 1983).

## SUBDURAL HEMATOMAS

Subdural hematoma was among the earliest described indicators of child abuse and is the most common intracranial sequela of abuse (Cameron, 1978; Sato et al., 1989; Merten & Carpenter, 1990). A rupture of the bridging veins between the brain and the sinuses of the dura can be caused by either direct blows to the head or shaking, with its rotational shearing forces. Subdural hematomas are most common under 24 months of age, with peak occurrence at 6 months (Reece & Grodin, 1985) (**Figure 2-14**). They are most often located within the interhemispheric fissure, given the frequent involvement of the sagittal sinus veins, and can extend over the cerebral convexity. Posterior fossa subdural hematomas can be difficult to evaluate on CT due to technical factors. The shape will depend on the amount of blood, the speed of hemorrhage, and the location within the brain. As blood accumulates at the site of the tear, it can widen the subdural space, causing further tearing and making the adjacent veins susceptible to more tearing.

The high frequency of bilateral subdural hematomas in child abuse corresponds with the picture expected from the shaking theory of injury. As the child is often grasped symmetrically by the limbs, the shearing forces tend to act symmetrically on the bridging veins (Guthkelch, 1971; Reece & Grodin, 1985).

Small hematomas may be difficult to visualize when at the base of the brain or the vertex. Larger subdural hematomas can easily be identified by the crescent configuration between the brain and the skull. These larger hematomas are encountered less often than the more typical intrahemispheric subdural hemorrhage. With time, subdural hematomas have been known to calcify (Kleinman, 1987). Chronic subdural hematomas are not uncommon, being typically located over the frontal convexities and associated with progressive ventricular enlargement. Cerebral atrophy can develop within a month after injury (Kleinman, 1987; Sato et al., 1989). MRI is superior for the detection of small subdural hematomas, especially in the posterior fossa (Merten & Carpenter, 1990).

MRI assists in dating subdural age by following the levels of hemoglobin breakdown products. Determining the presence of these breakdown products aids in distinguishing subdural collections from atrophy and communicating hydrocephalus. Multiple posttraumatic fluid collections of varying ages indicate repetitive trauma (Sato et al., 1989; Merten & Carpenter, 1990) (**Figure 2-15**). Ultrasound is not helpful for evaluation of small subdural hematomas, but it can be used to follow the progressive changes of large subdural hematomas. Varying echogenicity of extra-axial fluid may indicate injuries of different ages (Kleinman, 1987).

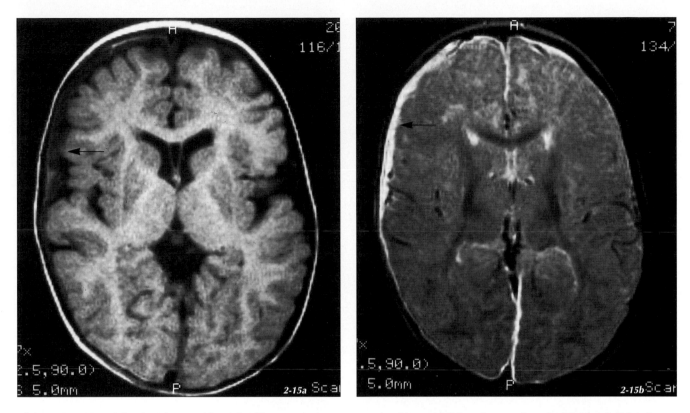

**Figure 2-15a.** *T1-weighted axial scan with subdural hematoma demonstrates signal (arrow) brighter than cerebrospinal fluid and slightly less intense than parenchyma (arrow).* **b.** *T2-weighted axial image showing bright subdural signal consistent with subarachnoid hemorrhage (arrow).*

## EPIDURAL HEMATOMAS

Epidural hematomas are not often found in the setting of child abuse. If present, they are typically associated with a skull fracture. Large epidural hematomas have a lenticular shape with mass effect. Small epidural hematomas may resemble subdural hematomas. It may be helpful in differentiating between the two to note that epidural hematomas can cross midline in contrast to subdural fluid collections, which do not. Due to arterial bleeding, epidural hematomas constitute neurosurgical emergencies (Kleinman, 1987; Merten & Carpenter, 1990) **(Figure 2-16)**.

## SUBARACHNOID HEMORRHAGES

Subarachnoid hemorrhages and subdural fluid collections frequently coexist. It can be difficult to differentiate between the two. MRI and CT are equally well-suited to detect subarachnoid hemorrhages. The association of subarachnoid hemorrhage with cerebral edema should raise the possibility of child abuse for the clinician if no other signs of trauma are present (Alexander et al., 1986, 1990; Cohen et al., 1986).

## INTRACRANIAL HEMORRHAGES

Intracranial hemorrhages on CT, though not specific for child abuse, can result from either direct trauma or vigorous shaking. These superficial or deep cerebral contusions/hematomas are not unusual in inflicted trauma and are frequently associated with other intracranial injuries. Contusional tears are often noted in the white matter adjacent to the gray/white matter junction.

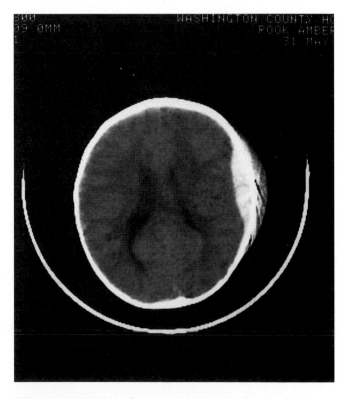

**Figure 2-16.** *CT section demonstrating left parietal epidural hematoma with lenticular shape. Associated fracture cannot be seen without alterations in window settings. Mass effect on left lateral ventricle.*

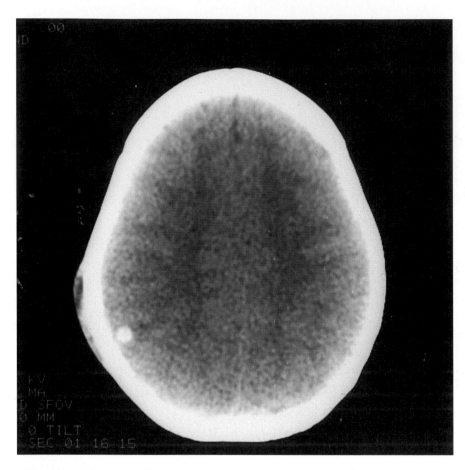

*Figure 2-17. A focal area of high density in the right parietal lobe is consistent with hemorrhagic contusion at gray/white matter interface. Right parietal skull fracture is visible on bone windows adjacent to subgaleal hematoma.*

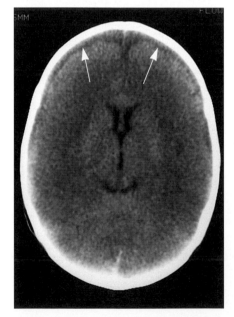

*Figure 2-18. Seven-month-old infant presenting in full arrest with bilateral subdural hematomas (arrows) and cerebral edema demonstrated by loss of gray/white matter differentiation.*

Little bleeding is associated with these changes, which are often microscopic (Reece & Grodin, 1985; Cohen et al., 1986; Kleinman, 1987; Merten & Carpenter, 1990) (**Figure 2-17**).

## CEREBRAL EDEMA

In one study of child abuse, cerebral edema occurred in 65% of patients (Guthkelch, 1971). The overall pattern and appearance of cerebral edema varies, depending on the time between examination and injury. Initially, no findings may be seen; delayed images, days later, may show cerebral edema with a mass effect. A small number of cases with diffuse edema have been described as having a "reversal sign," with the white matter having a higher attenuation than the gray matter on CT, reflecting severe diffuse edema. The reversal sign indicates irreversible brain damage (Cohen et al., 1986).

More typically, cerebral edema results in obliteration of the ventricles from mass effect and loss of the gray/white matter differentiation (**Figure 2-18**). Cerebral edema results from endothelial damage with resultant increased vascular permeability, possibly related to the child's higher level of vasoreactivity. These edema patterns may be focal or general. The presence of focal edema has a higher specificity for abuse. Cerebral edema or infarction may reflect altered cerebral blood flow as a result of vascular injury, as well as hypoxia from asphyxia, smothering, and strangulation (Guthkelch, 1971; Kleinman, 1987; Merten & Carpenter, 1990). Shaking appears to be a more common mechanism of injury for the marked cerebral edema seen without fracture in child abuse (Kleinman, 1987).

## CHRONIC SEQUELAE

Intracranial injury can result in focal or diffuse atrophy. Focal atrophy can be seen as ventricular dilatation with ipsilateral enlargement of the extra-axial spaces. Atrophic changes from abuse may be seen 1 month after injury, with encephalomalacic and porencephalic changes evident on follow-up, consistent with severe injury. The presence of diffuse ventricular enlargement with widening of the extra-axial spaces can be difficult to distinguish from communicating hydrocephalus or the normally prominent cerebrospinal fluid spaces in infants. The presence of blood within the ventricles is a marker for severe intracranial injury (Kleinman, 1987; Merten & Carpenter, 1990).

## SKULL FRACTURES

Statistically, fractures to the skull are the second most common bony injury in child abuse. History suspicious for child abuse and the presence of a skull fracture increase the likelihood of intracranial injury (Harwood-Nash, 1992). Most skull fractures are linear and nondepressed, with comminuted, depressed, and diastatic fractures being less common. The parietal and occipital bones are most typically involved. Depressed fractures, occiput fractures, and fractures crossing the midline carry a greater specificity for nonaccidental injury than simple linear fractures (Merten & Osborne, 1983; Harwood-Nash, 1992) (**Figure 2-19**).

Fractures to the skull may be imaged with CT, bone scan, and plain films. CT is sensitive for detection of fractures, given appropriate slice thickness and window settings. However, fractures in the plane of CT section can be missed. The standard method for evaluation is the two-view skull; radiographs must always be obtained in addition to bone scans to evaluate the abused child.

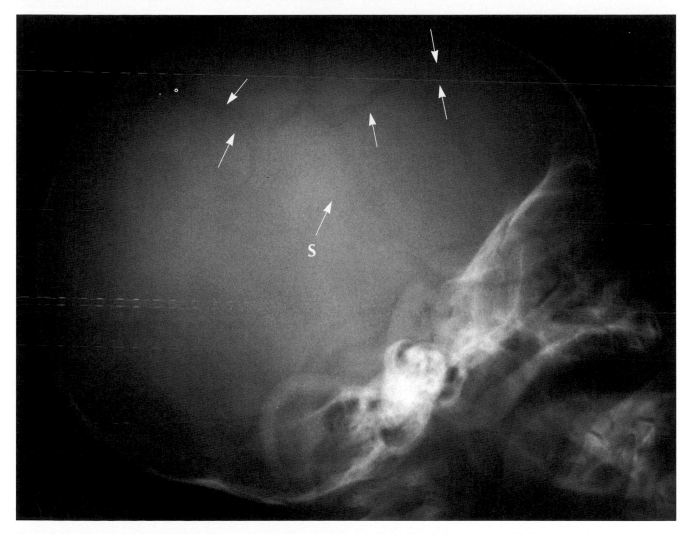

**Figure 2-19**. *Depressed right parietal skull fracture crosses the coronal suture. Depression is evident on the AP view. Fractures crossing sutures(s) are more common in child abuse than in accidental injury.*

Sutural widening is one radiographic sign of increased intracranial pressure, as might be seen in chronic subdural hematomas. In cases of psychosocial dwarfism, however, an interesting variation is seen. The deprived child at the time of diagnosis will have normal-appearing sutures. After successful treatment for neglect, the child's brain may grow faster than the skull, resulting in sutural splitting. This widening may be mild to 4 mm in width (Kleinman, 1987) (**Figures 2-20 and 2-21**).

## MAXILLOFACIAL INJURIES

Maxillofacial abnormalities are rare, manifesting most often as facial soft tissue injuries. Typically, when fractures occur, they involve older children and are mandibular. Unexplained facial fractures in infants and children suggest abuse (Kleinman, 1987; Merten & Carpenter, 1990). Blows to the mouth can cause

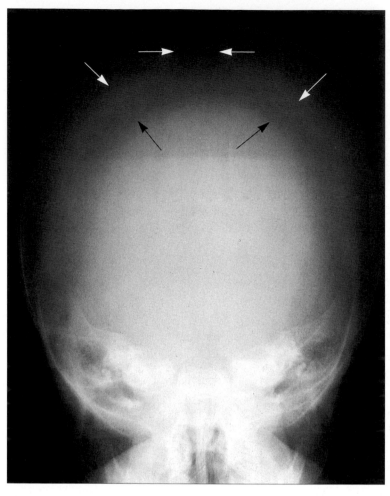

**Figure 2-20**. *Towne's view of the skull demonstrating sutural diastasis (arrows) suggesting increased intracranial pressure. This 4-month-old infant had bilateral chronic subdural hematomas on CT.*

missing teeth or fractures of the mandible. Nasal septal deviation may result from direct trauma to the nose. The only clinical sign might be hemorrhage from the nose (McNeese & Hebeler, 1977). Injuries to the ear often involve the pinna. Subgaleal hematomas or cephalhematomas may result from cases of severe hair-pulling and can be visible on skull films if the soft tissues are hot-lighted (McNeese & Hebeler, 1977; Kleinman, 1987; Merten & Carpenter, 1990). Soft tissue injuries around the orbit called "black eyes" may look identical to the "raccoon eyes" in basilar skull fractures. Appropriate imaging is essential for these situations, as bilateral periorbital hematomas seldom occur without a unique history in the accidental setting (Reece & Grodin, 1985).

Retinal hemorrhage is a specific finding in child abuse not easily explained by impact and is a well-described result of shaking. Specifically, subdural hematomas with retinal hemorrhage should be regarded as the shaking syndrome of child abuse unless another plausible etiology can be determined (Rekate, 1985; Alexander et al., 1990; Swischuk, 1992).

### NEUROIMAGING

The modalities of CT, MRI, and ultrasound are available to evaluate intracranial injuries. CT is both sensitive and specific in defining the acute and chronic intracranial abnormalities of abuse. MRI is the most sensitive mode of detecting intracranial injuries (especially shaking trauma). In acute situations, CT is the modality of choice, as it allows the rapid evaluation of both intracranial and calvarial abnormalities in an unstable patient.

The strengths of MRI are apparent in cases of subacute and chronic neural trauma. MRI effectively evaluates the posterior fossa, as it lacks beam-hardening artifact and possesses multiplanar capability. MRI is better than CT at showing nonhemorrhagic contusions of the white matter and other deep cerebral injuries. It is also better than CT in determining the age of extra-axial fluid collections by following changing MRI signals of hemoglobin breakdown products. CT is the primary screening method, with MRI obtained in cases highly suspicious for abuse but with negative head CTs (Alexander et al., 1986; Kleinman, 1987; Sato et al., 1989; Merten & Carpenter, 1990). Neurosonography is of limited use in CNS injury and is best used for follow-up of ventricle size and gross parenchymal involvement in those patients with open fontanelles (Merten & Carpenter, 1990).

### ◆ ABDOMINAL INJURIES

In cases of nonaccidental trauma, the abdomen is involved less than the skeleton or the brain. What abdominal injury lacks in frequency it makes up in mortality, with visceral injuries producing a mortality of 50% in child abuse (Touloukian, 1968). Visceral injuries rank second only to head trauma as the leading cause of death from child abuse (Kleinman, 1987).

Abdominal injuries typically occur after the child is ambulatory, that is, older than 2 years. As age increases, a shift occurs in the site of fatal injury from the brain to the abdomen (Kleinman, 1987). Surveys have shown that truly accidental injuries differ in site and severity from inflicted abuse. Accidental injuries usually have specific histories and are brought promptly for treatment. In abuse, the history is more general, such as a fall. In combination with the typically vague symptoms of abdominal injury, this lack of accurate history increases the morbidity and mortality by delaying essential treatment. CT examination has helped bring to light the true prevalence of abuse-related abdominal injury.

## LIVER

The liver is the solid visceral organ most often involved in child abuse due to its exposed location next to the epigastric region. This is the site of most direct blows, the usual mechanism for hepatic injury (Merten & Carpenter, 1990). Trauma subsequent to compression and crushing is less common, but it has been known to produce burst injuries to the liver. Hepatic injury from rib fracture is rarely seen. In infants, hepatic injuries are not common, as direct blows are rarely administered to children of that age (Cameron, 1978; Kleinman, 1987).

Hepatic contusion, subcapsular hematoma, and hemorrhage occur in child abuse. CT is the study of choice if clinical findings are highly suspicious for hepatic injury. Ultrasound can be used as an initial screening evaluation because it will provide adequate evaluation of the biliary system, hepatic parenchyma, and the presence of ascites (Kleinman, 1987) (**Figure 2-22**).

Historically, the liver/spleen scan has been used to evaluate the abdomen. However, the radionuclide study is of relatively low sensitivity and specificity in child abuse. The frequent difficulty in obtaining an emergent liver/spleen scan also renders it less desirable as an imaging modality in this setting.

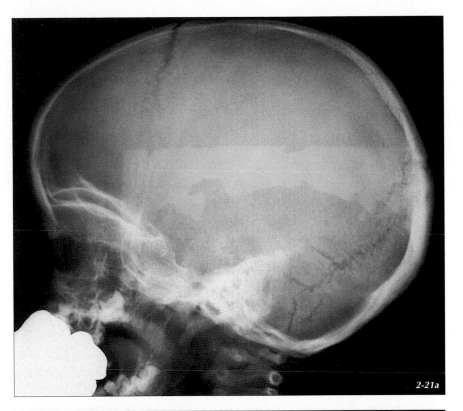

2-21a

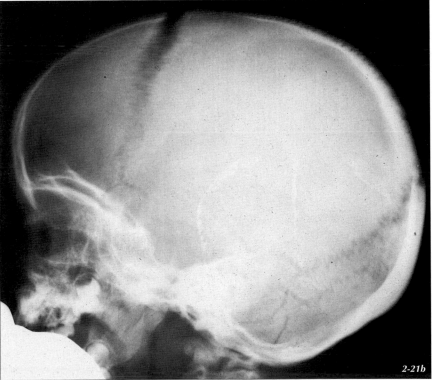

2-21b

***Figure 2-21a,b***. *Initial skeletal survey demonstrated normal sutures in this case of neglect/abuse. Follow-up at 1 month after placement in foster care revealed sutural diastasis from accelerated intracerebral growth and lagging calvarial development, not from raised intracranial pressure.*

### SPLEEN

The spleen is rarely involved in child abuse, secondary to its distance from the epigastric region. Direct blows with their resultant decelerating force are the most common mechanism of splenic injury (Kirks, 1983). Contusions of the spleen and subcapsular hematomas are more common than splenic lacerations in nonaccidental trauma. Ultrasound provides a rapid and safe method of screening; however, CT is more sensitive and specific (**Figure 2-23**).

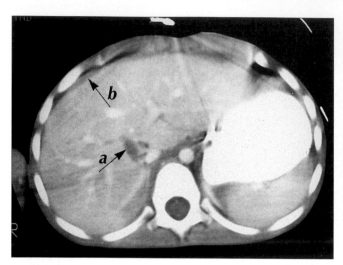

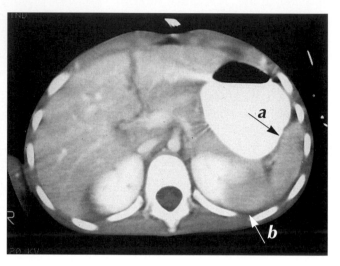

**Figure 2-22**. CT scan demonstrates hypodensity in the inferomedial right hepatic lobe, consistent with laceration (arrow a). A small subcapsular hematoma shows as a crescent of low density along the anterior right hepatic lobe (arrow b).

**Figure 2-23**. Normal-appearing spleen (arrow a). Area of low density indenting upper left kidney, consistent with splenic hematoma visualized on ultrasound (arrow b).

### PANCREAS

Pancreatic disease in children is rare. The pancreas lies over the spine in the epigastrium and is susceptible to compression by a direct blow with subsequent release of pancreatic enzymes due to acinar or ductal rupture. This causes autonecrosis and inflammation of the organ. A resultant mass of necrotic tissue may form a firm, fibrous capsule known as a pancreatic pseudocyst. This may develop rapidly within days of the injury, or it may be gradual and insidious (Kirks, 1983; Kleinman, 1987). In children under 3 years of age, pancreatitis is highly suspicious for abuse (Tolia et al., 1990) (**Figure 2-24**). Symptoms can be mild or severe, and additional physical findings may include elevated serum amylase and ascites. A normal amylase measurement does not exclude a pseudocyst, since amylase levels can return to normal with time (Kleinman, 1987).

Abdominal trauma causes more than half of reported cases of pseudocysts in children, with 30% of these showing concurrent evidence of abuse (Merten & Carpenter, 1990). Radiographic changes of pancreatitis are the well-described, nonspecific sentinel loops and colon cut-off signs. Pancreatic pseudocyst may generate mass effect on adjacent bowel, such as the duodenum or stomach. If the pseudocyst obstructs the bowel, radiographic changes of obstruction may be seen.

Ultrasound is the diagnostic method of choice to evaluate the pancreas and pseudocysts in both the initial and follow-up phases. CT can also be helpful in evaluating injuries to adjacent organs in the retroperitoneum.

In cases of pancreatic involvement, lytic bone lesions from medullary fat necrosis can occur 2 to 10 weeks after injury. Pancreatic enzymes break down medullary fat in bone, producing lytic lesions of variable appearance. The lower extremities, specifically the small bones in the foot, are most often involved, with associated pain and swelling. Spontaneous resolution occurs, with residual changes evident up to 1 year later. These lesions should not be mistaken for the bone lesions of leukemia and metastatic neuroblastoma (Wilner, 1982; Kleinman, 1987).

## KIDNEY

Nonaccidental trauma rarely results in direct renal injury. In abuse, renal disease is most commonly due to a metabolic imbalance from major trauma, such as shock or myoglobinuria following muscle breakdown. Renal trauma, as in the liver, is rarely caused by rib fracture. Direct blows to the kidney can result in parenchymal tearing and discontinuity of the collecting system, hemorrhage, or extravasation into the retroperitoneum. Ectopic renal location can make the kidney more susceptible to injury. If the kidney overlies the spine, as in cross-fused ectopia or horseshoe kidney, it is susceptible to the same mechanism that injures the pancreas. CT is the most sensitive and the most specific modality. However, gross screening can be cost-effectively performed with ultrasound.

## BLADDER AND URETHRA

The rare occurrence of bladder or urethral involvement may relate to the protected intrapelvic location of these organs (Kleinman, 1987). Perforating injury to the bladder is rare. Urethral injury could occur as a result of sexual abuse or inflicted straddle injury.

## ESOPHAGUS

Esophageal involvement in child abuse often relates to Munchausen Syndrome by Proxy. Children have been forced to consume dangerous foreign bodies, such as safety pins or glass. Force-feeding lye or hot water can cause esophageal ulceration and spasm on the barium swallow with resultant strictures. Such occurrences are rare (Kleinman, 1987).

## STOMACH

Stomach distensibility usually spares it from injury caused by a direct blow or compression. If distended, such as after a meal, perforation can occur, usually along the anterior stomach wall, with resultant pneumoperitoneum. However, this is uncommon, as only 2% of bowel ruptures involve the stomach. Radiographically, findings are nonspecific, except for massive amounts of intraperitoneal air. The clinical presentation is very serious and may be associated with other visceral injury (Kleinman, 1987; Merten & Carpenter, 1990).

Most commonly, the stomach is indirectly involved, relating to either duodenal obstruction or gastric atony from starvation or neglect. This atony is a paralytic phenomenon, not a result of mechanical obstruction. In a child who is neither postoperative nor medicated, marked gastric dilatation should raise the suspicion of chronic starvation or neglect (Kirks, 1983).

## DUODENUM

The duodenum is often involved in nontraumatic injury because its location over the spine allows it to be trapped and compressed. Involvement of the descending duodenum, which lies to the side of the spine, may result from its firm fixation, making it susceptible to compressive blows (Kleinman, 1987).

Being well-vascularized, the duodenum has multiple potential bleeding sites, and intestinal hematoma without appropriate trauma history is classic in cases of child abuse. The areas of hematoma may be diffuse or localized with bleeding in a subserosal location, sparing the mucosa. The majority of small bowel hematomas are found in the duodenum and proximal jejunum, immediately distal to the ligament of Treitz. Duodenal hematomas are typically antimesenteric in location, in contrast to the mesenteric location of jejunal and ileal hematomas (Kleinman, 1987).

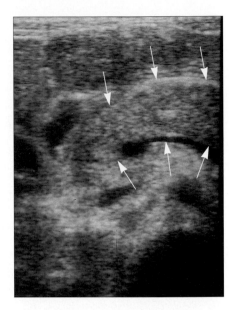

**Figure 2-24**. *Transverse ultrasound view through pancreas demonstrates thickening and inhomogeneity consistent with pancreatitis. The amylase level was 263 IU/L.*

A hematoma frequently appears on upper gastrointestinal (GI) examinations as a large, smooth, intramural mass that narrows the lumen. In the presence of duodenal hematoma, the plain film may be normal or may show a dilated stomach with a large air/fluid level. Free air or ascites may also be seen from separate concurrent injuries. Circumferential, diffuse bleeding may produce fold-thickening without focal mural defect, known as the stacked coin appearance. This sign is of lower specificity for duodenal hematoma related to abuse.

Over time, the hematomas resolve with varying degrees of mural nodularity. This later stage finding on an upper GI examination may be the only indicator of previous abuse. Ultrasound can help in acute trauma, but upper GI examination is recommended for confirmation of findings (**Figure 2-25 a,b**).

Direct crushing or compressive forces to the abdomen of the abused child can result in small bowel perforation. Sites susceptible to injury and/or perforation from shearing forces are those fixed in position or at the junction of bowel segments with

**Figure 2-25a**. *Following a direct mid-abdominal blow, this patient presented with emesis. Initial upper GI examination shows wall thickening and duodenal hematomas (arrows).*

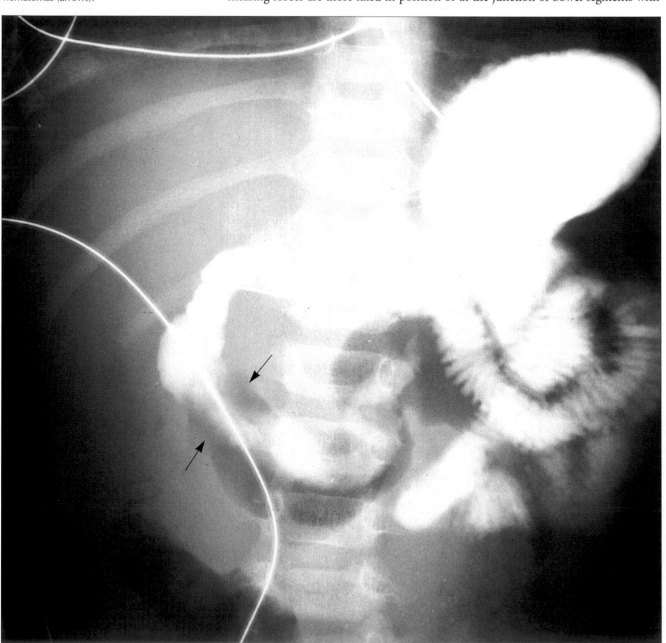

varying degrees of mobility. This explains why 60% of perforations occur in the proximal jejunum and 30% in the duodenum, followed by the ileum (Kleinman, 1987). Because of the duodenum's retroperitoneal location, plain film signs of free air are often absent (**Figure 2-26**).

The bowel wall can be torn in abuse, allowing gas-forming bacteria to enter the wall. The resultant curvilinear lucency or mottled radiographic appearance of intramural air, pneumatosis intestinalis, can also result from anoxic injury to the wall in abuse (Kleinman, 1987).

## COLON

Colonic involvement in nonaccidental injury is most often due to sexual abuse. Rectal perforation may result in free intraperitoneal air evident on plain films. Sexual assaults may utilize foreign objects that may be seen on plain films, and, on rare occasions, free intraperitoneal air can be seen following rape. In cases involving major genitorectal trauma, radiology can help assess the acute injury and any resultant sequelae. Sexually abused children may present with vague or unusual abdominal complaints, and it is in the course of evaluating these that the radiologist may meet the patient. The radiologist needs to be aware of physical signs suggesting anogenital trauma, as these may be appreciated when performing examinations for GI or voiding disorders.

Colonic injuries from blunt trauma are rare. This may relate to the mobility of the colon and its location either on the edge of the abdomen or in the pelvis. Colonic hematomas and perforation following abuse have been described. This most commonly involves the transverse colon (Kleinman, 1987).

CT examination is the modality of choice for assessing blunt abdominal trauma. Ultrasound is most useful as a screening examination of the abdomen and in pancreatic assessment and follow-up. MRI has limitations in evaluation of

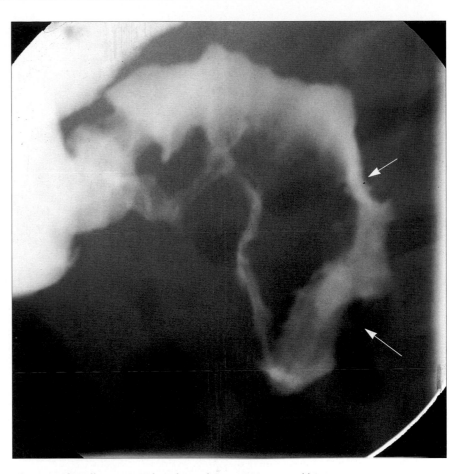

***Figure 2-25b***. *Follow-up in 5 days shows decrease in intramural hematomas on antimesenteric border.*

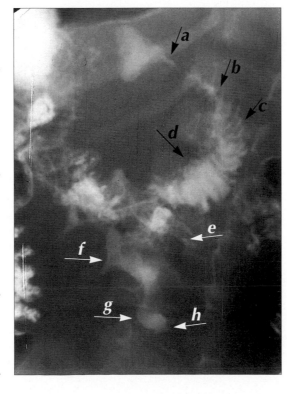

***Figure 2-26***. *A 26-month-old male presented with vague abdominal complaints; previous lower GI examination was negative. Upper GI examination shows duodenal perforation into a walled-off cavity (arrows a,b,c,d indicate duodenum, arrows e,f,g,h delineate walled-off cavity).*

the abdomen related to motion artifact. Children with unusual or unexplainable abdominal bruising should always be evaluated for visceral injuries, regardless of whether other injuries are apparent (Cameron, 1978; Kirks, 1983).

## ◆DIFFERENTIAL CONSIDERATIONS IN CHILD ABUSE

In diagnosing child abuse, it is important to keep in mind several congenital and acquired diseases that can mimic the bony lesions of nonaccidental injury. Failure to consider these possibilities and eliminate them can result in false diagnosis. These disease entities can usually be differentiated from child abuse by careful physical examination and a thorough history. Certain laboratory tests may also be required to eliminate them from the differential diagnosis.

Accidental trauma can cause fractures that mimic abuse. The toddler's fracture is a well-known example. The rotational stress from a newly walking child may result in a minimally displaced fracture, indistinguishable from an oblique fracture caused by applied stress in abuse. The bone appearance and appropriate history and age help distinguish this specific fracture from abuse. Clavicle fractures are also common injuries that might be mistaken for abuse. Well-described in the perinatal period as a result of birth trauma, these fractures show healing reaction by 14 days. Absence of callus in a clavicle fracture after this time strongly suggests nonaccidental cause (Kleinman, 1987).

Rib fractures related to delivery are uncommon. Those found incidentally weeks after birth when the callus becomes palpable are usually due to abuse unless a plausible history of severe direct trauma is present (Kleinman, 1987). Epiphyseal injuries have been associated with birth trauma related to a breech delivery. These injuries are usually noted in the neonate because of abnormal or absent movement of the afflicted joints. Most long bone fractures from delivery are in the humeral mid-shaft. Fractures of the lower extremity long bones and fractures in varying stages of repair in the newborn are most often related to infection, rickets, or neuromuscular diseases (Radkowski, 1983; Kleinman, 1987).

Many normal variants exist that can be confused with child abuse in infants. Standard radiographic texts or atlases of radiographic variants are helpful to avoid misdiagnosis. A commonly encountered variant is the periosteal reaction due to new bone formation and spurring of the metaphyses in healthy, unabused infants. While the periosteal changes mimic traumatic periostitis, the metaphyseal spurs are not suspicious for abuse unless fragmentation is present. These bony changes occur between 2 and 8 months of life (Kleinman, 1987).

Osteogenesis imperfecta is a frequently mentioned disease entity in the differential diagnosis of child abuse. Abnormalities of collagen production result in weak bones. Four types of osteogenesis imperfecta are recognized, with types I, III, and IV most often implicated, as type II is the lethal perinatal form with multiple fractures, blue sclerae, and recessive inheritance. The diagnosis is not complicated by the more severe forms, like type II, but by the types with delayed presentation and subtle bone change. Metaphyseal fractures are typically absent, with long bone fractures more common. Osteopenia with thin bone cortices is typical. Extraskeletal manifestations such as blue sclerae, dentinogenesis imperfecta, or familial inheritance may be of help in the differential diagnosis in infancy (Radkowski, 1983; Kleinman, 1987). The possibility of intentional injury cannot be disregarded in osteogenesis imperfecta, since even children with this disease can be abused (Cameron, 1978).

Children with congenital insensitivity to pain may demonstrate metaphyseal and shaft fractures and periosteal reaction, mimicking abuse even though mineralization is normal. A careful neurologic examination and history are required for this diagnosis. A similar radiographic appearance can occur in children with spinal defects. For example, patients with meningomyeloceles may have altered or absent sensation from the lower extremities and varying degrees of motor involvement, allowing repetitive injury resembling abuse (Radkowski, 1983; Kleinman, 1987).

Congenital syphilis produces diffuse symmetric bone changes very similar to child abuse. However, erosions on the medial aspect of the proximal tibia (Wimberger sign) with periosteal new bone formation are diagnostic for syphilis. The spine and epiphyseal ossification centers are spared. Serologic analysis is helpful in eliminating this from consideration (Radkowski, 1983; Kleinman, 1987).

Osteomyelitis can imitate abuse not only by producing periosteal reaction and metaphyseal irregularity, but it can also be multifocal in infancy. Corner fractures are not a part of the radiologic presentation. Clinical tests such as joint tapping and blood cultures can help differentiate this from abuse. Also, infantile meningococcemia has been described as resulting in metaphyseal abnormalities years after the infection. The postulated mechanism is ischemic injury. This makes the presence of infantile meningococcemia an important historical question along with metaphyseal abnormalities (Patriquin et al., 1982; Kleinman, 1987).

Infantile cortical hyperostosis (Caffey's disease) is a rare occurrence in young infants, producing painful periosteal reaction. Infants 2 to 3 months of age present with red and edematous extremities at multiple locations. The periosteal reactions spare the metaphyses. Both flat and tubular bones can be involved. The etiology is unknown, and complete healing occurs. The mandible is involved in more than 95% of cases, making mandibular involvement and the sparing of the metaphyses useful differentiators. A careful and thorough history is also an essential component in differentiating Caffey's disease from abuse (Radkowski, 1983; Radkowski et al., 1983; Reece & Grodin, 1985).

Methotrexate therapy has been known to produce periosteal reactions and metaphyseal-epiphyseal fractures with osteopenia. With current therapy regimens, this is less likely to occur. Long-term prostaglandin-E therapy is used to prevent closure of a patent ductus arteriosus. It can produce cortical proliferation in these patients. Bony sequelae involve the long bones and the ribs; patient history can differentiate it from traumatic periostitis (Radkowski, 1983; Radkowski et al., 1983). Vitamin A toxicity can show diaphyseal periosteal reaction; however, metaphyseal-epiphyseal lesions are absent. Epiphyseal abnormalities (cone-shaped epiphyses) may occur with associated limb shortening. Hypervitaminosis A can be a cause of increased intracranial pressure with sutural widening. Vitamin A blood levels and history of abnormal intake can assist in differentiation from traumatic periostitis (Radkowski et al., 1983; Kleinman, 1987).

Infantile rickets can manifest the bony changes seen in child abuse, but with the addition of osteopenia. Metaphyseal fraying and multiple fractures are common. A typical radiographic finding in rickets is Looser's zones, symmetric transverse stress fractures not found in nonaccidental injury. Diffuse osteopenia with epiphyseal widening and poor epiphyseal definition is typical in rickets and not found in abuse. Radiographic changes of rickets can also be seen in the diseases of biliary atresia, hypophosphatasia, and osteopetrosis (Radkowski, 1983; Radkowski et al., 1983; Kleinman, 1987).

Vitamin C deficiency (scurvy) is less common than rickets and rarely occurs before 6 months. Metaphyseal irregularities and periosteal reaction can simulate abuse, but the associated osteopenia is atypical. The presence of dense metaphyseal bands along with thin dense rings around the epiphyses helps differentiate scurvy from abuse. Long bone fractures are also rare (Radkowski et al., 1983; Kleinman, 1987).

Menkes' kinky hair disease is an abnormality of copper absorption with metaphyseal fractures that can mimic the changes of abuse. Periosteal reaction of long bone diaphyses can also be seen. Distinguishing features from child abuse are the presence of multiple wormian bones, kinky hair, and low serum copper levels.

A significant factor in the misdiagnosis of child abuse is the suboptimal radiograph. This can take the form of an incomplete skeletal survey, poor positioning, and underexposure or overexposure of the radiograph (Merten & Carpenter, 1990). Careful attention must be paid in the initial evaluation to the overall bone density and architecture. Most of the disease entities mentioned above can be eliminated through careful histories, which include social, medical, and dietary assessments. Physical examination and laboratory data can then be useful, especially in patients with a baseline chronic illness. In addition, it is important to remember that a child with a chronic disease can be abused as easily as a healthy child and, in fact, is even more prone to abuse (Radkowski, 1983).

## ◆CONCLUSION

A certain set of diagnostic guidelines emerges from the literature on radiology's role in child abuse. Its strength lies in detecting type, extent, and age of injury. The motivating force for radiology's contribution is that without recognition and intervention, the abused child "will almost always be abused again, and statistics show that by the third hospitalization, he will be either dead or dying" (Elliot, 1979). A frequent occurrence, often overlooked, is the contribution of the radiologic technologist, who sees both patient and caretaker in a nonthreatening, physician-free environment. The technologist's observations may often assist the radiologist's interpretation, ranging from reports of cutaneous injury to notes on abnormal behavior by the patient or caretaker.

Perhaps the radiologist's greatest advantage in diagnosing abuse has been stated by Dr. Michael Weller, Department of Radiology, Miller Children's Hospital, Long Beach, California: "The radiologist has black and white film before him and is not swayed by knowledge of the family and preconceptions about them."

## ◆BIBLIOGRAPHY

Alexander, R, Sato, Y, Smith, W, and Bennett, T: Incidence of impact trauma with cranial injuries ascribed to shaking, *Am J Dis Child* 144(6):724-726, 1990.

Alexander, RC, Schor, DP, and Smith, WL: Magnetic resonance imaging of intracranial injuries from child abuse, *J Pediatr* 6:975-979, 1986.

Ball, WS, Jr: Nonaccidental craniocerebral trauma (child abuse): MR imaging, *Radiology* 173:609-610, 1989.

Brodeur, AE, Silberstein, MJ, and Graviss, ER: *Radiology of the Pediatric Elbow*, GK Hall Medical Publishers, Boston, 1981.

Cameron, JM: Radiological pathological aspects of the battered child syndrome. In SM Smith, ed: *The Maltreatment of Children*, University Park Press, Baltimore, 1978, pp. 69-81.

Cohen, RA, Kaufman, RA, Myers, PA, and Tobin, RB: Cranial computed tomography in the abused child with head injury, *Am J Radiol* 146:97-102, 1986.

Edwards, IK: Court testimony in cases of nonaccidental trauma. In SVW Hilton, DK Edwards, and JW Hilton, eds: *Practical Pediatric Radiology*, WB Saunders Co, Philadelphia, 1984, pp. 487-496.

Ellerstein, NS, and Norris, KJ: Value of radiologic skeletal survey in assessment of abused children, *Pediatrics* 74:1075-1078, 1984.

Elliot, DS: Child abuse: The radiologist's pivotal position, *Appl Radiol* 74-79, 1979.

English, PC, and Grossman, H: Radiology and history of child abuse, *Pediatr Ann* 12(12):870-874, 1989.

Feldman, KW, and Brewer, DK: Child abuse, cardiopulmonary resuscitation, and rib fractures, *Pediatrics* 73(3):339-342, 1984.

Garrow, I, and Werne, J: Sudden apparently unexplained death during infancy. III. Pathologic findings in infants dying immediately after violence, contrasted with those after sudden apparently unexplained death, *Am J Pathol* 29:833-851, 1953.

Gross, RH: Child abuse: Are you recognizing it when you see it? *Contemp Orthop* 92:676-678, 1980.

Guthkelch, AN: Infantile subdural hematoma and its relationship to whiplash injuries, *Br J Med* 2:430-431, 1971.

Harcke, HT, Jr: Bone imaging in infants and children: A review, *J Nucl Med* 19:324-329, 1978.

Harwood-Nash, DC: Abuse to the pediatric nervous system, *Am J Neuroradiol* 13(2):569-575, 1992.

Keats, TE: *Atlas of Roentgenographic Measurement*, Year Book Medical Publishers, Inc, Chicago, 1985, p. 116.

Kirks, DR: Radiological evaluation of visceral injuries in the battered child syndrome, *Pediatr Ann* 12:888-893, 1983.

Kirks, DR: Practical pediatric imaging. In HL Abrams, ed: *Diagnostic Radiology of Infants and Children*, Little, Brown & Co, Boston, 1984, p. 277.

Kleinman, PK: *Diagnostic Imaging of Child Abuse*, The Williams & Wilkins Co, Baltimore, 1987.

Leonidas, JC: Skeletal trauma in the child abuse syndrome, *Pediatr Ann* 12(12):875-881, 1983.

Matin, P: Bone scintigraphy in the diagnosis and management of traumatic injury, *Semin Nucl Med* 13:104-122, 1983.

McClain, PW, Sacks, JJ, Froehlke, RG, and Ewigman, BG: Estimates of fatal child abuse and neglect, United States, 1979 through 1988, *Pediatrics* 91(2):338-343, 1993.

McClelland, CQ, Rekate, H, Kaufman, B, and Perse, L: Cerebral injury in child abuse: A changing profile, *Childs Brain* 7:225-235, 1980.

McNeese, MC, and Hebeler, JR: The abused child—a clinical approach to identification and management, *Clin Symp* 29(5):1-36, 1977.

Meller, JL, Little, AG, and Shermeta, DW: Thoracic trauma in children, *Pediatrics* 74:813-819, 1984.

Merten, DF: Introduction: The battered child syndrome: The role of radiological imaging, *Pediatr Ann* 12:867-868, 1983.

Merten, DF, and Carpenter, BL: Radiologic imaging of inflicted injury in child abuse syndrome, *Pediatr Clin North Am* 37(4):815-836, 1990.

Merten, DF, and Osborne, DS: Craniocerebral trauma in the child abuse syndrome, *Pediatr Ann* 12:12, 1983.

Miller, DS: Fractures among children. I. Parental assault as causative agent, *Minn Med* 42:1209-1213, 1959.

Patriquin, HC, Antoni, T, Jacquier, S, and Marton, D: Late sequelae of infantile meningococcemia in growing bones of children, *Radiology* 141:77-82, 1982.

Perper, JA, and Wecht, CH, eds: *Microscopic Diagnosis in Forensic Pathology*, Charles C Thomas, Springfield, IL, 1980, pp. 3-16.

Radkowski, MA: The battered child syndrome: Pitfalls in radiologic diagnosis, *Pediatr Ann* 12:894-903, 1983.

Radkowski, MA, Merten, DR, and Leonidas, JC: The abused child: Criteria for the radiological diagnosis, *Radiographics* 3:262-297, 1983.

Reece, RM, and Grodin, MA: Recognition of nonaccidental injury, *Pediatr Clin North Am* 32:41-60, 1985.

Rekate, HL: Subdural hematomas in infants, *Neurosurgery* 62:316-317, 1985.

Sato, Y, Yuh, WT, Smith, WL, Alexander, RC, Kao, SC, and Ellerbroek, CJ: Head injury in child abuse: Evaluation with MRI imaging, *Radiology* 173:653-657, 1989.

Silverman, FN, and Kuhn, JP, eds: *Caffey's Pediatric X-ray Diagnosis: An Integrated Imaging Approach*, The CV Mosby Co, St. Louis, 1992, pp. 1814-1816.

Sivit, CJ, and Taylor, BA: Visceral injury in battered children: A changing perspective, *Radiology* 173(3):659-661, 1989.

Starbuck, GW: Recognition and early management of child abuse, *Pediatr Ann* 5:27-41, 1976.

Swischuk, LE: Radiographic signs of skeletal trauma. In S Ludwig and A Kornberg, eds: *Child Abuse: A Medical Reference*, ed 2, Churchill Livingstone, New York, 1992, pp. 151-174.

Teng, CT, Singleton, EB, and Daeschner, CW, Jr: Skeletal injuries of the battered child, *Am J Orthop* 6:202-207, 1964.

Tolia, V, Patel, AS, and Amundson, GM: Pancreatic fracture secondary to child abuse: The role of computed tomography in its diagnosis, *Clin Pediatr* 29(11): 667-668, 1990.

Touloukian, R: Abdominal visceral injuries in battered children, *Pediatrics* 42(4):642-646, 1968.

Tredwell, SJ, Van Peteghem, K, and Clough, M: Pattern of forearm fractures in children, *J Pediatr Orthop* 4:604-608, 1984.

Tufts, E, Blank, E, and Dickerson, D: Periosteal thickening as a manifestation of trauma in infancy, *Child Abuse Negl* 6:359-364, 1982.

Wilner, D: *Radiology of Bone Tumors and Allied Disorders*, WB Saunders Co, Philadelphia, 1982, p. 3621.

Zimmerman, RA, Bilaniuk, LT, and Genneralli, T: Computed tomography of shearing injuries of the cerebral white matter, *Radiology* 127:393-396, 1978.

# Oral Injuries of Child Abuse

Lynn Douglas Mouden, D.D.S, M.P.H, F.I.C.D, F.A.C.D.

## ◆ Background

It has long been recognized that the most common injuries of child abuse involve the head, neck, and mouth. Various studies have shown that the incidence of these injuries is from 50% (Cameron et al., 1966) to 65% (Becker et al., 1978) or even 75% (da Fenesca et al., 1992) of all physical injuries of child abuse. All such studies are hampered by being retrospective in nature and are based on children admitted to a medical facility. However, the vast number of these studies clearly shows that injuries of the head and facial regions are the most common of all physical child abuse injuries.

Injuries to the mouth and oral structures are a common factor in child abuse cases. Assault on the communicative "self" of the child is often the compelling reason behind abuse directed at the mouth, along with the adult's easy accessibility to the child's head (Schwartz et al., 1977). Furthermore, any physical or emotional discomfort to the child, or other abusive injuries to any part of the child's body, may elicit a cry. Efforts to silence a crying child often result in injuries to the mouth.

Recognition of abusive injuries to the mouth is necessary in the medical as well as the dental setting. Although treatment of oral injuries is usually referred to the general dentist or oral surgeon, it should be emphasized that proper evaluation of an abused child is not complete without a thorough visual oral examination and referral to the dentist as necessary.

The types of oral injuries that may be encountered in child abuse include trauma not only to the teeth, but also to supporting and surrounding oral tissues. According to a nationwide survey of pediatric dentists, the principal oral injuries of child abuse include missing and fractured teeth (32% of reported cases), oral contusions (24%), oral lacerations (14%), jaw fractures (11%), and oral burns (5%) (Malecz, 1979).

## ◆ Oral Injuries To Infants

Abuse injuries to oral structures of the edentulous infant should be considered separately from those of older children. Infants are likely to be edentulous because eruption of the lower incisor teeth does not usually occur before 4 to 6 months of age. The clinician must remember that the eruption pattern of primary teeth varies widely and is not usually important in the differential diagnosis of child abuse. However, delayed eruption of primary teeth may indicate a pattern of child neglect resulting from poor nutrition either for the child or for the mother during pregnancy.

The difficulties and frustrations surrounding an infant's feeding may lead to abuse associated with the feeding itself. Intra-oral lacerations have long been recognized as possible indicators of forced feeding (Kempe, 1975). The injury occurs when excessive pressure is used while feeding with a nursing bottle (Kempe, 1971) or

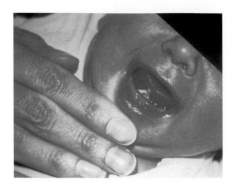

***Figure 3-1.*** *Torn lingual frenum from forced feeding.*

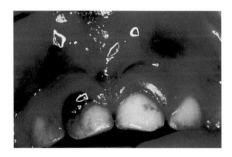

***Figure 3-2.*** *Torn frenulum, lacerated lip, and subluxated central incisor in an 8-year-old struck with an open-handed slap. The injuries include an upper lip lacerated by the upper incisors, ecchymosis of the upper lip and vestibule, and subluxation of the permanent right central incisor, as evidenced by bleeding of the periodontal ligament.*

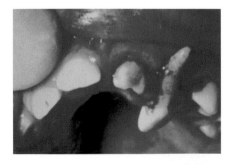

***Figure 3-3.*** *Displaced upper primary left cuspid with the root forced labially through the cortical plate.*

when a utensil is misdirected during feeding (Kittle, 1981). If the adult feels that the child is uncooperative during bottle feeding, he or she may use excessive force to introduce the latex nipple into the child's mouth or press too firmly against oral structures. This can cause contusions of the alveolar ridge, the frenum, or the nonkeratinized tissue of the vestibule. Pushing the bottle against the infant's mouth can also cause tearing of the labial frenum because of the lateral displacement of the lip. Forced feeding with a utensil can lead to laceration of the lingual frenum, the floor of the mouth, or the labial frenum (**Figure 3-1**). Lacerations to the alveolar ridge during forced feeding of infants are not common.

## ♦ INJURIES TO TEETH

All injuries to teeth and supporting structures should be referred to a dentist as soon as possible. The injuries to teeth can include luxation, displacement, fracture, or avulsion. Any trauma to a tooth that does not result in loss of the tooth may, however, result in loss of the tooth's vitality. Even relatively minor trauma may disrupt the neurovascular supply to the tooth and cause the tooth to be nonvital. Immediately after trauma to the tooth, disruption of the tooth's enervation can only be diagnosed by thermal or electrical pulp testing. However, after several weeks, a nonvital tooth appears discolored or markedly darker than unaffected surrounding teeth.

### LUXATION

A luxated tooth has been moved within the alveolar socket but not avulsed. The tooth may not appear to have been displaced from the dental arch. Luxation often results in tearing of the periodontal ligament and may exhibit bleeding around the tooth (**Figure 3-2**). Luxated teeth may also be mobile within their socket. Because of the elasticity of the periodontal ligament, normal primary and permanent teeth have some mobility within the socket. However, palpation using two instruments placed on opposite sides of the tooth should show no more than 0.5 mm of movement in any direction. Mobility beyond this limited scope may indicate luxation or displacement of the tooth.

### DISPLACEMENT

Displacement of a traumatized tooth can occur in any direction and happens with accidental injuries as well as in abuse. Contact directly on the tooth or a blow to the face that transmits force to the tooth can cause the displacement. Either the abuser's hand or an object can deliver sufficient force to displace one or several teeth.

The most common displacement is in the lingual or palatal direction. The tooth may be moved markedly from its normal position within the dental arch. The tooth may either be moved bodily or rotated in a facial-lingual direction. With the alveolar crest serving as the fulcrum, the tooth's crown can be displaced lingually while the root is rotated facially, thus perforating the alveolar bone and overlying gingival tissue (**Figure 3-3**).

Other directions of displacement are less common. In some instances the tooth can be displaced facially, but this is rare in abuse injuries. In addition, a blow to the tooth can result in intrusion of the tooth. If the tooth has fully erupted and is in the plane of occlusion, the intrusion makes it appear shorter than the surrounding, unaffected teeth. An intruded tooth is often accompanied by trauma to the surrounding structures and bleeding from the gingiva and periodontal ligament. The clinician must be aware that a normal, partially erupted tooth also may not be in the plane of occlusion. Comparison of contralateral teeth may be useful in determining if the tooth was fully erupted before the trauma. Displacement of a tooth in a mesial or distal direction can occur if the adjacent teeth are missing or avulsed.

## AVULSION

Avulsion is the forceful expulsion of the entire tooth from alveolar bone. The tendency for any tooth to be avulsed during trauma is related to both the force and the direction of the trauma as well as the anatomy of the root(s). Avulsions from abusive injuries are almost exclusively limited to anterior teeth because they are supported by a single root. A traumatic blow to the alveolar bone apical to the tooth's crown may impart sufficient force to the root to expel the tooth from its socket (**Figure 3-4**). Multirooted teeth are less susceptible to avulsion, both because of their location in the posterior part of the mouth and because of the physics of forcing the tooth out bodily. Because the root anatomy of a primary tooth is likely to be less conical than that of a permanent tooth, avulsion of teeth during physical violence is less common in children with primary dentition.

The more conical root anatomy of permanent anterior teeth allows for easier tooth extraction, not only by the dentist but also in cases of abuse by tooth removal. At least two cases have been reported of children abused by having permanent teeth "extracted" by the parents (Carrotte, 1990). In these cases, one adult held the child while another removed the intact teeth without any form of anesthesia.

Traumatic tooth avulsion requires immediate dental consultation. The tooth must be kept moist using isotonic saline solution or even milk. The chances for successful reimplantation are best if the procedure is accomplished within 30 minutes of the avulsion. No effort should be made to cleanse the tooth or to remove any tissue fragments before the dentist reimplants it. Attempts to clean the tooth may result in the loss of tissue important to periodontal tissue regeneration. Reimplanted teeth must be stabilized for a minimum of 7 to 10 days (Andreason, 1975).

## TOOTH FRACTURES

Fractures of teeth can involve the crown, the root, or both. While tooth fractures are sometimes seen in abusive injuries, they are more likely to result from accidental injury. Fractures occur either when the tooth is struck with a hard object or when the tooth comes into contact with a hard surface. Coronal fractures can involve only the enamel, extend into the dentin, or involve the tooth's pulp. Timely referral to a dentist is mandatory for treatment of tooth fractures. Modern restorative materials and bonding procedures can save teeth with fractures that only a decade ago would have required full crowns or even extraction. If the pulp is involved in the fracture, a bleeding point is often evident where the pulp is exposed. Immediate dental treatment with appropriate pulp capping materials may obviate the need for subsequent restorative dental procedures.

Evidence of root fractures or displaced roots may also indicate abuse. Fractures of tooth roots may be seen on radiographic examination, but usually an intra-oral or panoramic radiograph is required. Radiographs may also be useful in distinguishing abnormal tooth development or eruption from the signs of trauma.

## ♦ ABUSE INJURIES TO ORAL SOFT TISSUES

### GINGIVA

Trauma that affects teeth is also likely to affect the surrounding gingiva. In addition, trauma from a hard object striking the child can produce contusions or laceration of the gingiva without apparent trauma to the adjacent teeth. Periapical radiographs are indicated in all cases of gingival trauma to properly diagnose any damage to the teeth or alveolar bone.

### LINGUAL AND LABIAL FRENULA

Abuse trauma can cause mild to extensive damage of the fibrous tissue of the labial or lingual frenum. Along with the frenum lacerations caused by forced feeding that were discussed previously, many forms of abusive trauma can tear the frenum.

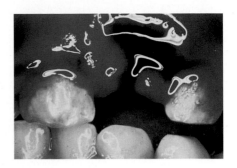

***Figure 3-4.*** *Avulsed permanent central incisor in a 14-year-old boy who was abused over several years with repeated beatings to the head and neck areas.*

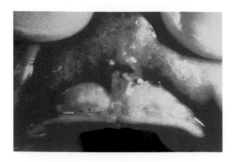

***Figure 3-5a.*** *Torn frenulum in a 5-month-old child who was force-fed due to a reluctance to take spoon feeding. The injury was done with a plastic "infant spoon."*

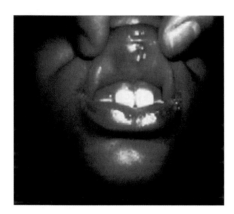

***Figure 3-5b.*** *Contusion of upper lip.*

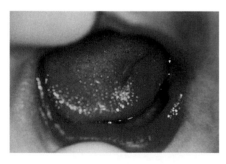

***Figure 3-6.*** *Infant's mouth with no teeth. The tongue shows a crescent shaped bite on left side.*

Blows to the face can displace the lip far enough to stretch the labial frenum beyond its elastic limit (**Figure 3-5a**). This can result in laceration of the frenum, usually at or near the insertion into the labialis muscle or at the insertion into the alveolar ridge. In addition, intrusion of a hard or sharp object into the mouth can also lacerate the frenum.

Laceration of the lingual frenum is seen less often from blows to the face and almost always results from trauma caused by a hard object. However, the tissue of the floor of the child's mouth is more friable than other, keratinized oral tissues, and extensive damage can result from trauma to this area.

## LIPS

Any force to the mouth can cause contusions or lacerations of the upper or lower lip (**Figure 3-5b**). Abuse injuries to the lips are evidenced by marks either from the offending object or from the child's own teeth. When a blow is directed at the face or lips, the oral mucosa can come into forceful contact with the child's teeth. Laceration of the lip mucosa may show "bite marks" from the child's own teeth. In addition, if the child is wearing either fixed or removable orthodontic appliances, these appliances may also damage the lips during trauma. The clinician must exercise caution when examining the child's mouth if orthodontic appliances are in place because the mucosa of the lips may become entrapped in the orthodontic wires or brackets. Disengaging the lips from the appliance may even require local anesthetic.

Another consideration is the presence of bruising or laceration at the commissures of the lips. These injuries could result from the use of a rope or other material to gag and silence the child.

## TONGUE

Although laceration of the tongue occurs with abuse involving a sharp or hard object in the mouth, most abusive injuries to the tongue are caused by biting the tongue. Any blow to the jaw can trap the tongue between the upper and lower teeth. These injuries most often involve the lateral borders of the tongue and usually exhibit the jagged indentations consistent with a bite mark in soft tissue. If the bite involves the posterior tongue, the marks may appear as crushed tissue because of the broad occlusal surface of the posterior teeth.

Bite marks to the tongue inflicted by the child's own dentition are likely to show a curvature consistent with the child's own arch form. A bite mark on the tongue from an abuser may show a curve in the direction opposite to the child's dental arch (**Figure 3-6**).

## HARD AND SOFT PALATE

Lacerations or contusions of the palate are often seen in accidental injuries when the child falls with an object in the mouth. Abusive injuries to the hard and soft palate are reported exclusively from the introduction of a foreign object into the mouth or when the child is struck while an object is already in the mouth.

Forced oral sex can also cause contusions to the palate. These injuries tend to be a diffuse distribution of contusions, palatal petechiae, or ulcerations and may involve the hard palate, soft palate, tonsillar pillars, or posterior pharynx (**Figure 3-7**). Reported cases of repeated forced fellatio have included sufficient erosion of the palatal mucosa to expose underlying cortical bone (Heitzler et al., 1994).

## BURNS

Any oral soft tissue can be burned. The burns reflecting child abuse can include the introduction of a hot object into the mouth, forced feeding of a food or liquid that is too hot, or the use of caustic or acidic fluids (chemical burns).

# ♦DENTAL IMPLICATIONS OF CHILD NEGLECT

Dental neglect has been defined as lack of care that (1) makes routine eating impossible, (2) causes chronic pain, (3) delays or retards a child's growth, or (4) makes it difficult or impossible for a child to perform daily activities (Vadiakas et al., 1991). It is well accepted in health care that untreated dental problems are as serious as an untreated wound in any other part of the body because neglecting dental treatment can lead to complications that affect the entire body (Blain & Kittle, 1989). Dental neglect is usually just one manifestation in the general neglect of a child.

Just as attitudes toward neglect in general vary throughout society, as reflected in the child abuse reporting statutes, the practical definitions of dental neglect in specific locations also differ based on local economic conditions (Mouden & Bross, 1995). The American Academy of Pediatric Dentistry has defined dental neglect as the caregiver's failure to seek treatment for untreated rampant caries, trauma, pain, infection, or bleeding. Rampant caries is generally defined as decay involving every tooth, including the lower anterior teeth, which are typically the most resistant to decay. Because gross decay of the anterior teeth is so obvious, rampant caries is easily discernible to everyone who sees the child's smile.

Also included in the Academy's definition is the failure to follow up on treatment needs once the caregiver has been informed that these conditions exist (Schmitt, 1986). Many parents have told practitioners that they were totally unaware of the conditions in their child's mouth before receiving the dentist's diagnosis. Therefore parents' failure to follow through with treatment is probably more important in determining dental neglect than is their lack of knowledge. Also, most practitioners would agree that no neglect may exist if parents are providing for their children's needs in a manner consistent with their own financial situation or available economic assistance.

The Academy's definition serves as neither a law nor a standard of practice. It is merely a guideline for those practitioners evaluating a patient's oral health in light of societal norms. It is up to the health care professional to weigh the guidelines and legal definitions against regional or local norms and access-to-care issues.

The most common form of dental neglect is failure to provide treatment for carious teeth. Multiple carious teeth can debilitate an otherwise healthy child, while caries that have led to pulpal necrosis and suppuration cause not only pain, but also fever, malaise, and lethargy. Pulpal necrosis may exhibit as suppuration from the carious tooth or as a parulis where the infection has penetrated alveolar bone and entered the gingiva, usually near the tooth's apex.

Baby bottle tooth decay (BBTD), a type of early childhood caries, is a severe form of rampant caries resulting from the habit of putting a child to bed with a nursing bottle, and can also occur from falling asleep at the breast. If the milk or another sugar-containing liquid remains in contact with the teeth for extended periods, serious tooth decay can result. In BBTD, all teeth may be affected and carious amputation of the tooth crowns may occur. While failure to provide treatment for such severe carious involvement can be considered neglect, some Native American tribal councils have considered BBTD as a form of child abuse, not child neglect, because it is a direct result of actions taken by the adult.

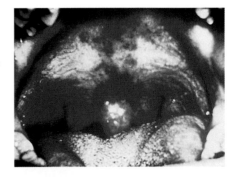

*Figure 3-7.* Palatal contusions from forced oral sex.

Other conditions may constitute dental neglect if left untreated. These include severe malocclusions, abnormal tongue positions, cleft palate or lip, missing teeth, or other malformations that may lead to speech or eating disorders (Badger, 1982).

Over the past several decades, the dental community has had difficulty getting child protective service (CPS) agencies to recognize and deal with reported dental neglect.

However, recent efforts at educating CPS workers have led to a greater willingness for CPS agencies to recognize dental neglect as a form of child maltreatment.

## ◆ DENTISTRY'S INVOLVEMENT IN PREVENTING CHILD MALTREATMENT

The attitude of dental professionals with regard to child maltreatment has been slow to change. However, the American Dental Association (ADA) has added the required recognition and reporting of suspected child abuse to the *Principles of Ethics and Code of Professional Conduct*. In 1993 this code of ethics was amended to state as follows: "Dentists shall be obliged to become familiar with the perioral signs of child abuse and to report suspected cases to the proper authorities consistent with state laws" (Minutes of House of Delegates, 1994). Official ADA policy further states that dentists should "become familiar with all physical signs of child abuse that are observable in the course of the normal dental visit" (Minutes of House of Delegates, 1994).

Over the years, some health care providers have shown a reluctance to diagnose or report suspected child abuse and neglect, and, despite legislative and ethical mandates, dentists often fail to comply with their professional responsibilities in this matter (Sanger, 1984). Data from states that track cases by the reporter's profession indicate that although as much as 75% of the physical injuries of child abuse involve the head, neck, and mouth, dentists have made less than 1% of all reports (Mouden & Bross, 1995).

Surveys have shown that dentists are hesitant to report a suspected case of child abuse because of a lack of adequate history, lack of knowledge about child abuse and the dentist's role in reporting, concern about the effect that reporting might have on the practice, and lack of time caused by a busy practice schedule (Kassebaum et al., 1991). However, recent efforts by the dental profession aimed at addressing these concerns have led to remarkable advances in dentistry's efforts to prevent child maltreatment.

In 1995 the ADA published its third edition of *The Dentist's Responsibility in Identifying and Reporting Child Abuse and Neglect* to help educate its members about their role in preventing child maltreatment (Council on Dental Practice, 1995). In addition, the ADA offers a continuing education seminar to promote awareness about child abuse prevention. This seminar, "Dentistry's Role in Preventing Child Abuse and Neglect," includes clinical recognition, diagnosis, documentation, reporting, and related social issues.

Other efforts have also succeeded in taking this message directly to dental professionals. The most notable effort to date has been Missouri's Prevent Abuse and Neglect through Dental Awareness (P.A.N.D.A.) Coalition. The P.A.N.D.A. Coalition is a public-private partnership between the dental community, social service agencies, and a dental insurance company, Delta Dental of Missouri. Previously, cooperation between CPS agencies and the dental community had not been widely promoted. During discussions aimed at forming dental education efforts, CPS staff are often surprised to learn that dentists can become a valuable resource in preventing child maltreatment (Larkin, 1992).

The success of the P.A.N.D.A. program is evidenced by dentists' increased reporting since the program's inception in 1992. Since the educational and awareness program began, although total reports to CPS have increased by 16%, the number of reports from dentists has increased 160% (Mouden, 1996). The success of the P.A.N.D.A. program has led to its replication in 34 additional states in the United States and two coalitions in Romania. Interested individuals and organizations from each remaining state of the United States, from Canada, from Israel and from the territory of Guam and Belgium are also working toward forming P.A.N.D.A. coalitions.

Initiatives such as P.A.N.D.A. and the ADA's educational efforts continue to show positive results. Using data collected at the 1994 ADA Annual Session, an ADA/Colgate Health Survey reported that the number of dentists making an initial diagnosis of child abuse or neglect rose 74% from 1993 to 1994. It is hoped that a greater awareness of dentistry's legal and ethical obligation to protect children will lead to a greater involvement in preventing child abuse and neglect. At the same time, dental professionals must strive to educate other members of the health care team about the importance of quality dental care for children and how dentistry can help prevent child abuse and neglect.

## ◆ BIBLIOGRAPHY

Andreason, JO: Periodontal healing after reimplantation of traumatically avulsed human teeth, *Acta Odontol Scand* 33:325, 1975.

Badger, GR: Dental neglect: A solution, *J Dent Child* 49:285-287, 1982.

Becker, D, Needleman, HL, and Kotelchuck, M: Orofacial trauma and its recognition by dentists, *JADA* 97:24-28, 1978.

Blain, SM, and Kittle, PE: Child abuse and neglect—dentistry's intervention (update), *Pediatr Dent* 2:1-7, 1989.

Cameron, JM, Johnson, HR, and Camps, FE: The battered child syndrome, *Med Sci Law* 6:2-21, 1966.

Carrotte, PV: An unusual case of child abuse, *Br Dent J* 168:444-445, 1990.

Council on Dental Practice: *The Dentist's Responsibility in Identifying and Reporting Child Abuse and Neglect,* ed. 3, American Dental Association, Chicago, 1995.

da Fenesca, MA, Feigal RJ, and ten Besel, RW: Dental aspects of 1248 cases of child maltreatment on file at a major county hospital, *Pediatr Dent* 14:152-157, 1992.

Heitzler, GD, Cranin, AN, and Gallo, L: Sexual abuse of the oral cavity in children, *NY State Dent J* 60:31-33, 1994.

Kassebaum, DK, Dove, SB, and Cottone, JA: Recognition and reporting of child abuse: A survey of dentists, *General Dent* 39:159-162, 1991.

Kempe, CH: Pediatric implications of battered baby syndrome, *Arch Dis Child* 46:28-37, 1971.

Kempe, CH: Uncommon manifestations of the battered child syndrome, *Am J Dis Child* 129:1265, 1975.

Kittle, PE: Two child abuse/neglect examinations for the dentist, *J Dent Child* 48:175-180, 1981.

Larkin, S: Child abuse on the rise, *MO Dent J* 72:18-31, 1992.

Malecz, RE: Child abuse, its relationship to pedodontics: A survey, *ASCD J Dent Child* 46:193-194, 1979.

Minutes of House of Delegates, November 6-10, 1993. In *1993 Transactions of the 134th Annual Session*, American Dental Association, Chicago, 1994.

Mouden LD: How dentistry succeeds in preventing family violence. (Accepted for publication, J, *Mich Dent Assoc,* January 1996.)

Mouden, LD, and Bross, DC: Legal issues affecting dentistry's role in preventing child abuse and neglect, *JADA* 126:1173-1180, 1995.

Sanger, RG: Professional responsibility in child abuse and neglect. In RG Sanger and DC Bross, editors: *Clinical Management of Child Abuse and Neglect*, Quintessence Publishing Co., Chicago, 1984.

Schmitt, BD: Types of child abuse and neglect: An overview for dentists, *Pediatr Dent* 8(special issue):67-71, 1986.

Schwartz, S, Woolridge, E, and Stege, D: Oral manifestations and legal aspects of child abuse, *JADA* 95:586-591, 1977.

Vadiakas, G, Roberts, MW, and Dilley, DCH: Child abuse and neglect: Ethical and legal issues for dentistry, *J Mass Dent* Soc 40:13-15, 1991.

# THORACOABDOMINAL INJURIES ASSOCIATED WITH CHILD ABUSE

RICHARD C. BARRY, M.D.
THOMAS R. WEBER, M.D.

*Case One: A 10-month-old male presented to the Emergency Room (ER) with cough and wheezing, and on a routine chest X-ray there were noted multiple healing rib fractures (**Figure 4-1**). Reexamination noted badly bruised buttocks with the outline of a hand. Appropriate further assessment was completed, and the case referred immediately to the Division of Family Services for further investigation.*

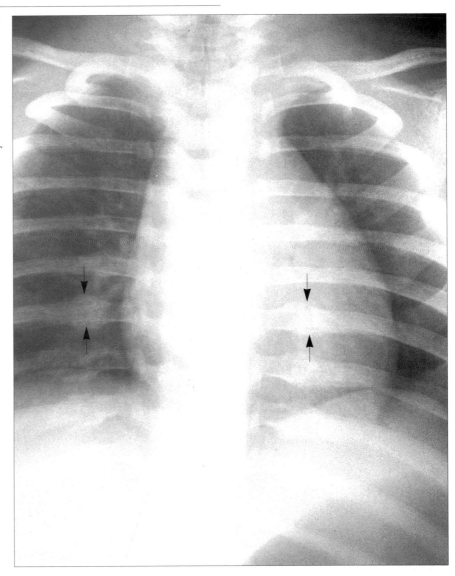

***Figure 4-1***. *Multiple posterior rib fractures.*

*Case Two: A 19-year-old mother rushed into the ER with a pale, lifeless 1-year-old whom she reported would not wake up. The physical examination revealed an obtunded, pale male with extremely precarious vital signs and ecchymotic upper and lower right eyelids as well as old scars on the buttocks in the configuration of an electric cord loop. Further assessment revealed marked anemia and elevated liver enzymes; a computed tomography (CT) scan of the abdomen showed a liver laceration and a duodenal hematoma (**Figure 4-2c**). The Division of Family Services (DFS) was immediately notified for further investigation.*

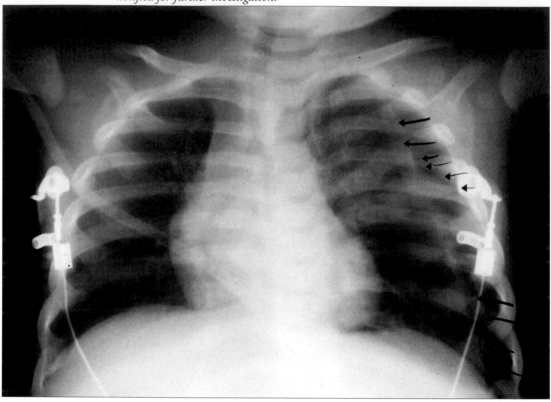

**Figure 4-2a**. *Multiple posterior rib fractures with pneumothorax on left (arrows).*

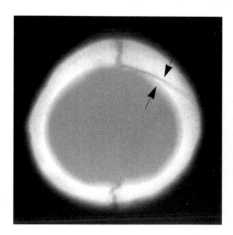

**Figure 4-2b**. *CT scan of head with skull fracture.*

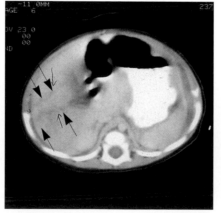

**Figure 4-2c**. *Liver laceration (arrows).*

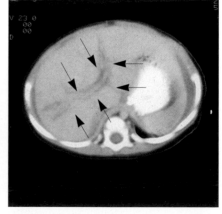

**Figure 4-2d**. *Blood in peritoneum (arrows).*

**Figures 4-2a** through **4-2d** represent the extremes of thoracoabdominal trauma associated with child abuse. The latter case, although not common, is much more serious and life-threatening. The importance of early recognition of an abuse-prone environment cannot be overstressed, not only to prevent the terrible result shown in the second case but also to protect other children who may be in the same immediate setting.

# ◆ UNINTENTIONAL VERSUS ABUSIVE INJURIES

Blunt trauma has been, and continues to be, the primary type of kinetic force (90% to 95% of the cases) associated with thoracoabdominal injury in the pediatric patient, both with accidental and with abusive injuries. Although visceral injuries account for only 2% of all child abuse cases, they are the second leading cause of death after central nervous system trauma. However, many emergency rooms, especially in the inner cities, are seeing an increasing incidence of penetrating injuries primarily due to gunshot wounds and stabbings. In the young patient, up to preteen years, the situation is usually a child caught in the crossfire of a dispute. These truncal penetrations can be rapidly life-threatening and are prone to significant morbidity and mortality. Unfortunately, young children are actually becoming the intended target of gunshots and stabbings as revengeful acts against a parent or relative and, occasionally, due to the impulsive reaction to a child's behavior.

In the preteen and teen years, a significant number of blunt truncal injuries are associated with risk taking, a perceived sense of indestructibility, and the additive use of alcohol, drugs, and motor vehicles. However, it is also in this age group that we see an alarming increase in the number of penetrating wounds, whether inflicted against self or another individual to resolve a dispute, or as an act of revenge. The easy accessibility of weapons, drug activity, and the promise of money are all enticing to the socioeconomically deprived or bored, unsupervised teenager.

Several notable differences in the usual presentation patterns (**Table 4-1**) may be helpful in determining abuse as the cause of thoracoabdominal trauma. In accidental truncal injury due to motor vehicle injury, the child is often brought immediately to the emergency room by ambulance. The child is accompanied by emergency medical services personnel, and usually everyone involved in the incident, including the child, if alert, willingly gives a reasonable and useful history. This is in marked contrast to the abusive setting in which there is often a delay, sometimes until even the caretaker recognizes that the child has reached a life-threatening stage. Unfortunately, the history given by the caretaker in these latter instances will frequently be one of trivial trauma or no history of trauma. This leaves the physician in an extremely difficult position, with a child in a tenuous cardiovascular status, perhaps comatose, and with little or no historical information.

| Table 4-1. Differences in Usual Presentation Factors in Child Abuse Versus Accidental Thoracoabdominal Injury | | |
|---|---|---|
| **Presentation Factor** | Accidental | Abuse |
| Time of presentation after injury | Immediate | Delayed |
| History | | |
|   Present | Available and reliable | Often unavailable or unreliable or inconsistent with the injury |
|   Past | Unremarkable | Previous abusive episodes and 50% known to DFS |
| Age | 7.8 years (mean) | 2.5 years (mean) |
| Old inflicted bruises | 0% | 50% to 90% |
| Old fractures | Very infrequent | Frequent |
| Most frequent abdominal organ injured | Spleen | Liver |
| Multiple visceral injuries | Infrequent | Frequent |
| Intestinal injury | Infrequent | Frequent |
| Death | 4.5% to 12.5% | 12% to 60% |

Pediatric child abuse occurs at all ages but primarily in children less than 6 years of age with the peak age range being infancy to about 3 years of age. The older toddler (mean age, 2.5 years) is most likely to be exposed to visceral trauma. On the other hand, accidental blunt thoracoabdominal trauma occurs more often in school-aged children (mean age, 7.8 years), and the majority are related to motor vehicle accidents.

In both accidental and abusive settings, males outnumber females 2:1 to 3:1. In general, the skin is the most common organ to call attention to abuse. Since abuse is usually a repetitive activity, about 50% to 90% of the patients with visceral injuries have multiple old scars or bruises in various stages of healing. The locations and configurations often clearly indicate inflicted injuries. When it comes to the visceral organs, the liver is more likely to be injured with abuse and the spleen with accidental injury; however, there is a fair amount of overlap among solid organ injuries. Abusive settings are more likely to produce multiple organ injuries. Gastrointestinal injuries such as intraluminal hematomas, perforations, and shearing mesentery injuries are more common in abuse (40% to 65%) than in accidents (8% to 15%). This type of injury is more frequently due to a punch or kick to the mid-epigastrium, leading to compression of the liver and the fixed retroperitoneal portion of the duodenum (**Figures 4-3 and 4-4**). These types of injuries can also occur in accidents associated with seat belt injuries or by hitting the handlebars of a bicycle. Mortality rates associated with visceral injuries range from 12% to 60% in the abusive setting; this relates primarily to the late presentation and the poor or absent history of trauma, leading to further delay in making a final diagnosis. Death rates due to accidental visceral injuries are much lower, ranging from 4.5% to 12.5%. Of course, if head injury is associated with either situation, the death rate markedly increases.

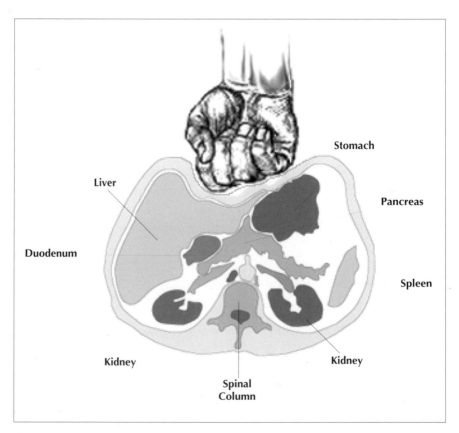

**Figure 4-3**. *Dynamics of blunt trauma to the abdomen.*

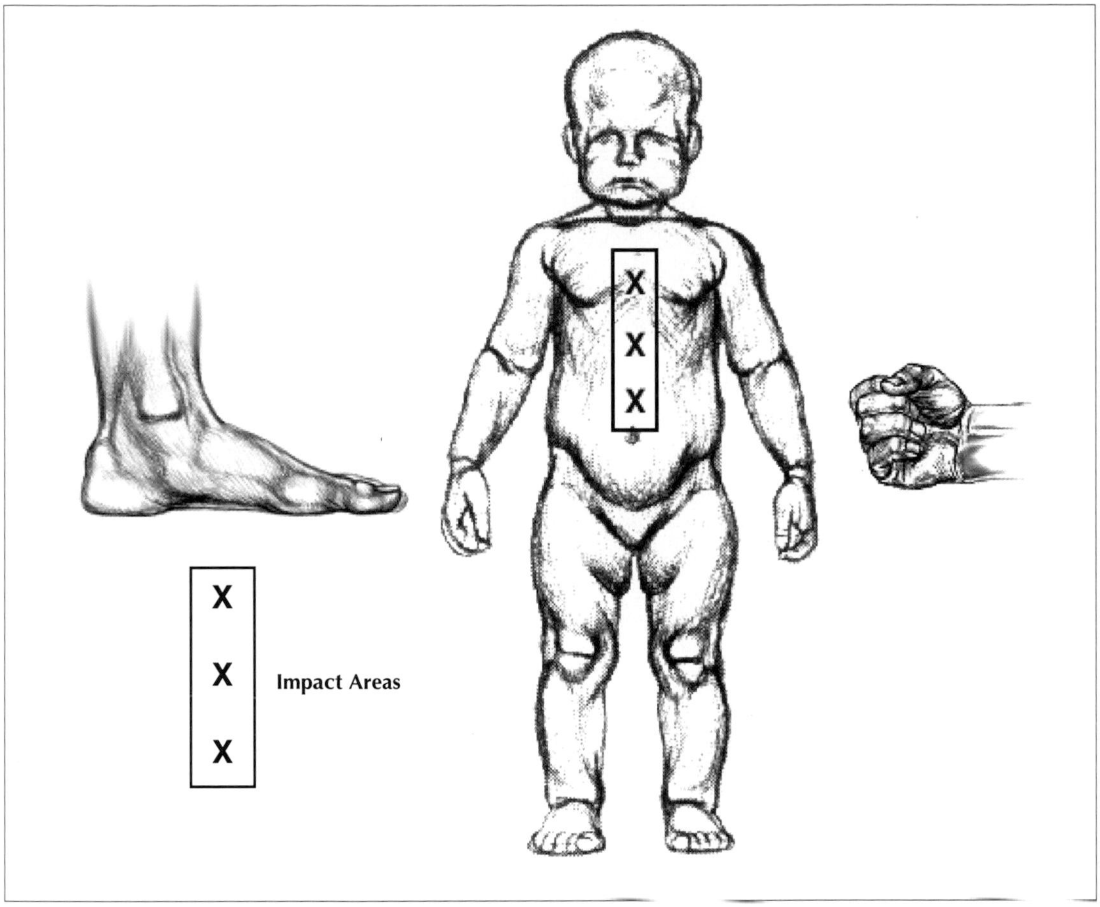

***Figure 4-4**. Areas of impact with blunt trauma.*

Impact Areas

## ♦HISTORY

To reiterate, in significant accidental truncal injuries, presentations are usually immediate and a consistent, reasonable history is given by observers and the caretaker. This is not the case with abuse and, frequently, the accompanying adult, usually the mother, will not be responsible for the injury and may or may not know about the incident. She may not disclose this information out of fear of recrimination or to protect the father or boyfriend. Although the history may not be correct, it often focuses on the site of injury. For example, if there was abdominal trauma, the mother may report that the child has had bilious emesis or report one or more of the following symptoms in her child: stomach pain, swollen abdomen, difficulty in breathing, or tarry, black stools. One should focus on the history to be sure it is consistent with the injury and the child's developmental level. If there are multiple historians, one needs to pay attention to inconsistencies in the histories. Likewise, one should check with other medical personnel to ensure that they received the same information. Multiple instances of changing or varied stories may be the first clues that the child is the victim of abuse. The alert child may not be old enough to verbalize details of what has happened or may not describe the abusive episode because he fears further abuse and trusts the abusive adult caretaker more than unfamiliar medical personnel.

Past family history may actually be more helpful in some situations and may be willingly offered by the mother. For example, she may volunteer that a sibling was previously removed from the home for neglect. The present, abused child may have been seen many times in the past. The records of previous visits should always be reviewed, looking for multiple previous episodes of trauma. Some institutions have computer programs that tabulate the number of visits for trauma each time a patient is seen. This system is to alert the practitioner that this could be an "at-risk" child. One can also assess if the caretaker is meeting minimal health maintenance care by getting routine immunizations and screening studies. It is advisable to contact the hospital social services department and/or the state Division of Family Services (DFS) to check on previous reports. Approximately 50% of patients with major abusive events, including truncal injuries, are already known to the DFS. It should be emphasized that responsibility is not only to the immediate patient in medical care but also to other children who may be exposed to these abusive caretakers.

## ♦ GENERAL APPROACH AND CLINICAL ASSESSMENT

Although the main objective of this chapter is to discuss the approach and evaluation of thoracoabdominal injuries associated with abuse, it should be noted that, not infrequently, other sites may be injured as well, influencing the ability to provide an adequate clinical assessment. A good example is an associated head and neck injury in a child who has been violently shaken with vigorous holding of the trunk, and also has visceral injury as a result of trauma to the trunk. The child's level of consciousness and responses may be markedly depressed due to the head and neck injury, making examination of the truncal area essentially unreliable. All patients, especially those brought to an emergency room setting, should have a rapid cardiopulmonary assessment to determine hemodynamic stability. If the patient is unconscious, obtunded, or pale with poor cardiovascular status, these abnormalities must be rapidly addressed and reversed. Only then should one proceed with further assessment of the child. Unfortunately, abused patients who present at this stage, with truncal injury and associated shock, frequently have a very poor outcome and a significant rise in mortality due to the long delay in seeking medical help. Since the history is often unreliable, one must do a complete clinical assessment, including a good physical examination. The child should be unclothed during that examination, and all surfaces should be viewed.

Examination of the skin is often helpful, even in thoracoabdominal injuries where there may not be obvious fresh or old bruises over the site of actual visceral injury. The presence of scars and bruises in other areas, representing repetitive abuse by their location or patterns, for example, old and recent burns, loop marks, handprints, and other patterns, suggests an abusive situation and further leads the physician to a thorough evaluation of the child.

Alert children who are young and frequently upset and frightened must be made as comfortable as possible to allow for a reliable examination. Often these children appreciate being held in their mothers' laps, which is reassuring and gives a sense of security. A complete physical examination should be performed and, if one suspects there is thoracoabdominal injury, that part of the examination should be performed last. It is important to visualize, listen to, feel, and percuss all appropriate anatomical sites, including soft tissues, solid organs, and bony skeleton, looking for clues to present and previous abuse. If the child is alert and old enough to walk, it is a good idea to see the patient walk, while looking for signs of discomfort and abnormal gait. This is particularly valuable in the toddler and preschool child. When significant physical findings are noted or there is strong suspicion of truncal abuse, these areas should be assessed with appropriate laboratory and imaging studies.

## LABORATORY STUDIES

Some or all of the trauma laboratory studies (**Table 4-2**) are frequently obtained on patients suspected of visceral injury due to abuse. Many times these studies are strongly encouraged and freely obtained to provide direction regarding further testing and imaging.

## Table 4-2. Laboratory Studies

| CBC | Result | Clinical Significance |
|---|---|---|
| Hg/Ht | ↓ | Blood loss versus anemia of other cause |
| MCV | WNL | Blood loss |
| | ↓ | Anemia from previous blood loss or other etiology |
| WBC | ↑(left shift) | Stress reaction versus infection (i.e., peritonitis with perforated bowel) |
| Guaiac | ⊕Stool | Intraluminal gastrointestinal bleeding |
| | ⊕Gastric | Intraluminal gastrointestinal bleeding |
| Urine RBC/hemoglobin | > 10 | Genital/urinary injury |
| Myoglobin | ⊕ | Rhabdomyolysis |
| AST/ALT | ≥ 450/250 IU | Liver injury |
| Amylase | ↑ | Pancreatic and/or contiguous bowel/spleen injury |
| Lytes/BUN/BS | ↑BS | Stress response |
| Creatinine | Abnormal K | Necrotic bowel, etc. |
| Blood gases | Persistent decreased $CO_2$ | |
| | Persistent metabolic acidosis | |
| PT/PTT | ↑ | Potential bleeding problems |
| CPK - MB bands | ↑ | Cardiac injury |
| Drug screen (urine/serum) | Positive | Caretaker neglectful or intentional poisoning |

*CBC, Complete blood count; HG/Ht, hemoglobin/hematocrit; WBC, whole blood cells; RBC, red blood cells; AST/ALT, aspartate amino transferase; Lytes, electrolytes; BUN, blood urea nitrogen; BS, blood sugar; PT/PTT, prothrombin time/partial thromboplastin time; CPK, creatinine phosphokinase with MB bands. CPK specific for brain; WNL, within normal limits; ⊕, present; IU, international units; K, potassium; $CO_2$, carbon dioxide.*

The complete blood count (CBC) and indices will give a baseline hemoglobin, hematocrit, and white blood cell count; when these are abnormal, blood loss or infection, such as peritonitis, may be present. However, iron deficiency anemia and lead toxicity are common in this age group and, therefore, the total hemogram should be examined to determine if the abnormalities are due to blood loss, lack of production of blood, or both. A strongly positive stool and/or gastric aspirate guaiac test suggests that there is intraluminal gastrointestinal bleeding. Red blood cells or hemoglobin in the urine can suggest renal injury, but their absence does not negate this possibility. The kidneys, because of their location, are relatively well-protected; therefore, if they are damaged, this suggests a vigorous abusive assault.

Aspartate amino transferase (AST) and alanine amino transferase (ALT) can be useful predictors of liver injury. Oldham et al. (1984) found that 44 of 100 patients with blunt abdominal trauma had elevated liver enzymes (AST/ALT). Nineteen of the 44 with abnormal elevation of liver enzymes had abdominal CT scan–proven injuries to the liver. None of the children in this series with negative abdominal CT scans had elevated liver enzyme studies. This suggests that these are extremely reliable tests. Hennes et al. (1990) further refined the predictability of liver enzymes with abdominal trauma by showing that an AST and ALT level equal to or greater than 450 and 250 IU, respectively, identified all patients with liver injury proven by CT scan.

An elevated amylase level indicates traumatic pancreatitis, which is the most common type of pancreatitis seen in the young child, but also may suggest injury to the duodenum and spleen due to the proximal location of these structures and their closeness to the pancreas. Child abuse is the most common etiology for duodenal hematoma and is associated with signs and symptoms of duodenal obstruction. Serum electrolytes, blood urea nitrogen (BUN), blood glucose, creatinine, and blood gases should be measured to assess the total clinical status of the child. A child who remains persistently acidotic, hyperkalemic, and obtunded after appropriate fluid resuscitation suggests possible necrotic bowel, waiting to perforate, or significant rhabdomyolysis. Prothrombin time (PT) and partial thromboplastin time (PTT) are probably not helpful if the child has no history of bleeding disorders and if a reliable history is obtained. However, these studies might help in assessing liver injury and preparing for appropriate infusion therapy if the patient requires operative intervention.

In the child suspected of having cardiac injury, serial creatinine phosphokinase (CPK) isoenzymes with MB bands will often be more useful than repeated electrocardiograms (EKGs). Cardiac injury occurs far less frequently than both abdominal and pulmonary insult. In general, chest trauma is much less common than abdominal injury but should be suspected when respiratory distress is noted. The chest contents can be injured without fracture of the thoracic cage due to the marked plasticity and flexibility of the ribs of the young child. However, if fractured ribs are present, the probability of injury to the chest viscera, as well as to the abdominal contents, is much higher.

| Table 4-3. Imaging Studies | |
|---|---|
| **Plain Radiographs** | Spine |
| | Chest |
| | Abdomen |
| | Pelvis |
| | Detailed skeletal survey |
| **CT Scans** | Abdomen |
| | Head |

Drug screens of urine and serum are often necessary in obtunded or comatose patients without an adequate history. A child may have been given an overdose of a sedative or barbiturate after excessive crying from the pain associated with abusive blows to the abdomen, which might be detected only by laboratory studies.

## Imaging Studies

Chapter 2 reviews the studies that are useful in the assessment of individual organs. Some or all of the imaging studies listed in **Table 4-3** can be obtained based on the clinical assessment and relevant correlation of other studies obtained. Spinal, chest, abdominal, and pelvic radiographs are obtained because of their rapid accessibility and are primarily used to find fractures, dislocations, and major abnormalities of the chest and to suggest the need for evaluation of soft tissue structures and organs using more sophisticated imaging. The primary practitioner, who may see this patient in an after-hours setting or in an emergency room and who might be required to make an initial reading of the radiographs, must pay particular attention to the presence of old rib fractures and metaphyseal fractures. Often films of the chest and abdomen will include parts of the appendicular skeleton. However, if there is serious concern regarding appendicular skeletal injuries, then detailed skeletal films and, occasionally, even a radioisotope bone scan may be necessary. It should be remembered that fractures are the next most common sign of abuse after bruises and skin findings. A useful technique in reading the radiographs is to evaluate the X-rays as individual segments, that is, bones, soft tissues, and air shadows, and then assess the whole picture. If one traces and visualizes each skeletal part with a finger, one is less likely to miss old rib fractures or the coincidental healing of a spiral humeral fracture on a chest film. In general, soft tissue integrity of both chest and abdomen is most reliably evaluated by CT. For the abdomen, the use of intraluminal and intravenous contrast allows identification of organ structural integrity, gastrointestinal tract obstruction, perforation, and shearing injury. This imaging modality is helpful in identifying the site of injury and allows for appropriate monitoring and preparedness in incidences of nonoperative management. Diagnostic peritoneal lavage has been relegated to a minor position in pediatric trauma. Although it reliably identifies bleeding, it does not delineate which organ(s) may be involved and whether the patient needs an operation. Most of the care is supportive, with close observation. Diagnostic peritoneal lavage is still used when the patient requires emergency neurosurgical operative intervention and there is no time available for an abdominal CT. Arteriography is used for the rare chest vascular injury.

**It must be emphasized that in a comatose child, even after abusive head injury is recognized, the abdomen must still be aggressively evaluated to detect major injury, which can suddenly lead to unexpected deterioration.**

## ♦ SUMMARY

Thoracoabdominal injury secondary to child abuse is relatively rare but can have very high mortality and morbidity. *Consequently, it is important to be aware of this possibility and to remember the following clues:*

1. Delayed presentation with nonspecific complaints, usually related to the abdomen and chest, with either multiple stories or reports that are inconsistent with the physical findings or the child's development.

2. Past history of that abusive or neglectful incident and previous report to the Division of Family Services.

3. Mean age of 2.5 years.

4. Old inflicted bruises or scars (present in 50% to 90% of cases). Consequently, all young children with nonspecific complaints or injuries should have a rapid but thorough complete physical examination.

5. Generous use of screening trauma laboratory studies, especially serum glutamic oxaloacetic transaminase, serum glutamic pyruvic transaminase, amylase, stool guaiac, hemoglobin, hematocrit, and urine analysis to give direction with regard to the need for CT imaging or other diagnostic studies.

## ♦ BIBLIOGRAPHY

Coant, P, Kornberg, A, Brody, A, and Edwards-Holmes, K: Markers for occult liver injury in cases of physical abuse in children, *Pediatrics* 89(2):274-278, 1992.

Cooper, A, Floyd, T, Barlow, B, Niemirska, M, Ludwig, S, Seidl, T, O'Neill, J, Templeton, J, Ziegler, M, Ross, A, Gandhi, R, and Catherman, R: Major blunt abdominal trauma due to child abuse, *J Trauma* 28(10):1483-1487, 1988.

Evers, K, and DeGaeta, LR: Abdominal trauma, *Emerg Med Clin North Am* 3(3):525-539, 1985.

Feldman, KW, and Brewer, DK: Child abuse, cardiopulmonary resuscitation, and rib fractures, *Pediatrics* 73(3):339-342, 1984.

Fossum, RM, and Descheneaux, KA: Blunt trauma of the abdomen in children, *JFSCS* 36(1)47-50, 1991.

Gornall, P, Ahmed, S, Jolleys, A, and Cohen, S: Intra-abdominal injuries in the battered baby syndrome, *Arch Dis Child* 47:211-214, 1972.

Grosfeld, JL, and Ballantine, TVN: Surgical aspects of child abuse (trauma-x), *Pediatr Ann* 106-120, 1976.

Haller, JA: Injuries of the gastrointestinal tract in children: Notes on recognition and management, *Clin Pediatr* 5(8):476-480, 1966.

Haller, JO, Bass, IS, and Sclafani, SJA: Imaging evaluation of traumatic hematuria in children, *Urol Radiol* 7:211-218, 1984.

Haller, JO, Kleinman, PK, Merten, DF, Cohen, HL, Cohen, MD, Hayden, PW, Keller, M, Towbin, R, and Sane, SM: Diagnostic imaging of child abuse, *Pediatrics* 87(2):262-265, 1991.

Hennes, HM, Smith, DS, Schneider, K, Hegenbarth, MA, Duma, MA, and Jona, JZ: Elevated liver transaminase levels in children with blunt abdominal trauma: A predictor of liver injury, *Pediatrics* 86(1):87-94, 1990.

Hernanz-Schulman, M, Genieser, NB, and Ambrosino, M: Sonographic diagnosis on intramural duodenal hematoma, *J Ultrasound Med* 8:273-276, 1989.

Kaufman, RA, and Babcock, DS: An approach to imaging the upper abdomen in the injured child, *Semin Roentgenol* 14(4):308-320, 1984.

Kaufman, RA, Towbin, R, Babcock, DS, Gelfand, MJ, Fuice, KS, Oldham, KT, and Noseworthy, J: Upper abdominal trauma in children: Imaging evaluation, *AJR* 142:449-460, 1984.

Kirks, DR: Radiological evaluation of visceral injuries in the battered child syndrome, *Pediatr Ann* 12(12):888-893, 1983.

Kleinman, PK, Brill, PW, and Winchester, P: Resolving duodenal-jejunal hematoma in abused children, *Radiology* 160:747-750, 1986.

Kleinman, PK, Marks, SC, Adams, VI, and Blackbourne, BD: Factors affecting visualization of posterior rib fractures in abused infants, *AJR* 150:635-638, 1988.

Kleinman, PK, Raptopoulos, VD, and Brill, PW: Occult nonskeletal trauma in the battered-child syndrome, *Pediatr Radiol* 141:393-396, 1981.

Ledbetter, D, Hatch, E, Feldman, K, Fligner, C, and Tapper, D: Diagnostic and surgical implications of child abuse, *Arch Surg* 123:1101-1105, 1988.

Mayer, T, Walker, M, Johnson, D, and Matlak, M: Causes of morbidity and mortality in severe pediatric trauma, *JAMA* 245(7):719-721, 1981.

McEniery, J, Hanson, R, Grigor, W, and Horowitz, A: Lung injury resulting from a nonaccidental crush injury to the chest, *Pediatr Emerg Care* 7(3):166-168, 1991.

Meller, J, Little, A, and Shermeta, D: Thoracic trauma in children, *Pediatrics* 74(5):813-819, 1984.

Merten, D, and Carpenter, B: Radiologic imaging of inflicted injury in the child abuse syndrome, *Pediatr Clin North Am* 37(4): 815-837, 1990.

Oldham, K, Guice, K, Kaufman, R, Martin, L, and Noseworthy, J: Blunt hepatic injury and elevated hepatic enzymes: A clinical correlation in children, *J Pediatr Surg* 19(4):457-461, 1984.

O'Neill, JA, Meacham, WF, Griffin, PP, and Sawyers, JL: Patterns of injury in the battered child syndrome, *J Trauma* 13(4):332-339, 1973.

Pena, SDJ, and Medovy, H: Child abuse and traumatic pseudocyst of the pancreas, *J Pediatr* 83(6):1026-1028, 1973.

Philippart, AI: Blunt abdominal trauma in childhood, *Surg Clin North Am* 57(1)151-163, 1977.

Ramenofsky, ML: Pediatric abdominal trauma, *Pediatr Ann* 16(4)318-326, 1987.

Reece, RM, and Grodin, MA: Recognition of nonaccidental injury, *Pediatr Clin North Am* 32(1):41-60, 1985.

Rodgers, B: Trauma and the child, *Heart Lung* 6(6):1052-1056, 1977.

Sivit, C, Taylor, G, and Eichelberger, M: Visceral injury in battered children: A changing perspective, *Radiology* 173(3):659-661, 1989.

Taylor, GA, and Eichelberger, MR: Abdominal CT in children in neurologic impairment following blunt trauma, *Ann Surg* 210(2):229-233, 1989.

Taylor, GA, Fallat, ME, Potter, BM, and Eichelberger, MR: The role of computed tomography in blunt abdominal trauma in children, *J Trauma* 28(12):1660-1664, 1988.

Chapter

5

# Ophthalmic Manifestations of Child Abuse

Oscar A. Cruz, M.D.
Bradley V. Davitt, M.D.

In 1946 Caffey suggested that multiple fractures in the long bones of several infants with chronic subdural hematoma were secondary to trauma (Caffey, 1974). Two of these children also had retinal hemorrhage. Caffey recognized that only trauma could explain this spectrum of injuries, yet he failed to implicate intentional trauma and stated that the injuries could be the result of forgotten or relatively minor traumatic episodes.

It was not until 1964 that ophthalmologists began to describe the ocular manifestations of child abuse. The first report of abusive injuries in the ophthalmic literature was made by G. T. Kiffney. Kiffney reported an abused child who presented with multiple skull fractures, intracranial hemorrhage, and leukocoria (Kiffney, 1964). The child had bilateral cataracts and total retinal detachments. Retrospectively, the diagnosis of child abuse was made.

## ◆ Presenting Signs

From 4% to 6% of child abuse cases present with ophthalmic manifestations (Friendly, 1971; Jensen et al., 1987), and the spectrum of ocular findings in the battered child syndrome is vast. An ocular injury may be as minor as periorbital edema or as severe as a ruptured globe (Table 5-1). The ocular sequelae of abuse can include amblyopia on the basis of monocular cataract, strabismus, or anterior segment injury. Detection of eye injury is difficult when the examination takes place several days after the abuse has occurred. Because nearly 40% of physically abused children have associated ocular trauma, it is imperative that all children suspected of being abused have a thorough dilated ophthalmic examination (Friendly, 1971; Jensen et al., 1987). The presence of positive ocular findings often indicates that the child should have prompt neuroimaging (MRI).

| Table 5-1. Ocular Manifestations of the Two Most Common Forms of Child Abuse | |
| --- | --- |
| Physical Abuse | Intraocular retinal hemorrhages |
| | Periorbital ecchymosis |
| | Vitreoretinal injury other than hemorrhage |
| | Cataract or subluxated lens |
| | Hyphema |
| | Subconjunctival hemorrhage |
| | Optic nerve injury |
| | Strabismus or gaze palsy |
| Sexual Abuse | Sexually transmitted infections |

79

## ◆Nonabusive Ocular Injuries

Nonabusive ocular injuries are often seen in newborns, infants, and children. Examples of nonabusive injuries include retinal hemorrhage resulting from the birth process or those associated with thoracic compression needed in cardiopulmonary resuscitation (CPR) (**Table 5-2**). These nonabusive hemorrhages may appear similar to those retinal hemorrhages resulting from abusive-inflicted injury. Other nonabusive ophthalmic injuries include periorbital edema and subconjunctival hemorrhages.

| Table 5-2. Common Nonabusive Causes of Retinal Hemorrhage | |
|---|---|
| **Medical Procedures** | Birthing process<br>Extracorporeal membrane oxygenation (ECMO)<br>blood dyscrasias; hemoglobinopathies |
| **Accidental Trauma** | Subdural or subarachnoid hemorrhages secondary<br>to accidental trauma |

### Retinal Hemorrhage

Retinal hemorrhages can occur in any layer of the retina without being the result of child abuse. However, the presence of retinal or vitreous hemorrhages in a child younger than 3 years of age who has no medical risk factors has been considered by some to be pathognomonic of nonaccidental injury until proven otherwise (Levin, 1991).

### Result of Birth Process

Head trauma resulting from birthing has been found to cause retinal hemorrhages in 8% to 50% of otherwise healthy newborns (Von Barsewisch, 1979). Giles found retinal hemorrhages in 40 of 100 newborns examined on the first day of life, but only 20% of these infants still had retinal hemorrhages on the third day of life (Giles, 1960). If retinal hemorrhages are detected in infants over 1 month of age, a cause other than the birth process must be considered (Friendly, 1983).

### Result of CPR

Retinal hemorrhages rarely occur when CPR is administered. Goetting and Sowa studied 20 resuscitated children and found 2 with retinal hemorrhages in the absence of other recognized injuries (Goetting & Sowa, 1990). Gilliland and Luckenbach performed postmortem ocular examinations on 169 children following unsuccessful resuscitation attempts and did not find one case to support the hypothesis that retinal hemorrhages are caused by resuscitation attempts (Gilliland et al., 1993). It is postulated that sufficient thoracic compression can cause an acute rise in retinal venous pressure and subsequent hemorrhage. Caution must be used when interpreting fundus findings in children who have undergone CPR, as the findings could be the result of nonaccidental trauma.

### Result of Ruptured Vascular Malformations

A ruptured vascular malformation masquerading as Battered/Shaken Baby Syndrome has been reported (Weissgold et al., 1995). Abuse was originally suspected because of an unusual parental reaction to the child's death, acute intracranial hemorrhage, and discovery of optic nerve sheath hemorrhages at necropsy. However, careful microscopic study uncovered an unusual subarachnoid vascular malformation, the rupture of which was felt to cause the infant's death.

### Periorbital Edema and Subconjunctival Hemorrhage

Periorbital edema and subconjunctival hemorrhage are common ocular manifestations of nonaccidental injury. These injuries are frequently accompanied

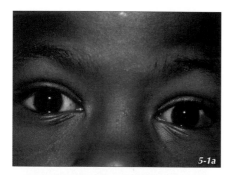
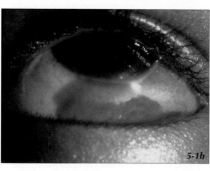

*Figure 5-1a.* Subconjunctival hemorrhage occurs in 2% to 4% of abused children with ocular manifestations. Direct trauma or increases in thoracic pressure by chest compression can be the cause. *b.* This is the presumed mechanism of subconjunctival hemorrhage in attempted strangulation.

by bleeding from forehead and scalp contusions. The ophthalmologist then faces the challenge of determining if the physical findings of periorbital edema or subconjunctival hemorrhage (**Figure 5-1 a,b**) are consistent with the history of an accidental injury.

The pattern of bruising can be a secondary aid in determining if the injury is nonaccidental. Signs of bilateral ocular trauma suggest inflicted injury because accidents usually involve only one eye (Nelson & Parlato, 1993). With these particular injuries, the large volume of potential tissue space in the periorbital area can lead to significant blood accumulation, and this in turn can lead to marked ecchymotic eyelid swelling. This accumulation of blood often makes the ecchymosis look darker than bruises at other sites, causing the injury to appear older than it actually is. In addition, the increased volume of blood leads to a slower resolution (Levin, 1991).

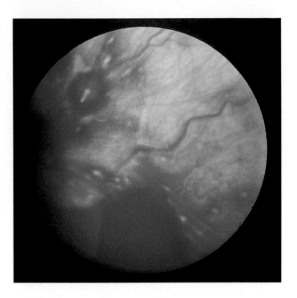

*Figure 5-2. Retinal hemorrhage.*

## ◆ ABUSIVE OCULAR INJURIES

The single most common ocular manifestation in child abuse is the presence of these retinal hemorrhages (**Figure 5-2**), which have been found in 5% to 23% of physically abused children (Friendly, 1971; Levin, 1990). Eisenbrey's study of victims of head trauma found retinal hemorrhages in 15 of 26 (62%) abused children and in only 1 of 32 (3%) nonabused children. The one child with retinal hemorrhage in the nonabused group was a "newborn infant following a traumatic delivery" (Eisenbrey, 1979).

### CURRENT RESEARCH

Retrospective studies of children with retinal hemorrhages have been flawed by lack of matched controls. They have been limited by the fact that cases of retinal hemorrhages easily could have been missed if routine funduscopic examinations were not performed on all the children. Buys et al. (1992) have produced the only published report of prospective retinal examination of children who suffered head trauma. They performed dilated, indirect ophthalmoscopy on 78 children between the ages of 4 weeks and 3 years within 48 hours after their head trauma occurred. Seventy-five children in their study sustained accidental head injuries and had normal funduscopic examinations. It was determined that three children sustained inflicted head injuries. These children all had varying degrees of retinal hemorrhage.

Billmire and Myers (1985) did a retrospective study of infants younger than 1 year of age who were admitted to the hospital with a head injury. They reported that retinal hemorrhages occurred in 89% of 28 abused infants but that none occurred in 54 infants with accidental injuries.

These data support the conclusion that retinal hemorrhages occur only rarely in children younger than 36 months of age after severe head trauma and not at all after moderate or mild head trauma. When a child presents with a head injury and retinal hemorrhages without an obvious cause, an investigation for child abuse must be considered.

### SHAKEN BABY SYNDROME

In infants with shaken baby syndrome (SBS), the incidence of retinal hemorrhage is 50% to 100% (Ludwig & Warman, 1984; Billmire & Myers, 1985; Duhaime et al., 1987). Ludwig and Warman reported that 50% of babies determined to have been shaken had gaze disturbances. These hemorrhages often involve the posterior pole and are bilateral in 58% to 100% of cases (Levin, 1990), although they can be asymmetric. Retinal hemorrhages can be subretinal or intraretinal, predominantly in the bipolar layer or in the nerve fiber layer. Increased severity of retinal

*Other Vitreoretinal Injuries Resulting From Shaken Baby Syndrome*

*Retinal dialysis (disinsertion of the retina from its insertion at the ora serrata)*

*Retinal edema (commotio retinae) in the photoreceptor layer*

*Central retinal artery occlusion*

*Exudate*

*Traction from scarring (gliosis)*

hemorrhages in shaken baby syndrome has been correlated with acute neurologic findings (Wilkinson et al., 1989). Additionally, the presence of dense vitreous hemorrhages in infants with shaken baby syndrome predicts poor visual and neurological prognosis (Matthews et al., 1996).

## PATHOGENESIS

The pathogenesis of retinal hemorrhages in the shaken baby syndrome is a matter of dispute. Many authors believe that the intraocular hemorrhages occur secondary to a sudden rise in retinal venous hydrostatic pressure, which is produced by intracranial hypertension. Greenwall et al. have proposed that hemorrhages secondary to internal splitting of the retina, or traumatic retinoschisis, are caused by tractional forces transmitted from the vitreous, which oscillates violently as the head is shaken (Greenwall et al., 1986). There is both clinical and pathological evidence to support this view (Rao et al., 1988). The time of onset of symptoms occurs quite variably. There can be a delay between the occurrence of an intraocular hemorrhage and the subsequent development of subdural hemorrhage or effusions.

Terson syndrome is caused by a sudden rise in intracranial pressure due to acute subdural or subarachnoid hemorrhage and is generally characterized by preretinal and vitreous hemorrhage. Purtscher retinopathy, characterized by cotton-wool exudates and retinal hemorrhages, is thought to be produced by increased orbital venous pressure secondary to thoracic compression. This type of hemorrhagic retinal angiopathy occurs with pulmonary compression or contusions/fractures of long bones. When it is seen in association with child abuse, there is a paucity of intracranial hemorrhages (Tomasi & Rosman, 1986). Positive ocular findings indicate that the child should have prompt neuroimaging (CT) or magnetic resonance imaging (MRI).

## VITREOUS HEMORRHAGE

Vitreous hemorrhage can also occur in shaken baby syndrome, although its appearance is usually delayed from 2 days to 2 weeks after the shaking episode occurs. Vitreoretinal injury, like retinal hemorrhage, is a vision-threatening injury. Vitreous hemorrhage is acutely associated with retinal or subhyaloid hemorrhage.

## PHYSIOLOGY

The repeated violent shaking described in shaken baby syndrome can result in repeated severe acceleration/deceleration of the vitreous, which causes trauma to the retina and retinal blood vessels. Chorioretinal atrophy in the extreme periphery of the retina, particularly the inferior temporal quadrant, has been demonstrated in child abuse victims. Fundus examination demonstrates scalloped areas of the retinal pigment epithelial atrophy that are associated with pigment proliferation and atrophic choroidal changes (**Figure 5-3**). They are nonprogressive and are not associated with any other retinal defect (Nelson & Parlato, 1993).

This mechanism has been proposed as the cause of traumatic retinoschisis (Levin, 1990), while retinal folds arise from the more common retinal hemorrhages (Gaynon et al., 1988; Massicotte et al., 1991). Macular folds have been shown to occur where previous large subhyaloid hemorrhages have resolved (Han & Wilkinson, 1990). Unilateral and bilateral retinal detachment due to abuse is most often rhegmatogenous or due to a tear or a hole in the retina that allows fluid vitreous to track underneath the retina and separate it from the sclera. When a giant retinal tear results in vitreous hemorrhage, the visual prognosis is dismal.

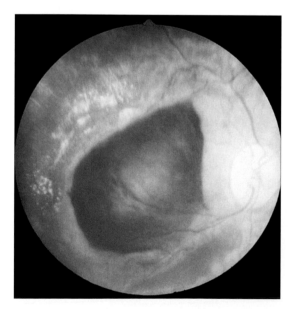

*Figure 5-3*. Scattered retinal hemorrhages are a benchmark feature of child abuse.

## LENS SUBLUXATION OR DISLOCATION

Trauma is the most common cause of lens subluxation or dislocation in childhood, and there have been a number of reported cases involving abuse (Friendly, 1971). The first step, of course, is to rule out nontraumatic displacement — such as that associated with Marfan syndrome, homocystinuria, aniridia, and congenital glaucoma. Traumatic dislocation is usually unilateral, as opposed to spontaneous ectopia lentis, which is usually bilateral, although it can be markedly asymmetric. The lens is displaced in any direction except upward in reported cases resulting from child abuse. Upward displacement is the most common lens displacement direction seen in Marfan syndrome, which is also the most common cause of spontaneous ectopia lentis. Findings associated with subluxation of the lens include marked astigmatism, monocular diplopia, cataract, and amblyopia in unilateral cases. Dislocation can also cause all of these complications with the addition of glaucoma.

## ANTERIOR CHAMBER INJURY

The anterior chamber includes the cornea, iris, and trabecular meshwork (the outflow system for the aqueous humor); essentially it is the area between the crystalline lens and the cornea. Anterior chamber trauma occurring in abused children ranges from 0% to 5%. Hyphema, or blood in the anterior chamber, is caused by injury to the vessels of the peripheral iris or the anterior ciliary body. Other anterior segment injuries, as well as hyphema, are usually caused by direct blunt trauma and are not the result of shaken baby syndrome.

## INJURY TO CORTICAL PATHWAYS

The cortical visual pathways can be injured as a result of child abuse and are most commonly seen in shaken baby syndrome. These injuries result in a poor visual outcome even when there is no permanent vitreoretinal injury. Cortical injuries result in visual field deficits or reduced visual acuity.

Optic atrophy can be unilateral or bilateral. It can result from direct injury, increased intracranial pressure, or injury secondary to cortical injury with retrograde transsynaptic degeneration. Acute papilledema, almost exclusively bilateral, is a poor prognostic sign. The finding of optic nerve sheath hemorrhages suggests that the hemorrhages found surrounding the optic disc could have originated in the subarachnoid space (Lambert et al., 1986).

## OCULAR MANIFESTATIONS IN SEXUAL ABUSE

No case of either isolated ocular manifestations or of ocular manifestations in conjunction with findings at another site have been reported in sexually abused children. However, periorbital ecchymosis, retinal and vitreous hemorrhages, papilledema, and subconjunctival hemorrhage have been reported in children who were beaten *and* sexually abused (San Martin et al., 1981). A more likely ophthalmologic manifestation of sexual abuse, however, is the onset of functional visual loss or other functional ocular complaints such as blindness, transient visual obscurations, and photophobia (Catalano et al., 1986; Vrabec et al., 1989). An ocular manifestation of sexually transmitted disease, such as gonococcal conjunctivitis, should be considered a possible indicator of covert sexual abuse (Levin, 1990).

Gonococcal conjunctivitis is characterized by the acute onset of copious mucopurulent conjunctivitis. Corneal involvement can lead to corneal damage or perforation. Evaluation of the child with gonococcal conjunctivitis must include genital and anal inspection, cultures of the rectum, vagina, or male urethra, and a culture of the throat for *Neisseria gonorrhoeae* and other sexually transmitted disease organisms.

## CHILD NEGLECT

The most common form of child neglect encountered by the ophthalmologist includes medical noncompliance. Failure to obtain glasses, adhere to patching regimens, or keep follow-up appointments is a frequent and frustrating experience in the practice of pediatric ophthalmology. Some parents also do not seek medical attention for their child when obvious ocular symptoms are present. It is often difficult to determine whether noncompliance is abusively neglectful or whether inadequate financial or social resources are responsible (Levin, 1991).

## ♦ TEAM APPROACH

The ophthalmologist must be a part of the multidisciplinary team caring for possible child abuse victims. All ophthalmologists must consider the possibility of child abuse in the differential diagnosis, especially when in the role of primary care provider or when ocular manifestations are the only visible signs of abuse. Whether the trauma sustained is accidental or deliberate, the physical findings in these children should be carefully documented. Riffenburgh and Sathyavagiswaran (1991) recommend that indirect ophthalmoscopy be included as part of the autopsy in all children who die without an obvious cause of death. The ophthalmologic findings often provide confirmatory evidence in cases where abuse is suspected. Specifically, histopathologic analysis of optic nerve sheath and intraocular hemorrhages may be helpful in distinguishing traumatic from non-traumatic causes of infants deaths (Budenz et al., 1994). The ophthalmologic findings must not be reported in isolation; they need to be documented in conjunction with all of the other physical findings in these children.

## ♦ BIBLIOGRAPHY

Alexander, RC, Schor, DP, and Smith, WL, Jr: Magnetic resonance imaging of intracranial injuries from child abuse, *J Pediatr* 109:975-979, 1986.

Billmire, ME, and Myers, PA: Serious head injury in infants: Accident or abuse? *Pediatrics* 75:340-342, 1985.

Budenz DL, Farber, MG, Mirchandani, HG, et al: Ocular and optic nerve hemorrhages in abused infants with intracranial injuries, *Ophthalmology* 101:559-565, 1994.

Buys, YM, Levin, AV, Enzenauer, RW, et al: Retinal findings after head trauma in infants and young children, *Ophthalmology* 99:1718-1723, 1992.

Caffey, J: The whiplash shaken infant syndrome: Manual shaking by the extremities with whiplash-induced intracranial and intraocular bleedings linked with residual permanent brain damage and mental retardation, *Pediatrics* 54:396-403, 1974.

Catalona, RA, Simon, JW, Krobel, GB, et al: Functional visual loss in children, *Ophthalmology* 93:385-390, 1986.

Duhaime, AC, Alario, A, Lewander, W, et al: Head injury in very young children: Mechanism, injury types and ophthalmic findings in 100 hospitalized patients younger than 2 years of age, *Pediatrics* 90:179-185, 1992.

Duhaime, AC, Gennarelli, TA, Thibault, LE, et al: The shaken baby syndrome: A clinical, pathological, and biomechanical study, *J Neurosurg* 66:409-415, 1987.

Eisenbrey, AB: Retinal hemorrhage in the battered child, *Childs Brain* 5:40-44, 1979.

Elner, SG, Elner, VM, Arnall, M, and Albert, DM: Ocular and associate systemic findings in suspected child abuse: A necroscopy study, *Arch Ophthalmol* 108:1094-1101, 1990.

Friendly, DS: Ocular manifestations of physical child abuse, *Trans Am Acad Ophthalmol Orolaryngol* 75:318-332, 1971.

Friendly, DS: Ocular aspects of physical child abuse. In RD Harley, ed: *Pediatric Ophthalmology*, WB Saunders Co, Philadelphia, 1983.

Gaynon, MW, Koh, K, Marmor, MF, and Frankel, LR: Retinal folds in the shaken baby syndrome, *Am J Ophthalmol* 106:423-425, 1988.

Giangiacomo, J, and Barkett, KJ: Ophthalmoscopic findings in occult child abuse, *J Pediatr Ophthalmol Strabismus* 22:234-237, 1985.

Giles, MJ: Retinal hemorrhages in the newborn, *Am J Ophthalmol* 49:1005-1011, 1960.

Gilliland, MG, Luckenbach, MW: Are retinal hemorrhages found after resuscitation attempts? A study of the eyes of 169 children, *Am J Forensic Med Pathol* 14:187-192, 1993.

Goetting, MG, and Sowa, B: Retinal hemorrhage after cardiopulmonary resuscitation in children: An etiologic re-evaluation, *Pediatrics* 85:585-588, 1990.

Greenwall, MJ, Weiss, A, Oesterle, CS, and Friendly, DS: Traumatic retinoschisis in battered babies, *Ophthalmology* 93:618-625, 1986.

Han, DP, and Wilkinson, WS: Late ophthalmic manifestations of the shaken baby syndrome, *J Pediatr Ophthalmol Strabismus* 27:299-303, 1990.

Hobbs, CJ: When are burns nonaccidental? *Arch Dis Child* 61:357-361, 1986.

Jensen, AD, Smith, RE, and Olson, MI: Ocular clues to child abuse, *J Pediatr Ophthalmol* 8:270-272, 1987.

Kanter, RK: Retinal hemorrhage after cardiopulmonary resuscitation or child abuse, *J Pediatr* 108:430-432, 1986.

Keen, JH, Lendrum, J, and Wolman, B: Inflicted burns and scalds in children, *Br Med J* 4:268-269, 1975.

Kiffney, GT, Jr: The eye of the battered child, *Arch Ophthalmol* 72:231-233, 1964.

Kleinman, PK: Diagnostic imaging in infant abuse, *AJR* 155:703-712, 1990.

Lambert, SR, Johnson, TE, and Hoyt, CS: Optic nerve sheath hemorrhages associated with the shaken baby syndrome, *Arch Ophthalmol* 104:1509-1512, 1986.

Levin, AV: Ocular manifestations of child abuse, *Ophthalmol Clin North Am* 3:249-264, 1990.

Levin, AV: Ophthalmologic manifestations. In S Ludwig, ed: *Child Abuse, A Medical Reference*, Churchill Livingstone, New York, 1991.

Ludwig, S, and Warman, M: Shaken baby syndrome: A review of 20 cases, *Ann Emerg Med* 13:104-107, 1984.

Massicotte, SJ, Folberg, R, Torczynski, E, et al: Vitreoretinal traction and perimacular retinal folds in the eyes of deliberately traumatized children, *Ophthalmology* 98:1124-1127, 1991.

Matthews, GP, Das, A: Dense vitreous hemorrhages predict poor visual and neurological prognosis in infants with shaken baby syndrome, *J Pediatr Ophthalmol Strabismus* 33:260-265, 1996.

Neinstein, LS, Goldenring, J, and Carpenter, S: Nonsexual transmission of sexually transmitted diseases: An infrequent occurrence, *Pediatrics* 74:67-76, 1984.

Nelson, LB, and Parlato, CJ: Systemic and ophthalmic manifestations of child abuse. In W Tasman, ed: *Duane's Clinical Ophthalmology*, JB Lippincott Co, Philadelphia, Volume 5, Chapter 44, 1993.

Ommaya, AK, Faas, F, and Yarnell, P: Whiplash injury and brain damage: An experimental study, *JAMA* 204:285-289, 1968.

Podgore, JK, and Holmes, KK: Ocular gonococcal infection with minimal or inflammatory response, *JAMA* 246:242-243, 1981.

Rao, N, Smith, RE, Choi, JH, et al: Autopsy findings in the eyes of fourteen fatally abused children, *Forensic Sci Int* 39:293-296, 1988.

Riffenburgh, RS, and Sathyavagiswaran, L: The eyes of child abuse victims: Autopsy findings, *J Forensic Sci* 36:741-747, 1991.

San Martin, R, Steinkuller, PG, and Nisbert, RM: Retinopathy in the sexually abused battered child, *Ann Ophthalmol* 13:89-91, 1981.

Tomasi, LG, and Rosman, NP: Purtscher retinopathy in the battered child syndrome, *Am J Dis Child* 93:1435-1437, 1986.

Von Barsewisch, B: *Perinatal Retinal Hemorrhages*, Springer-Verlag, Berlin, 1979.

Vrabec, TR, Levin, AV, and Nelson, LB: Functional blinking in childhood, *Pediatrics* 83:967-970, 1989.

Weissgold, DJ, Budenz, DL, Hood, I, et al: Ruptured vascular malformation masquerading as battered/shaken baby syndrome: A nearly tragic mistake, *Surv Ophthalmol* 39:509-512, 1995.

Wilkinson, WS, Han, DP, Rappley, MD, and Owings, CL: Retinal hemorrhage predicts neurologic injury in the shaken baby syndrome, *Arch Ophthalmol* 107:1472-1474, 1989.

# HEAD INJURY IN CHILD ABUSE

Mary E. S. Case, M.D.

In a 1946 paper, Caffey called attention to a correlation between the findings of multiple skeletal fractures and subdural hemorrhage in children he believed to have suffered inflicted trauma (Caffey, 1946). In 1962 Kempe stressed the same correlation Caffey found, and the term "battered child syndrome" was applied to describe the medicosociological phenomenon discovered (Kempe et al., 1962).

Since the early 1960s, considerable data have accumulated concerning abusive pediatric head injuries. Recognition of inflicted versus accidental injuries is accomplished in the light of a vast body of literature and knowledge. This chapter will overview the findings in relation to types of head injury and signs to be sought by the practitioner; Chapter 25 will review head injuries from the perspective of a pathologist.

Head injury resulting from abuse is a significant cause of disability and death in children. It is the leading cause of death from abuse, playing a role in 40% to 75% of abusive deaths. Children with nonfatal head injuries often suffer permanent neurological impairments, previously incorrectly attributed to prenatal or perinatal disorders (Oliver, 1975).

Because head injuries in children differ greatly in many aspects from those occurring in adults, particular mention will be made of these differences in describing the various injuries.

## ♦EXTERNAL FINDINGS IN ABUSIVE HEAD AND FACE INJURIES

Because of the great disparity in size and strength between the adult and child, an adult does not need a weapon or instrument to inflict injury on the child. Many injuries to the head are inflicted by manual violence and result in observable blunt trauma lesions, particularly bruises or contusions and abrasions; less often lacerations may occur. Instruments may also be used, and gunshot wounds, stab wounds, or impact marks from objects such as hammers, boards, or choppers may be seen in children.

A bruise or contusion is an impact site on the skin's surface over subcutaneous or deeper bleeding. Small blood vessels are torn by the impact, yielding the site of hemorrhage. On the surface, bruises undergo progressive color changes—purple/blue to green to yellow and then to brown—before fading away. When injury is inflicted by belts, cords, hands, bites, or hairbrush bristles, bruises appear in distinctive patterns.

| Table 6-1. Population Distribution/St. Louis Study *(January 1977-June 30, 1985)* | | |
|---|---|---|
| Homicide 70 children | Accident 63 children | Undetermined 27 children |
| **Age** | **Homicide*** | **Accident†** |
| Under 1 year of age | 45% | 39% |
| 1 to 2 years of age | 19% | 28% |
| 2 to 3 years of age | 18% | 8% |
| Older | 18% | 22% |

*82% of the homicide group were under 3 years of age.
†75% of the accident group were under 3 years of age.

| Table 6-2. Accidents—Marks of Injury Other than Point of Lethal Impact | | |
|---|---|---|
| **Contusions** | | |
| *Face* | 1 on each of 2 children | <1% |
| **Abrasions** | | |
| *Scratch on nose* | 1 child | <1% |
| **Scars** | | |
| *Face* | 1 child | <1% |

Bruises on the face, scalp, or neck of a child are significant lesions that should be noted on physical examination. Fewer than 1% of children who die of accidental causes have bruises unrelated to the lethal injury (**Tables 6-1 and 6-2 and Figures 6-1 and 6-2**). In contrast, 65% of children with lethal inflicted injuries have bruises in areas other than those involved in the fatal injury (**Table 6-3**). When bruises appear on physical examination, the parent or caregiver should be questioned regarding their cause. If the explanation does not adequately account for the bruises, abuse should be suspected. The presence of more than one unexplained bruise on a child's head correlates highly with abuse.

The absence of an external lesion on a child's head does not preclude massive internal injury. A child's scalp is extremely elastic, so even massive impacts may leave no external marks. Clinicians can inspect only the external scalp; when the child dies, a pathologist can evaluate sites of hemorrhage into the subgaleal scalp tissues, noting points of impact (**Figure 6-3a,b**). Microscopic sections from these sites can be evaluated to establish the age of the injury; it is especially important to establish the age if gross differences in age between various sites are noted.

It should be noted that on rare occasions the child's head may be massively impacted (e.g., due to direct impact on, swinging, or throwing the child), yet no

**Figure 6-1.** *Bruises to head and face of abused victim.*

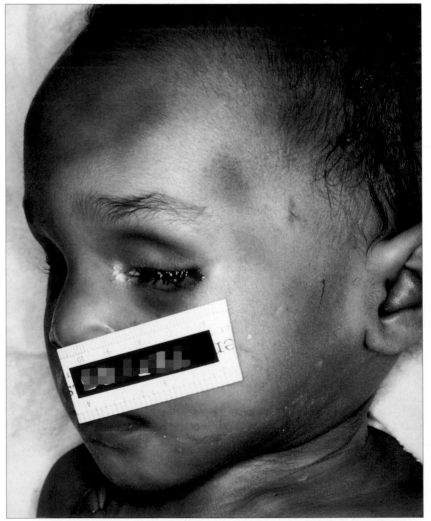

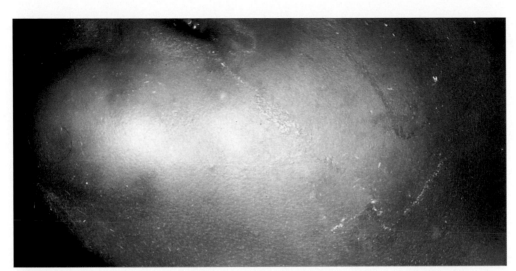

**Figure 6-2.** *Bruises to face of abused victim seen in Figure 6-1.*

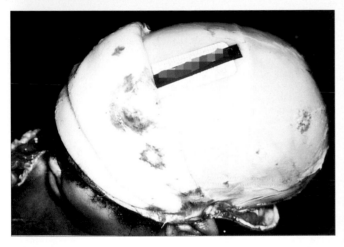

**Figure 6-3a.** *Multiple areas of subgaleal hemorrhage visible on inner surface of scalp. These were not evident externally on the scalp.*

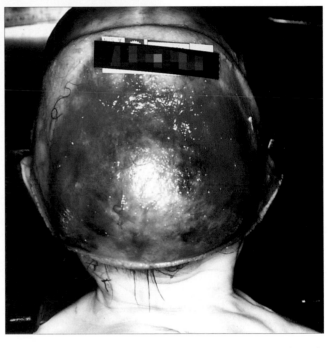

**Figure 6-3b.** *Large area of subgaleal hemorrhage on inner surface of scalp in which can be discerned multiple overlapping impact sites. No external bruise was evident on the scalp.*

impact site is discernible on the inner surface of the scalp. When this occurs, the impacting surface is usually broad based. When the scalp and brain show extensive damage, however, further evidence is unnecessary.

## ◆ IMPACT INJURIES

Impact injuries result from a blow to the head by a hand, fist, foot, or other object or by throwing or swinging the child so that the head impacts with a surface. Impacts can be single or multiple and can cause skull fractures, epidural hemorrhage, subdural hemorrhage, and contusions.

### SKULL FRACTURES

Approximately 50% of children with fatal abusive head injuries sustain skull fractures (O'Neill et al., 1973). Accidental injuries in children that produce skull fractures can be divided into two categories: significant event injuries and trivial falls.

1. Children may be injured as passengers or pedestrians in motor vehicle accidents, falls from second-story or higher windows, or in disasters such as structural collapses due to tornadoes or earthquakes. These injuries produce skull fractures comparable to what is seen in abusive injury, but the well-documented accidental nature of the event shows that it is not abuse.

2. Falls occur frequently in and around the home. Such falls are commonly from beds, cribs, tables, or couches. Minor falls should not produce major injury, and the physician must be certain that the degree of damage correlates with the reported fall. Studies reveal that fewer than 1% of children involved in these trivial home falls sustain a skull fracture. Fractures that do occur are small, linear, and usually parietal; they generally cause no loss of or decrease in consciousness, seizures, or intracranial injury.

| Table 6-3. Homicide—Marks of Injury | | |
|---|---|---|
| **Contusions** | | |
| *Face (26 children)* | | 37% |
| 2 to 5 contusions | 13 children | |
| 6 to 30 contusions | 6 children | |
| *Neck* | 4 children | |
| *Scalp (35 children)* | | 50% |
| 2 to 5 contusions | 19 children | |
| 6 to 21 contusions | 6 children | |
| **Abrasions** | | |
| *Face (26 children)* | | 37% |
| 2 to 5 abrasions | 8 children | |
| Broom marks (metal wires) on child, multiple sites | 1 child | |
| Comb | 1 child | |
| Hair brush | 1 child | |
| Zipper | 1 child | |
| *Neck (5 children)* | | |
| *Scalp (7 children)* | | |
| 2 to 5 abrasions | 4 children | |
| **Scars** | | |
| *Face (13 children)* | | 19% |

An exception to the benign nature of a minor home fall occurs when a toddler sitting or standing in a walker or heavy toy falls together with the object down a flight of stairs. The added weight of the walker or heavy toy increases the potential for serious or fatal head injury. This type of fall is rare and usually can be verified by the damage done to the walker or toy and often to the stairs.

Two recent studies reviewed skull fracture characteristics to distinguish between accidental and abusive origins (Hobbs, 1984; Meservy et al., 1987). Hobbs concluded that it was possible to predict an inflicted injury if one or more of the following were present when a minor fall was alleged:

1. Depressed fracture

2. Diastatic fracture (**Figure 6-4**)

3. Fracture width greater than 3 mm (**Figure 6-5**)

4. Complex configuration fractures

5. Multiple fractures

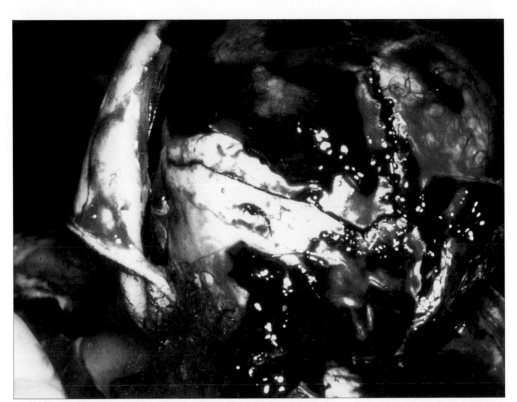

**Figure 6-4.** *Fractures of the left parietal calvaria associated with a very wide diastatic fracture of the sagittal suture.*

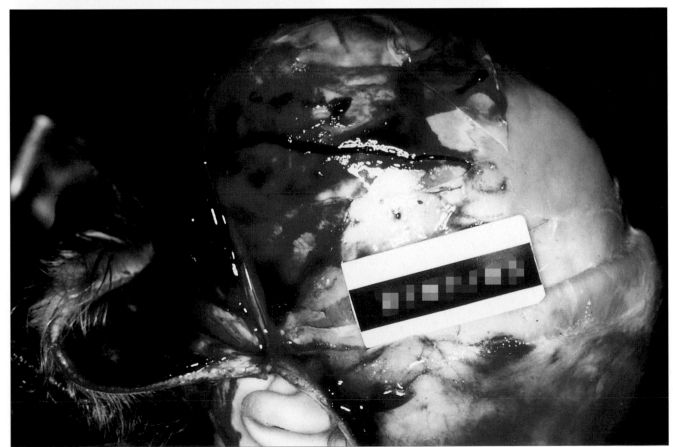

**Figure 6-5.** *Linear fracture 3 to 4 mm wide, above which is a craniectomy site for removal of subdural blood.*

**Figure 6-6.** A 9-month-old child's skull base with fractures on each side of the posterior fossa.

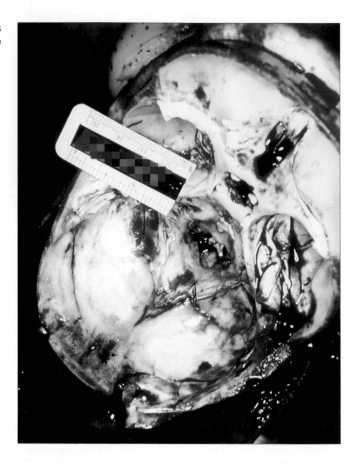

**Figure 6-7.** Skull base with very wide fracture, 5 to 6 mm, extending from the occipital bone into the posterior fossa.

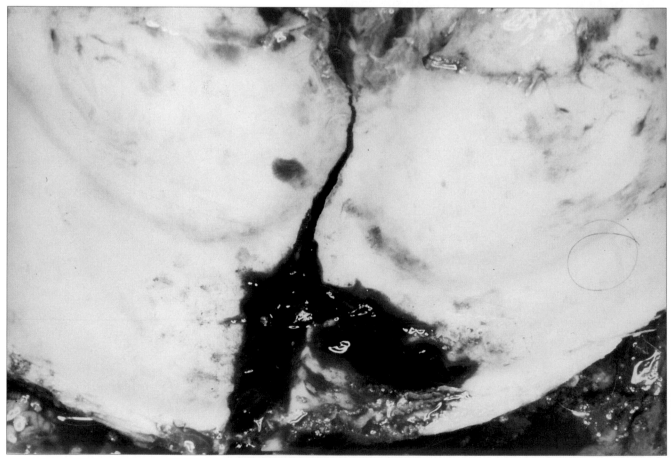

6. Bilateral fractures (**Figure 6-6**)

7. Nonparietal fractures (**Figure 6-7**)

8. Associated intracranial injury

Meservy's study concurred with Hobbs' in finding a much higher correlation of multiple fractures, bilateral fractures, and diastatic fractures with abusive injuries than with those caused accidentally.

## EPIDURAL HEMORRHAGE

Epidural hemorrhage is less common in children than in adults. Whereas epidural hemorrhage in the adult is usually associated with a fracture that lacerates vessels on the inner table of the skull, in children it may occur when the pliable and poorly ossified skull is deformed in a way that pulls the dura away from the inner table of bone. Vessels may be torn without an associated fracture, with bleeding into the epidural space. Significant force is required to produce such deformation of the skull. Unless a significant accidental event, such as a motor vehicle collision, is reported, epidural hemorrhage in the child is highly suggestive of abuse (Leestma, 1988).

## SUBDURAL HEMORRHAGE

Ninety percent of children with fatal inflicted head trauma have subdural hemorrhage. Only 20% of children who sustain massive accidental trauma have subdural hemorrhage; 60% of these have massive crushing injuries with skull fractures and brain lacerations (**Table 6-4**). Therefore in the absence of a major accidental event, subdural hemorrhage in a child is highly indicative of abusive injury. Of those children who sustain massive abusive impacts to the head, the most common intracranial injury is subdural hemorrhage, which is accompanied by skull fracture in 50% of cases (**Figure 6-8**).

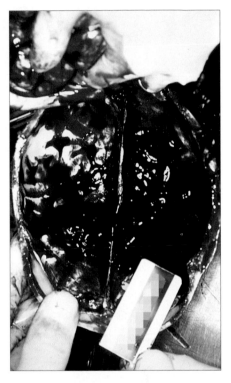

*Figure 6-8. Photograph of the calvaria removed and reflected backward into which a large volume of fresh subdural blood has run off the cerebral convexities to be collected in the skull cap.*

| Table 6-4. Fatally Head-Injured Children | | |
| --- | --- | --- |
| **Homicide (70 cases)** | | |
| *Head injury* | | |
| Subdural with fracture | 11 (39%) | 93% |
| Subdural without fracture | 15 (54%) | |
| Brain contusions (fracture) | 7 | |
| Contusion-tears | 2 | |
| Shaking injury | 5 | |
| **Accident (63 cases)** | | |
| *Head injury (10 cases or 16%)* | | |
| Subdural with fracture | 2 | 20% |
| Subdural without fracture | 0 | |
| Cervical spine trauma | 2 | |
| Penetrating wound | 1 | |
| Massive crushing fractures and brain lacerations | 6 (60%) | |

*NOTE: Some children had more than one type of injury.*

## CONTUSIONS

The adult patterns of coup and contrecoup contusions are not commonly seen in children younger than 3 or 4 years. The incomplete myelination of the brain,

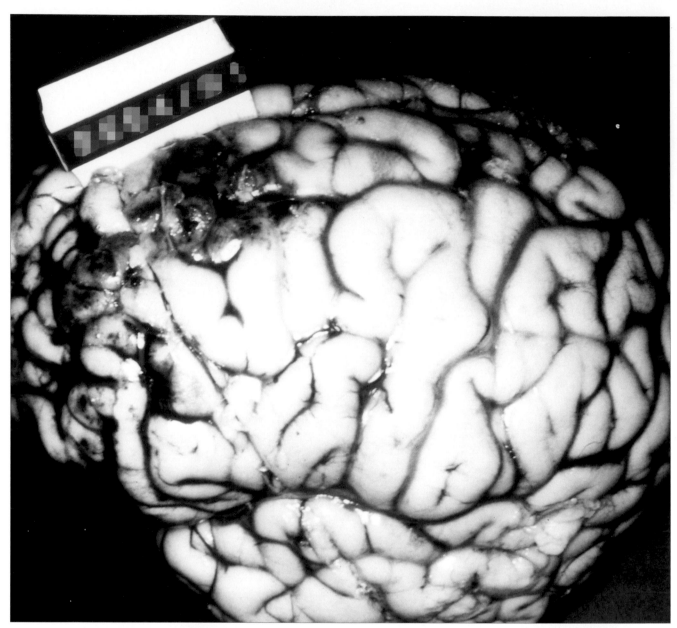

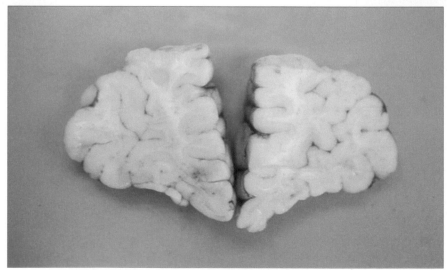

**Figure 6-9.** *An 18-month-old child who was struck on the head with a heavy ceramic figure, producing frontoparietal fracture with an underlying fracture contusion.*

**Figure 6-10.** *Coronal section of brain of 7-month-old infant with contusion tears of left orbital gyrus within the subcortical white matter. The lesion grossly appears as a cluster of small hemorrhages at the interface between cortex and white matter.*

94

pliable skull, and very shallow cranial fossae typical of children under 3 years of age account for this paucity of cortical contusions (Merten & Osborne, 1983). When contusions are seen in children as young as 1 1/2 to 2 years old, they are usually associated with overlying fractures and should be considered fracture contusions rather than coup contusions (**Figure 6-9**).

Lindenberg described lesions referred to as contusion tears that usually occur in infants 5 months of age or younger but can be seen up to age 12 months (Lindenberg & Freytag, 1969). These tears result from an impact that deforms the flexible skull and separates the cortex and subcortical white matter or produces a separation within the cortical layer itself. Tears occur anywhere in the cerebral hemispheres, but most commonly in the frontal and temporal lobes. The tears are poorly delineated by hemorrhage and may be overlooked in a poorly fixed brain (**Figure 6-10**). Since these lesions result from forceful deformation of the head, unless a massive accidental event is associated, their presence is highly suggestive of abusive force.

## ◆ SHAKEN INFANT SYNDROME

In 1972 Caffey described the practice now known as shaking an infant and the associated findings resulting from this behavior (Caffey, 1972). Although this syndrome is described in Chapters 1 and 25, those aspects related to head injury will be reviewed here.

A child's head and brain differ from those of an adult. First, the child's head represents about 10% of the total body weight compared to about 2% for an adult head (Calder et al., 1984). Also, a child's incompletely myelinated brain is softer in consistency and the thin axonal processes are more vulnerable to shearing forces than the better protected, larger adult brain. The neck muscles of a child are relatively weak and cannot adequately protect against forced whiplash movements of the head. Therefore the top-heavy head can be violently shaken in a whiplash fashion, and there is little protection from the neck musculature to resist such movements. Because the skull is not fully ossified, vigorous whiplash movements of the head can cause the head to actually elongate by molding it with the forces of acceleration-deceleration during shaking.

Shaking can occur in several ways. The child is grasped by the trunk or arms and violently shaken back and forth, causing the head to move forward until the chin strikes the chest and then to move backward until the occiput strikes the upper back. The child can also be shaken by grasping the ankles or legs and either shaking or swinging him in a circular motion.

Children at greatest risk for injury from shaking are under 4 years old. Fatal injuries have been observed in children up to 4 years old, but most of these occur in children 2 years or younger.

The pathophysiological consequences of shaking primarily consist of diffuse axonal injury produced by the acceleration of the head as it moves rapidly forward and backward (Vowles et al., 1986). As the brain is elongated in a sagittal plane, axonal processes, particularly those that run perpendicular to the sagittal plane, are stretched and can eventually tear. Small blood vessels are also stretched and torn. The structures most affected are the corpus callosum, fornix, corona radiata, and rostrolateral quadrants of the brainstem. The lesions that result from these injuries appear grossly as hemorrhagic foci; microscopically, axonal retraction bulbs or spheroids can be seen (**Figure 6-11**). Silver stains demonstrate varicosities in axonal processes that are damaged but not torn completely, allowing axoplasm to escape and form retraction bulbs. Changes can be observed immediately by electron microscopy or within 12 hours of injury by light microscopy. After several weeks, microglial clusters are seen in these areas. With long-term survival there is loss of white matter by wallerian degeneration of the long tracts.

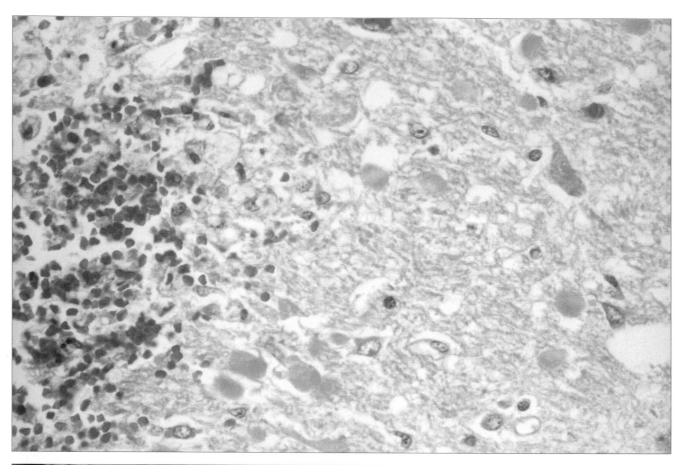

**Figure 6-11.** *Photomicrograph of a section of the superior cerebellar peduncle with numerous retraction bulbs or spheroids. (Hematoxylin & eosin stain, x200.)*

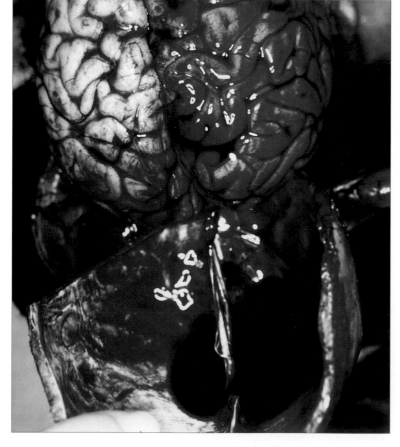

**Figure 6-12.** *This photograph demonstrates the few milliliters of subdural blood from over the cerebral convexities collected in the reflected calvarium in a fatally shaken infant.*

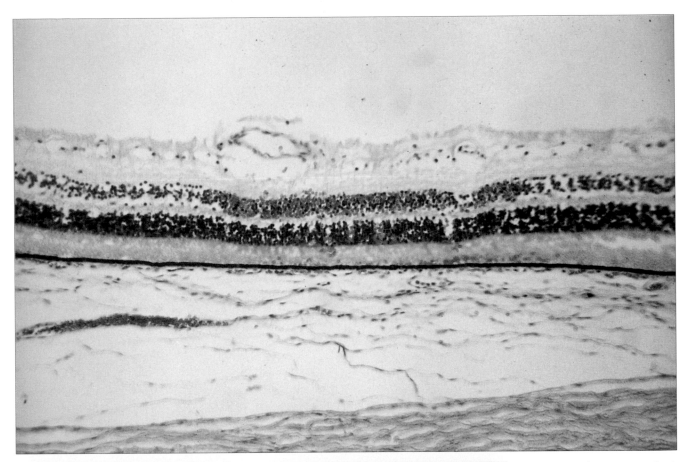

**Figure 6-13.** Photomicrograph of the retina with hemorrhage from a fatally shaken infant. (Hematoxylin & eosin stain, x100.)

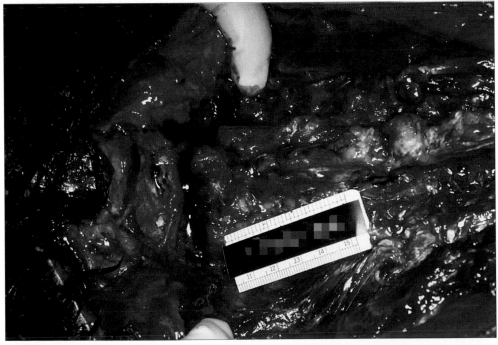

**Figure 6-14.** Photograph of a posterior neck dissection demonstrating fracture dislocation of C1-2 in a shaken infant.

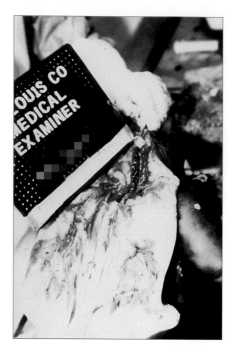

**Figure 6-15.** *Photograph of a posterior neck dissection in a fatally shaken infant (same child as Figure 6-10) illustrating epidural hemorrhage over the upper cervical cord.*

Another finding in shaking is subdural hemorrhage resulting from tearing of the bridging veins between the cortex and dura (**Figure 6-12**). Hemorrhage can be unilateral or bilateral and varies from only a few milliliters to larger amounts. Subdural hemorrhage does not cause the brain injury as a space-occupying mass might, but indicates that there has been brain acceleration. Experimental studies demonstrate that acceleration without impact can produce subdural hemorrhage (Adams et al., 1985).

Retinal hemorrhages are also found in about 80% to 85% of shaken infants. Hemorrhages occur commonly in the retina but also in the uvea or vitreous. In nonfatal suspected abuse cases the eyes should be examined by an experienced ophthalmologist (Greenwald et al., 1986). In fatal cases the eyes are removed at autopsy to document these hemorrhages (**Figure 6-13**).

The whiplash action of the head can also damage the upper cervical spinal cord. On rare occasions, fracture of a cervical vertebra occurs (**Figure 6-14**). At autopsy a posterior neck dissection is done to reveal epidural or subdural hemorrhage of the upper cervical cord (**Figure 6-15**). A recent report demonstrated upper cervical cord contusion from shaking (Hadley et al., 1989).

The act of shaking a child can also result in bruises on the arms or trunk from fingers grasping the child. In addition, there can be avulsion of metaphyseal periosteum in the arms.

## ♦ Level of Consciousness

Another area in which the child differs from the adult is the rapid development of neurological impairment with severe or fatal head injury. Severely head-injured children very rapidly become unconscious or exhibit a marked decrease in level of consciousness, quickly progressing to unconsciousness. This sequence identifies when the injury occurred, since the caretaker should immediately become aware of such a drastic change in the child. It also provides a clue as to whom the perpetrator could be, narrowing the focus to those persons present when the injury and change occurred. In the study of fatally head-injured children shown in Table 6-3, none was conscious on arrival at the hospital and many were already dead.

In children who are shaken to a less than fatal degree, the history frequently includes description of a seizure following the shaking episode. Many children who are neurologically impaired from infancy and were thought to represent prenatal or perinatal hypoxic damage actually suffered repeated shaking to a less than lethal degree but sufficiently to result in the loss of extensive axonal connections, leading to permanent brain damage (Benstead, 1983; Frank et al., 1985).

### Mechanisms and Pathophysiology of the Young Child's Head Injury

Injuries to the young child's brain are unique in that the trauma occurs to an organ that is in the process of maturing; the mechanisms and the types of injury differ from those which affect the older child or adult (Gjerris, 1986; Graham, 1989). At birth, the brain is enclosed in a pliable skull which allows the head to easily pass through the birth canal as well as to accommodate the rapidly developing brain. The skull is pliable because of the unfused sutures, the open fontanelles, and a thin unilaminar skull. The young brain grows rapidly, reaching 75% of its weight by age 2 years and almost adult weight by 5 or 6 years (Friede, 1975). The brain of the young child is very soft because the myelination of the cerebral hemispheres is just beginning at birth and then rapidly progresses during the next 2 years (Norton, 1972). Also contributing to the softness of the brain is the much greater water content of the young brain, 87% for cortex and 89% for white matter at birth compared to 83% and 69%, respectively, in the second decade (Katzman, 1973).

The skull at birth is disproportionately large compared to the rest of the skeleton and the largeness is due primarily to the calvarium; the face of the child is small and in proportion to other parts of the skeleton (Warwick, 1973). At birth, the weight of the child's head is about 15% of its body weight, compared to only 2% to 3% in adult life; it is a large heavy head (Friede, 1975). The bone of the infant calvarium is thin and the double layer of the diploe does not develop until the fourth year (Warwick, 1973). The base of the skull of the infant is relatively flat and shallow and lacks the development yet to come of the orbital roof shelf, sphenoid bone, and middle cranial fossae (Mann, 1986). These distinct bony compartments in later life help to prevent easy rotational movement of the brain within the cranial cavity. In the infant, the brain is freer to rotate within the relatively smooth skull base. The last factor of importance is the weak undeveloped neck muscles of the child, which allows the head to move without much resistance on shaking or impact.

Children under age 2 years are particularly vulnerable to shearing injury of the brain (Zimmerman et al., 1978; Zimmerman, 1987; Kriel et al., 1989). Impact to the immature brain is more likely to produce shearing injury rather than the contusions seen in older children and adults (Vowles, 1986). First, the incomplete degree of myelination and small axonal size predispose to shearing brain injury. Second, impact force is readily transferred through the thin pliant skull and across the shallow subarachnoid space of a young child's head to produce shearing brain injury. Third, the large heavy head and weak neck of a young child account for an unstable head that produces greater movement of the head and brain when acted on by acceleration-deceleration forces. Finally, the shallow skull base allows the young child's brain to turn readily in response to head acceleration or deceleration.

The mechanical forces important in head injury are translational and rotational forces (Merten, 1983). Translational forces are generated by a direct blow or impact to the head, which may produce focal injury to the skull, but the only effect on the brain is to produce linear movement, a type of brain movement that is quite benign. The trivial falls that children sustain in the home generate translational forces and, although they occasionally result in a skull fracture, generally these falls tend to be very benign.

Rotational forces are generated by either impact or nonimpact injuries that produce a sudden acceleration or deceleration of the head (Sahuquillo-Barris, 1988). Whiplash shaking is one nonimpact mechanism that produces an acceleration and deceleration of the head (Guthkelch, 1971; Caffey, 1972, 1974). Rotational injuries result in rotational movement of the brain within the cranial cavity; they cause the brain to turn abruptly on its axis or attachment at the brainstem-cerebrum junction. Extensive clinical and experimental data demonstrate that such rotational movement of the brain results in a type of injury referred to as shearing injury or diffuse axonal injury (Strich, 1956; Adams et al., 1980, 1982). As the brain turns or rotates within the cranial cavity, different portions of the brain differentially rotate so that tears occur as some parts rotate further or more rapidly than other parts (Holbourn, 1945; Ommaya, 1974). In young children, both impact and shaking result in the same brain injury—diffuse axonal injury or shearing injury—as both mechanisms cause rotation of the brain (Merten et al., 1984; Vowles et al., 1986; Hanigan et al., 1987; Duhaime, 1987, 1992; Hahn, 1988).

There is some experimental evidence that shaking alone may not be forceful enough to develop the angular acceleration necessary to sustain shear injury (Duhaime et al., 1992). The perpetrator of a child's injury may admit to only shaking, but often there is also a final throwing of the child against another surface or onto a couch or bed. Such impacts may not be reflected on the scalp if the surface is padded or even if it is firm because a child's scalp is elastic and stretches on impact. It may not be helpful to try to distinguish a child's head injury as resulting from either impact or shaking because the pathology is identical in both. If there are focal injuries such as skull fractures or scalp bruises, certainly impact can be assumed. In the absence of such impacts, however, shaking only should not be presumed.

The pathology of young children's head injuries of rotation or acceleration-deceleration type consists of the lesions or *markers* of shearing injury: subarachnoid hemorrhage, subdural hemorrhage, and retinal hemorrhages. The subarachnoid hemorrhage occurs in patches especially over the parasagittal regions and possibly elsewhere over the cerebrum; it is present in 100%, although the amount may be small. Subdural hemorrhage results from tearing of the bridging veins that run from the brain surface to the dura and that shear off as the brain rotates within the cranial cavity (Barris, 1988). The same shearing forces that tear the bridging veins also disrupt adjacent leptomeningeal vessels and cause the subarachnoid hemorrhage. Subdural hemorrhage is also probably present in 100% of cases but is readily evident in about 90% to 95% at autopsy (**Table 6-2**). By CT scan, small amounts of interhemispheric subdural blood can be detected, which may be missed at autopsy (Zimmerman et al., 1979; Merten et al., 1984). At autopsy, the amount of subdural hemorrhage observed may be only 2 to 3 ml of blood and will be hard to see if the prosector does not remove the calvarium himself or herself. The amount of subdural hemorrhage may vary up to 100 ml or even more but usually is much less and is important as a marker of shearing injury rather than as a mass lesion. Retinal hemorrhages are found in 70% to 85% of the cases of shearing brain injuries. Their mechanism is not precisely understood, but their presence correlates highly with a shearing injury.

While the subarachnoid hemorrhage, subdural hemorrhage, and retinal hemorrhages are markers of the shearing injury, the underlying pathology is that of diffuse axonal injury. The pathology of diffuse axonal injury consists of tears of axonal processes and small blood vessels and actual tissue tears in certain areas of the brain (Adams, 1980; Adams, 1989). These injured areas are the corpus callosum, periventricular areas, and dorsal lateral quadrants of the rostral brainstem. The axonal tears are microscopic lesions and are visible by light microscopy 18 to 24 hours after injury as retraction balls. Retraction balls are accumulations of axoplasm that appear as a pink bulb or swelling where axons have been severed. These are very difficult to see in young children because of the small size of the axonal processes. The blood vessel tears are seen grossly as linear or punctate hemorrhages. The tissue tears are visible grossly and usually are found in children under the age of 1 year as the lesion Lindenberg described as a contusion tear. These are tiny tears that occur at the cortex–white matter junction or within the layers of the cortex and reflect the rotational movement of the brain as some parts slip away from other parts as the brain rotates (Lindenberg, 1969; Vowles, 1986).

One of the implications of the diffuse brain injury in these young children is that these injuries become symptomatic immediately if there is a significant neurological outcome or death (Ommaya, 1974; Bruce, 1979; Gennarelli, 1982; Levin, 1988; Rosenthal, 1989). A significant neurological outcome refers to a moderate or severe degree of head injury. Diffuse axonal injury of these degrees causes immediate disruption of many axonal processes in the deeper gray structures and mesencephalon, and such disruptions will cause immediate loss of consciousness. The symptoms are those of an immediate decrease in the level of consciousness accompanied by respiratory difficulty and frequently seizures.

Children who sustain repetitive episodes of mild injury of diffuse type gradually accumulate deficiencies and the exact timing of those injuries is not possible.

The distinction between nonaccidental and accidental head injuries in children is an area of concern for many. The injuries described above as shearing or diffuse injuries require such extremes of rotational force that they occur in accidental head injuries only in obvious incidents such as motor vehicle accidents. Most other serious or fatal accidental childhood head injuries are crushing head injuries or penetrating head injuries. The usual trivial home accidents result only in translational forces, which do not significantly injure brain tissue, although they may occasionally produce a simple skull fracture.

## ♦BIBLIOGRAPHY

Adams, JH, et al: Brain damage in fatal non-missile head injury, *J Clin Pathol* 33:1132-1145, 1980.

Adams, JH, Graham, DI, and Gennarelli, TA: Contemporary neuropathological considerations regarding brain damage in head injury. In D Becker and JT Povlishock: *Central Nervous System Trauma Status Report*, prepared for the National Institute of Neurological and Communicative Disorders and Stroke, NIH, Bethesda, MD, 1985, Chapter 4.

Adams, JH, et al: Diffuse axonal injury due to non-missile head injury in humans: An analysis of 45 cases, *Ann Neurol* 12:557-563, 1982.

Adams, JH, et al: Diffuse axonal injury in head injury: Definition, diagnosis and grading, *Histopathology* 15:49-59, 1989.

Benstead, JG: Shaking as a culpable cause of subdural hemorrhage in infants, *Med Sci Law* 23:242-244, 1983.

Bruce, DA: Scope of the problem: Early assessment and management. In Rosenthal M, Griffith ER, Bond M, and Miller JD (eds

): *Rehabilitation of the Adult and Child with Traumatic Brain Injury*, Philadelphia, FA Davis Company, 1990, pp 521-537.

Bruce, DA, et al: Pathophysiology, treatment and outcome following severe head injury in children. *Childs Brain* 5:174-191, 1979.

Caffey, J: Multiple fractures in the long bones of infants suffering from subdural hematoma, *AJR* 56:163-173, 1946.

Caffey, J: On the theory and practice of shaking infants, *Am J Dis Child* 24:161-169, 1972.

Caffey, J: The whiplash shaken infant syndrome: Manual shaking by the extremities with whiplash-induced intracranial and intraocular bleedings, linked with residual brain damage and mental retardation, *Pediatrics* 54:396-403, 1974.

Calder, IM, et al: Primary brain trauma in non-accidental injury, *J Clin Pathol* 37:1095-1100, 1984.

Choux, M, et al: Extradural hematomas in children: 104 cases, *Childs Brain* 1:337-3476, 1979.

Courville, CB: Contrecoup injuries of the brain in infancy, *Arch Surg* 90:157-165, 1965.

Duhaime, AC, et al: The shaken baby syndrome: A clinical, pathological and biochemical study, *J Neurosurg* 66:409-415, 1987.

Duhaime, AC, et al: Head injury in very young children: Mechanisms, injury types and ophthalmologic findings in 100 hospitalized patients younger than 2 years of age. *Pediatrics* 90:179-185, 1992.

Frank, Y, et al: Neurological manifestations in abused children who have been shaken, *Dev Med Child Neurol* 27:312-316, 1985.

Friede, R: *Developmental Neuropathology*, Springer-Verlag, New York, 1975.

Gennarelli, TA, et al: Diffuse axonal injury and traumatic coma in the primate, *Ann Neurol* 12:564-574, 1982.

Gjerris, F: Head injuries in children—special features, *Acta Neurochirurgica, Suppl* 36:155-158, 1986.

Graham, DI, et al: Fatal head injury in children, *J Clin Pathol* 42:18-22, 1989.

Greenwald, MJ, et al: Traumatic retinoschisis in battered babies, *Ophthalmology* 93:618-625, 1986.

Guthkelch, AN: Infantile subdural hematoma and its relationship to whiplash injury, *Br Med J* 2:430-431, 1971.

Hadley, MN, et al: The infant whiplash-shake injury syndrome: A clinical and pathological study, *Neurosurgery* 24:536-540, 1989.

Hahn, YS, et al: Head injuries in children under 36 months of age, *Child's Nerv Sys* 4:34-40, 1988.

Hanigan WC, et al: Tin ear syndrome: Rotational acceleration in pediatric head injuries. *Pediatrics* 80(5):618-620, 1987.

Hobbs, CJ: Skull fracture and the diagnosis of abuse, *Am J Dis Childhood* 59:246-252, 1984.

Holbourn, AHS: The mechanism of brain injuries, *Br Med J* 3:147-149, 1945.

Katzman, R, et al: *Brain Electrolytes and Fluid Metabolism*, Williams & Wilkins Co, Baltimore, 1973.

Kempe, CH, et al: The battered child syndrome, *JAMA* 181:17-24, 1962.

Kriel, RL, et al: Closed head injury: Comparison of children younger and older than 6 years, *Pediatr Neurol* 5:296-300, 1989.

Leestma, JE: Neuropathology of child abuse. In *Forensic Neuropathology*, Raven Press, New York, 1988.

Levin, HS, et al: Relationship of depth of brain lesions to consciousness and outcome after closed head trauma. *J Neurosurg* 69:861-866, 1988.

Lindenberg, R, and Freytag, E: Morphology of brain lesions from blunt trauma in early infancy, *Arch Pathol* 87:298-305, 1969.

Mann, KS, et al: Skull fractures in children: Their assessment in relation to developmental skull changes and acute intracranial hematomas, *Child's Nerv Syst* 2:258-261, 1986.

Merten, DF, and Osborne, DR: Craniocerebral trauma in the child abuse syndrome, *Pediatr Ann* 12:882-887, 1983.

Merten, DF, et al: Craniocerebral trauma in the child abuse syndrome: Radiological observations, *Pediatr Radiol* 14:272-274, 1984.

Meservy, CJ, et al: Radiographic characteristics of skull fractures resulting from child abuse, *AJR* 149:173-175, 1987.

Norton, WT: Formation, structure and biochemistry of myelin. In Siegel GJ et al., (eds): *Basic Neurochemistry*. Little, Brown & Co., Boston, 1972, pp 74-99.

Oliver, JE: Microcephaly following baby battering and shaking, *Br Med* J 2:262-264, 1975.

Ommaya, AK, and Gennarelli, TA: Cerebral concussion and traumatic unconsciousness. Correlation of experimental and clinical observation on blunt head injury. *Brain* 97:633-654, 1974.

O'Neill, JA, et al: Patterns of injury in the battered child syndrome, *J Trauma* 13:332-339, 1973.

Rosenthal, BW, and Bergman I: Intracranial injury after moderate head trauma in children, *J Pediatr* 115:346-350, 1989.

Sahuquillo-Barris, J, et al: Acute subdural hematoma and diffuse axonal injury after severe head trauma, J *Neurosurg* 68:894-900, 1988.

Strich, SJ: Diffuse degeneration of the cerebral white matter in severe dementia following head injury, *J Neurol Neurosurg Psychiatry* 19:163-185, 1956.

Vowles, D, et al: Diffuse axonal injury in early infancy, *J Clin Pathol* 108:185-189, 1986.

Warwick R, and William P (eds): In *Gray's anatomy,* ed 35, WB Saunders, Philadelphia, 1973, pp. 310-312.

Zimmerman, RA, et al: Computed tomography in pediatric head trauma, *J Neuroradiol* 8:257-271, 1981.

Zimmerman, RA, et al: Computed tomography of shearing injuries of the cerebral white matter, *Radiology* 127:393-396, 1978.

Zimmerman, RA, et al: Computed tomography of craniocerebral injury in the abused child, *Radiology* 130:687-690, 1979.

# Burns and Child Maltreatment

Anthony J. Scalzo, M.D., F.A.A.P., A.C.M.T.

When reviewing the literature on the subject of child maltreatment by burning or while providing direct care to a victim of this form of abuse, one is impressed with the notion that "to burn is to brand." Children who are abusively burned are marked or branded with the outward manifestation of parental violence, emotional imbalance, impulsivity, educational and cultural deprivation, and poverty. To intentionally burn a child implies a sustained anger or hostility and appears to be a controlled, premeditated, or even sadistic action (Fowler, 1979).

Others echo these sentiments and suggest that social intervention mechanisms be mobilized to address the multiple problems of the abusively burned child. In terms of severity among the varying forms of abuse, abusive burns should be handled as top priority. The severity of subsequent injuries in burned children suggests that the abusive pattern may be well-ingrained by the time of the burning episode.

The literature attests not only to the physical and emotional trauma but also to the psychological sequelae of abusive burning (Bernstein & Cahners, 1979; Leeder, 1979; Green, 1984; Libber & Stayton, 1984; McLoughlin & Crawford, 1985; Benians, 1988; Weimer et al., 1988; Hammond et al., 1989; Tarnowski et al., 1989; Renz & Sherman, 1992; McMahon et al., 1995). Many victims of house fires die, but victims of scalds often survive with permanent disfigurement, motion disabilities due to contractures, and psychological sequelae. Children who were victims of burns can exhibit aggressive behavior ranging from biting another child to attacking a sibling with an axe. Depression can be manifest by crying without reason, refusal to socialize, or overt attempts at suicide. Withdrawal and other behavioral problems are all aspects of posttreatment adjustment in severely burned children, which was described by a group from the Burn Unit, Cape Town, South Africa, that studied children up to 11 years after the burn event (deWet et al., 1979).

The stigma of the burn does not end when the child is removed from the home of the abusing parent or discharged from the hospital; it may persist for years.

## ◆ Incidence and Epidemiology

Children 1 to 5 years old comprise the peak age category when burns occur (Demling, 1985). In a study of 30 deliberately scalded children with buttock involvement, mean age was 22.5 months (Renz & Sherman, 1993). Furthermore, bath scalds in children under 5 years of age were the cause of 14.7 per 100,000 children admitted to the unit in a year (Yeoh et al., 1994). Statistics from the U.S. Consumer Products Safety Commission reveal that 37,000 children under 14 years of age were treated for hot liquid or food and tap water scalds in 1988; nearly half, 16,000 of these children, treated in emergency departments were under 5 years of age. Of the above children, 5,000 were scalded by hot tap water, most often in the

**Table 7-1. Location and Type of Pediatric Burns**

*Baltimore Regional Burn Center*

**Place of Accident**

| | |
|---|---|
| Home | 84.6% |
| Outside | 7.6% |
| Boat/Auto | 3.4% |
| Other | 4.0% |

**Type of Burn**

| | |
|---|---|
| Scald | 47.6% |
| Flame | 29.6% |
| Grease | 6.5% |
| Flash | 5.6% |
| Contact | 5.6% |
| Electrical | 3.9% |
| Chemical | 1.1% |

bathtub. A U.K. study of 68 children admitted to a specialized burn unit for bath related scald injuries revealed 4 (5.9%) were due to non-accidental immersion (Yeoh et al., 1994). Although flame injury usually results in a burn involving a larger surface area and therefore is more severe, it is not seen as frequently as scalds. In a study of 520 children treated at a major burn center, most burns were of the scald type (47.6%) and occurred in the home (84.6%) (Spear & Munster, 1987) (**Table 7-1**).

The National Safe Kids Coalition estimates that burns are the third most common form of childhood accidental death in the United States. In *Accident Facts* (National Safety Council, 1979), burns were noted to cause more than 1,300 childhood deaths per year in the United States and ranked behind only motor vehicle and drowning accidents. In 1985 the National Center for Health Statistics (NCHS) revealed that death due to fire and/or burns occurred in 1,461 children ranging in age from birth to 19 years. Other estimates note that 23,638 children were hospitalized and 440,000 were treated for burns, bringing the total cost to society from childhood burn deaths and injuries to approximately $3.5 billion (McLoughlin & McGuire, 1990). Approximately 100,000 children in the United States are hospitalized for the treatment of burn injuries, and several hundred thousand are seen and treated as outpatients (Otherson, 1983). The number of burns not brought to medical attention and those that go unreported as abuse are probably significant.

It is apparent from review of the literature that the victim of abusive burning is usually a young child, 3 to 4 years of age or younger. In one study of 142 inflicted burns (number of patients examined = 892), the average age of the intentionally burned child was 32 months (Hight et al., 1979). The peak age of victims was 13 to 24 months. In one review of burns at Emory University in Atlanta Georgia, up to 26% of pediatric burn admissions were the result of abuse (Renz & Sherman, 1992).

Various studies have also linked educationally or culturally deprived maternal background, single or divorced marital status, unemployment, physical abuse of mother (wife battery), and other maternal characteristics, such as isolation, suspiciousness, rigidity, dependence, and immaturity, to increased incidence of abusive burning of children (Ayoub & Pfeifer, 1979; Hight et al., 1979; Joseph & Douglas, 1979; Rosenberg et al., 1982; Libber & Stayton, 1984; Rosenberg & Marino, 1989; Hunmel et al., 1993). In fact, a comparative study of children suspected of being scalded intentionally were statistically more likely to be from a broken home, belong to a single parent and have a younger mother than were those in a control group of nonabused scalded children (Hunmel et al, 1993).

Of all burns, 70% to 90% occur in the home (Feldman, 1980). It is believed that these burns may occur at peak times of stress in the parents' day. In a study of 464 burned children, the risk for burns was highest between 6 p.m. and midnight (Parish et al., 1986). Another study found that the peak hours are in the late afternoon and morning (Feldman, 1980).

Regardless of parental educational deprivation, scald burns occur more often in poorer socioeconomic housing or multi-unit buildings, where units close to the complexes' heating plant receive hotter water than those more distant from the heat source. With poor insulation and inefficient heat sources, the hot water heater's temperature may be increased to satisfy the demands in more distant units, meaning that those units close to the source can receive dangerously hot water. Often these dwellings lack other safety devices, such as smoke detectors, and the families lack the knowledge or resources to install such devices. In the way of prevention, strategies have been presented in such communities to avoid burning episodes (Haddon, 1980; Gallagher, 1982; Libber & Stayton, 1984; Micik & Miclette, 1985; Maley & Achauer, 1987; Murray, 1988; Katcher et al., 1989; Webne et al., 1989; McLoughlin & McGuire, 1990; National Safe Kids Campaign, 1990). Burn prevention issues are discussed later in this chapter.

## ◆TYPES OF BURNS AND PHYSICAL CONCEPTS

There are six categories of burn injuries: flame, scald, contact (with hot object), electrical, chemical, and ultraviolet radiation (sun) (McLoughlin & Crawford, 1985). Abusive burns are generally concentrated in the scald and contact categories, although rarer reports of flame (matches, cigarette lighters, or stove), chemical, microwave (actually placing an infant inside a microwave), or even hair dryer-inflicted burns have been reported (Ayoub & Pfeifer, 1979; Reece & Grodin, 1985; Alexander et al., 1987; Prescott, 1990). In reviewing hospital burn admissions, scalds are the most common type of thermal injury seen in children (Feldman et al., 1978). However, if all burn abuse cases are included in the studies, contact burns are more common (Keen et al., 1975; Johnson & Showers, 1985; Showers & Garrison, 1988).

Scald burns result from exposure to a hot liquid. Scalds were the predominant type of burn in both Lenoski and Hunter's (1977) series and Johnson and Showers' (1985) series. Others report that immersion scald burns are more frequently seen than splash, pour, or contact burns.

Scald burns can be superficial, partial, or full thickness; however, the presence of full-thickness, sharply demarcated or symmetrical burns on the buttocks, perineum, genitalia, and distal ends of limbs should alert the professional to the likelihood of child abuse.

Since scalds are the most common cause of burn morbidity, attention must be given to some specific details as to why scalds occur (Caniano et al., 1986). More scald burns occur in the bathroom than in the kitchen (Showers & Garrison, 1988); therefore hot water temperature in the bathtub, as a physical characteristic, is important. Time of thermal contact and repeated exposure are also important factors in many of these burns. At 49°C (120°F), the lowest setting on most gas water heater thermostats, it takes 5 to 10 minutes to cause full-thickness transepidermal injury to adult skin. However, at 51°C (124°F) it takes 4 minutes. At 52°C (125°F) it takes 2 minutes, and at 54°C (130°F) it takes only 30 seconds to result in a scald. Water at 60°C (140°F), an average temperature for most households, will take 5 seconds to produce a scald burn (Moritz & Henriques, 1947). It is interesting to note that 140°F is generally the recommended intake temperature for many home dishwashers, although some commercial dishwashing detergents will dissolve and sanitize at 130°F. At 70°C (158°F), which is found in some homes, a transepidermal burn will occur in less than 1 second (Robinson & Seward, 1987). Temperature versus time-to-scalding data are given in **Table 7-2 and Figure 7-1**.

| Table 7-2. Temperature Versus Time Burn Chart | | |
|---|---|---|
| Temperature °C | °F | Time to Produce Scald Burn in Adult (less time in children) |
| 49° | 120° | 5-10 minutes |
| 52° | 125° | 2 minutes |
| 54° | 130° | 30 seconds |
| 57° | 135° | 10 seconds |
| 60° | 140° | 5 seconds |
| 63° | 145° | 3 seconds |
| 66° | 150° | 1-5 seconds |
| 68° | 155° | 1 second or less |
| 70° | 158° | < 1 second |

*Adapted from Scald Burn Prevention Strategy Manual, Washington, D.C., 1990.*

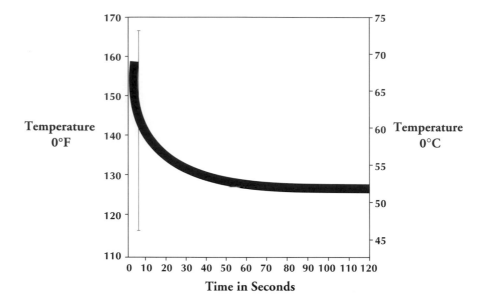

It is helpful to remember that children's skin is thinner than adult's skin, so serious burning occurs more rapidly and at lower temperatures. Furthermore, hot water exposures of subthreshold time and temperature will result in significant burns if the contact is repeated with little time between exposures. Water at 49°C applied to skin for 3 minutes can be tolerated, but an application of 9 minutes' duration can result in a full-thickness burn (Moritz & Henriques, 1947).

## ♦ DIAGNOSING THE ABUSIVE BURN

The differentiation of inflicted versus accidental injury must begin with definitions. These definitions have both medical and legal implications. The requirement that physicians report abuse, which is law in all 50 states, depends on the physician's ability to recognize abuse and on having a reasonable definition of abuse.

> *The definition of physical abuse offered here does not exclude reasonable corporal punishment by parents. Physical abuse is: An injury to a child caused by a caretaker, for any reason, including injury resulting from a caretaker's reaction to an unwanted behavior. Injury includes tissue damage beyond erythema or redness from a slap to any area other than the hand or buttocks. Physical discipline should not be used on children who are under 12 months of age. The child should be normal developmentally, emotionally, and physically. Tissue damage includes bruises, burns, tears, punctures, fractures, ruptures of organs and disruption of functions. The use of an instrument on any part of the body is abuse. The injury may be caused by impact, penetration, heat, a caustic, a chemical or a drug (Johnson, 1990).*

This definition leaves no confusion defining any physical abuse situation, including burns. An instrument is defined to include devices, gadgets, and implements and mediums of delivery.

All suspicious cases of abuse by burning must be thoroughly investigated. Suspicious burns in a child with prior history of abuse or other physical stigmata of abuse places that child at high risk for lethal abuse.

### INCIDENCE OF ABUSIVE BURNS

The incidence of abusive burns ranges from 4% (Stone et al., 1970) of hospitalized childhood burns to 10% in a more recent study (Showers & Garrison, 1988) or to 28% in specific burn injuries such as tap water scalds (Feldman et al., 1978). During a 12-month period, 84 of 431 burned children (19.5%) were suspected to be abused or neglected (Rosenberg & Marino, 1989). During a 6-year period, 142 of 872 cases of children admitted to a burn center at Children's Hospital of Michigan were found to be nonaccidental (Hight et al., 1979). However, in a study of all pediatric emergency department patients less than 1 year of age, the authors found no incidence of abuse or neglect (Rivara et al., 1988). (It should be noted that most studies reveal the peak age for abusive burning to be over 1 year of age.) Large nationwide studies of overall burns, without specific attention to type, yield 9% to 10% of cases resulting from abuse or neglect.

Comparing it to other forms of abuse, maltreatment by burning has ranked as high as 28% of all types of batterings (Feldman et al., 1978). In a 4-year study at Children's Hospital of Philadelphia, burns accounted for 13% of cases of physical abuse (Ludwig & Fleisher, 1983). More recently, of 256 patients hospitalized for child abuse at a major pediatric center, 56 suffered burns (22%), 53 central nervous system (CNS) injuries (22%), 66 failure-to-thrive (26%), and the remainder various other forms of abuse and neglect (Caniano et al., 1986).

Review of the literature over the last 10 to 15 years and clinical experience indicate that the victim of abusive burning is usually 3 to 4 years of age or younger. In Hight's study of 142 of 892 inflicted burns, the average age of the intentionally burned child was 32 months (Hight et al., 1979). The peak age group of victims was 13 to 24 months. Most studies reveal higher rates among male infants and children as compared to adults. One study showed a male:female ratio of 2.5:1 (Libber & Stayton, 1984), while others report a more even distribution (Hight et al., 1979; Showers & Garrison, 1988). The data shown in **Figure** 7-2 reveal that although males are more likely to be physically abused (60% compared to 49%), females account for more cases of overall abuse (368,600 compared to 252,500), largely due to the higher incidence of sexual abuse among females.

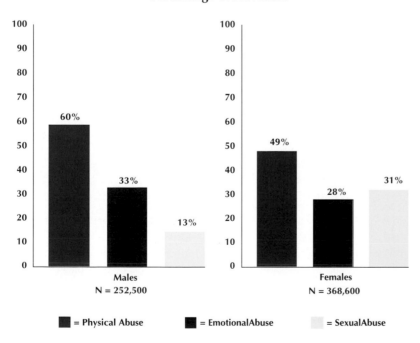

**Percentage of All Abuse**

*Figure 7-2*. Distribution of reported forms of abuse by child's sex. (Data from the U.S. Department of Health and Human Services Study of the National Incidence and Prevalence of Child Abuse and Neglect, 1988.)

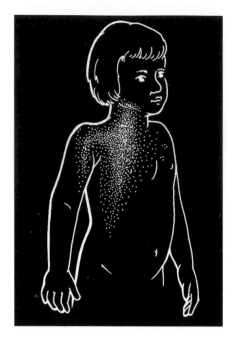

**Figure 7-3.** *Pattern of accidental burn with distribution on anterior trunk. Note that the cooling pattern as water descends results in an "arrow"-shaped configuration.*

## HISTORY AND COMPREHENSIVE EVALUATION

Care for the burn patient's primary medical needs is discussed in books and journals devoted to burn treatment. While these needs are vital, the focus of this book is on identifying abuse and integrating the findings into a plan of action.

Once the patient's medical needs are met, the practitioner directs efforts toward obtaining a careful history outlining the time, nature, extent, and location where the burn occurred. Photographs should be obtained early and a radiologic skeletal survey (humanogram) performed if abuse is suspected, lest the abusive party claim the injuries occurred in the health care facility.

The clinician should attempt to determine if the burn is abusive, accidental, or pseudoabusive (due to folk medicine practices) (Sandler & Haynes, 1978; Asnes & Wisotsky, 1981; Feldman, 1995), comparing the history with the physical evidence. First, the patient's developmental skills must be evaluated. Second, the physical aspects of the burn should be analyzed with respect to body anatomic location and compared to the reported cause of the burn. For example, scald burns on the anterior body with a pattern of cooling as it descends (**Figure 7-3**) are consistent with a child pulling a hot liquid from a vessel onto himself. However, a burn located behind the ear, not involving the submental area of the jaw and also avoiding the axilla and back of the shoulder, suggests a liquid thrown from behind (Lung et al., 1977). Scald burns on the buttocks usually occur from forced immersion in hot water, so a history of an accidental fall into the bathtub is suspect. Full-thickness scald burns with a stocking or glove pattern of sharp demarcation on a limb (**Figures 7-4 and 7-5**) or immersion lines with circular or ovoid patterns on the buttocks are not likely to be accidental.

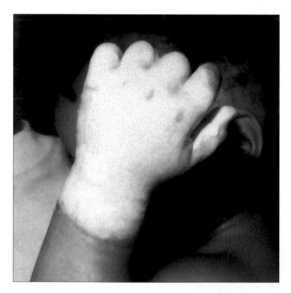

**Figure 7-4.** *Uniform scald of the hand in a 9-month-old girl. This "glove-like" distribution was caused by intentional immersion.*

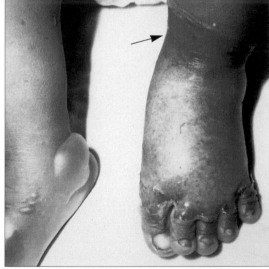

**Figure 7-5.** *"Stocking" type burn to the foot. Note the sharp demarcation of the immersion line.*

The professional must consider the physical injuries or findings in the context of the history offered. Reliance on a single source for the history or information regarding the injuries can limit the professional's ability to correctly differentiate accidental from suspicious or intentional burns. A cooperative effort between law enforcement, social services, and medical staff is needed. All involved should consider the plausibility of the parents' or guardian's description of how any given injury occurred. This includes scene investigation of serious burns, photographs of the child and the scene of the event, history obtained by several professionals (law enforcement, social workers, nurses, and medical personnel), physical examination, and diagnostic imaging.

In suspicious burns, it may be necessary to visit the scene of the burn or analyze photographs taken by police to ascertain if the burn could have occurred in the manner reported. A visit by trained social workers and detectives to the home or scene of the incident can reveal valuable data. This procedure should be requested by medical personnel before final conclusions regarding the etiology of the burn are made. Having the caretaker review the events while walking through the area and demonstrating with a doll the child's position, describing the depth of the water, and so on, helps medical personnel to determine whether the injury was accidental.

*An interdisciplinary approach was used in the following case:*

## CASE HISTORY

A 5-month-old female was admitted through the emergency department. She was in respiratory arrest and required immediate intubation. The mother stated that 2 days before coming to the hospital an adult was pouring hot water near the baby and accidentally spilled it on the child. She treated the burn with cocoa butter. It seemed to be improving. The child's father stated that while he was cleaning the burn with alcohol the baby stopped breathing and had no heart rate. He said that he performed CPR for 2 hours while waiting for the mother to return home so that she could call an ambulance.

## PHYSICAL AND LABORATORY FINDINGS

On examination the child was noted to have a deep partial thickness burn of the anterior chest (**Figure 7-6**) with smaller involvement of the chin and forearm. Further examination revealed a distended abdomen, retinal hemorrhages, and a stellate laceration to the vaginal posterior fourchette. Laboratory and radiologic investigation revealed elevated liver transaminases, fracture of the distal femoral metaphysis, fracture of the distal tibial metaphysis (classic "bucket-handle" type fracture), and healing fractures of the left sixth through ninth ribs. Computed tomography of the brain revealed a subarachnoid hemorrhage.

## EVALUATION

This history is not believable; it is obviously false. Furthermore, such a severe burn in a young infant normally causes a caretaker to seek medical attention immediately. Thinking beyond the emergency at hand and the history given, the emergency staff were able to define a constellation of physical injuries, as well as laboratory and diagnostic imaging findings that could only point to one cause—child abuse.

In another case, emergency department staff were given the history that a 23-month-old boy, while riding his tricycle, was caught between a space heater and a wall. The child sustained full thickness (third-degree) burns to his buttocks and partial thickness (second-degree) burns to his posterior legs. The family did not seek medical attention for 2 1/2 weeks. After the parents dropped the child off to leave on vacation, he was taken to the emergency department by his grandparents when they noted the injury while bathing him. Analysis of the information gathered at the scene as well as other points of the history led to the conclusion that the burn could not have occurred in the manner reported. The child was unable to ride a tricycle. The temperature of the space heater at the level of the burn would have required 20 minutes to develop a full-thickness burn; only the top of the heater had temperatures hot enough to cause a burn that severe. Using a doll, no position could explain the combination of the buttock and leg burns and their configuration. Investigation revealed that a better source for the burn was the kitchen stove. Measuring the size of the burn and noting its circular configuration, it could be deduced that the circular heating plate of the stove was most likely the

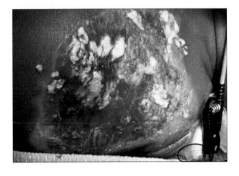

***Figure 7-6.*** *Deep burn of the anterior chest in a 5-month-old infant who was intubated secondary to respiratory arrest.*

source of the buttocks injury. Assuming that the child was intentionally placed on the stove, his calves would align with the hot front door of the stove. This coincided with the tape measurements of the stove and the patient's limb length. In addition, other facts supported abuse as the cause: the child was being toilet trained, the area was typical for disciplinary abuse, there was a long delay before seeking medical assistance, and only a third party, the grandparents, sought help (see Stone's criteria on the following page).

## PROTOCOLS AND CRITERIA FOR DETERMINING ABUSE

Many states have comprehensive protocols for determining the likelihood of child abuse. The report of the Task Force for the Study of Non-Accidental Injuries and Child Deaths convened by the Illinois Department of Children and Family Services, and the Office of the Medical Examiner, Cook County, gives specific details for professionals involved in child health care (Illinois Department of Children and Family Services, 1986). Descriptions should be as detailed and as precise as possible, such as "4x6 cm ovoid-shaped scald of the right posterior buttock with sharp demarcation of edges and uniform burn depth" as opposed to "moderate size burn on the bottom."

Burns themselves are often emotionally as well as physically devastating to the child. Therefore extreme care must be exercised to avoid contributing to the emotional trauma by *incorrectly* accusing a parent of abuse. To effectively develop and use criteria for diagnosing intentional burns, professionals should be familiar with the common manifestations of child abuse and neglect along with those of inflicted burns.

The instruments used to injure children are varied and depend, to some extent, on what is available. A belt, strap, or an adult's hand slapping, grabbing, choking, or pinching accounts for up to 45% of inflicted injuries (Johnson, 1990). Even hairdryers have been implicated in abusive burns of children (Sudekoff & Young, 1994). When hot objects or water is readily available, the abusive parent chooses these modes.

The full constellation of family psychosocial factors, child's developmental milestones, physical diagnosis, and associated laboratory or radiologic findings may be difficult to collate initially. Identification and reporting of possible cases of physical maltreatment in children by a variety of professionals are crucial antecedents to intervention with abusive families. Unfortunately, not all physically abused children are identified or reported to authorities (Warner & Hansen, 1994; Dublin & Reynolds, 1994). Several authors have developed guidelines for the clinician, social worker, or nurse to differentiate accidental from abusive or neglectful burns (Stone et al., 1970; Ayoub & Pfeifer, 1979; Rosenberg & Marino, 1989; Hammond et al., 1991).

*When a child comes for treatment of a burn and one or more of the following are found to be present, one should consider abuse:*

1. Multiple hematomas or scars in various stages of healing

2. Concurrent injuries or evidence of neglect such as malnutrition and failure to thrive (especially suspicious are bone injuries such as old rib fractures and distal tibial, metaphyseal, or spiral fractures)

3. History of multiple prior hospitalizations for "accidental" trauma

4. An inexplicable delay between time of injury and first attempt to obtain medical attention (In some cases, if the parent has medical training, such as an R.N. or M.D., the delay may be because the parents tried to initially care for the burn on their own.)

5.  Burns appearing older than alleged day of the accident, similarly indicating ambivalence about seeking care and possibly risking exposure of the abuse

6.  An account of the incident not compatible with age and ability of child (An example is that of an infant who "crawled into the hot bathtub" when the infant is only a few months old and developmentally incapable of doing so.)

7.  The responsible adults allege that there were no witnesses to the "accident" and the child was merely discovered to be burned, thus hoping to discourage any further inquiry

8.  Relatives other than the parents bring the injured child to the hospital or a nonrelated adult brings the child (unless there is good explanation for the parents' absence, such as when a child is being cared for by a baby sitter while the parents are out of town)

9.  The burn is attributed to action of a sibling or other child (though this is often a false explanation for abusive burns, it should be noted that siblings can indeed be abusive [Green, 1984])

10. The injured child is excessively withdrawn, submissive, or overly polite, or does not cry during painful procedures

11. There are scalds of the hands or feet, often symmetrical, appearing to be full thickness in depth, suggesting that the extremities were forcibly immersed and held in hot liquid

12. There are isolated burns of the buttocks or perineum and genitalia or the characteristic doughnut-shaped burn of the buttocks, which in children can hardly ever be produced by accidental means

13. The responsible adults give different stories as to the cause of the burn or change their story when questioned

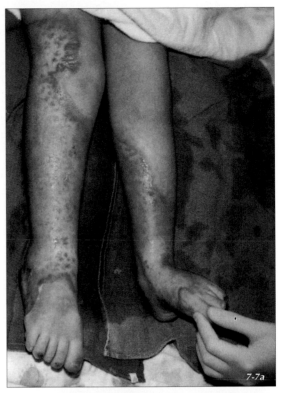

Stone and associates developed this set of criteria after reviewing 26 cases of burn abuse in Chicago (Stone et al., 1970). They noted that males were the victims in 20 of the 26 cases. A large percentage of burns were on the buttocks, perineum, and lower extremities (25 of the 26 cases). Hot liquids were the cause in 15 cases, hot metal surfaces in five, flame in four, and inflicted cigarette burns in one. In a more contemporary study of the predictive value of historical and physical characteristics of burns for the diagnosis of child abuse, the authors found that the presence of two or more of the 13 factors increased the yield in identification of child maltreatment to more than 60% (Hammond et al., 1991).

Since the palm of the hand and the sole of the foot are thick and relatively resistant to thermal damage, full-thickness burns seen here suggest prolonged immersion and hence inflicted injury (Hight et al., 1979). An exception might be handicapped children, in whom the anesthetic or hypoesthetic areas are thinner skinned and the child may burn unexpectedly and more easily (**Figure 7-7a,b**). However, handicapped children are at increased risk of abuse (Feldman et al., 1981). Sometimes burns or decubitus sores in handicapped children fall into the neglect or pseudoabusive category.

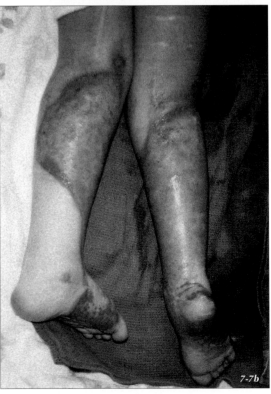

***Figure 7-7a,b.*** *Accidental burn to the legs of an 8 1/2-year-old handicapped child.*

## ♦ ACCIDENTAL BURNS AND CONDITIONS THAT ARE NOT ABUSE

When determining whether an injury is accidental or inflicted, unusual causes of burn injuries should be considered. Unsuspecting parents may expose their children to burn injuries unintentionally.

There were an estimated 656 cases of vaporizer-related injuries in 1979. Two cases of steam vaporizer burns with respiratory involvement have been reported (Colombo et al., 1981). Thermal injury to the lungs from flame or dry hot air is rare; usually the toxic gases from products of pyrolysis (i.e., smoke and other gases) cause inhalation injury. However, inhalation of steam can produce severe pulmonary injury (Moritz et al., 1945) as well as burns to the skin (Colombo et al., 1981).

Another unexpected accidental burn may occur secondary to deck floor tiling such as that used around outdoor pools. These tiles can become very hot after long exposure to the sun (Sheldon & Woodward, 1983).

Inside the home, children have been injured accidentally on hot registers (grating) for floor furnaces (Berger & Kalishman, 1983). In a study conducted on floor register temperatures, a group from New Mexico found that four of the five registers tested exceeded 250°F or 121°C (Berger & Kalishman, 1983). A burn can occur virtually instantaneously at temperatures of this degree. Wall registers may also be sources of accidental burns to children. It may be more likely that hot floor grate registers are sources for accidental rather than inflicted injury. **Tables 7-3 and 7-4** list the estimated sources of burn (U.S. Consumer Product Safety Commission, 1989).

| Table 7-3. Heating Units Related to Injury and/or Burns in Children 0 to 4 years of Age (1989)* | |
| --- | --- |
| **Type of Unit** | **Estimated Number of Children Treated in U.S. Hospital Emergency Departments** |
| Home radiators | 8,925 |
| Fireplaces (all types) | 7,174 |
| Kerosene or oil heaters | 4,151 |
| Heating systems, not specified | 3,948 |
| Coal or wood-burning stoves | 2,941 |
| Water heaters | 347 |

Other consumer safety and/or convenience items impact childhood burning. Infant automobile restraint systems are lifesaving and in no way should be discouraged. However, many adults — and health care workers — are not aware how hot the metal parts of the infant car seat can become when left exposed to direct sunlight in hot weather. A 12-week-old infant sustained a 3 cm partial thickness burn to the exposed portion of the anterior thigh from the hot metal turnbuckle adjustment of a car seat (Hankin & Vermeulen, 1980). This case, as well as others cited in the literature of car seat burns (Saitz, 1975; Schmitt et al., 1978), point to the need for advocates for child safety to be aware of unexpected dangers that can cause injuries which may be misdiagnosed as abuse.

The worker must also be aware of unique religious and cultural practices as well as unexpected injuries. Called "pseudoabusive" injuries, burns may be incurred within certain folk medicine customs. For example, in Vietnamese or Cambodian cultures the practice of rubbing a coin or alternatively applying a cup, spoon, or shot glass heated in oil to the skin of an ill child's neck, spine, back, or ribs is termed "coining" ("Cao Gio") or cupping, respectively (Sandler & Haynes, 1978; Asnes & Wisotsky, 1981; Johnson, 1990). These cultures believe that this folk medicine treatment will diminish pain, restore appetite, draw out the fever, and strengthen a weak stomach (Asnes & Wisotsky, 1981). Managing these situations involves education of the families.

| Table 7-4. Agents Related to Injury and/or Burns in Children 0 to 4 Years Age (1989)* | |
| --- | --- |
| **Burn Source** | **Estimated Number of Children Treated in U.S. Hospital Emergency Departments†** |
| Irons | 11,745 |
| Hair curlers and curling irons | 11,362 |
| Hot water | 10,495 |
| Cigarettes, pipes, cigars, or tobacco | 6,468 |
| Ranges not specified | 5,423 |
| Household products, caustics, drain cleaners, ammonia, oven cleaner | 3,155 |
| Gasoline and gasoline cans | 2,832 |
| Electrical wiring, outlets, receptacles, and extension cords | 2,814 |
| All other ovens | 2,690 |
| General home or room fires† | 1,592 |
| Light bulbs | 1,410 |
| Electric and gas ranges | 1,116 |
| Fireworks | 1,002 |
| Microwave ovens | 817 |
| Cigarette or pipe lighters | 713 |
| Hairdryers | 368 |
| Matches | 209 |

*Estimates based on U.S. Consumer Products Safety Commission: National Electronic Injury Surveillance System: Product Summary Report—1989, National Injury Information Clearinghouse, Washington, D.C., 1989.*

*†Does not include those who die at the scene and never arrive at emergency departments.*

Common infectious or occasional bullous dermatologic disorders should also be investigated. Most physicians should be familiar with the appearance and associated findings of common impetigo, but sometimes cigarette burns become infected and are difficult to differentiate from circular impetiginous lesions (Raimer et al., 1981). Cigarette burns are usually in clusters and in various stages of healing. Impetiginous lesions usually do not scar, whereas accidental cigarette burns do. Intentional cigarette burns are usually deeper and scar more extensively.

Staphylococcal scalded skin syndrome may be confused with abusive burning, especially since it often involves the inguinal and perigenital area. Scalded skin syndrome is usually generalized rather than localized as in an intentional scald. Also, identifying the staph organism and its response to antibiotics aids in differentiation.

Ischemic, hypoxic-induced injury from various causes can result in the formation of bullae. Innocent pressure injuries can be confused with inflicted dry contact burns (Feldman, 1995). Although epidermolysis bullosa and related disorders are rare in childhood, they may be present and the clinician should seek dermatologic consultation upon encountering unusual blistering or bullous lesions that lack the other associated features of burns.

Adolescents with preexisting psychiatric illness may come for treatment with burns that are self-inflicted, although suicide by this means is rare in Western cultures (Hammond et al., 1988).

## ♦ABUSIVE BURN PATTERNS

### SCALD AND IMMERSION BURNS

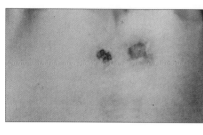

**Figure 7-8.** *Two circular burns of skin overlying pubic area in a young toddler. These were caused by inflicted injury from cigarettes.*

Although one study of 131 cases involving abusive forms of burn injury found that contact burns were more common than scald or immersion burns (56% versus 38%) (Showers & Garrison, 1988), the scald is generally considered the most common type of abusive burning (Keen et al., 1975; Johnson & Showers, 1985; Showers & Garrison, 1988). Inflicted scald burns are most frequently caused by hot tap water; a smaller percentage (6%) of the time the liquid is coffee, tea, or cooking grease (Feldman et al., 1978; Joseph & Douglas, 1979; Bradshaw et al., 1988).

Immersion burns to the buttocks or genitals are often inflicted by the perpetrator to punish the child for soiling or wetting his or her pants. This occurs in families where the caretakers are rigid in toilet training beliefs. Cigarette burns inflicted in the pubic area as well as blows to the penis with hair brush bristles have also been used to discipline a child during toilet training (**Figure 7-8**).

Depending on the depth of the water, whether in the bath or in the sink, burns may involve the back, buttocks, perineum, and genitalia or may spare these areas and involve "stocking" or "glove-like" burns of the extremities. Children held in a bathtub of shallow water may raise up on their hands and feet or "tripod" themselves in an attempt to protect their buttocks and perineum (Feldman, 1980). This may leave characteristic patterns of full-thickness burns to the distal parts of the extremities, especially if the water temperature exceeds 150°F

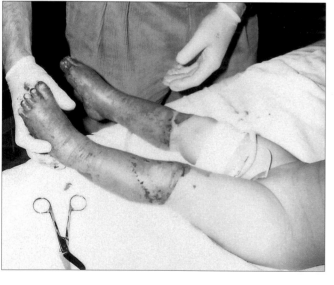

**Figure 7-9.** *A 32-month-old girl with uniform thickness burns to the lower extremities caused by immersion dipping. This child was burned because she soiled her pants.*

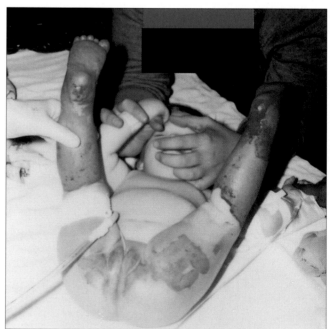

**Figure 7-10.** *Posterior aspect of the legs demonstrating a "stocking/like" distribution of the burn in the same child as Figure 7-9. Also note the burns to the genital area.*

(**Figures 7-9 and 7-10**). Sometimes the child is held by the head and legs and immersed back first into hot water. A scald as shown in **Figure 7-11** may occur.

Additionally, the child may be forced down against the vessel (tub or sink) and sustain an immersion line burn to the back, part of the buttocks and side, but with a spared area centrally on the buttocks. This so-called doughnut-shaped burn is seen infrequently (**Figures 7-12a,b and 7-13**).

Knowledge of distinctive patterns of burning lead the child protection team to correctly suspect abuse and pursue the correct history for the injury. Phaedrus in 8 A.D. said, "Things are not always what they seem." In the field of child abuse, "things may actually be what they seem" if one questions and obtains the true explanation.

## SPLASH BURN INJURIES

Splash burns occur when a hot liquid is thrown or poured onto a victim. The depth of burning is usually less than with the immersion type due to the cooling effect of the liquid as it spreads out or falls secondary to gravity. Splash burns often involve the back, the lateral side of the face, and the posterior shoulder (Lung et al., 1977). The anterior lower side of the face, neck, and shoulder, as well as the front of the chest and trunk, outline a common distribution following an accidental spill from a kettle or saucepan (Yiacoumettes & Roberts, 1977; Reece & Grodin, 1985; Coren, 1987; Rosenberg & Marino, 1989). As the hot liquid drips downward, it often burns in the shape of a "V" ("arrow sign"). This burn pattern occurs when the hot liquid initially contacts the skin and then spreads down the body, cooling as it goes. The edges cool faster than the central tract of hot fluid (**Figure 7-14a,b**). The direction of the "arrow" or combination of "arrow signs" seen with burns in more than one area can aid in making the diagnosis of child abuse. By studying the flow pattern of the hot liquid, clues can be gained that indicate the direction the liquid came from as well as the position of the patient (Feldman, 1980). If the history does not coincide with these physical characteristics, child abuse should be suspected.

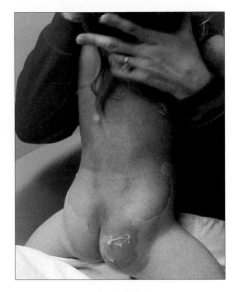

**Figure 7-11.** *Uniform thickness scald burn of the entire back on a 2 1/2-year-old girl who was immersed in hot water at 155°F as punishment for soiling her pants.*

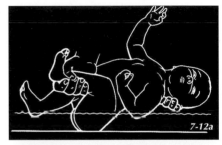

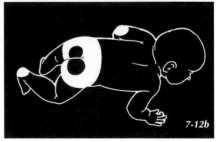

**Figure 7-12a,b.** *Drawing depicts mechanism by which a child is forcibly held against the bottom of a tub and is burned by hot water in the vessel but has a central area of sparing on the buttocks where skin is in contact with the cooler surface of the vessel.*

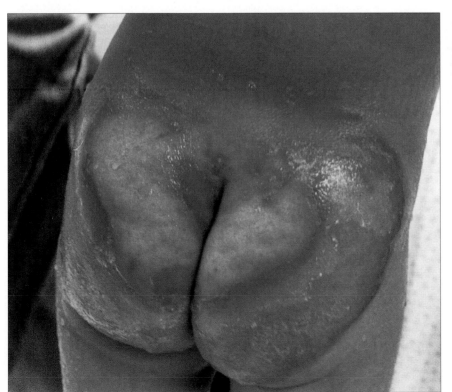

**Figure 7-13.** *Doughnut-shaped burn of the buttocks in 3 1/2-year-old girl. Note the central area of noninvolved skin. This occurred when the child was forcibly held against the relatively cooler bottom of a sink while hot water burned the area surrounding the center.*

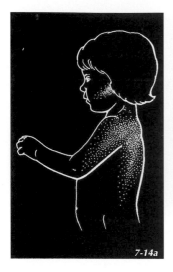
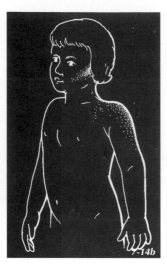

**Figure 7-14a,b.** *Drawing depicting the pattern of burn forming "arrow" signs on the cheek and back. This may occur when hot water is thrown from behind.*

The classic arrow sign may not be present, however, with hot grease spills. Grease becomes hotter than water and sticks to the skin rather than running off the surface (Othersen, 1983). It may cause a full-thickness burn to a subcutaneous depth of 0.04 inches (Coren, 1987). The arrow sign may also be absent in forced exposure to running hot water from a faucet. The continuous flow of hot water from the faucet serves as a constant source of heat energy, referred to as an "energy sink." This may cause uniform full-thickness burns without a cooling pattern, as described above. If the child is developmentally old enough to turn on the hot water faucet, he may accidentally sustain such a burn on the anterior surface of his lower trunk and legs. Therefore, when given that history, one must analyze the patterns of the burn, the child's developmental skills, and the presence of other associated findings in order to differentiate abusive from accidental causes of injury.

### FLEXION BURNS

Another pattern of abusive burning seen in either of the two types discussed above (immersion or splash) is the flexion burn. In one study this was seen in 5 of 43 burn patients from a series of 712 child abuse cases (Lenoski & Hunter, 1977). This type of burn pattern may occur when a hot liquid is intentionally poured onto the body or the victim is immersed in a hot liquid with the hips or other body parts maximally flexed. The skin within the flexed body area, such as the inguinal crease or popliteal fossa behind the knee, is spared from contact with the burning agent (**Figure** 7-15).

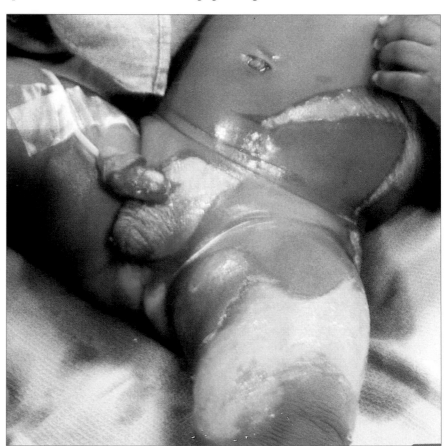

**Figure 7-15.** *Scald burn of 1-year-old child showing spared skin in the inguinal area due to flexion at the hip when the burn occurred.*

This may occur in one area or in several areas parallel to each other, yielding alternating areas of burn and spared skin or a "zebra" pattern. Partial contact with grills or repeated application of curling irons to the skin on an area of the body may also give an alternating "zebra" pattern. Additionally, hot water scalds to limbs partially protected by clothes such as socks may yield alternating patterns of burned and spared skin (**Figure 7-16**). These, however, have patterns distinct from scald immersion lines.

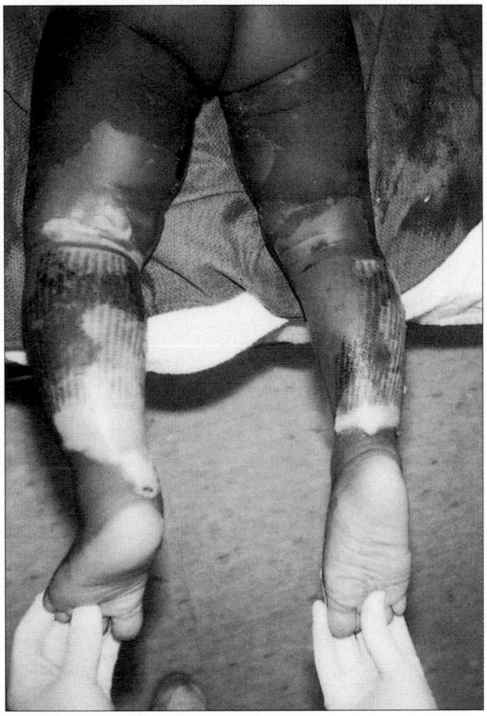

## CONTACT BURNS

Contact burns comprise a unique group of pattern burns. The health care worker may need to assume the role of a detective in order to accurately diagnose the cause of these inflicted burns. In our experience, curling irons (**Figure** 7-17), steam irons (**Figure** 7-18), cigarettes (**Figure** 7-19) and cigarette lighters, and space heater grills (**Figure** 7-20) are a few of the implements used in abusive burning. Hot plates, light bulbs, and knives also have been used (Stone et al., 1970; Lenoski & Hunter, 1977; Feldman, 1980; Green, 1984; Johnson, 1990).

*Figure 7-16. Hot water scald to the posterior legs of a child who was wearing socks. Note the ribbed pattern from the sock "branded" on the skin.*

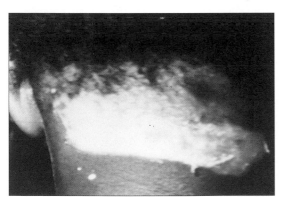

*Figure 7-17. Curling iron burn on the back of the neck of a 3-year-old girl.*

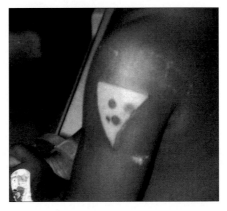

*Figure 7-18. Inflicted steam iron burn on the lateral surface of the left arm of a 2-year-old child. Note the sharply demarcated edges and the pattern of steam vent holes "branded" onto the skin. The father claimed that the burn was accidental, but he admitted to spanking the child for "messing her pants."*

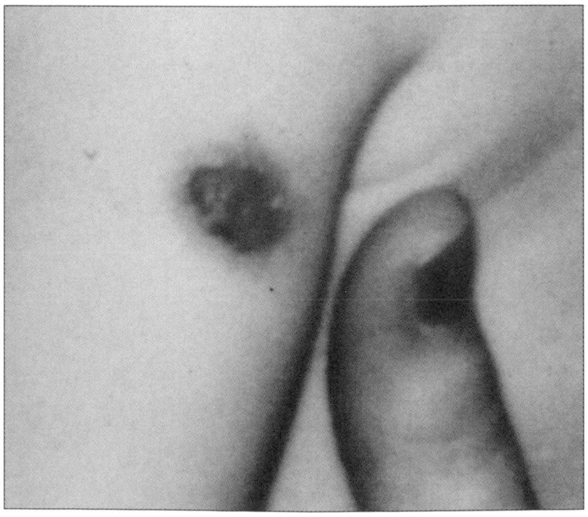

*Figure 7-19. Cigarette burn to the posterolateral arm of a child. This area is unlikely to have been injured accidentally.*

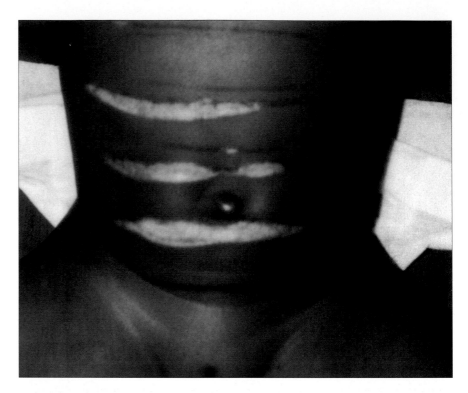

**Figure 7-20.** *Linear pattern of burns caused by a space heater grill intentionally placed on the child's abdomen.*

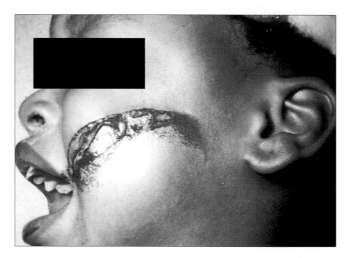

**Figure 7-21.** *Burn on the left lateral cheek of a child who pulled a hot clothes iron down onto her face by pulling on the cord. Note the irregular shape of the lower half of the burn, which is consistent with a hot object contacting the patient's face but then causing a glancing type of injury as it falls.*

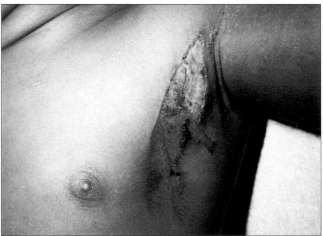

**Figure 7-22.** *Same child as in Figure 7-21. The hot iron fell downward and caused a burn to the anterolateral chest.*

The shape of the object is branded on the child's skin. Tissue destruction, mediated by conduction of heat, in the case of inflicted burns is often uniform in all directions. The shape or pattern of the object or the end of the object is faithfully reproduced in the burn pattern. Such objects can also cause accidental burns, but the patterns are generally nonuniform and appear to be a glancing (brushing against) type of injury. The child in **Figures 7-21 and 7-22** sustained a glancing type injury with a nonuniform burning pattern when she pulled on the cord of an iron, causing it to accidentally fall onto the skin. Here the child

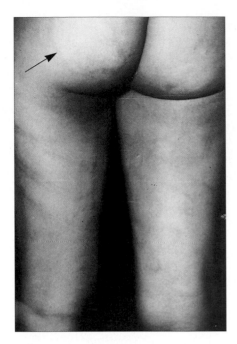

**Figure 7-23.** *Old clothes iron burn scar of the left buttock with depigmentation. Also note the whip and lash marks on the posterior legs.*

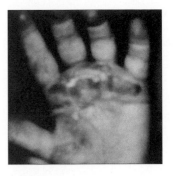

**Figure 7-24.** *Burn to the palm of the hand in a toddler who reached up to a hot oven door.*

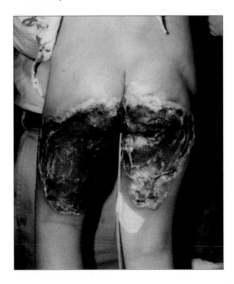

**Figure 7-25.** *Third-degree burn of the buttocks in an 18-month-old boy who was intentionally set on a hot wood-burning stove as punishment for wetting the bed.*

sustained a partial and irregular burn to the face and then, as the iron continued its fall, to the anterior axilla and chest area. A careful history and analysis of the burn as well as recognition of accidental patterns of burning is essential in a case such as this. This must be compared to the clearly demarcated and inflicted burn pattern seen in Figure 7-18. Additionally, one should be aware of what well-healed iron burns look like years later. **Figure 7-23** shows a well-healed, depigmented iron-shaped burn scar on the left buttock of a child being evaluated for additional signs of abuse, such as old loop and lash marks.

The developmental skill of the child must be considered when evaluating contact burn injuries. Johnson (1990) described the case of a 7-month-old infant with a knife-shaped full-thickness burn to the sole of the foot. The parents said the child accidentally stepped on the hot object. The unlikely occurrence of a hot knife lying on the floor is made even more incredulous by the claim that the 7-month-old stepped on it when the infant could not even stand without support, let alone walk on his own. Similarly, in reference to scald burns, the ability to turn a circular faucet for hot water is achieved beyond infancy and early toddler age; it is unlikely that an accidental burn could be caused this way unless the child is approximately 18 to 24 months old.

Wood-burning stoves are another cause of contact burns, one that is quite prevalent in some areas; it is estimated that 13 million wood stoves are used in the United States (Yanofsky & Morain, 1984). The location of the burn on the body aids in the evaluation of suspected abuse versus accidental injury. The functional position of the hand at the time of the burn yields a recognizable burn pattern (**Figure 7-24**). However, **Figure 7-25** shows a boy who is obviously a victim of abuse with severe burns to the buttocks from a woodstove.

Oppressive toilet training practices account for many abusive burns; for example, an 18-month-old was forced to sit on a hot wood-burning stove for having wet the bed. Occasionally, open flames are used to inflict punishment on a child, as shown in **Figure 7-26**. In some older homes, floor heaters made in the 1950s stand approximately 3 feet high with a grid or grill on the top surface. One was involved in the case of an 18-month-old girl with a serious burn (**Figure 7-27**). The history given by her caretaker was that she climbed up and accidentally sat on the heater. This history is not consistent with the burn pattern nor the physics of how the human body sits. The "sitting" part of the buttocks near the inferior gluteal creases and posterior thighs is not burned at all, and there are no burns to the child's hands or knees, as would be expected during climbing. However, the upper buttocks, posterior iliac crest, and sacral areas are "branded" with the grid pattern of the heater's top cover, indicating the child was forcibly held against the hot surface.

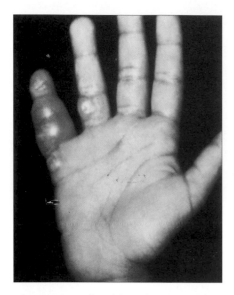

**Figure 7-26.** *Bullous blister formation on the fourth and fifth fingers of a 2-year-old child whose hand was held over an open flame as punishment.*

Sometimes burns are isolated events, but not infrequently a child will come for treatment with multiple old stigmata indicative of child abuse. In addition to the obvious scars, the child may suffer from psychological, emotional, and sexual abuse, as shown in the following case (**Figures 7-28 through 7-30**).

## CASE HISTORY

A 3 1/2-year-old girl was referred to the sexual abuse management clinic after child protection workers in conjunction with a child psychologist discovered evidence of possible sexual abuse. While in day care, she was sexually acting out with the other children and the staff and was constantly masturbating. The child was severely developmentally delayed. With counseling, the child disclosed sexual abuse.

On examination she was noted to have a constellation of old scars from a variety of agents. The child's grandmother stated that the mother had severely disciplined the child and used a graded system of increasingly severe punishment to match the desired level of discipline. First, she used a cigarette to inflict burns or bit the child; next she would burn her repeatedly with a curling iron; and finally she inflicted scalding hot water immersion burns.

## ◆ PREVENTION

Several authors have presented strategies for injury prevention in the community and in the home (Haddon, 1980; Gallagher, 1982; Libber & Stayton, 1984; Micik & Miclette, 1985; Maley & Achauer, 1987; Murray, 1988; Katcher et al., 1989; Webne et al., 1989; McLoughlin & McGuire, 1990; National Safe Kids Campaign, 1990). Accident prevention theorists conceptualize injury as a disease that is predictable rather than a random event (Haddon, 1980). In 1972 Haddon first described the 10 classic intervention strategies for systematic analysis of injuries; these included the "reduction in the amount of a given hazard brought into being" (Micik & Miclette, 1985). When considering an object as a hazard, one must take into account the triple axis of the injury phenomenon: the host (victim), the vehicle (vector), and the environment. Placing these main points into the context of abusive burns, one would expect fewer bathtub scald burns if there was a maximum water heater temperature of 125°F built into all manufactured units. Antiscald devices are available, which, if installed at the faucet or shower head, will instantly shut off the flow of water if the temperature exceeds a preset value (McLoughlin & McGuire, 1990). Some authors suggest using liquid crystal thermometers to check bathtub water temperature in order to prevent scalds (Katcher et al., 1989). Others who distributed educational pamphlets and liquid crystal thermometers to 12 families found no statistically significant reduction in hot water temperature as a result of the intervention (Webne et al., 1989). This led to the notion that the best preventive measure may be to have hot water heaters installed with preset safe temperatures.

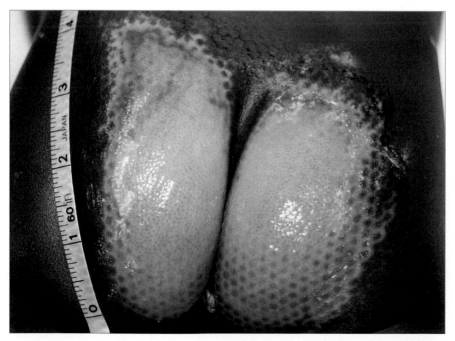

**Figure 7-27.** *Inflicted pattern burn to the buttocks and sacral area of an 18-month-old girl who was forcibly held against the grid cover of a floor heater.*

Unfortunately, the human host or child victim cannot be modified physically to resist injury, unlike head injury prevention whereby some host modification occurs by using a bicycle helmet. It is also doubtful that we can change the environment for some burns, as people still cook food and boil water in the kitchen and are unlikely to install barriers around such areas to protect small children. However, parents can be educated to unexpected dangers, such as burns from liquids heated in microwave ovens (Puczynski et al., 1983), where skin scalds (James, 1989) and palatal burns (Hibbard & Blevins, 1988) have occurred. Interestingly, water heated in microwaves may not cool off to a safe temperature until some 10 minutes after water that is heated conventionally (James, 1989).

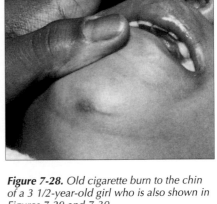

*Figure 7-28.* Old cigarette burn to the chin of a 3 1/2-year-old girl who is also shown in Figures 7-29 and 7-30.

More importantly, we may and should continue to try to change the vector of the trauma, namely the abusive parent. Obviously, this can be an extremely difficult and complex task. Even though studies show a relationship between socioeconomic status and the incidence of burn injuries (Slater et al., 1987; Graitcer & Sneizek, 1988), research is needed in effective ways of rehabilitating the abusive parent. Our system of adjudication may successfully remove children from the home of an abusive parent, but this is certainly not ideal. The child then not only struggles with his or her physical imperfections as a result of the burning process but may also suffer further emotional turmoil due to parental separation.

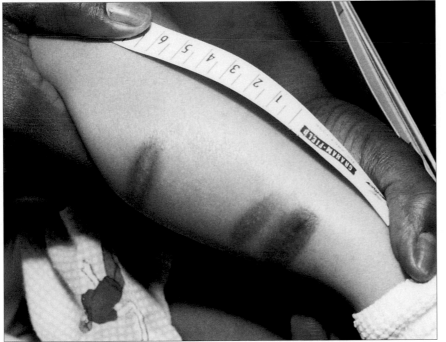

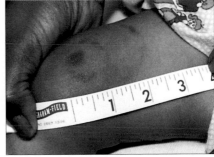

*Figure 7-30.* Human bite mark on the thigh just above the knee in the child shown in Figure 7-29.

*Figure 7-29.* Multiple linear curling iron burns on the lower posterior leg (more likely non-accidental) of a 3 1/2-year-old girl.

One suggestion is to offer parents anticipating having children a course on child development at a level they can understand. Reporting on their results with a group of well-child classes, some authors found that 76% of the subjects in the experimental group (those whose child care instruction included home fire and burn safety) set their hot water heaters at a safe level, compared to only 23% of those in the control group (Thomas et al., 1984). Such classes might also include counseling regarding child temperament characteristics.

Parents should be discouraged from using infant walkers because children have been able to approach hot objects such as oven doors; reach and pull on cords to pots, fryers, and irons; and pull on tablecloths, thereby sustaining serious burns

(Johnson et al., 1990). Infant walkers have also been related to numerous falls down staircases when parents fail to secure doors or open stairwells.

In cases of accidental trauma, a child's temperament may determine what he does (the "how" of behavior), his motivation (the "why" of behavior), and his competencies or physical abilities (the "what" of behavior) (Zuckerman & Duby, 1985). However, the child's rhythmicity, or lack thereof, with regard to sleep, hunger, or elimination functions as well as the quality of his or her mood (i.e., crying or displeasing behavior) may play even greater roles in abuse or nonaccidental injuries.

It has been suggested that high-risk populations should be targeted for abuse prevention strategies (Webne et al., 1989). These strategies include education and counseling of parents to achieve realistic expectations for themselves and their children, income supplementation, employment counseling, and provision of day-care services (Reece & Grodin, 1985).

Secondary prevention is also important. High-risk parental signals such as teenage pregnancy, unwanted pregnancy, or substance abuse as well as infant prematurity and childhood developmental disorders should be noted (Johnson, 1990). Furthermore, early intervention may be indicated if one notes undue concern over an unborn baby's sex, a mother's denial of pregnancy or severe depression, lack of eye contact or holding of a baby, parental complaints that diapers are messy and repulsive to clean, and numerous emergency department visits. With regard to the latter, an important caveat in emergency medicine is to always be aware of a "hidden agenda." The parent may present repeatedly to the emergency room with seemingly trivial complaints because she may be asking for help in the only way she knows how. Pediatricians, family practitioners, obstetricians, nurses, and social workers who come into contact with parents and children should be cognizant of these high-risk signals. When possible, they should intervene with counseling, education, and/or referrals to child protection agencies. Nevertheless, the ability of the emergency department caregivers to recognize the intentionally injured child is critical because immediate intervention may be required to prevent further harm to the physical or psychological well being of a child (Hyden & Gallagher, 1992).

One must appreciate the value of *anticipating* injury. Prevention should be the goal toward which our ultimate achievement should aim. When we expect injurious acts or prevent further abuse to a child, we complete the triad of *Anticipation, Recognition,* and *Treatment* and thereby realize the true *ART* of medicine.

## ◆BIBLIOGRAPHY

Alexander, RC, Surrell, JA, and Cohle, SD: Microwave oven burns to children, an unusual manifestation of child abuse, *Pediatrics* 79:255-260, 1987.

Asnes, RS, and Wisotsky, DH: Cupping lesions simulating child abuse, *J Pediatr* 99:267, 1981.

Ayoub, C, and Pfeifer, D: Burns as a manifestation of child abuse and neglect, *Am J Dis Child* 133:910, 1979.

Benians, RC: The influence of parental visiting on survival and recovery of extensively burned children, *Burns Incl Therm Inj* 14:31-34, 1988.

Berger, LR, and Kalishman, S: Floor furnace burns to children, *Pediatrics* 71:97-99, 1983.

Bernstein, N, and Cahners, SS: Rehabilitating families of burned children, *Scand J Reconstruct Surg* 13:173-175, 1979.

Bradshaw, C, Hawkins, J, Leach, M, et al: A study of childhood scalds, *Burns Incl Therm Inj* 14:21-24, 1988.

Caniano, DA, Beaver, BL, and Boles, ET: Child abuse: An update on surgical management in 256 cases, *Ann Surg* 203:219-224, 1986.

Colombo, JL, Hopkins, RL, and Waring, WW: Steam vaporizer injuries, *Pediatrics* 67:661-663, 1981.

Coren, CV: Burn injuries in children, *Pediatr Ann* 16:328-339, 1987.

Demling, RH: Burns, *N Engl J Med* 313:1389, 1985.

Devlin, BK, and Reynolds, E: Child abuse. How to recognize it, how to intervene, *Am J Nursing* 94(3):26-31, 1994.

deWet, B, Cywes, S, Davies, MRQ, et al: Some aspects of post-treatment adjustments in severely burned children, *Burns Incl Therm Inj* 5:321-325, 1979.

Feldman, KW: Child abuse by burning. In CH Kempe and RE Helfer: *The Battered Child*, University of Chicago Press, Chicago, 1980.

Feldman, KW: Pseudoabusive burns in Asian refugees, *Child Abuse & Neglect* 19(5):657-8, 1995.

Feldman, KW: Confusion of innocent pressure injuries with inflicted dry contact burns, *Clinical Pediatrics* 34(2):114-5, 1995.

Feldman, KW, Clarren, SK, and McLaughlin, JF: Tap water burns in handicapped children, *Pediatrics* 67:560-562, 1981.

Feldman, KW, Schaller, RT, Feldman, JA, et al: Tap water scald burns in children, *Pediatrics* 62:1-7, 1978.

Fowler, J: Child maltreatment by burning, *Burns Incl Therm Inj* 5:83-86, 1979.

Gallagher, SS: A strategy for the reduction of childhood injuries in Massachusetts: SCIPP, *N Engl J Med* 307:1015, 1982.

Graitcer, PL, and Sneizek, JE: Hospitalizations due to tap water scalds, 1978-1985, *MMWR* 37:35, 1988.

Green, AH: Child abuse by siblings, *Child Abuse Negl* 8:311-317, 1984.

Haddon, W, Jr: Advances in the epidemiology of injuries on a basis for public policy, *Public Health Rep* 95:411-421, 1980.

Hammond, J, Nebel-Gould, A, and Brooks, J: The value of speech-language assessment in the diagnosis of child abuse, *J Trauma* 29:1258-1260, 1989.

Hammond, J, Perez-Stable A, and Ward, CG: Predictive value of historical and physical characteristics for the diagnosis of child abuse, *Southern Med J* 84(2):116-8, 1991.

Hammond, JS, Ward, CG, and Pereira, E: Self-inflicted burns, *J Burn Care Rehabil* 9:178-179, 1988.

Hankin, F, and Vermeulen, F: Infant automobile restraint systems: Beware of the sun, *Pediatrics* 65:625-626, 1980.

Hibbard, RA, and Blevins, R: Palatal burn due to bottle warming in a microwave oven, *Pediatrics* 82:382-384, 1988.

Hight, DW, Bakalar, HR, and Lloyd, JR: Inflicted burns in children, *JAMA* 242:517-520, 1979.

Hummel, RP 3d, Greenhalgh, DG, Barthel, PP, DeSerna, CM, Gottschlich, MM, James, LE, and Warden, GD: Outcome and socioeconomic aspects of suspected child abuse scald burns, *J Burn Care & Rehabilitation* 14(1):121-6, 1993.

Hyden, PW, Gallagher, TA: Child abuse intervention in the emergency room, *Pediatr Clin North Am* 39(5):1053-81, 1992.

Illinois Department of Children and Family Services, and The Office of the Medical Examiner, Cook County: Protocol for determining if an injury is a result of child abuse or neglect, The Task Force for the Study of Non-Accidental Injuries and Child Deaths, State of Illinois, 1986.

James, MI: Burns from fluid heated in a microwave oven (letter), *Br Med J* 298:1452, 1989.

Johnson, CF: Inflicted injury versus accidental injury, *Pediatr Clin North Am* 37:791-814, 1990.

Johnson, CF, Ericson, AK, and Caniano, D: Walker-related burns in infants and toddlers, *Pediatr Emerg Care* 6:58-61, 1990.

Johnson, CF, and Showers, J: Injury variables in child abuse, *Child Abuse Negl* 9:207-215, 1985.

Joseph, TP, and Douglas, BS: Childhood burns in South Australia: A socio-economic and aetiological study, *Burns Incl Therm Inj* 5:335-342, 1979.

Katcher, ML, Landry, GL, and Shapiro, MM: Liquid crystal thermometer use in pediatric office counseling about tap water burn prevention, *Pediatrics* 83:766-771, 1989.

Keen, JH, Lendrum, J, and Wolman, B: Inflicted burns and scalds in children, *Br Med J* 4:268, 1975.

Leeder, CJ: Families of burn victims receive help through regular group meetings, *Burns* 5:89-91, 1979.

Lenoski, EF, and Hunter, KA: Specific patterns of inflicted burn injuries, *J Trauma* 17:842, 1977.

Libber, SM, and Stayton, DJ: Childhood burns reconsidered: The child, the family, and the burn injury, *J Trauma* 24:245-252, 1984.

Ludwig, S, and Fleisher, G, eds: *Textbook of Pediatric Emergency Medicine*, The Williams & Wilkins Co, Baltimore, 1983.

Lung, RF, Miller, SH, Davis, TS, et al: Recognizing burn injuries as abuse, *Am Fam Physician* 15:134-135, 1977.

Maley, MP, and Achauer, BM: Prevention of tap water scald burns, *J Burn Care Rehabil* 8:62-65, 1987.

McLoughlin, E, and Crawford, JD: Burns, *Pediatr Clin North Am* 321:61-75, 1985.

McLoughlin, E, and McGuire, A: The causes, cost, and prevention of childhood burn injuries, *Am J Dis Child* 144:677-683, 1990.

McMahon, P, Grossman, W, Gaffney, M, and Stanitski, C: Soft-tissue injury as an indication of child abuse, *J Bone & Joint Surgery- Am Vol* 77(8):1179-83, 1995.

Micik, S, and Miclette, M: Injury prevention in the community: A systems approach, *Pediatr Clin North Am* 32:251-265, 1985.

Moritz, AR, and Henriques, FC: Study of thermal injury: The relative importance of time and surface temperature in the causation of cutaneous burns, *Am J Pathol* 23:695-720, 1947.

Moritz, AR, Henriques, FC, and McLean, R: The effects of inhaled heat on the air passage and lungs, *Am J Pathol* 21:311, 1945.

Murray, JP: A study of the prevention of hot tapwater burns, *Burns Incl Therm Inj* 14:185-193, 1988.

National Safe Kids Campaign, Children's Hospital National Medical Center, Washington, DC, 1990.

National Safety Council: *Accident Facts,* Washington, DC, 1979.

Otherson, HB: Burns and scalds, *Pediatr Ann* 12:753, 1983.

Parish, RA, Novack, AH, Heimbach, DM, et al: Pediatric patients in a regional burn center, *Pediatr Emerg Care* 2:165-167, 1986.

Prescott, PR: Hair dryer burns in children, *Pediatrics* 86:692-697, 1990.

Puczynski, M, Rademaker, D, and Gatson, RL: Burn injury related to the improper uses of a microwave oven, *Pediatrics* 72:714-715, 1983.

Raimer, BG, Raimer, SS, and Hebeler, JR: Cutaneous signs of child abuse, *J Am Acad Dermatol* 5:203-214, 1981.

Reece, RM, and Grodin, MA: Recognition of non-accidental injury, *Pediatr Clin North Am* 32:41-60, 1985.

Renz, BM, and Sherman R: Abusive scald burns in infants and children: a prospective study, *Am Surgeon* 95(5):329-34, 1993.

Renz, BM, and Sherman R: Child abuse by scalding, *Journal of the Medical Association of Georgia* 81(10):574-8, 1992.

Rivara, FP, Kamitsuka, MD, and Quan, L: Injuries to children younger than one year of age, *Pediatrics* 81:93-97, 1988.

Robinson, MD, and Seward, PN: Thermal injury in children, *Pediatr Emerg Care* 3:266-270, 1987.

Rosenberg, NM, and Marino, D: Frequency of suspected abuse/neglect in burn patients, *Pediatr Emerg Care* 5:219-221, 1989.

Rosenberg, NM, Meyers, S, and Shackleton, N: Prediction of child abuse in an ambulatory setting, *Pediatrics* 70:879, 1982.

Saitz, EW: Seat belt buckle burns, *Am J Dis Child* 129:1456, 1975.

Sandler, AP, and Haynes, V: Non-accidental trauma and medical folk belief: A case of cupping, *Pediatrics* 61:921-922, 1978.

Schmitt, BD, Gray, JD, and Britton, HL: Car seat burns in infants: Avoiding confusion with inflicted burns, *Pediatrics* 62:607-609, 1978.

Sheldon, SH, and Woodward, C: Burn injuries secondary to hot floor tiling (letter), *Clin Pediatr* 22:658, 1983.

Showers, J, and Garrison, KM: Burn abuse: A four-year study, *J Trauma* 28:1581-1583, 1988.

Slater, SJ, Slater, H, and Goldfarb, JW: Burned children: A socioeconomic profile for focused prevention programs, *J Burn Care Rehabil* 8:566, 1987.

Spear, RM, and Munster, AM: Burns, inhalation injury and electrical injury. In MC Rogers, ed: *Textbook of Pediatric Intensive Care Medicine*, The Williams & Wilkins Co, Philadelphia, 1987.

Stone, NH, Rinaldo, L, Humphrey, CR, et al: Child abuse by burning, *Surg Clin North Am* 50:1419-1424, 1970.

Sudikoff, S, and Young, RS: Burn from hairdryer: accident or abuse?, *Pediatrics* 93(3):540, 1994.

Tarnowski, KJ, Rasnake, LK, Linsheid, TR, et al: Behavioral adjustment of pediatric burn victims, *J Pediatr Psychol* 14:607-615, 1989.

Thomas, KA, Hassanein, RS, and Christophersen, ER: Evaluation of group well-child care for improving burn prevention practices in the home, *Pediatrics* 74:879-882, 1984.

US Consumer Product Safety Commission: National electronic injury surveillance system: *Product summary report,* National Injury Information Clearinghouse, Washington, DC,1989.

Warner, JE, and Hansen, DJ: The identification and reporting of physical abuse by physicians: a review and implications for research, *Child Abuse & Neglect* 18(1):11-25, 1994.

Webne, S, Kaplan, BJ, and Shaw, M: Pediatric burn prevention: An evaluation of the efficacy of a strategy to reduce tap water temperature in a population at risk for scalds, *J Dev Behav Pediatr* 10:187-191, 1989.

Weimer, CL, Goldfarb, W, and Slater, H: Multidisciplinary approach to working with burn victims of child abuse, *J Burn Care Rehabil* 9:79-82, 1988.

Yanofsky, NN, and Morain, WD: Upper extremity burns from wood stoves, *Pediatrics* 73:722-726, 1984.

Yeoh, C, Nixon, JW, Dickwon, W, and Sibert, JR: Patterns of scald injuries, *Archives of Disease in Childhood* 71(2):156-8, 1994.

Yiacoumettes, A, and Roberts, M: An analysis of burns in children, *Burns Incl Therm Inj* 3:195-201, 1977.

Zuckerman, BS, and Duby, JC: Developmental approach to injury prevention, *Pediatr Clin North Am* 32:17-29, 1985.

# SEXUAL ABUSE: AN OVERVIEW

JAMES A. MONTELEONE, M.D.
SHEILAH GLAZE, M.S.W., L.C.S.W.
KAREN M. BLY, R.N., B.S.N., M.A., M.ED.

*A 1-month-old boy was admitted to the nursery. The child had been seen by his private pediatrician because of respiratory distress. A routine chest film revealed the child had marble bone disease. The child's mother was 14 years old.*

*Shortly after admission, the hospital social service department received an anonymous phone call stating that the infant was the result of an incestuous relationship. Since marble bone disease is a rare autosomal recessive disorder, consanguinity was definitely a possibility. The mother was interviewed and she denied the possibility. The Division of Family Services was notified, and it stated the family had previously been anonymously reported and the allegation was unsubstantiated.*

*The infant was scheduled for a bone marrow transplant, and, when selecting possible donors, the infant's "grandfather" was a perfect match. The odds of a grandfather being a perfect match are very slim unless he is also the father. With that information, the child's mother was removed from the home. While out of the home, with counseling, she acknowledged that she had been sexually abused by her father and the father subsequently admitted that he had abused her.*

This chapter is the first of three dealing with the management of cases involving sexual abuse. These chapters present an overview *(Chapter 8)*, the physical examination procedure *(Chapter 9)*, and the specifics of interviewing these children *(Chapter 10)*. It is the purpose of this chapter to identify and define the components of sexual abuse and to propose a working philosophy for dealing with these cases.

## ♦DEFINITION OF SEXUAL ABUSE

Sexual abuse occurs between a child and an adult or older child and is defined as sexual contact or interaction for sexual stimulation and gratification of the adult or older child, who is a parent or caretaker and responsible for the child's care. Sexual abuse is a form of child abuse and must be reported to state child protective services. If the perpetrator is not a caretaker, the sexual activity is sexual assault and may not fall into the category of behaviors reportable to state protective services, but must be reported to a local law enforcement sex crimes unit. The sex crimes unit deals with perpetrators of sex crimes who have no role in the child's care, but are usually known to the victim or the victim's family. The sex offender often pursues this practice as a career and will abuse many children over the course of time.

The long-term effects of sexual abuse are not clearly known (Brassard, 1983). Some children appear to suffer lasting psychological problems, while others are able to cope effectively. Intrafamilial abuse may be passed from one generation to another (American Humane Society, 1981).

### ABUSIVE OR ASSAULTIVE ACTS

Sexual abusive or assaultive acts include sexual intercourse, sodomy or anal penetration, oral genital contact, fondling, masturbation, digital penetration or manipulation, and exposure. The acts can be reciprocal or one-sided. Of the acts listed, exposure can be the most difficult to define. Some families are comfortable with nudity in the home; they share bathrooms, share bedrooms, or live in small quarters where privacy is at a premium. Exposure becomes sexual abuse when the person exposing is sexually aroused by the event and does it specifically for that purpose.

### CLASSIFICATION OF SEXUAL ABUSE

The acts of sexual abuse can be divided into three categories: assault, incest, and exploitation. Assault and incest are somewhat self-explanatory; exploitation includes prostitution and pornography.

### *ASSAULT*

The perpetrator of a sexual assault is usually male. Sexual assault is usually a one-time event in which the perpetrator forces himself on the child. If the child is examined within a short time of the assault, there is generally physical evidence of trauma, such as tears, blood, and bruises, which constitute dramatic, acute findings of abuse. When dealing with an assault case the child is at greatest risk because the molester is often emotionally unstable. One must make certain the child is protected and does not return to the situation in which the assault took place; the perpetrator must not have access to the child.

### *INCEST*

Incest is defined as sexual intercourse between persons so closely related that they are forbidden by law to marry. Incestuous abuse usually occurs over a long period of time and often involves a conditioning process. The perpetrator is usually male, although female perpetrators are possible and probably underreported. The abuser may not necessarily be related to the child; he may be a stepfather or paramour, but generally is the father figure or provider in the home. Although the classical incestuous relationship involves father and daughter, other common liaisons form between older brother and younger sister, uncle and niece or nephew, and grandfather and granddaughter or grandson.

Classically, there is no evidence of trauma or acute injury. The physical findings are subtle or nonexistent, unless there has been complete penile penetration over a long period. The child usually does not make a disclosure until the abuse has gone on for a number of years, beginning when the child was an infant and continuing with her becoming conditioned and manipulated over many years to accept this as a way of life. Several children in the home may be involved in the abuse.

There is disagreement among authorities, in the classical incestuous situation, whether the child and the perpetrator should be separated during therapy or during the investigation. Some therapists advocate separation. Others believe that as long as the perpetrator admits to the abuse, it is acceptable to allow the abuser to remain in the home and keep the family intact. If possible, the child should remain in the home to avoid being blamed or blaming herself for the disintegration of the family. She may perceive being removed as punishment. The victim must also receive counseling. She often faces alienation, denial, and hostility from mother, father, and siblings. As a result, she may deny that the abuse took place and retract her disclosure.

If the perpetrator does not admit to the abuse, he should be removed from the home so that he cannot manipulate the child further and convince her to retract her disclosure and thus allow the abuse to continue. If the other parent does not accept that the child has been abused, the child should be taken out of the home again so that she will not be influenced to change her mind and deny the truth.

## EXPLOITATION

Sexual exploitation, involving prostitution and pornography, is unique in that it often involves a group of participants. It can occur within a family or outside of the home, involving several adults and nonrelated children; then it is referred to as a sex ring. In cases involving families, the whole family—mother, father, and children—can be involved, and the children must be protected and removed from the home situation. This is a pathologic situation in which both parents are often sexually involved with the children and are using the children for prostitution or for pornography. **Exploited children need the greatest intervention and psychiatric help.**

## RISK FACTORS

In a review of the data from the 1987 National Survey of Children (Moore et al., 1989), social settings were identified that increased the risk of sexual abuse. Those social conditions are listed in **Table 8-1.** The incidence of abuse was 6% of girls with no risk factor, 9% of girls with one risk factor, 26% of girls with two risk factors, and 68% of girls with three or more risk factors.

## ♦ SEXUAL ABUSE VICTIMS

Three-fourths of the crimes against children are sex crimes. The American Humane Association estimates that about 4,000 cases of sexual abuse occur annually in each city in the United States. The usual cases of child sexual abuse involve young female children and male caretakers, older male relatives, or other older males with whom they are acquainted. The age difference between the abuser and the victim is 5 years or more. Sex play between age-mates, unless there is coercion, is usually normal. In older studies, females were reported as victims 10 times more often than males (DeVine, 1980). The offenders are male 97% of the time; 50% to 80% are known by the victims. Parents and other relatives are the offenders in 30% to 50% of the cases.

DeFrancis (1969) noted that the average age of female victims, under the age of 16, was 11. The American Humane Association (1981) reported that 72% of incest victims were 13 years or older. In my experience, in over 5,000 victims under 18, the average age was around 5. This may reflect a greater awareness of child sexual abuse in the 1980s, cultural issues, or other, as yet undefined, trends.

**Table 8-1. Social Conditions Increasing Risk of Sexual Abuse**

**Social condition**

Lived apart from both biological parents
Raised in poverty
Child handicapped
Alcoholic family member
Drug-abusing family member
Prostitution at home
Transient adults living at home
Mentally ill caretaker
AIDS-related disability of caretaker

Victims of child sexual abuse come from all races, creeds, and socioeconomic levels. Boys are more commonly victimized by someone outside the home, whereas girls are often abused by someone within the home. The children are often threatened with punishment if they do not cooperate. They are told that the activity is a game or something special and fun, but that it must be kept secret.

## MALE VICTIMS

A study of 100 patients at the Mayo Clinic (Greenwood et al., 1990) revealed that one in six of the females interviewed admitted to being a victim of sexual abuse; none of the males in a comparable population admitted to abuse. It is possible that a young boy who has a sexual relationship with an adult female may consider it manly and acceptable. If that relationship is with an adult male, the stigmata of homosexuality may arise, so he may not want anyone to know about it or to misinterpret his role in the encounter. Therefore the true incidence of sexual abuse of males is difficult to estimate; many experts feel that it is at least as frequent as the incidence in females, if not higher. Reports suggest that males are 10 times less apt to be abused as females. It is hoped that the true incidence of this problem will be revealed with time.

## *CHILD VULNERABILITIES*

Children have characteristics that make them ideal victims. They are endowed with natural curiosity, even about sex, a taboo subject with which they generally have no experience. A clever child molester can exploit this trait to lower the child's inhibitions and seduce the child into sexual activity. Parents instruct their children to respect and obey adults, so children are easily led by adults. Also, the adult is bigger, stronger, and wiser in the child's eyes. The adult uses these suppositions to influence and control the child's behavior. Most importantly, children crave attention, affection, and approval. Children from broken homes and victims of emotional abuse and neglect are at greatest risk of victimization, trading sex for the missing affection and attention in their lives.

Adolescents can also be exploited by the child molester. An adolescent boy who has been victimized because he rebelliously defies guidelines set by his parents is very unlikely to admit erring.

## RESPONSES TO BEING ABUSED

Children who have been sexually abused often act seductively toward adults or act out sexually. A child molester may say that the child seduced him (see later discussion of perpetrators). For this reason, when social services place a sexually abused child in a foster home, the home should be selected with great care and the foster parents must be alerted to the fact that the child has been sexually abused and may behave seductively and act out sexually with others in the home, whether adults or children. The family should be instructed how to deal with the child when he or she demonstrates these behaviors.

## ADOLESCENT PREGNANCY AND SEXUAL ABUSE

Sexual abuse affects children in many areas of their development. They have delays in cognitive, social, emotional, and psychological functioning. Victims of sexual abuse may be at higher risk for mental health and social functioning problems. The interpersonal problems and coping patterns of young women with a history of sexual abuse are conditioned by long-term negative effects on self-esteem, self-concept, and sexual adjustment (Conte & Schuerman, 1987).

These effects of child abuse may be linked to adolescent pregnancy. Boyer and Fine (1992) conducted a study between 1988 and 1992 examining the relationship between sexual victimization in childhood and adolescent pregnancy and also child maltreatment by adolescent parents. Data were collected in three phases: baseline surveys, a follow-up survey, and a review of Child Protective Services (CPS) case records. The sample included 535 pregnant and parenting adolescents recruited from school and community programs.

The most important finding from the survey data was the prevalence of sexual victimization experienced by the young women in the study. Of the sample, 62% had experienced contact molestation, attempted rape, or rape before their first pregnancy. Overall, 55% of the sample had been sexually molested. The average age of the respondents was 9.7 years old at first molestation, with 24% reporting that their first such experience occurred at age 5 or younger. The mean age of the offender was 27.4 years. Seventy-seven percent of those molested were molested more than once, and 54% were victimized by a family member. Forty-two percent of the sample had experienced at least one attempted rape, and 44% had been raped. The average age at the first rape was 13.3; the age of the perpetrator was 22.6. One half of the respondents who had been raped were raped more than once.

When they compared abused and nonabused groups, the young women who had been sexually victimized before their first pregnancy had begun voluntary intercourse earlier and were more likely to have used drugs and alcohol. Their sexual partners were older and were also more likely to be using drugs and alcohol. The age of the first pregnancy was the same for both groups; however, the partners of those who were abused were older. The young women who had been abused were less likely to use contraception and were more likely to have had an abortion and second and third pregnancies. Those girls who had been abused were more likely to have been in a violent relationship. The abused young women reported more emotional abuse and physical abuse in childhood. They were more likely to have experienced repeated victimization in the previous year, to have had a sexually transmitted disease, and to have problems with drugs or alcohol. The abused young women were more likely to report that their children had been abused.

The prevalence of childhood sexual abuse among adolescent mothers must be addressed in teen pregnancy prevention programs. Sexual abuse treatment programs should also consider the long-term effects of victimization. Programs must plan prevention and intervention strategies to identify young girls who have had the dual experience of victimization and teen pregnancy.

## ◆ THE PERPETRATOR OF SEXUAL ABUSE

The phenomenon of having a sexual attraction for prepubertal children has been defined as **pedophilia** and having a sexual attraction for pubertal children as **ephebephilia**. The term *ephebephile* is rarely used today. For the purpose of this chapter, a pedophile will be defined as an adult who prefers to have sex with children. The pedophile has recurrent, intense sexual urges and sexually arousing fantasies involving children. Although pedophiles prefer to have sex with children, they can and do have sex with adults. Some even have sex with adults specifically to gain access to children.

About 85% of all reported perpetrators are male, and they may come from any profession or trade. It should be noted that this figure may be inaccurate due to the belief that most female child molesters are not reported.

*While little is known about female perpetrators, two assumptions are made:*

1.  Males may be less traumatized by sexual abuse, seeing it as part of coming of age rather than an abusive act.

2.  Female/female abuse is probably underreported, with the victims finding the female abuser less frightening than a male abuser and subsequently being less likely to report the abuse. Those females who have been reported were baby-sitters, younger girls, and occasionally older women.

Pedophiles and child molesters are not necessarily the same. A child molester sexually molests children, whereas a pedophile has a sexual preference for children and fantasizes about having sex with them, but if he does not act it out, he is not a child molester. Some pedophiles act out their fantasies in legal ways by engaging in sexual activity with adults who look, act, or dress like children. Not all child molesters are pedophiles. A person who prefers to have sex with an adult may decide to have sex with a child. If the sexual fantasies of these individuals do not focus on children, they are not pedophiles.

Groth et al. (1982) divided child molesters into two groups, **regressed** and **fixated**. A regressed individual has a primary sexual orientation toward adults of the opposite sex. Under conditions of stress, this individual may psychologically regress to an earlier psychosexual age and engage in sex with children. Dietz (1983) included the regressed abuser as part of his situational group. The fixated child molester (preferential group of Dietz) has a primary sexual orientation toward children.

Approximately 75% to 80% of abusers are known to their victims. They may be surrogate father figures, especially in families where the father is absent, either physically or emotionally. The child molester usually slowly, consciously or unconsciously, conditions the child. Most do not want to hurt the child. The amount of force or aggression used in their abuse differs. They may be involved in a wide variety of other variant paraphilias, such as exhibitionism, voyeurism, frotteurism, masochism, or sadism.

*Araji and Finkelhor (1985) reviewed existing research on pedophilia and noted the following:*

1. Children have a special meaning to pedophiles because children lack dominance. They called this emotional congruence.

2. Pedophiles have an unusual pattern of sexual arousal toward children, which they called deviant sexual arousal.

3. Pedophiles seem blocked in their social and heterosexual relationships. This they labeled blockage.

4. Many pedophiles use alcohol or other drugs to lower their inhibitions before abusing children. This was termed disinhibition.

The median age of the pedophile at first conviction is reported as 34.5 years for heterosexuals and 30.2 for homosexuals (Bancroft, 1989). Many begin to abuse children at much younger ages. Lanyon (1986) noted that the child molester is usually a respectable, otherwise law-abiding person, who, because of that respectability, may escape detection and prosecution. Abel et al., (1987) reported that the average child molester is a young, well-educated, middle-class, married, Caucasian (61%) male who is employed in a stable job at a good salary.

Among child molesters, Dietz (1983) proposed two broad categories: **situational** and **preferential**. Lanning (1991) prepared a monograph for law-enforcement officers investigating cases of child sexual exploitation. He reviewed the literature and, following Dietz's recommendations, classified child molesters (**Table 8-2**).

## SITUATIONAL CHILD MOLESTERS

The **situational child molester** does not have a true sexual preference for children; sexuality with children may range from a single act to numerous encounters. He abuses not only children but also other vulnerable individuals, such as those who are elderly, sick, or disabled. Four major patterns of behavior are recognized in this category *(see Table 8-2).*

The **regressed** offender, a subcategory of the situational molester, has low self-esteem and poor coping skills. He turns to children as a sexual substitute. His main criterion is availability. He coerces the child into having sex.

---

**Table 8-2. Classification of Child Molesters**

Situational child molesters
    Regressed
        Morally indiscriminate
        Sexually indiscriminate
        Inadequate

Preferential child molesters
    Pedophile

---

The **morally indiscriminate** individual sexually abuses children as part of a general pattern of abuse. He uses people, and abuses everyone he comes in contact with. He lies, cheats, or steals when it is to his advantage and whenever he thinks he can get away with it. His main criteria are vulnerability and opportunity. He uses force, lures, or manipulation to obtain his victims. His victims usually are strangers or acquaintances, but they can also be his own children.

The **sexually indiscriminate** individual is discriminating in his behavior except when it comes to sex. He is willing to try anything sexual. His main criterion is sexual experimentation. He has sex with children because they are new and different. The children may be his own, and he may also provide them for other adults as part of group sex.

The **inadequate** individual belongs to a group whose pattern of behavior includes psychoses, personality disorders, mental retardation, and senility; he can be classified as the social outcast, the withdrawn, or the unusual. This person becomes sexually involved with children out of insecurity or curiosity. He finds children nonthreatening and ideal for use in fulfilling his sexual fantasies. His sexual activity with children is impulsive.

## PREFERENTIAL CHILD MOLESTERS

Preferential child molesters focus their sexual fantasies on children. They have sex with children because they are sexually attracted to and prefer children. Their specific character traits vary, but their sexual behavior is highly predictable. Their problem is a need for frequent and repeated sex with children, so they have the potential to molest large numbers of victims. Three patterns of behavior are recognized in this category (**Table 8-3**).

| Table 8-3. Patterns of Behavior |
| --- |
| Seduction |
| Introversion |
| Sadism |

### SEDUCTION

This offender seduces his victims. He courts them, giving them attention, affection, and gifts over a period of time, gradually lowering their sexual inhibitions. His victims are willing to yield to sex for the attention, affection, and gifts they have received. These offenders are often involved with multiple victims at once, in essence a child sex ring, including a group of children in the same class at school, in the same scout troop, or in the same neighborhood. This individual is a master seducer of children because he is able to identify with them. He knows how to talk to children and, more importantly, he knows how to listen to them. He frequently selects children who are already victims of emotional abuse or neglect. His adult status and authority are important in the seduction process.

### INTROVERSION

This offender has a preference for children but lacks the personality skills necessary to seduce them. He uses little verbal communication, and usually molests strangers and very young children. He is likely to frequent areas where children congregate, watching them and hoping to find an opportunity to engage them in a sexual encounter. To have access to children, he might marry a woman with children or have his own children.

### SADISM

This preferential offender, in order to be aroused and gratified, must inflict pain on the victim. He uses lures or force to access his victims. He is more likely than other preferential child molesters to abduct and murder his victims.

## IDENTIFYING PEDOPHILES

A pedophile's sexual behavior is repetitive and predictable. The four major characteristics of the pedophile and the indicators of each are shown in **Table 8-4**. These characteristics can help identify the pedophile, but they are not diagnostic.

**Table 8-4. Characteristics of the Pedophile**

1. Long-term and persistent patterns of behavior.
    - Sexual abuse in background
    - Limited social contact as a teenager
    - Premature separation from military
    - Frequent and unexpected moves
    - Prior arrests
    - Multiple victims
    - Planned, repeated, or high-risk attempts

2. Children as preferred sexual objects.
    - Over 25, single, never married
    - Lives alone or with parents
    - Limited dating relationships if not married
    - If married, "special" relationship with spouse
    - Excessive interest in children
    - Associates and circle of friends are young
    - Limited peer relationships
    - Age and gender specificity
    - Refers to children as objects

3. Well-developed techniques in obtaining victims.
    - Skilled at identifying vulnerable victims
    - Identifies with children
    - Has access to children
    - Activities with children often excluding adults
    - Seduces with attention, affection, and gifts
    - Skilled at manipulating children
    - Has hobbies and interests appealing to children
    - Shows sexually explicit material to children

4. Sexual fantasies focusing on children.
    - Youth-oriented decorations in house or room
    - Photographing of children
    - Collecting child pornography or child erotica

*(After K. V. Lanning, 1991.)*

As in any profile of indicators, no single indicator or group of indicators is sufficient for an absolute identification. Knowledge of the case and common sense should prevail. If enough of these indicators are present, there is cause to believe that the individual is a pedophile. However, it must be reemphasized that not all pedophiles are child molesters.

1. **Long-Term and Persistent Patterns of Behavior.** Most of these indicators are self-evident. Several need expanding.
    a. **Sexual abuse in background.** Fortunately the great majority of victims of child sexual abuse do not become offenders; however, most offenders were victims. The pedophile's sexual preference for children usually begins in early adolescence. The pedophile often parallels the patterns of his own abuse on his victims, for example, choosing a victim of the same age as he was when he was abused or choosing the same acts. For this reason, all victims of sexual abuse must receive counseling. This should also include any child who is a perpetrator in order to, hopefully, through therapy, abort a career of abuse.
    b. **Frequent and unexpected moves.** Pedophiles frequently show a pattern of living in one place for several years with a good job and then suddenly moving and changing jobs. When identified, pedophiles are often forced to leave town; this was, and still is, a common way to deal with the problem.
    c. **Multiple victims.** This, along with collecting child pornography, is one of the most important indicators. If a pedophile is caught molesting one child, chances are great that he has molested or attempted to molest other children. A concerted effort should be made to identify the multiple victims.

    In 1987 Abel and associates asked 377 child molesters, who had committed sexual acts against children outside of their homes, to reveal the sexual crimes they had committed. The researchers assured confidentiality and immunity from prosecution. These 377 adults had victimized a total of 4,435 girls and 22,981 boys. They acknowledged 5,197 acts of abuse against the girls and 43,100 against the boys. The study also included 203 perpetrators who were sexually involved with children within the home (incest). These 203 incest perpetrators accosted 286 female victims and 75 male victims. They committed a total of 12,927 incestuous acts against the girls and 2,741 against the boys. Fuller (1989) confirmed these findings. Obviously, a single child molester has the potential of committing hundreds of sexual acts on hundreds of children. To stop one abuser can save hundreds of future victims.

2. **Age and Gender Specificity.** Most pedophiles prefer children of a specific sex in a specific age range. Pedophiles attracted to young children such as toddlers may not show sex specificity.

3. **Well-Developed Techniques in Obtaining Victims**
    a. **Access to children.** This is one of the most important indicators of a pedophile. The pedophile will have a method of gaining access to children. A pedophile may seek employment where he will be in contact with children or where he can specialize in dealing with children.
    b. **Shows sexually explicit material to children.** This is done to misrepresent standards and try to convince the child that these acts are normal.

4. **Sexual Fantasies Focusing on Children**
    a. **Collecting child pornography or child erotica.** As mentioned earlier, this indicator is one of the most significant characteristics of a pedophile. Pedophiles almost always collect child pornography or child erotica. Their collection is their most cherished possession. A search for child pornography is therefore urgent. As soon as legally possible, law enforcement must obtain a warrant to search for child pornography or erotica. If there is a long delay, the

pedophile will learn of the investigation and move or hide his collection.

Another characteristic to be noted about his collection is constancy—he never has enough and he never throws anything away. It is also well-organized. He maintains detailed, neat, orderly records. He is not likely to destroy the collection. He is concerned about the security of his collection, so he hides it in a safe place where he has easy access to it.

## THE PEDOPHILE'S DEFENSES

In dealing with pedophiles, the practitioner must be aware of their orientation and their responses to the situation. Evaluation of these responses may be helpful in determining whether abuse has indeed taken place.

### DENIAL

Usually the first reaction of a child molester to discovery will be denial. He may act shocked, surprised, or indignant about the allegations. Alternatively, he might admit to an act but deny the intent was sexual gratification.

### MINIMIZATION

If the evidence against him rules out denial, the offender may attempt to minimize what he has done. He might claim that it happened on one or two isolated occasions or that he only touched or caressed the victim.

### JUSTIFICATION

A child molester typically attempts to justify his behavior, usually blaming the victim and claiming that the victim seduced him, or initiated the sexual activity, or is promiscuous or a prostitute.

### FABRICATION

The child molester may create ingenious stories to explain his behavior and dispel any misunderstanding that he is an abuser. The stories range from ludicrous to believable.

### MENTAL ILLNESS

The child molester may claim mental illness, stating that he had no control over his actions. He may state that he did not choose to be what he is; it was an act of God and he is the victim.

### SYMPATHY

Here the offender expresses regret for what happened. He tries to convince his accusers that he is a good person — law-abiding, God-fearing, and all-American. He pleads for another chance based on his good record and swears that it will never happen again.

### ATTACK

The pedophile may decide that the best defense is a good offense. He may harass, threaten, or bribe victims and witnesses. He may attack the reputation of the investigating officer or the motives of the prosecutor. He may become violent.

## GUILTY, BUT NOT GUILTY

This defense involves a plea of nolo contender. The offender states that he is pleading guilty to spare the children the trauma of having to testify or because he has no money to defend himself. This plea saves the offender from acknowledging responsibility for his acts.

**It should be noted that after arrest or conviction the offender is at risk for suicide. Family and friends of the accused frequently blame the investigators for the perpetrator's death should a suicide attempt be successful.**

## ◆JUVENILE SEX OFFENDERS

The importance of identifying juvenile offenders is becoming increasingly more apparent. Changing one's sexual preference is not an easy task, but if it is possible, it makes sense to begin at an early age. In one research project on 411 adult offenders, 58% reported the onset of deviant sexual interest in adolescence (Abel et al., 1985). In another report (Groth et al., 1982) 60% to 80% of adult offenders admitted that they began their deviant sexual behaviors as adolescents. Rogers and Tremain (1984), in a study of 401 child sex abuse cases, reported that 56% of the male child victims and 28% of the female child victims reported being abused by a juvenile offender. Two other studies had similar results (Showers et al., 1983; Faber et al., 1984).

A national database (Ryan, 1991) on 1,600 juvenile offenders indicates that juvenile sexual offenders range in age from 5 to 19 years of age, with a median age between 14 and 15. These offenders represent all ethnic, racial, and socioeconomic classes; 90% are male, and more that 60% of the sexual offenses involve penetration. Ninety percent select a victim known to them, and the most common age of the victim is 7 to 8 years of age.

The juvenile offender is characterized as lacking assertive and social skills and having low academic performance, learning problems, and learning disabilities. Depression can also be a major characteristic in the juvenile sex offender (Becker, 1994). One study of 293 male adolescent offenders (Fehrenbach et al., 1986) reported that 44% committed nonsexual offenses before their first sexual offense.

## ◆PATTERNS OF ABUSE

Suzanne Sgroi was the first to point out that sexual encounters between adults and children usually follow a predictable progressive pattern involving engagement, sexual interaction, secrecy, disclosure, and suppression. Perpetrators look for opportunities to be alone with children and engage in sexual activity. After victimization, most perpetrators impose secrecy, which eliminates accountability and enables repetition of the behavior. A suppression phase often follows the disclosure. Others have modified and expanded Sgroi's original theory.

### RITUALISM AND SATANIC WORSHIP

Child protection workers often see children who tell of being subjected to sadistic and perverted acts that frequently accompany sexual abuse. They attribute these acts to ritualism or satanic worship.

Jonker and Jonker-Bakker (1991) reported the results of interviews of 98 children 4 to 11 years of age, and Young et al., (1991), in the same journal, reported the results of interviews of 37 adults who described similar abuse as children. They described sadistic activity such as passing sticks or objects into the vagina, anus, or penis.

The children told of severe physical violence and threats of violence. The children were young when first initiated into these activities. Sex between children was promoted by the abusers. The children described defecation and urination during sexual activity and reported that they were given drugs and/or alcohol before and during these activities. Some children said that the abusers dressed up with masks, robes, and other unusual clothes. Often the abuse involved more than one child. Pornography was frequently a prominent feature. These acts were coordinated into a satanic ritual and belief system. The children told of being tortured, witnessing animal and human sacrifice, ingesting body parts and fluids, and taking part in burial ceremonies.

The 37 adults in the Young et al. (1991) report were dissociative disorder patients who came from separate clinical settings and geographical locations. The most frequently reported types of ritual abuse are listed in **Table 8-5.** The clinical syndrome includes dissociative states with satanic overtures, severe post-traumatic stress disorder, survivor guilt, bizarre self-abuse, unusual fears, sexualization of sadistic impulses, indoctrinated beliefs, and substance abuse.

Many child protection workers are skeptical of this form of abuse. Lanning (1991) states that the problem of discussing the ritualistic abuse of children is how to define it. He does not use the term "ritualistic abuse" because he feels it is misleading and counterproductive, as is the use of the word satanic.

Lanning goes on to state that not all ritualistic activity is spiritually motivated and that not all spiritually motivated ritualistic activity is satanic. When a victim describes what might be determined ritualistic activity, several possibilities must be considered. The activity may be part of the excessive religiosity of mentally disturbed offenders, it may be a part of sexual ritualism, or it may be incidental to any real abuse. The offenders may be engaging in ritualistic activity as part of child abuse and exploitation. The motivation may not be to indoctrinate the child into a belief system, but to lower the inhibitions of, control, manipulate, or confuse the child. Lanning warns that labeling this abuse as ritualistic means to apply the same definition to all acts within all spiritual belief systems.

Lanning further states that the idea of secretive individuals regularly killing people as part of a ritual or ceremony and getting away with it is possible but the number of alleged cases has grown so that there are hundreds of victims alleging that thousands of offenders have murdered tens of thousands of people, and there is little or no corroborative evidence. One cannot ignore the lack of physical evidence, that no bodies have been found, or that no other physical evidence has been left following alleged violent murders. It would be difficult to successfully commit a large-scale conspiracy crime because the more people involved in any crime conspiracy, the more difficult it is to get away with it. Intra-group conflicts, resulting in individual self-serving disclosures, are likely to occur in any group involved in organized kidnapping, baby breeding, and human sacrifice. The U.S. Department of Justice estimates that 52 to 158 children, the majority between 14 and 17 years of age, are kidnapped and murdered by strangers each year (Lanning, 1991). There is no evidence, however, to support claims that hundreds to thousands of children are being sacrificed or abused in satanic rituals.

Why would victims describe events that cannot be true? Some of the allegations are impossible. They tell of victims who were cut up and put back together and of sustaining severe injuries that leave no scars. Reports of human sacrifice, cannibalism, and vampirism, although possible, are highly improbable. There may be a genuine phenomenon to explain these allegations with different mechanisms responsible in different cases. The explanation for these claims probably lies in a complex set of dynamics. Ganaway (1989) discusses the psychological issues that might be involved in satanic allegations by adults. Putnam (1991) feels that the material generated by children may be influenced and/or misinterpreted by interviewers. Alternative explanations might involve misperception, offender trickery, or symbolism.

No one can prove with absolute certainty that ritualistic, satanic abuse has not occurred. To totally dismiss these allegations as impossible would be a mistake. Some of the allegations of child pornography are probable, and some have been corroborated by medical evidence and by offender confessions.

American law enforcement has been aggressively investigating the allegations of victims of ritualistic abuse. There is little or no evidence of large-scale baby breeding, human sacrifice, and organized satanic conspiracies.

There is great need for research in which criminal, health, and social service agencies are coordinated to study these allegations. It is up to mental health professionals to explain why victims are alleging things that cannot be proven. This area desperately needs study and research by rational, objective social scientists.

| Table 8-5. Percentage of 37 Patients Reporting 10 Ritual Abuses in Childhood | |
|---|---|
| **Abuse Reported** | **Patients (%)** |
| Sexual abuse | 100 |
| Witnessing and receiving physical abuse/torture | 100 |
| Witnessing animal mutilations/killings | 100 |
| Death threats | 100 |
| Forced drug usage | 97 |
| Witnessing and forced participation in human adult and infant sacrifice | 83 |
| Forced cannibalism | 81 |
| Marriage to Satan | 78* |
| Buried alive in coffins or graves | 72 |
| Forced impregnation and sacrifice of own child | 60* |

Total number of patients = 37. Total female patients = 33. Total male patients = 4.
*Percentages based on 33 female patients.
(From Young et al., 1991.)

This chapter will offer some general tenets that should guide the decisions involved in following a sexual abuse case. Specifically, we will cover principles involved in the history and medical evaluation, behavioral indicators, and the role and philosophy of the sexual abuse management clinic.

## ♦ THE HISTORY AND MEDICAL EVALUATION

There are three components to consider in evaluating the child suspected to be a victim of sexual abuse. The first, and most important, component is the history or the child's statement of what happened. The second component of the evaluation is assessing the behavioral patterns of the child, comparing them with the behavioral indicators typical of abused children, and then deciding which indicators the child is demonstrating, their importance, and their specificity. The third component of the evaluation is the physical examination. **Neither the physical examination nor the behavioral indicators should stand on their own; they can only support the history given by the child.**

In most medical assessments the history is the most important part of the evaluation of the patient. This is particularly true in the evaluation of a child suspected to be the victim of sexual abuse. Obtaining the child's statement requires an experienced individual who is patient and able to assess the child's developmental skills and the child's credibility. This individual must be able to resist the urge to find out all the details of the abuse before knowing more about the child and the family. **This is both the most difficult phase of the evaluation and the most important.** Every decision that follows hinges on a credible disclosure.

Too much emphasis has been placed on the physical examination. Most sexually abused children show no physical findings, so if one concludes that only those children with positive physical findings are credible, he will be doing a disservice to 60% to 70% of children claiming to be abused. Several physical findings, such as pregnancy in a child under 12 years of age and semen in the vagina, clearly diagnose abuse, but, without a clear statement from the child identifying the perpetrator, the investigation is stymied. The child may even deny abuse. The best option in this situation is to arrange for long-term supportive therapeutic intervention for the child with an experienced therapist who is skilled at talking with abused children. The practitioner must not make the mistake of becoming too anxious and aggressive with this child, or being too eager to learn all the details of the case, thus placing the child in a situation where she has to give an answer. She may give the wrong answer. Patience is essential because it may take several sessions before she is ready to trust the investigator and disclose information about abuse. Alternatively, she may never disclose. The primary concern at this point must be for the safety of the child and the extension of services to ensure that the child receives treatment, if necessary. While the practitioner might prefer to know the identity of the perpetrator, it may be best to be patient and wait for the child to disclose voluntarily.

The nature of the disclosure is important. When gathering background information, it is important to find out the circumstances of the child's disclosure, specifically why she disclosed the information, where the statement was given, and when it was disclosed.

*The following vignette illustrates:*

> Two siblings are sent to play in the yard. The older boy, Jimmy, is 15 years old, and the younger, Johnny, is 7. Their mother admonishes, "Jimmy, take care of Johnny. I expect you to behave and not to fight. Jimmy, I hold you responsible." There is a disagreement and Jimmy punches Johnny, leaving a considerable bruise. Johnny runs into the house, crying "Jimmy hurt me. He punched me. Look at my arm." Their mother can be certain that Johnny was hurt and that Jimmy was involved. She may not know all of the details, but with time and patience she will soon know.

Use the same set of circumstances and the same disagreement with the same results, but this time the mother is not home. When the upset and injured Johnny runs into the house, he finds no one there. Jimmy follows him into the house and pleads, "Please, don't tell Mom, she'll kill me, she'll ground me." Johnny calms down and Jimmy rewards him with a piece of candy. When Mom comes home, she is none the wiser about the incident until that night, when putting Johnny to bed she sees the bruise left by Jimmy. "How did you get that bruise?" she asks. Johnny, having promised his brother not to tell about the incident, responds, "I don't know, I don't remember." The mother pressures him for an explanation. What does Johnny do? The odds are he will keep his promise and protect Jimmy. If Mom persists, he may well lie. This does not imply that, under similar circumstances, all children will lie. But with these circumstances, with pressure for an answer from the mother, the optimum conditions for disclosure are compromised and the child is placed in a situation in which he may give an improper answer.

*An actual case involved the following circumstances:*

> A child was brought to the sexual abuse management clinic by the police. She had disclosed that, while at a day care center, a teenage boy employed by the center had injured her when he put a ballpoint pen into her vagina. She made a consistent and convincing disclosure of the incident. On physical examination the vaginal mucosa was erythematous with a small abrasion of the posterior fourchette. There was, to the right of the hymen, a blue dot. The examiner felt there was good evidence that someone had put a ballpoint pen in the child's vagina, as the child had said, leaving a blue dot. The police had the panties she had worn to the center the day before and there was a large spot of blood. It was the blood on the panties which had alerted the mother of the injury. The mother called the police, who arrested the boy. The boy denied he abused the child. Others working with him at the center said that the boy was never alone with the child, or in the bathroom, in which the abuse allegedly occurred. They further said that it would have been impossible to do what the child had described without being seen. The police investigated the bathroom scene and agreed with the center staff that it would have been difficult, if not impossible, to abuse the child in that location. The police and the sexual abuse management team felt certain the child was abused but wondered if the child might be protecting someone. The

mother was asked about the circumstances of the disclosure. She said that she had noted the blood on the child's panties when putting her to bed. The mother asked the child what had happened and who had hurt her. When the child refused to answer, the mother told her that if she did not tell who had hurt her, the child would not be allowed to go to bed. The child then gave her the boy's name and told of the incident. After further investigation, the police felt that the perpetrator was most likely the child's father.

While the nature of the disclosure is important, the nature of the questioning is equally important. Leading, demanding questions can distort the disclosure. Chapter 9 explores this in greater detail, focusing on specific preparation and questions that can be used in interviewing the child.

The investigator must be aware of the child's developmental level, verbal skills, and experiences and realize that young children think in concrete terms. Depending on the age, a child may have limited concepts regarding numbers and times. In addition, children generally have had limited experiences and their vocabulary will reflect this. If the child says, "He peed in my mouth," or "he got pee on me," he may be talking about urine, but he is most likely describing an ejaculation. Depending on the child's age, the child knows only one function for the penis—to urinate; therefore anything coming out of the penis must be urine. The child may say that "he cut me down there with a knife." She may not have been cut with a knife. The child knows how it feels to be cut with a knife and that was how it felt, so she feels that she must have been cut with a knife. What was it that hurt her? It may have been a finger, a fingernail, or a penis, but to the child it felt like a knife.

When a child relates the circumstances of an incident, he concentrates on central or core activity and has limited recollection of peripheral happenings and objects. For example, a 5-year-old girl stated that she had climbed up on an air conditioner and saw the father of a neighbor, her playmate, sexually abusing the child. She described what she saw happening. When asked where this had happened, she said it was in the bedroom. During the investigation of the home it was noted that the air conditioner from which the 5-year-old stated she had observed the abuse overlooked the kitchen. The investigators concluded the child was lying. That may be so, but most likely the child was relating central information and any incidental or peripheral information escaped her attention and memory. The longer the time since the event, the more peripheral details will escape memory. To a lesser degree, even adults miss details of an event.

Children may also have difficulty with number concepts and with how many times something happened. A child may readily count to 10, but when asked to count a number of objects, may not be able to do so. Days of the week, months, and seasons frequently mean nothing to them. The investigator must not depend on either what day of the week the incident happened or how many times when related by a child.

Children do purposely lie. Any parent or teacher can attest to this. Children usually lie to get out of trouble or to avoid trouble. However, the probability that children lie about sexual abuse has been greatly exaggerated. Jones (1986) studied 576 cases of sexual abuse reported to the Denver Department of Social Services; a total of 7.81% of the reports were determined to be fictitious: 6.25% of the total number were fictitiously made by an adult and a mere 1.56% by a child. Children may lie to protect, to deny, or to minimize what has happened. In a related sense, they may withhold information, giving a little bit at a time. Children may also lie with coercion or coaching, more often to deny abuse than to admit it, and with repeated questioning by different interviewers. The child who has been interviewed multiple times may interpret that as disbelief. She tires of telling the same story over and over and may embellish the facts, hoping to convince or please her interrogators.

## ◆ BEHAVIORAL INDICATORS OF SEXUAL ABUSE

A number of behavioral indicators reveal the possibility of abuse; most are nonspecific and can be seen in any child under stress. No behavioral indicator can provide absolute certainty that abuse has occurred, although several present strong supportive evidence for abuse.

Age-inappropriate knowledge of sex is at the top of the list. If a 3-year-old child gives explicit details of sexual activity, describing ejaculation, fellatio, or anal sex, or states that the abuser used a lubricant such as Vaseline or saliva, the investigator can be confident that the child learned this firsthand. Children may have fantasies that have sexual connotations, but those fantasies do not contain explicit detail regarding sexual acts. Children do not fantasize sexual abuse.

Other strong indicators of abuse are running away and attempting suicide. Platt and Kroth (1979) identified sexual abuse as one of the three main reasons why children run away from home. These authors also reported that 70% of adolescent drug addicts were involved in some form of family sexual abuse, that 75% of adolescent prostitutes were involved in incestuous relationships, and that 50% of the children in a reformatory in Maine and nearly all the children in a Chicago reformatory had been sexually molested before commitment.

Dissociative reaction or multiple personality, a controversial area of child sexual abuse, may explain memory loss and denial. Indications of dissociative reaction may be subtle. At the genital examination the child may suddenly become passive and distant after having been outgoing and relating well. Dissociative reaction can also explain why the child may have trouble remembering details; he has learned to block out unpleasant experiences.

Many children who have been abused show no behavioral indicators. It may be years after the abuse before the child, now an adult, manifests behavior indicators, frequently becoming aggressive or angry and having problems with interpersonal relationships.

## ◆ THE SEXUAL ABUSE MANAGEMENT CLINIC

The main purpose of the sexual abuse management clinic is to help abused children, make certain the child is safe from further abuse, and help the child and the family cope with and recover from the assault, both emotionally and physically. Too much emphasis has been placed on the legal aspects of abuse and prosecution of the perpetrator. Confessions aside, less than 3% of abuse cases go to trial (Peach, 1991). In my experience, less than 10% of rape kits are recovered by the police for use in prosecution, yet great emphasis has been placed on gathering evidence and following legal protocols for interviewing abused children and their families. **It is not appropriate to compromise the child's evaluation and therapy for the slim possibility of legal involvement. The first priority is to take care of the child. Evidence gathering must take second place.**

### EMERGENCY ROOM RESPONSIBILITIES

Sexual abuse cases do not belong in the emergency room, an often chaotic environment. Sexually abused children need a calm, nonthreatening environment, as do the parents. Unfortunately, they frequently come to the emergency room in the evening, the busiest time for emergency room personnel. The child usually has just made a statement about the abuse, but the parents cannot reach their physician for advice and therefore they panic. The emergency room should not turn them away, but rather should deal with the situation in an efficient, sensitive manner.

The physical examination should not be postponed if the abuse has occurred recently. If the child has been abused within the past week, it is advisable to arrange for the child to be seen while still in the emergency room or an emergency evaluation may be done in the sexual abuse clinic. If the abuse happened within 72 hours of the examination, a rape kit should be prepared. Rape kits are provided by police forensic departments with standard instructions for their preparation. Any clinic where victims of sexual abuse may be examined should have these kits immediately available.

If the abuse occurred longer than 7 days before, there is no need for an emergency examination, and the evaluator may delay the examination as long as there is certainty that the child is safe.

Personnel in the emergency room may show dismay when they realize there is no advantage to performing a physical examination and no way to obtain physical evidence. They must understand that they may be dealing with a psychiatric emergency, and the family is in crisis and needs reassurance.

*The emergency room personnel have the following responsibilities:*

1. Be certain the child is safe and will return to a safe environment.

2. Treat any condition that must be treated now; examples include pelvic inflammatory disease, *Neisseria gonorrhoeae* infection, other sexually transmitted diseases, or unrelated infections.

3. Help the family through the crisis. The child may have just disclosed and the family requires immediate emotional support.

4. Make a report to the child abuse hot line, if one has not already been made. If the assault was not by a caretaker, the case should be reported to a sex crimes unit.

5. Involve hospital social services. They will follow up with state services and the hot line, or, if necessary, will initiate the hot line call.

6. Schedule the child to be seen in the sexual abuse management clinic.

The most important considerations are *(1)* the child is kept safe, *(2)* the perpetrator will not have access to her, *(3)* she will receive emergency psychiatric therapy if needed, and *(4)* any trauma or infection is noted and treated.

## ◆ PHILOSOPHY OF CARE FOR SEXUALLY ABUSED CHILDREN

To do an effective job when caring for the potentially sexually abused child and feel confident with decisions, it is important that one develop a sound philosophy. Each team should develop a protocol as a guide, including a mission statement and a working philosophy, or position.

*The following statements of philosophy were taken from a sexual abuse management protocol. Several have been expanded to provide clarification:*

1. The sexual abuse management team is primarily concerned with identification of sexual abuse, crisis intervention, evidence gathering, and long-term therapy for the child and the family.

2. The workup of the sexually abused child is a team effort and should involve all team members. Communication between all team members is essential to ensure a favorable outcome.

3. The team is *not* an arm of the legal system; it is a resource for that system as well as for the state social system and the community.

   The team's function is not to put people in jail or take children away from families; these are functions of the court system. If the team provides the court with good information, the court can make good decisions.

4. Team personnel must guard against having blinders on regarding the possibility of sexual abuse, or they will miss all but the most obvious cases. On the other hand, they must also guard against being too hasty to diagnose sexual abuse. One must remain objective and open-minded in both directions.

5. Sexual abuse management requires special skills. Sexual abuse can have long-lasting psychological effects on the victim and family. Every effort should be made to lessen these sequelae. The sexual abuse clinic experience should not be worse than the actual sexual abuse.

6. Although sexual abuse is unique, it is still similar to other medical problems. Each team member must respect the other's role and allow the process to evolve as in any other medical situation.

7. The evaluation is patient-oriented. The team needs first to deal with the acute situation and to help the patient, yet the needs of others affected by the situation must not be forgotten. At all times, confidentiality must be maintained.

8. Sexual abuse is also a medicolegal problem involving gathering evidence. Although this is an important component, it must take second place to the needs of the child and family.

9. No matter how good a team is, it cannot resolve all problems and it cannot be all things to all people. Events and circumstances are not black or white, but are generally gray.

   A significant number of cases, especially those involving preverbal or nonverbal children, fall into a gray zone; the team may be able to decide that something happened but may not be able to determine whether it was sexual abuse or a misunderstanding of a benign event. Although the team may perceive the event as "gray," the family may view it otherwise and will require help in understanding and coping with the situation. Patience is essential.

10. The team cannot expect "justice" in all cases. The legal system must work with, among other things, the reality of admissible evidence and credible witnesses.

    Although everyone, from the family to the medical team to law enforcement personnel to the prosecutor, may believe a child has been abused, for a number of good reasons, not all cases go to court. No sensible prosecutor accepts a case for trial that he does not believe has a reasonable chance for a successful outcome. Families can become so caught up in seeking justice that they become dysfunctional; they can also drag the team into the mire of their cause.

11. Continuous education is a must.

    This can be accomplished in a number of ways, for example, intradepartmental and extradepartmental conferences and meetings, journals, and texts.

12. When dealing with the family and the perpetrator, the team must not judge or confront them.

    Judgment belongs in the courtroom, and confrontation is best handled by state social services and law enforcement personnel.

## ♦ ADDITIONAL CONCERNS IN CRISIS CENTERS

### REGIONAL CENTERS FOR ABUSE MANAGEMENT

The workup of the sexually abused child requires special skills. Just as these children do not belong in an emergency room, neither do they belong in a practitioner's office or in a general medical clinic. Ideally they should be seen in regional centers or child advocacy centers where there is a team of specialists. In that locale one person who is an expert at interviewing the abused child conducts the interview. The center should be equipped so that protective agencies, juvenile court, police, medical personnel, and the prosecuting attorney can witness the interview and have input. All interviews, even those involving the parents and the perpetrator, are carried out in the same setting, with one person asking the questions for all interested parties. The interviews can also be videotaped. In addition, this center should have facilities so that the medical evaluation can be conducted there. Ideally, each state should have enough of these units that they are easily accessible to all and provide 24-hour coverage.

| Table 8-6. Sexual Abuse Management Protocol |
| --- |

**Table of Contents**

I. **Mission Statement**
II. **Philosophy**
III. **Statement of Services**
IV. **Referral Process**
V. **Clinical Process**
    A. Physical Examination
    B. Follow-up Referrals
    C. Parent/Caregiver Interview
    D. Child Interview
        *1. Initial interview*
        *2. Subsequent interviews*
        *3. Use of dolls and other aids*
        *4. Videotaping*
        *5. Probability and Credibility Assessment*
VI. **Decision Making**
    A. Pre-evaluation
    B. Case Review
    C. Documentation
    D. Recommendations and Follow-up
VII. **Special Considerations**
    Multiple Victims/Multiple Suspects
VIII. **Training of Professionals and Others**
IX. **The Legal System and Testifying**

**Appendix**

I. **Colposcopic Protocol**
II. **Film Processing and Chain of Custody**
III. **Polaroid Photos**
IV. **Videotaping**
    A. Legal Guidelines
    B. Video Cassette Processing and Chain of Custody
    C. Medical Record Protocol on Videotape Cassettes
        *1. Protocol for viewing videos*
        *2. Preparing copies of videos*

**Clinic Forms**

    *1. State Form*
    *2. Parent Interview Form*
    *3. Child Interview Form*
    *4. Telephone Screening/Referral Form*

## PROTOCOL

To standardize procedures, it is advisable to employ a protocol that covers all aspects of the evaluation. It should be noted that no protocol is perfect and followed without exception, and no two cases are alike. Informed judgment must be employed in all evaluations. Nevertheless, a protocol sets the pace for the evaluation. The attorneys involved in the case often request a copy of the protocol that is to be followed and expect the practitioner to defend it.

A suggested protocol table of contents is shown in **Table 8-6**. While this can serve as a guide, each institution must develop a protocol that satisfies the clinic's needs and provides for local laws, hospital practices, etc.

## SCREENING PATIENTS

It is often necessary to screen which patients are to be evaluated in the clinic, especially if the number of patients that can be evaluated is limited. The schedule could be filled with patients who are only mildly suspected to have been abused—patients with nonspecific physical and behavioral indicators who have not disclosed information about being abused or who even deny abuse. A common complaint that must be handled comes from a divorced or separated parent, fighting custody, who calls after each visitation because the child cries when seeing the other parent and refuses to go with him or her. On return from visitation if the child gives any signs or symptoms, such as "a red vagina or anus," burning on urination, or suspicious acting-out, the parent demands a complete evaluation. While it is important to respond to cases appropriately, in my experience it is best to handle these calls by phone, employing an experienced person who can evaluate the situation and make referral to the family physician or pediatrician if appropriate. Other referrals that can be made by the abuse center in order to use their resources most effectively include parental counseling to supply education concerning the abuse problem and child or family counseling to handle other problems. As stated earlier, without a credible disclosure from the child, the case may well end up in frustration for all.

The sexual abuse management clinic at my institution accepts no walk-in patients. All cases are screened and the essentials noted. The team meets on a regular basis to discuss each case and prepare a plan before the patient is evaluated. The clinic evaluates only those children who have made a disclosure or who are symptomatic and recommended by a physician who requests further evaluation. Those patients who have specific behavioral indicators and who have not made any disclosure are interviewed by our therapist or recommended to another experienced counselor before a physical examination is performed.

# ◆QUESTIONS OFTEN ASKED REGARDING CHILDREN'S CREDIBILITY

## ARE CHILDREN'S MEMORIES RELIABLE?

Although children recall less than adults do, what they can recall can be accurate. Young children spontaneously recall less information than older children and adults; their developing memories are not as proficient at the complex task of free recall (Myers et al., 1989). However, if the child understands and is more familiar with a particular event than an adult is, the child may be more accurate (Goodman & Helgeson, 1985).

The questioner must consider the characteristics of children's accounts of abuse. As already noted, children are more likely to correctly answer questions about the main actions that took place (central actions) than those about the peripheral details. As a result, it may be difficult for a child to describe the perpetrator, especially if he is an unfamiliar person. Children also have trouble answering questions requiring abstract conclusions, such as a person's motivations—the "why" questions.

Consistency is often lacking in children's stories. Developmentally younger children are less able to relate a story consistently (Austin et al., 1977). Memories in children and adults contain inaccuracies and distortions of the details recalled. Children are not sophisticated enough to protect themselves against the appearance of inconsistency (Myers et al., 1989). They have difficulty evaluating their reports for possible errors, omissions, inconsistencies, or contradictions. However, it is not the small details (the exact age, the number of incidents, the time) that are essential, but rather the validation of the abuse that is critical. **The question is not whether there are inaccuracies in memory, but whether memory retains essential truths** ( Austin et al., 1977).

Young children do not understand that they can ask for clarification when they do not understand what is being asked of them (Myers et al., 1989). They often will not ask for a question to be repeated or clarified, even if they do not understand what is being asked. Instead, they are apt to give an answer. Thus adults must not only try to ask questions children can understand, but they must also make certain that the child does in fact understand the question.

The fact that children may not disclose abuse until months or years after the assault increases the chance that they will have forgotten part of what occurred. Whether children's memories fade more quickly than adults' memories is not known. If they do, children are at a relative disadvantage. Children are less likely than adults to fill memory gaps with inferred information. Adults who have forgotten part of what happened will attempt to relate a believable, coherent story. Because a child may be less able to do so, his or her testimony may appear less coherent, even if it is more accurate, than the adult's (Goodman & Helgeson, 1985).

Lenore Terr (1988) studied the verbal and behavioral remembrances of 20 children who suffered psychological trauma before age 5 years. She reported that short, single traumatic events are more likely to be remembered in words, and, at any age, behavioral memories of trauma remain quite accurate and true to the events that stimulated them.

## ARE CHILDREN SUGGESTIBLE?

Children's answers, like those of adults, can be altered by suggestion. Children usually say so little in response to questioning that adults are tempted to ask suggestive questions. However, this can lead to inaccurate answers. Examples of suggestive questions include those phrased as follows: "John taught you that, didn't he?" or "The car was speeding, wasn't it?" These types of questions should be avoided. In addition, if the questioner is a person of high status as perceived by the child, such as a policeman in uniform, the child can be suggestible.

Although research indicates that children can be more suggestible than adults, it is important to note that in most of these studies the children and adults were asked suggestive questions about relatively *peripheral* information. It is more difficult to lead a child into making a false statement about *central* information. No recent studies indicate that children can be led to fabricate an entire event (Goodman & Helgeson, 1985).

## IS THERE A FALSE MEMORY SYNDROME?

Scientific findings do not support a simplistic explanation that disclosures of childhood abuse are the result of therapist suggestion. This idea may be more indicative of a wish to find another explanation for these terrible stories and a need to locate the problem outside of ourselves (Olio, 1994).

Herman (1992) said that a focus on a false memory "syndrome" exaggerates the role of memory in the determination of a diagnosis of post-traumatic stress disorder. Childhood abuse is confirmed by a constellation of symptoms, including memories, affective fragmentation, flooding and numbness, chronic patterns of denial and dissociation, and current life distress. These patterns, the hallmarks of childhood trauma, are of biological reactivity, with both constructive and intrusive symptoms, and are not a single memory that might have been suggested (Herman 1992).

## DON'T CHILDREN USUALLY LIE ABOUT SEXUAL ABUSE?

Children's reporting errors are more apt to be acts of omission than commission, meaning they are more likely to forget or deny information than to fabricate events that did not occur (Myers et al., 1989). Cantwell (1981) determined that children's allegations of sexual abuse were usually true, perhaps as much as 90% of the time. Nonetheless, one must be open-minded. It is possible that the allegation is a false statement arising in the mind of an adult and is imposed on the mind of the child through suggestion, indoctrination, or group contagion. The allegation can also be the result of a delusion or confabulation by the child or involve perpetrator substitution or lying by the child (Bernet, 1993).

For more information on these topics, see Chapters 11 and 12.

## ◆ BIBLIOGRAPHY

Abel, G, Becker, J, Mittleman, M, Cunningham-Rathner, J, Rouleau, J, and Murphy, W: Self-reported sex crimes of nonincarcerated paraphiliacs, *J Interpersonal Violence* 2:3-25, 1987.

Abel, G, Mittelman, M, and Becker, J: Sex offenders: Results of assessment and recommendations for treatment, In Ben-Aron, Hucker, and Webster, eds: *Clinical Criminology: Current Concepts*, M & M Graphics, Toronto, 1985.

American Humane Society: Sexual Abuse of Children, American Humane Society, 1981.

Araji, S, and Finkelhor, D: Explanations of pedophilia: Review of empirical research, *Bull Am Acad Psychiatry Law* 13:17-37, 1985.

Austin, VD, Ruble, DN, and Trabasso, T: Recall and order effects as factors in children's moral judgements, *Child Dev* 48:470-474, 1977.

Bancroft, J: *Human Sexuality and Its Problems*, Churchill Livingstone, London, 1989.

Becker JV: Offenders: Characteristics and treatments: Sexual abuse of children, *In The Future of Children,* Center For The Future Of Children, Vol 4, No 2, pp. 176-197, 1994.

Bernet, W: False statement and the differential diagnosis of abuse allegations, *J Am Acad Child Adolesc Psychiatry* 32:903-910, 1993.

Boyer, D, and Fine, D: Sexual abuse as a factor in adolescent pregnancy and child maltreatment, *Family Plan Perspect* 24:1, 4-11, 1992.

Brassard, MR: Sexually abused children: Identification and suggestions for intervention, *School Psychol Rev* 12:93-97, 1983.

Cantwell, HB: Sexual abuse of children in Denver, 1979: Reviewed with implications for pediatric intervention and possible prevention, *Child Abuse Negl* 5:75-85, 1981.

*Child molesters: A behavioral analysis*, ed 3, National Center for Missing and Exploited Children, 1992.

Conte, J, and Schuerman, J: Factors associated with an increased impact of child sexual abuse, *Child Abuse Negl* 11:201-211 1987.

DeFrancis, V: *Protecting the child victim of sex crimes committed by adults, final report*, American Humane Association, Children's Division, Denver, 1969.

DeVine, RA: *Incest: A review of the literature; Sexual abuse of children: Selected readings,* US Department of Health and Human Services, DHHS Publication No. (OHDS)78-30161, Nov 1980.

Dietz, PE: Sex offenses: Behavioral aspects. In SH Kadish et al., eds: *Encyclopedia of Crime and Justice*, New York Free Press, New York, 1983.

Farber, E, Showers, J, and Johnson, C: The sexual abuse of children: A comparison of male and female victims, *Clin Child Psychol* 13:294-297, 1984.

Fehrenbach, P, Smith, W, Monastersky, C, and Deisher, R: Adolescent sexual offenders: Offender and offense characteristics, *Am J Orthopsychiatry* 56:225-233, 1986.

Ganaway, GK: Historical truth versus narrative truth: Clarifying the role of exogenous trauma in the etiology of multiple personality disorder and its variants, *Dissociation* 2:205-220, 1989.

Goodman, GS, and Helgeson, VS: Child sexual abuse: children's memory and the law, *Univ Miami Law Rev* 40:181-208,1985.

Greenwood, CL, Tangalos, EG, and Maruta, T: Prevalence of sexual abuse, physical abuse, and concurrent traumatic life events in a general medical population, *Mayo Clin Proc* 65:1067-1071, 1990.

Groth, A, Longo, R, and McFadin, J: Undetected recidivism among rapists and child molesters, *Crime Delinquency* 28:450-458, 1982.

Groth, N, and Birnbaum, H: Adult sexual orientation and attraction to underage persons, *Arch Sex Beh* 7:175-181, 1978.

Herman, J: *Trauma and Recovery*, Basic books, New York, 1992.

Jones, DPH: Reliable and fictitious accounts of sexual abuse in children, *J Interpersonal Violence*, June 1986.

Jones, DPH: Ritualism and child abuse, *Child Abuse Negl* 15:163-170, 1991.

Jonker, F, and Jonker-Bakker, P: Experiences with ritualist child sexual abuse: A case study for the Netherlands, *Child Abuse Negl* 15:191-196, 1991.

Lanning, KV: Ritual abuse: A law enforcement view or perspective, *Child Abuse Negl* 15:171-173, 1991.

Lanyon, R: Theory and treatment in child molestation, *J Consult Clin Psychol* 54:176-182, 1986.

Moore, KA, Nord, CW, and Peterson, JL: Nonvoluntary sexual activity among adolescents, *Fam Plann Perspect* 21:110-114, 1989.

Myers, JEB, et al: Expert testimony in child abuse litigation, *Nebraska Law Review* 68:95-107, 1989.

Olio, KA: Truth in memory, *Am Psychologist,* pp. 442-443,  May 1994.

Peach, G: Personal communication, 1991.

Platt, JS, and Kroth, RL: The behavioral Q sort as an aid in the responsible modification of adolescent's behavior, *Adolescence* 14:241-246, 1979.

Putnam, FW: The satanic ritual abuse controversy, *Child Abuse Negl* 15:175-179, 1991.

Rogers, C, and Tremain, T: Clinical interventions with boy victims of sexual abuse, In Stuart and Greer, eds: *Victims of sexual aggression*, Van Nostrand Reinhold, New York, 1984, pp. 91-104.

Ryan G: Juvenile sex offenders: Defining the population, In Ryan and Lane, eds: *Juvenile Sexual Offending*, Lexington Books, Lexington, MA, 1991, pp. 3-8.

Showers, J, Farber, E, and Joseph, J: The sexual victimization of boys: A three-year survey, *Health Values: Achieving High-Level Wellness* 7:15-18, 1983.

Terr, L: What happens to early memories of trauma? A study of twenty children under age five at the time of documented traumatic events, *J Am Acad Child Adolesc Psychiatry* 27:96-104, 1988.

Young, WC, Sachs, RG, Braun, BG, and Watkins, RT: Patients reporting ritual abuse in childhood: A clinical syndrome. Report of 37 cases, *Child Abuse Negl* 15:181-189, 1991.

# PHYSICAL EXAMINATION IN SEXUAL ABUSE

JAMES A. MONTELEONE, M.D.
JOHN R. BREWER, M.D.
TIMOTHY J. FETE, M.D.

*A 9-year-old girl was admitted to the hospital via the emergency room. She had been struck by an automobile while running across the street. She had multiple acute abrasions to the hip, head, and arm. She had been unconscious for a short period, and it was decided to admit her for observation overnight. A routine urine sample was found to have live sperm. The child denied sexual contact.*

*Physical findings revealed vaginal changes consistent with chronic sexual abuse.*

*The family vehemently denied the possibility of abuse. The child was placed in a foster home and after several counseling sessions continued to insist she was never sexually abused. The case was never resolved, and the juvenile court returned her to her family.*

The physical examination of children suspected to be victims of sexual abuse is not difficult if the parents and child are properly prepared. To achieve this, several steps must be taken. First, the practitioner explains to the parents and child what will take place during the examination, giving them an overview of the process. Next, the child and parents, if appropriate, are shown the various instruments that will be employed, including the stethoscope, ophthalmoscope, otoscope, and colposcope. The child may be allowed to examine and even use them. When the child realizes the examination is much like a well-child examination in the family physician or pediatrician's office, he or she usually cooperates.

## ◆DEVELOPING RAPPORT

The examiner should spend time getting acquainted with the child to establish rapport. Helping the child talk about special interests, school, sports, or music lessens the tension and enables the child to relax, which is important for the vaginal and anal examinations. The examiner should be patient and friendly. Children are frightened by a hurried or demanding examiner, but they generally respond to and cooperate with one who is pleasant and fun. It is not necessary to wear a lab coat or other hospital and medical garb; such apparel may be frightening for younger children. **Take the time necessary to earn the child's confidence.** Pediatricians are particularly adept at this, having learned through their experience to communicate with children at the child's level and thereby effectively gaining their trust. Above all, **DO NOT make the examination experience worse than the abuse.**

If a nurse will be assisting with the examination, he or she should also help in preparing the child for the examination. The nurse spends time developing a relationship with the child and helps to explain to the child what is going to happen during the examination. This eases the child's fears and ensures better cooperation during the examination.

## ◆PROVIDING REASSURANCE

The examiner assures the child that the examination will not cause pain and that he will stop whenever the child wishes. The child must also be assured that the examination is important and necessary.

It is unusual for a child to be badly frightened about or resistive to the examination. **Examining a terrified, resistive child by force is not appropriate.** Rather than force the child to submit to the examination, the child should be sent home and instructions given to the caretaker to reassure the child and return on another day. On the next visit the child is often much more cooperative. However, children younger than 3 years of age frequently cry during any examination procedure.

## ◆REVIEWING PREVIOUS RECORDS

If another physician has seen the child, it is important to obtain those medical records. Records from previous hospitalizations can also provide valuable information. The object of such research is old injuries. In particular when the child has physical evidence of injury, it is important to document whether there was a previous accident, perhaps attended by another physician, which might explain the finding, such as a genital injury. This is especially true when you are faced with an impaling injury that evidently happened several years before.

## ◆CONDUCTING THE PHYSICAL EXAMINATION

The help of a calm, sympathetic nurse, experienced in the evaluation of the sexually abused child, is essential during the examination. As already stated, the nurse can effectively reassure the child as well as be an advocate for the child during the examination. One other factor must be considered. This examination is very sensitive and the actions of the examiner can be misinterpreted. **During the examination, there MUST always be one other professional in the room in**

**addition to the examiner.** If possible, the parent of the same sex as the child should also be present during the examination. Occasionally an older child may prefer not to have a parent present during the examination, and this request should usually be honored. All adolescents should be given the choice of having a parent present during the examination.

Children who are forced to lie on an examining table for long periods may become apprehensive. Therefore the examination must be conducted as efficiently as possible.

Since embarrassment is a normal reaction, the examiner must respect the child's need for modesty at all times. An examining gown and sheet are used to cover the child, and only the portion of the body that is currently being examined is exposed. In addition, the examination should proceed as quickly as possible. For mutual protection of practitioners and patient, both the examiner and the nurse assisting should wear gloves during the examination.

## Observation

The examination begins with an evaluation of the child's general appearance; this should include looking for evidence of other abuse, such as loop marks or scars from previous injuries or burns; evaluating the status of the child's hygiene; checking nutritional status; assessing congenital anomalies, muscular development, and central nervous system abnormalities; determining whether the child is obese; and measuring vital signs, height, and weight.

Children who have been sexually abused often show signs of physical and emotional abuse. Their demeanor should be observed for signs of depression or dissociative behavior. The child and parents should realize that the examiner is interested in the whole child.

A thorough physical exam should follow with examination of the head, eyes, ears, nose, chest, and abdomen. Details of this examination may be found in pediatric textbooks.

## Genital Examination

### Normal Female Anatomy

The female external genitalia comprise the mons pubis, the labia majora, the labia minora, the vestibule of the vagina, and the clitoris (O'Rahilly, 1986) (**Figures 9-1 and 9-27**).

The *mons pubis* is the rounded, median elevation in front of the pubic symphysis. It consists mostly of an accumulation of fat. After puberty, the skin over it is covered with coarse hairs.

The *labia majora* (**Figure 9-2**) are homologous with the scrotum of the male. They are two elongated folds that run downward and backward from the mons pubis. Their outer aspects are covered by pigmented skin containing many sebaceous glands; hair obscures them after puberty. Their inner aspects are smooth and hairless. The labia majora are usually united in front by an anterior commissure. They are not united behind, but the forward projection of the perineal body into the pudendal cleft sometimes gives the appearance of a posterior commissure. This posterior meeting often has a folding, asymmetrical appearance that has been mistaken for abuse.

The *labia minora* (**Figure 9-2**) are the two small folds of skin located between the labia majora, at either side of the opening of the vagina. They end behind by joining the medial aspects of the labia majora and are usually connected with each other by a transverse fold, called the frenulum of the labia. In front, each labium divides into a lateral and a medial part. The lateral parts meet to form a fold over the glans clitoris, called the prepuce of the clitoris. The two medial parts unite below the clitoris to form the frenulum of the clitoris. The labia minora are devoid

*Figure 9-1a,b. Normal-appearing genital exam (Category I). Crescent-shaped hymen (H) with smooth edge except for a small mound (C) with a transverse ridge or rugae behind it; the opposite ridge (R) is better exposed. Other structures shown are the anterior column (B), the anterior hymenal attachment (A), the labia minora (D), and the fossa navicularis (E).*

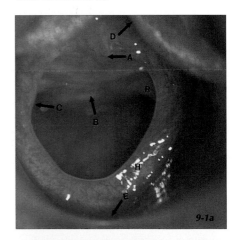

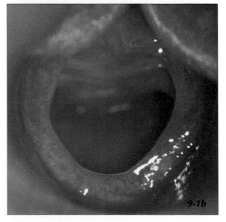

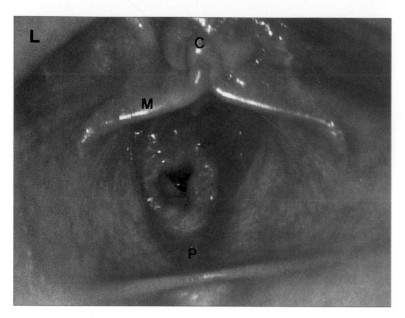

**Figure 9-2.** *Normal-appearing genital exam with a thickened, fimbriated hymen. Other structures shown are the labia majora (L), the labia minora (M), the clitoris (C), and the posterior fourchette (P).*

of fat, and the skin covering them is smooth, moist, and pink. They are hidden by the labia majora during childhood, when the labia majora contain less fat and are smaller. At puberty the labia minora change, become more pigmented, often protrude through the labia majora, and lose definition of the posterior ends when they elongate and blend into the vestibular mucosa.

The *vestibule of the vagina* is the area between the labia minora. It contains the openings of the vagina and the urethra. The external urethral orifice is a median slit situated behind the clitoris and immediately in front of the vaginal orifice. The vaginal orifice, larger than the urethral opening, is also a median cleft. Its size and appearance depend on the condition of the hymen. The fossa navicularis is a shallow depression in the vestibule between the vaginal orifice and the frenulum of the labia.

The *clitoris* (**see Figure 9-2**), like the penis, consists mainly of erectile tissue and is capable of enlargement as a result of engorgement with blood. Unlike the penis, it does not enclose the urethra. It is located behind the anterior commissure of the labia majora, and most of it is hidden by the labia minora.

The *vagina* has three layers: mucosa, muscular coat, and fibrous coat. The mucosa is lined by stratified squamous epithelium, which is influenced by hormonal change. The mucosa is thick and is marked by a number of transverse ridges, which are more prominent in the lower part of the vagina. These ridges are called vaginal rugae. A longitudinal ridge, termed the anterior column of the rugae, marks the anterior wall, and a similar ridge, termed the posterior column of the rugae, marks the posterior wall. A lower prominence of the anterior column is called the urethral carina or ridge, which is formed by the urethra.

The opening of the vagina into the vestibule is partially closed by the fold called the *hymen* (**see Figures 9-27 and 9-29**). The hymen varies in size and shape but is often concentric or less often annular (discussed later).

The *anal canal* is the part of the large intestine that extends from the level of the upper aspect of the pelvic diaphragm to the anus. The anus is the terminal orifice of the alimentary canal. Its circumference is called the anal verge. The pectinate line marks the lower limit of the anal valves around the circumference of the canal. The lower part of the anal canal differs in nerve supply, venous and lymphatic drainage, and type of epithelium above and below this line (**see Figure 9-24**).

Kellogg and Parra (1991) examined the genitalia of 123 normal nonabused female newborns to determine the incidence of variations of the posterior vestibule. The posterior vestibule was defined as the area above the perineum extending internally from the posterior commissure to the posterior hymenal border. They found that 93 (76%) of these children had no white spots or lines in the posterior vestibule, 17 (14%) had white spots in the posterior vestibule just internal to the posterior commissure, and 13 (10%) had white streaks extending from the posterior commissure into the posterior vestibule. In 10 (8%) of the 123 neonates the posterior vestibule was partially concealed by a lip formed by the perineum and posterior commissure positioned anterior to the vestibule.

They determined that such structures are normal anatomical variants and proposed that the white line be designated *linea vestibularis*. This structure is distinct from a median or perineal raphe. The raphe is a flesh-colored, slightly raised, perineal structure, whereas the linea vestibularis is an avascular, flat, posterior vestibule structure.

Posterior vestibule spots and lines are seen macroscopically and occur in the midline. No surrounding neovascularization or thickening of the structures is seen. The lines are distinct and without varying width. The spots occur just internal to the posterior commissure, whereas the line extends from the posterior commissure internally, but not up to the inferior hymenal border.

## FINDINGS IN STUDIES OF NONABUSED GIRLS

McCann et al. (1990) examined and photographed with the colposcope a sample of 93 nonabused prepubertal girls between the ages of 10 months and 10 years. Examination techniques included a supine labial separation approach, a supine labial traction method, and a prone knee-chest position. The findings in these children are summarized in **Table 9-1**. It should be noted that probably the only population one can be absolutely certain are not victims of sexual abuse are those in the newborn nursery. The report by Chadwick et al. (1989) was pivotal in describing what are clearly signs of abuse.

In one study of nonabused girls, Berenson et al. (1992) examined 211 girls. The study population consisted of 36% blacks, 33.6% white non-Hispanics, 29.9% Hispanics, and 0.5% Asians. Subjects had a mean age of $21 \pm 20.6$ (SD) months. Extensive labial agglutination was noted in 5% and partial agglutination in 17%. They noted a significant difference in hymenal configuration by age, with a fimbriated hymen the most common type (46%) in infants aged 12 months or younger and a crescentic hymen the most common (51%) in girls older than 24 months. No significant difference was noted in hymen configuration by race. Hymenal mounds were observed in 7%, hymenal tags in 3%, vestibular bands in 98%, longitudinal intravaginal ridges in 25%, and external ridges in 15% of subjects in whom the anatomy under study could be visualized. Hymenal notches (clefts) occurred superiorly and laterally on the hymenal rim but none were found interiorly on the lower half of the hymen. A narrow rounded hymenal ring with a transection was observed in 1 of 201 subjects and was not considered a normal finding. Transverse hymenal openings, measured only in annular and crescentic hymens, showed a mean that ranged from $2.5 \pm 0.8$ to $3.6 \pm 1.2$ mm and varied significantly with age.

Gardner (1992) examined the genitalia of 79 symptom-free young premenarchal girls not thought to have been sexually abused, aged between 3 months and 11 years, 7 months (mean, 5 years, 4 months). Gardner found increased vascularity (44%), midline avascular areas (27%), "ragged" posterior fourchette epithelium (18%), notch configuration of the posterior fourchette (10%), delicate tethers between the hymen and perihymen (14%), hymenal bumps between the 3 and 9 o'clock positions (11%), and asymmetry of the hymenal tissue (9%) **(Figures 9-3 and 9-4)**.

---

### Table 9-1. Genital Findings in Nonabused Girls

Genital findings
  Erythema of the vestibule (56%)
  Periurethral bands (50.6%)
  Labial adhesions (38.9%)
  Lymphoid follicles on the fossa navicularis (33.7%)
  Posterior fourchette midline avascular areas (25.6%)
  Urethral dilation
    With labial traction (90.5%)
    With the supine separation (79.3%)

Hymenal findings
  Mounds (33.8%)
  Projections (33.3%)
  Septal remnants (18.5%)

Intravaginal findings
  Vaginal ridges (90.2%)
  Rugae (88.7%)

*The cervix was visualized without a speculum in 69% of the children during the knee-chest examination.*

Unusual findings*
  Posterior fourchette friability (4.7%)
  Anterior hymenal clefts (1.2%), (1 child)
  Notches of the hymen (1.2%), (1 child)
  Hymenal septa (2.5%), (2 children)
  Vaginal discharge (2.6%), (2 children)
  Foreign body (1.3%), (1 child)

*The major concern in a study of this type is the lack of certainty about whether the sample contains only nonabused children. The children were screened for behavioral indicators but were not interviewed. (From McCann et al., 1990.)*

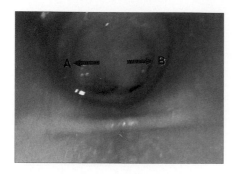

**Figure 9-3.** *Enlarged hymenal opening. Horizontal hymenal opening is measured from point A to B, the inner edges of the hymen from 9 to 3 o'clock.*

Normal hymens have three basic configurations or types: fimbriated (denticular, dentelle, or congenital frilly), circumferential (ring, annular, or concentric), and posterior rim (semilunar or crescentic) (Pokorny & Kozinetz, 1988; McCann et al., 1990). Rarer hymen types are cribriform, septate, imperforate, and hymens with lateral or high anterior or posterior openings. Redundant hymenal tissue may form cuffs, wings, or tags.

Dilations of existing blood vessels, which appear as increased vascularity or isolated, single blood vessels larger than the surrounding vessels located in an area that normally would not contain a large vessel, are usually normal. They should not be mistaken for the injection seen with irritation or infection.

A ridge or furrow may mark the line of union of the two halves of the perineum and is generally an embryonic remnant. Such ridges are usually narrow and can be slightly raised. Those which are extremely broadened can be the result of sexual abuse and stretching of the subcutaneous tissue.

A narrow, smooth, pale-appearing structure may be located in the midline of the posterior fourchette or the fossa navicularis or on the hymen. This can be mistaken for hymenal or vaginal scars. This structure can be identified by position (midline, contiguous with the perineal raphe) and uniformity in shape and contour (scars are usually thickened and retracted).

Small bands of tissue may be seen connecting two opposing surfaces, with the same color and texture as the surrounding tissue. These are periurethral and perihymenal bands. Periurethral bands were present in half of the nonabused children examined by McCann et al. (1990) and were bilateral in 91% of the children. These bands often have a semilunar appearance that creates a false pocket

**Figure 9-4.** *The points of measurement of the vertical hymenal opening: A the anterior hymenal attachment to B the hymenal edge at 6 o'clock.*

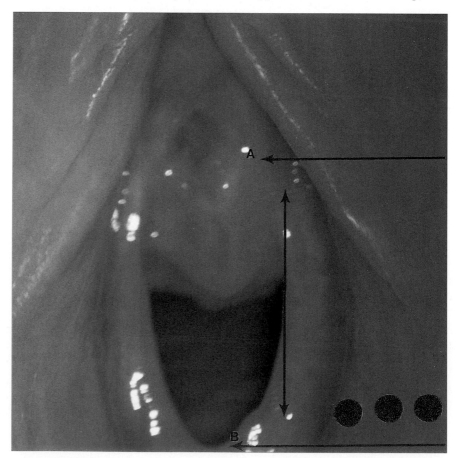

on either side of the urethral meatus. These bands are more commonly found anteriorly. They can appear throughout the vestibule and form an attachment to the hymen. The same structures can be seen in the posterior portion of the vestibule with asymmetry of the fossa navicularis. These bands can be mistaken for synechial bands.

Small (1 to 2 mm) vesicles (**Figure 9-5a,b**) or sacs on the hymen or surrounding tissues that appear to contain lymph-like material are termed *follicles*. The significance of follicles is unknown. McCann suggested that they could be related to irritation but could not confirm that premise because information on potential irritants was not available for their study.

The *hymenal septal remnant* is a small appendage, usually midline, attached to the edge of the hymen or lateral to the urethra (**Figure 9-6**). These remnants are detached pieces of septum and often dangle free of the hymen or, on the opposite position on the hymen, appear as a smooth mound on the hymen. They may be mistaken for free bits of torn hymen.

A localized, rounded, smooth-edged, and thickened area of tissue on the edge of the hymen is termed a *hymenal mound* (**Figures 9-1 and 9-5**). These small projections usually mark the spot of the attachment of an intravaginal ridge.

The *hymenal notch* or *cleft* is a concave, smooth-edged indentation on the edge of the hymen. These are usually midline but can also appear on other positions at the rim of the hymen. Their smooth-edged appearance differentiates them from old tears, which are angular at the base. The *anterior hymenal cleft* is a disruption of the usual curl-like configuration of the anterior hymenal attachment site of a crescent-shaped hymen that creates a shallow groove medially.

*Rolled hymenal edge* is the term applied to a narrow, rolled appearance at the edge of the hymen caused by a thickening of the hymenal rim or by a folding of a floppy hymen on itself (**see Figures 9-10 and 9-27**). These folds can be straightened out by placing traction on the hymen with labial traction or in the knee-chest position. These folds of the hymen can be mistaken for narrowing of the hymen. For that reason an effort should be made to be certain that any narrowing is not a rolled edge.

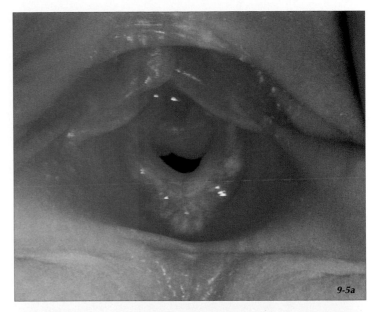

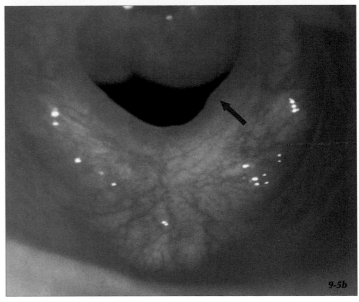

**Figure 9-5a.** *Normal vaginal exam demonstrating labial traction technique.* **b.** *Enlarged view of patient in* **a.** *Note small hymenal mound (arrow), smooth edge of hymen, and normal, lacy vascular pattern. The anterior column can be seen behind the hymen.*

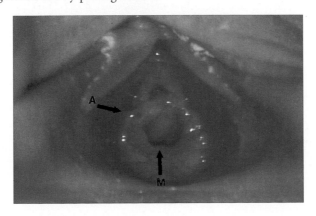

**Figure 9-6.** *Normal-appearing genital exam, crescent-shaped hymen with small midline mound (M) and hymenal band (A). There is a symmetrical band at 2 o'clock.*

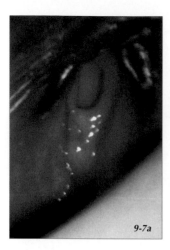

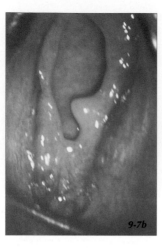

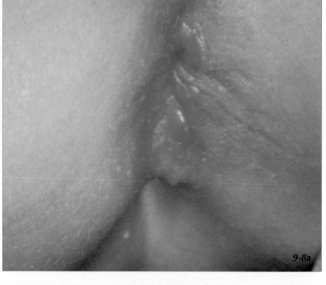

**Figure 9-7a,b.** *Abnormal genital exam with specific findings of abuse (Category III). In the first photo, simple separation technique is used. Without magnification this might appear as a normal exam. With labial traction technique the midline healing tear is clearly exposed. Note the follicles at the base of the hymen and the thickened avascular tissue around the injured area.*

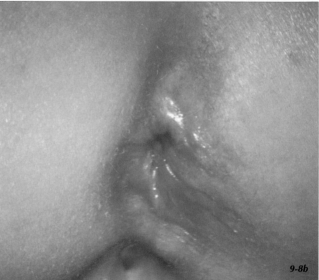

**Figure 9-8a,b,c.** *A progression of photos demonstrating the need to allow the child to relax. This is a 6-month-old chronically abused child with marked anal changes, loss of normal anal landmarks, and destruction of subcutaneous tissue. The child was also vaginally penetrated.*

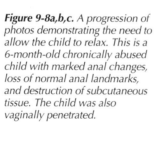

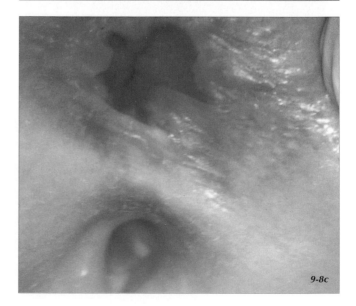

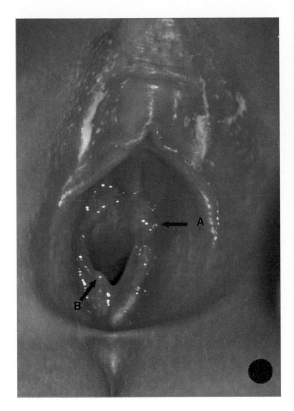

**Figure 9-9.** *Normal-appearing genital exam with septal remnants A and B. See Figure 9-10.*

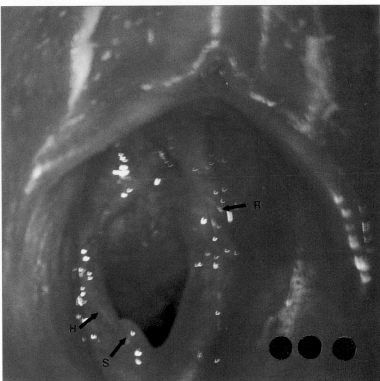

**Figure 9-10.** *Enlarged view of the patient in Figure 9-9. The mound (S) is the posterior attachment and (R) the filamentous anterior remnant of the septum. Note the rolled hymen edge (H).*

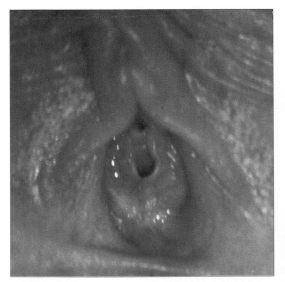

**Figure 9-11.** *Normal-appearing genital exam with boggy, estrogen-affected hymen in a 1-year-old child.*

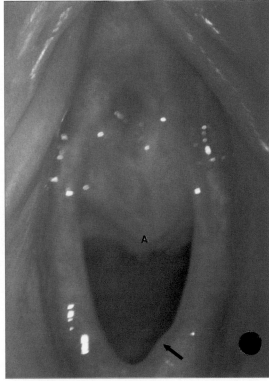

**Figure 9-12.** *Normal-appearing genital exam showing small hymenal mound (arrow) and the anterior column (A). The urethral opening diameter is normal.*

**Figure 9-13.**
*Abnormal genital exam, Category II, nonspecific findings. The vaginal mucosa and hymenal tissue are inflamed, a nonspecific vaginitis. The hymenal edge from 1 to 4 o'clock remains intact, while the limits of the rest of the hymenal edge are distorted and lost.*

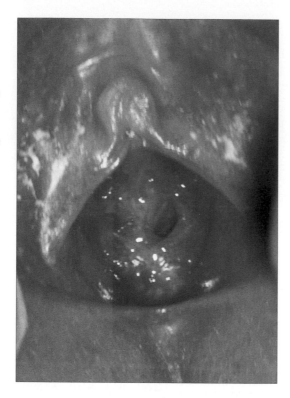

As already described, *intravaginal rugae* or *ridges* are narrow longitudinal ridges of mucosa-covered, fibrotic-like tissue that are attached to the inner surface of the hymen and located along either the lateral or the posterior-lateral wall of the vagina (**Figures 9-1 and 9-20**). Intravaginal rugae or ridges are present in most children. They coincide with the projections and mounds on the edges of the hymen. These ridges may be difficult to see without manipulation of the hymen and an attempt to see behind the membrane. The longitudinal ridges are located on the lateral and posterolateral vaginal walls.

*Intravaginal columns*, as noted, are wide midline longitudinal columns of mucosal tissue on the anterior and posterior walls of the vagina (**Figures 9-1, 9-5b, and 9-14**).

## CONDUCTING THE EXAMINATION

Because females are most often involved, the following discussion concerning the examination of the genitalia focuses on the female. A brief review of the male examination is given at the end.

An infant or small child can be examined either on the examining table or while on a parent's lap. During the genital and anal examination the nurse assistant or the mother positions the child and separates the child's thighs so that the examiner can see the genital and anal areas.

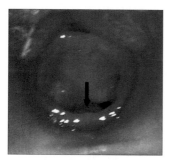

**Figure 9-14.** *Abnormal genital exam, Category III, specific findings. The hymenal opening is enlarged, hymenal tissue is narrowed, and posterior column (arrow) is visible.*

For a vaginal examination, girls 4 to 5 years of age or older are best examined while they are lying in a supine recumbent position, with knees flexed and heels against the buttocks, in a frog-leg position, on an ordinary examining table. The vulva and vestibule examination may be conducted using one of two techniques: *simple labial*

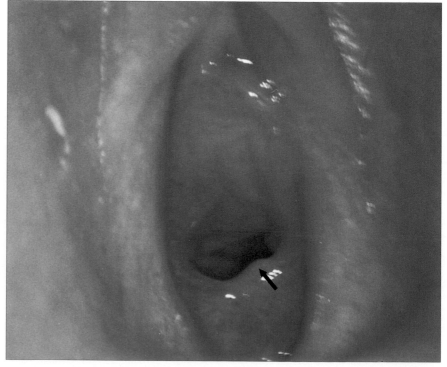

**Figure 9-15.** *Normal-appearing genital exam. Hymen is thickened, and there is a mound (arrow) at the hymenal edge.*

*separation,* in which light lateral and downward pressure is applied on each side of the perineum, and *labial traction* **(see Figure 9-7b),** in which the labia majora are gently grasped between the forefinger and thumb, separated, and pulled toward the examiner. The vulvar vestibule will not be visible if the labia minora are fused by adhesions. This condition may be confused with an imperforate hymen or vaginal agenesis. Adhesions of the labia majora may also limit the visibility of the vestibule. Lack of adequate hygiene is the most common cause of nonspecific vaginitis in girls. Girls with myelomeningocele and paralysis of the lower extremities will show marked vaginal laxity and an enlarged vaginal introitus (Steinhart & Monteleone, 1990). **Table 9-2** lists other conditions to note during the examination.

The vaginal and anal examination should be repeated with the child in the knee-chest position, knees flexed at a 90-degree angle, head turned, and back swayed. The supine knee-chest position, having the child flex her thighs on her abdomen, is often more comfortable for her and also gives excellent exposure.

Examination of a shy or anxious and resistive child can be accomplished with less apprehension if the child is placed in a modified Sims' position, with back to the examiner, head to the examiner's left, the child's left leg extended, and the right knee flexed and thigh drawn to the chest. The child is turned away from the examiner and does not see the examiner so feels less threatened.

| Table 9-2. Conditions to Note during the Physical Examination |
|---|
| Evidence of other abuse, such as loop marks and scars |
| General hygiene |
| Scars from other injuries |
| Nutritional status, including height and weight |
| Anatomic or congenital defects |
| Difficulty in walking or sitting |
| Semen on clothing |
| Grasp marks |
| Blood stains and/or discharge stains on underwear |
| Absent or suppressed gag reflex |
| Extreme compliance, child emotionally distant during examination |
| Child seductive |

The examiner should note the condition of the perineal and anal areas, common sites of dermatologic disorders, nonspecific bacterial inflammation, *Candida,* and eruptions that are part of a general skin disorder such as eczema. Perineal excoriations due to scratching may be evidence of pinworms. Inflammation and scratching may be the sequelae of poor perineal hygiene or nonspecific infection.

The examiner should note vulvar inflammations, eruptions, open lesions, tears, pain, and discharge. The patency of the hymenal orifice is determined, the size of the introital opening measured (if colposcopic photos are taken, this measurement can be determined from the photos), and the form and thickness of the hymen recorded. Usually there is one central opening with a crescent (53.5%) or concentric (34.9%) shaped hymen. There may be two openings, septate hymen (2.5%), or several small openings in the cribriform hymen (1.2%), or the membrane may be imperforate (1.2%) (McCann et al., 1990). McCann and associates were not able to determine the hymenal type in 8% of the study group. It should be noted that transhymenal widths taken with labial traction can be more than 50% wider than those with the supine separation approach.

The configuration and contour of the hymen vary with the age of the child and the method of examination. A redundant-appearing hymen can be changed with traction on the labia or through the use of the knee-chest position. The vertical and horizontal diameters of the introital opening increase with the age of the child (McCann et al., 1990). Maternal hormones also affect the hymen, causing it to be thick and redundant for as long as 2 years after birth and occasionally longer. Similar changes appear as the child reaches puberty, often before breast tissue changes and the appearance of pubic hair.

McCann et al. (1990) compared three separate methods used to examine 172 prepubertal girls for suspected sexual abuse. Their ages ranged from 10 months to 11 years, with a mean of 5 years, 8 months. The techniques used were the supine position with labial separation, the supine position with labial traction, and the knee-chest position. The knee-chest position (98%) and the supine traction method (96%) were superior to the supine separation technique (86%) in opening the vaginal introitus. The largest vertical transhymenal diameters were seen in the knee-chest position, and the greatest transverse horizontal diameters were seen in the supine traction procedure. Other soft tissue changes were noted but not quantified. McCann and associates recommended a multi-method approach to the examination of the sexually abused child to take advantage of the strengths of each technique.

If there is a discharge, the character, consistency, and color should be noted. The presence of any odor should also be recorded, since foreign bodies cause a foul-smelling, blood-streaked, purulent discharge. If there is evidence of infection, dry smears for bacteriologic studies, cultures, and wet slide preparations should be made. Fresh wet smears must be examined immediately for *Trichomonas vaginalis*, clue cells, and *Candida albicans*. The hymen is sensitive, and, when cultures are being procured, care should be taken to pass the culture swab beyond the hymen to a less sensitive area.

The examination of the male for sexual abuse is less difficult than the examination of the female. The positive findings in the male are limited to evidence of infection and injury, which are manifested by urethral discharge, bruises, lacerations, bites, ecchymotic areas, and petechiae of the penis. The anal examination of the male is the same as in the female.

## COLPOSCOPY

The colposcope has greatly aided the physical exam and enabled the retrieval of added physical findings in sexual abuse cases. It has allowed a better view of genital and anal areas, and, with a camera attached, provides an accurate means of documenting the findings of an examination. If the examiner does not have a colposcope, the naked eye will often suffice, or a magnifying lens or otoscope may be employed.

One additional advantage of colposcopic photographs is that they allow the examiner to share observations with colleagues and seek another opinion, sparing the child another examination. These photographs are also valuable as a teaching resource. It should be noted that because of technical difficulties and human error, photographs can be of poor quality, nonexistent, or lost. Therefore, immediately after the examination, drawings should be made and findings described in writing. Preprinted, large, fill-in drawings are useful in providing documentation.

## ◆ VAGINAL FINDINGS IN SEXUALLY ABUSED GIRLS

### ERYTHEMA, INFLAMMATION, AND INCREASED VASCULARITY

In sexual abuse cases the examiner may see redness of the skin or mucous membranes due to congestion of the capillaries. Normal vaginal mucosa has a pale pink coloration. McCann and associates noted erythema in 56% of the nonabused girls they examined.

### INCREASED FRIABILITY

A small dehiscence, or breakdown, with occasional oozing of blood, of the tissues of the posterior fourchette may be precipitated by the examination. This is usually associated with labial adhesions **(see Figure 9-16)**. McCann et al. (1990) noted this to be present in 39.9% of nonabused girls. When the adherent area is large, greater than 2 mm, the suspicion of abuse should be greater.

### ANGULATION OF THE HYMENAL EDGE

There may be V-shaped or angular configuration of the edge of the hymen. The hymenal edge should be smooth and round. Angulation often marks a healed old injury. The child with this finding should also be examined in the knee-chest position because if the angulation persists in this position, it is abnormal.

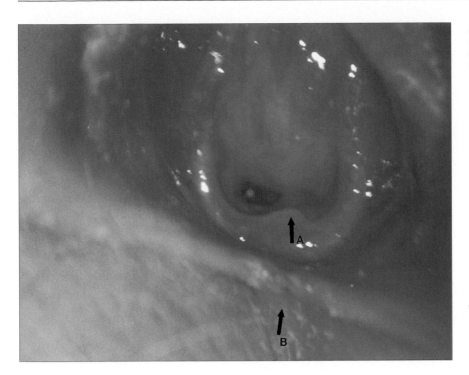

*Figure 9-16. Abnormal genital exam, Category III, specific findings. The hymen is attenuated, and the posterior column (A) is exposed. There is a breakdown of the friable labial adhesion (B).*

## LABIAL ADHESIONS

Adherent or fused labia majora are seen posteriorly as a thin central line of fusion. In McCann et al.'s (1990) sample of nonabused children, 38.9% had labial adhesions, more than half of which (19/35) were 2 mm or less in length. These minute adhesions explained the appearance of midline avascular areas and the increase in friability of the tissues of the posterior fourchette. These authors found that traction applied to these small labial adhesions caused them to blanch, producing an avascular appearance. Further traction occasionally caused them to dehisce, producing a small amount of bleeding.

While labial adhesions are a nonspecific finding often seen in girls with no history of sexual abuse, they may also be a manifestation of chronic irritation and can be seen in children who have been abused. McCann et al. (1990) stated that those found in the nonabused girls usually involved the posterior end of the labia majora and generally measured 2 mm or less in length.

## URETHRAL DILATATION

Urologists have described these changes in adults with urethral intercourse. Monteleone et al. (1988) reported urethral dilatation as an abnormal physical finding in several sexually abused females (**Figures 9-18 and 9-21**). They examined 1,014 children over a period of 2 years in the sexual abuse management clinic, and 234 of these included colposcopic examinations. They graded urethral opening as 1 to 2 mm, +1, up to greater than 8 mm, +4, with gradations between. Of the 234 patients examined colposcopically, 8 received a grade of +1, 8 were +2, 6

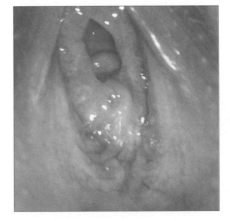

*Figure 9-17. Abnormal genital exam, Category III, specific findings. Healing injury of the lower half of the hymen and the posterior fourchette. There is early scar tissue along the midline of the hymen. The anterior half of the hymen, although boggy, is normal.*

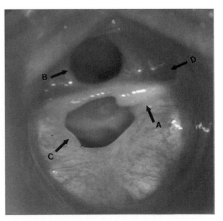

*Figure 9-18. Abnormal genital exam, Category III, specific findings. There is scar formation (A) of the hymen at the upper pole, raised and contracted. There is a small opening (D) communicating with the vagina. This may be mistaken for a septum. The mound (C) is normal. The urethral opening (B) is a little more than usually seen with the labial traction technique but is probably normal.*

were +3, and 2 were +4. They concluded that mild to moderate urethral dilatation (+1,+2) is probably normal and an artifact of the labial traction technique; higher grades were considered a manifestation of sexual abuse, probably the result of digital manipulation of the urethral orifice. However, they were not able to prove this was the mechanism of the insult. Although several of the children gave histories of digital insertion, none, as would be expected, could state that it involved the urethra. Several had a history of enuresis; none complained of incontinence.

## HYMENAL OR VAGINAL TEAR

Deep breaks in the mucosa of the vagina and hymen are referred to as tears (**see Figure 9-30**). These injuries can be seen with accidental injuries as well as with abuse. Often they occur when a history of impaling is given.

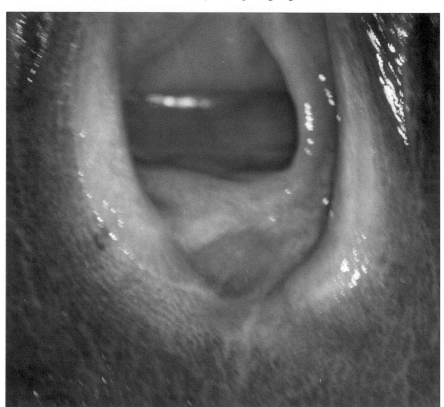

*Figure 9-19.* Abnormal genital exam, Category III, specific findings. Chronic sexual abuse, hymen at base is totally gone; labia minora show permanent thickening and devascularization.

As stated earlier, genital injuries are abuse until proven otherwise. Accidents such as straddle or impaling injuries, usually unilateral, injure anterior or lateral structures, not the interior vaginal introitus (Hobbs & Wynne, 1989). The bony pelvis and labia usually protect the hymen from accidental injury (Enos et al., 1986). Paul (1977) noted that in straddle injuries from falls onto a pointed object, the object rarely penetrates through the hymenal orifice into the vagina. The hymen is usually not torn, and penetration occurs at the lateral margins of the labia minora with the wound entering the vagina through its walls rather than through the hymen. Others concur (Herman-Giddens & Frothingham, 1987; Pokorny & Kozinetz, 1988). Paul stated that violent stretching injury, as seen when a child does a sudden, forceful split on a slippery surface, can cause midline lacerations. These injuries can also be caused during sexual abuse by forceful, sudden abduction of the legs.

In a recent multicenter report of young girls presenting to an emergency room because of accidental perineal injury, Bond et al. (1995) examined 56 preadolescent girls injured on a bicycle (39%), in other outdoor straddle and fall injuries (25%), and in indoor straddle and fall injuries (36%). The majority of the injuries were anterior or lateral to the hymen; 34% of the injuries were posterior to the hymen. Thigh injuries were observed only in older girls. In only one case was the hymen involved.

They concluded that abnormal hymenal findings are rarely the result of accidental injury. The presentation of a girl with hymenal injury should strongly suggest sexual abuse. Each other structure was injured in at least five girls. Thigh injuries were observed only in older girls engaged in bicycle riding or outdoor play. No anatomic pattern of injury was statistically associated with age or circumstance of injury.

Other previous studies (Wynne, 1980; West et al., 1989; Pokorny et al., 1992) included 47 girls. Six of these girls had vaginal or hymenal injuries. One was caused by a physician during a genital exam. One occurred in a severe auto accident and four when straddling or jumping on a penetrating object. It is important to note that all of the intravaginal injuries were dramatic and required immediate medical attention.

## DISCHARGE

Vaginal secretions are of various consistencies, colors, and odors. The usual cause of vaginal discharge is a nonspecific vaginitis. Nonspecific vaginitis yields a growth of mixed bacteria not related to a specific disease. Specific vaginitis is a bacterial infection involving such organisms as *Neisseria gonorrhoeae, Candida albicans*, and *Trichomonas vaginalis*. Nonspecific vaginitis is seen most often in children between 2 and 7 years of age. The causes of vaginitis are listed in **Table 9-3** (Huffman et al., 1981).

| Table 9-3. Etiologic Classification of Vaginitis | |
|---|---|
| *Vaginal Infections and Inflammations:*<br>**Bacterial Infections**<br><br>*Nonspecific Mixed Infections Secondary to:*<br>　Poor perineal hygiene<br>　Respiratory infections<br>　Skin infections<br>　Intestinal parasitic invasion of vagina<br>　Foreign bodies in vagina<br>　Urinary tract infection<br>　Unknown avenues of infection<br><br>*Specific infection due to:*<br>　The exanthemas<br>　*Hemophilus vaginalis*<br>　　*(Corynebacterium vaginalis)*<br>　Hemolytic streptococci<br>　*Corynebacterium diphtheriae*<br>　*Neisseria meningitidis*<br>　*Neisseria sicca*<br>　*Diplococcus pneumoniae*<br>　*Shigella flexneri*<br>　Chlamydia<br>　Gonorrhea (not all types are<br>　　sexually transmitted)<br><br>**Protozoal Infections**<br>　Trichomoniasis<br>　Amebiasis<br>　Other<br><br>**Mycotic Infections**<br>　*Candida*<br>　Other mycotic organisms<br><br>*(After Huffman et al., 1981.)* | **Mycoplasmas**<br><br>**Helminthiasis**<br><br>**Hirudiniasis**<br><br>**Viral Infections**<br>　Chickenpox<br>　Smallpox<br>　Vaccinia<br>　*Condylomata acuminata*<br>　Herpes<br><br>**Physical Agents**<br>　Sand<br>　Other foreign materials<br><br>**Chemical Agents**<br>　Bubble bath preparations<br>　Shampoo<br>　Medications<br>　Deodorant vulvar sprays<br><br>**Allergenic Agents**<br>　Nylon or rayon underclothing<br>　Medications<br>　Soaps, laundry detergents<br>　Other allergens<br><br>**Neoplasia**<br><br>**Granulomatous Diseases**<br><br>**Syphilis** |

Some genital discharges are not caused by infection or inflammation. It is important to distinguish between those that are inflammatory and those that are not. Most female babies will secrete vaginal fluid during the newborn period, caused by placental and maternal hormones. It is a thick, grayish white, mucoid material that not infrequently becomes blood-stained or grossly bloody. This discharge and bleeding disappear within a week or 10 days after birth. It is a physiologic condition requiring no treatment.

In early puberty, girls will have a discharge, usually first noted on the child's underwear. Examination will show vaginal fluid that is curded, thin, and milky or clear mucous in appearance. This is normal and requires no therapy. The menarcheal female often has a clear, sticky discharge during ovulation and a milky discharge before her cycle.

The signs of nonspecific vaginitis are vaginal inflammation and discharge. The child may or may not have symptoms. The only complaint may be a yellowish stain on the child's underpants, noticed by the mother. The character of the discharge, the appearance of the vaginal mucosa, and the child's symptoms do not help to identify the etiologic agent or the type of bacteria causing the infection.

Occasionally, nonspecific vaginitis has an acute onset and the vaginal tissues are inflamed and edematous with a profuse, purulent discharge and dysuria. On examination the vulvar mucosa and the outer third of the vagina look hyperemic with a small amount of light gray or clear mucoid discharge. A profuse, purulent, blood-streaked malodorous discharge is typical of a foreign body.

### FISSURES

Superficial breaks in the skin or mucous membranes, fissures may ooze blood and be painful. They heal completely and leave no sequelae unless they become infected, in which case they may result in a small scar or an anal tag.

### NEW OR HEALED LACERATIONS

Lacerations are deep breaks in the skin or mucous membranes of the vagina or anus. They often leave scar formation after healing. Fissures and lacerations with scar formation are discussed elsewhere in this chapter.

### ENLARGED HYMENAL INTROITAL OPENING

One criterion often used to make a diagnosis of sexual abuse is an enlargement of the hymenal introital opening (Heger & Emans, 1990) (**see Figure 9-28**). Cantwell (1983) stated that a hymenal diameter greater than 4 mm was associated with sexual abuse. White et al. (1989) reported similar findings when they studied 242 females, ages 1 through 12 years, to determine if the vaginal introital diameter was useful in evaluating a child for sexual abuse. The children were divided into three groups: Group I, history of sexual contact and/or *Neisseria gonorrhoeae*; Group II, no history of sexual contact but at risk; and Group III, nonabused. Forty-six percent of children who complained of fondling with penetration had a vaginal introital diameter greater than 4 mm as compared to 14% in those without a history of penetration. Fifty-eight percent of children with more than one encounter had a vaginal introital diameter greater than 4 mm as compared to 29% in those with one encounter. The greatest proportion of children with a vaginal introital

| Table 9-4. Size of Hymenal Opening | | |
|---|---|---|
| Group/Method | Vertical (mm) | Horizontal (mm) |
| Preschool (n=50) | | |
|    Separation | 6.1±2.6 (3.0-13.5) | 3.5±1.4 (1.0-7.0) |
|    Traction | 7.1±2.3 (3.0-14.0) | 5.7±1.6 (1.0-10.0) |
|    Knee/chest | 7.7±2.4 (3.5-14.0) | 4.7±1.5 (2.0-9.0) |
| Early School Age (n=52) | | |
|    Separation | 6.0±2.5 (1.0-15.5) | 4.0±1.6 (1.0-9.0) |
|    Traction | 6.7±2.2 (3.0-15.0) | 5.9±1.7 (2.5-10.0) |
|    Knee/chest | 7.8±2.2 (2.0-13.0) | 5.4±1.6 (2.5-8.0) |
| Preadolescent (n=42) | | |
|    Separation | 7.0±3.2 (2.5-18.0) | 5.0±2.0 (2.0-9.0) |
|    Traction | 7.7±2.8 (2.0-17.0) | 6.5±2.1 (3.0-10.0) |
|    Knee/chest | 8.8±2.5 (5.0-15.5) | 6.0±2.0 (2.5-11.0) |
| *Transhymenal diameter (n=144)* | | |
| *(From McCann et al., 1990.)* | | |

diameter greater than 4 mm was observed in the penile-vaginal contact group. These authors believed that a vaginal introital diameter of greater than 4 mm is highly associated with sexual contact in children less than 13 years of age.*

The size of the hymenal opening can vary with increasing age and pubertal development of the child. Other factors such as the position of the child during the measurement, the degree of traction placed on the external genitalia, and the degree of relaxation of the child can influence the measurements. The nature of the abuse and the time elapsed since the abuse can also change genital findings.

Studies by McCann et al. (1990) helped clarify this parameter as a sign of sexual abuse (**Table 9-4**). Horizontal diameters, measured with the labial traction technique or in the knee-chest position, of greater than 10 mm are beyond 2 standard deviations of normal range and can support a diagnosis of sexual abuse. Measurements obtained by simple separation are of limited value unless they are greater than 2 standard deviations beyond normal.

## ◆ SEXUALLY TRANSMITTED DISEASES

Transmission of sexually transmitted diseases outside the perinatal period by nonsexual means is rare (Paradise, 1989). Gonorrhea or syphilis infections are diagnostic of sexual abuse after perinatal transmission has been ruled out. Herpes type 2, *Chlamydia, Trichomonas,* and condyloma infections are extremely unlikely to be due to anything but abuse, particularly in children beyond infancy.

Chlamydial infections acquired at birth can persist 2 to 3 years in genital, anal, or pharyngeal sites. Untreated trichomonal infections can persist for several months, human papillomavirus can remain latent for up to 8 months or longer, and congenital human immunodeficiency virus (HIV) infection may not manifest for months to years. *Chlamydia* is an obligate intracellular organism, and fomite transmission has never been documented. Autoinoculation and fomite transmission may occur with genital warts.

If *Chlamydia, Trichomonas,* genital warts, or HIV infection is diagnosed, even in children younger than 3 years old, an evaluation for sexual abuse is indicated. In one study, 10 of 11 children who presented with venereal warts after age 1 year, including four children younger than 3 years, were proven to have been sexually abused (Herman-Giddens & Frothingham, 1987). Gutman et al. (1991) evaluated 96 children under the age of 13 years who tested positive for HIV and confirmed that 14 (14.6%) had been sexually abused.

*For more information on this topic see Chapter 15, Sexually Transmitted Diseases in Abused Children.*

### SPERM

If the abuse occurred within 72 hours, the examiner should look for the presence of sperm. The survival time of sperm is shortened in prepubertal girls because they lack cervical mucus; if there is a delay before an examination, the likelihood of finding sperm is diminished. Spermatozoa have rarely been detected in vaginal secretions from postpubertal rape victims longer than 12 hours after an assault, although longer survival times have been reported in older subjects. A Wood's lamp helps identify sperm on the clothing or skin. However, sperm is not the only substance that fluoresces under Wood's lamp, so fluorescence is a nonspecific finding. Wood's lamp is not a sensitive screening tool and should be used with caution.

To improve the detection of sexual abuse in children, Gabby et al. (1992) recommend that the p30-enzyme-linked immunosorbent assay be used because of its potential as a more sensitive assay than those in current clinical use. A semen glycoprotein of prostatic origin, p30 has been detected in vaginal fluid 47 hours

*Paradise (1989), in an editorial comment, although finding the study worthy of some praise, found fault because of methodologic uncertainties and limitations in three areas: identifying cases of sexual abuse, the nature of the control group, and the measurement of hymenal orifice diameters and a need to use different measurement techniques. The measurements were taken using supine labial separation only. McCann et al. answered the doubts when they suggested a means in which introital opening could be a reliable parameter in evaluating the abused child. Using the colposcope, they found significant differences in hymenal openings depending on position and methods used to make these measurements (**see Table 9-4**).*

*The significance of anteroposterior diameter is doubtful. Annular hymens with tissue encircling the vagina to a full 360 degrees cannot be compared with crescentic hymens in which the hymen is normally absent between 11 and 1 o'clock. Sleeve-like or fimbriated hymens should be excluded from comparisons of either horizontal or anteroposterior diameters because of the inability to measure the opening in this type of hymen. This is also true of septate and microperforate hymens.*

*Clinical reports have expanded our understanding of the healing process; with time, the hymen can completely heal or on occasion contract to a small opening as a result of scar formation.*

after intercourse. Herr et al. (1986) described the binding of a monoclonal antibody, mouse antihuman sperm-5 (MHS-5), to a sperm-coating peptide secreted by human seminal vesicles. This reaction does not depend on the presence of sperm and has been used to identify seminal fluid in forensic specimens as old as 6 months. Although MHS-5 binding decreases when diluted with cervical secretions, it is a specific and sensitive technique for detecting seminal fluid.

Acid phosphatase activity is also nonspecific unless the level is very high or specific for prostatic acid phosphatase. Prostatic acid phosphatase activity has been found up to 22 hours after sexual assault and up to 30 hours after voluntary intercourse (Graves et al., 1985). Testing for acid phosphatase should not be the only method used to screen for the presence of semen; sperm are detectable in specimens with no acid phosphatase activity.

A vaginal swab should be obtained and preps made for examination and for the rape kit. It is important to follow the instructions supplied with the kit exactly. Evidence should be stored securely and a written record kept to establish the chain of evidence, that is, every person-to-person transfer, to document that no tampering or mix-up occurs during the process. DNA fingerprinting, the isolation of a characteristic deoxyribonucleic acid in semen or blood, can establish the identity of a perpetrator with a high degree of certainty from these preparations (Kirby, 1990).

## ♦STUDIES OF VAGINAL FINDINGS IN SEXUALLY ABUSED CHILDREN

Muram (1989) examined female victims of sexual abuse in which the perpetrator confessed to the abuse. In this study, 30 individuals confessed to sexually assaulting 31 girls, mean age 9.1 years (range 1 to 17 years). In 18 cases (58%) the offender admitted to vaginal penetration. Specific findings were observed in 11 of these 18 (61%) girls. Only 3 of 13 (23%) girls in which penetration was denied showed specific findings. Importantly, in 2 of 18 girls (11%) in which penetration was admitted, the examiner described normal-appearing genitalia and 5 (28%) showed nonspecific abnormalities. Assuming that the perpetrators' reports of penetration are accurate, these data indicate that penetration is possible without leaving physical evidence. Muram classified his findings into the following four categories:

*Category 1. Normal-appearing genitalia.*

*Category 2. Nonspecific findings. Abnormalities of the genitalia that could have been caused by sexual abuse, but are also seen in girls who are not victims of sexual abuse. Included in this category are redness or inflammation of the external genitalia, increased vascular pattern of the vestibular and labial mucosa, presence of purulent discharge from the vagina, small skin fissures or lacerations in the area of the posterior fourchette, and agglutination of the labia minora.*

*Category 3. Specific findings. The presence of one or more abnormalities strongly suggesting sexual abuse. Such findings include recent or healed lacerations of the hymen and vaginal mucosa, hymenal opening of one or more centimeters, proctoepisiotomy (a laceration of the vaginal mucosa extending to involve the rectal mucosa), and indentations on the vulvar skin indicating teeth marks (bite marks). This category also includes patients with laboratory confirmation of a venereal disease (e.g., gonorrhea).*

*Category 4. Definitive findings. Any presence of sperm.*

A hymenal tear was the most common finding in girls who described penile or digital penetration. Of 18 girls who described vaginal penetration, 11 were found to have a hymenal tear, 5 had an irritated and inflamed perineal area, and 2 prepubertal girls had normal-appearing genitalia.

Normal-appearing genitalia was the most common finding in girls who denied penile or digital penetration. Of 13 girls who denied vaginal penetration, 7 were found to have normal-appearing genitalia, 3 were found to have an irritated and inflamed perineal area, and 3 were found to have a hymenal tear.

Of the 31 victims, 21 were evaluated within 1 week of the assault. Irritation and inflammation were noted in 9 of them. No inflammatory reaction was noted in any of the 10 victims who were evaluated 1 week or more after the assault, emphasizing the need for physical evaluation as soon after the assault as possible.

Woodling and Heger (1986) reported that 75% of children who told of painful genital or anal penetration by a penis, finger, or instrument had overt or subtle findings of sexual abuse. The acute findings included abrasions, avulsions, transections, contusions, ecchymoses, petechiae, and focal edema. Chronic or old injuries presented as focal scarring, hymenal deformity, healed microtransections, synechiae, hymenal thickening with scarring, and neovascularization. An additional 5% to 10% of cases were corroborated with colposcopic examination.

Finkel (1989) followed the healing process in 7 children who had experienced acute genital and anal trauma. He noted that superficial wounds which heal by the process of regeneration do not form granulation tissue and have a different healing chronology than wounds which form granulation tissue. Superficial lacerations and abrasions healing by regeneration progress through four stages: (1) thrombosis and inflammation, (2) regeneration of epithelium over denuded surface, (3) multiplication of new cells, and (4) differentiation of new epithelium. This process proceeds at a variable rate, but epithelium will generally cover a wound at a rate of 1 mm per 24 hours. Wound healing by the process of regeneration can be complete within 48 to 72 hours. Differentiation of new epithelium is usually complete by 5 to 7 days. When reexamined, 5 of the 7 children had epithelial healing and no changes apparent to the naked eye or at $10\times$ magnification. Superficial labial and anal trauma healed at similar rates.

When the injuries are more serious and deeper, the healing process involves repair, the formation of granulation tissue, and a subsequent scar. Wound healing by repair follows the same steps as regeneration but includes organization and wound contraction. Progressive contraction of the wound with time changes the appearance of the granulation tissue. Initially, the granulation tissue is red. With time, the cellular and vascular components of the forming scar tissue decrease, with color and volume changes of the scar tissue as it matures. Most scars will mature in 60 days. When scar tissue is seen in the process of maturing or having matured, a history of significant injury should be sought.

This study showed that if physical evidence of abuse is to be found in cases where superficial injuries are involved, the child must be examined within 5 to 7 days after the assault. Yet most children do not immediately disclose incidents of sexual abuse. Many victims do not have an examination for weeks, months, or even years after the abuse occurred. By then the injuries have healed and the physical examination reveals few abnormalities.

To emphasize this point, three children who incurred genital injuries as a result of sexual assaults were followed up on a longitudinal basis (McCann et al., 1992). The follow-up period ranged from 14 months to 3 years. Signs of the acute damage disappeared rapidly, and the wounds healed without complications. After resolution of the injuries, the changes remained stable throughout the prepubertal years. The most persistent findings were irregular hymenal edges and narrow rims at the point of the injury. Over time the jagged, angular margins smoothed off. Disruption of the hymen exposed underlying longitudinal intravaginal ridges whose hymenal attachments created mounds or projections. There was little scar formation. Injuries to the posterior fourchettes healed with minimal scar tissue and left slight evidence of trauma. With the onset of puberty, the hymenal changes were obscured by the hypertrophy of the membrane.

## ◆ PHYSICAL FINDINGS ASSOCIATED WITH ANAL SEXUAL ABUSE

Anal assaults comprise a significant proportion of child sexual abuse attacks. Genital injuries or abnormalities are more often recognized as possible signs of abuse, while anal and perianal injuries may be dismissed as being associated with common bowel disorders such as constipation or diarrhea.

The anal sphincter and anal canal are elastic and allow for dilatation. Digital penetration usually does not leave a tear of the anal mucosa or sphincter. Penetration by a larger object may result in injury varying from a little swelling of the anal verge to gross tearing of the sphincter. If lubrication is used and the sphincter is relaxed, it is possible that no physical evidence will be found. Even penetration by an adult penis can occur without significant injury. After penetration, sphincter laxity, swelling, and small mucosal tears of the anal verge may be observed as well as sphincter spasm. Within a few days the swelling subsides and the mucosal tears heal. Skin tags can form as a result of the tears. Repeated anal penetration over a long period may cause a loose anal sphincter and an enlarged opening.

In the differential diagnosis of anal sexual abuse the practitioner must be aware of nonabuse-related conditions. Perianal abnormalities are often seen in children with Crohn disease or Hirschsprung disease. The anal canal gapes in children with significant constipation. The distended rectum, with a normal anorectal reflex, initiates the gaping. Stool is often seen in the anal canal. Small fissures can also be seen. These children may have trouble with fecal soiling, which causes reddening of the perianal area. Unfortunately, children who were anally abused often suffer from functional constipation, which results in a damaged anal sphincter and fecal soiling. The pain and injury that follow the anal assault may cause spasm of the sphincter and result in functional constipation.

---

**Table 9-5. Anal and Perianal Findings in 310 Prepubertal Children Who Were Victims of Sexual Abuse**

| Finding | Frequency |
|---|---|
| Normal-appearing perineum | 206 (66%) |
| Abnormal findings | 104 (34%) |
|   Anal gaping* | 61 |
|   Skin tags | 44 |
|   Rectal tears | 33 |
|   Sphincter tears | 15 |
|   Human papillomavirus | 4 |
|   Perineal scarring | 2 |
|   Bite marks | 1 |

*Anal gaping–relaxation of the anal sphincter to a diameter ≥ 1 cm when the glutei were separated. (Most evaluators would use a diameter of > 2 cm when palpable stool in the rectum is absent on digital examination.)

Muram (1989) examined 310 prepubertal children who were determined to be sexually abused (**Table 9-5**). Muram found normal-appearing perianal and anal regions in 150 of 175 children (85%) who denied anal assault, and in 11 of 70 (16%) who described such assault. Giving a detailed history of anal abuse increased the likelihood of finding anal abnormalities, and anal and perianal abnormalities were found in 59 of the 70 children (84%) who gave a clear history of anal assault. The examination was most often normal when the child denied that anal assault had occurred; 25 of 175 (15%) who denied such abuse showed abnormalities. In this study, children who had normal results of the genital examination were more likely to have anal abnormalities. This was probably influenced by the large number of males in the study group. Muram showed that failure to document perianal abnormalities in two thirds of the patients demonstrates the limitations of the physical exam in validating allegations of sexual abuse and emphasizes the importance of the child's statement.

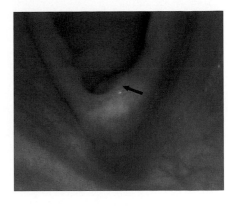

**Figure 9-20.** *Abnormal genital exam, Category III, specific findings. Narrowed hymen, exposing posterior ridge (arrow).*

## PERIANAL ERYTHEMA

Reddening of the skin overlying the perineum as well as the inner aspects of the thighs and labia generally indicates that there has been intracrural intercourse (penis between legs and laid along the perineum). Erythema in this area, however, also results from diaper rash or poor hygiene, and can occur after scratching and irritation from pinworms.

McCann et al. (1990) found perianal erythema in 40.5% of the children they examined. The mean radius of the erythema as measured from the interior edge of the anal verge to the outer border of the color change was 1.5 cm with a maximum width of 3 cm. They found a significant difference in the percentage of males (57%) with perianal erythema as compared to the females (32%).

## SWELLING OF THE PERIANAL TISSUES

Circumferential perianal swelling appears as a thickened ring around the anus and has been called the tire sign. It is an acute sign and can reflect traumatic edema.

## LAXITY AND REDUCED TONE OF THE ANAL SPHINCTER

Sphincter tone should be assessed by exerting gentle traction on the sphincter. While some doctors prefer digital examination when assessing children who have been abused and anally penetrated, it would seem unwise to assess anal sphincter tone by digital penetration.

## SHORTENING OR EVERSION OF THE ANAL CANAL

When there has been anal abuse the anorectal junction becomes approximated to the anal orifice. This is associated with laxity and reduced anal tone. This finding occurs only in the first 2 or 3 years of life and reflects repeated anal intercourse (**see Figure 9-8a,b,c**).

## ANAL DILATATION

Forensic physicians use various terms to describe anal dilatation, including reflex anal dilatation, reflex relaxation of the anus, the lateral buttock traction test, and the "0" sign. McCann et al. (1989) noted anal sphincter dilatation in 49% of the children they examined. The anteroposterior diameter of the orifice varied from less than 0.1 to 2.5 cm with a mean of 1.0 cm. In 91% of the subjects with anal dilatation the anteroposterior diameter was less than 20 mm. The percentage of children with anal dilatation of 20 mm or greater without presence of stool in the rectal ampulla was 1.2%. Stool was seen in 44% of the cases in which dilatation took place. The horizontal diameters of the anal orifice ranged from less than 0.1 to 2 cm with a mean of 0.57 cm.

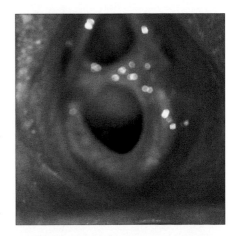

**Figure 9-21.** *Abnormal genital exam, Category III, specific findings. There is a loss of hymenal tissue at 10 to 11 o'clock. The urethral opening is abnormally enlarged and patulous.*

In those with dilatation, 30% opened within 30 seconds, 55% had their initial dilatation before 2 minutes, and 5% dilated after 4 minutes. None of the anuses

*Figure 9-22.* Abnormal genital exam, Category II, nonspecific findings. Hymen irregular and thickened, probably due to early estrogen effect. Hymenal opening slightly enlarged. Urethral opening +2, but rim is thickened and avascular.

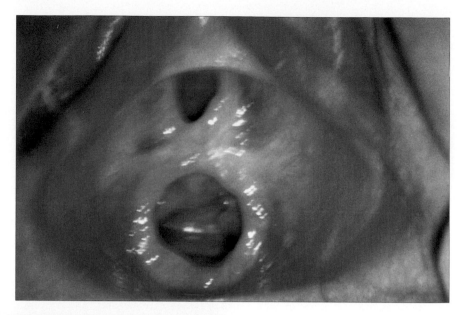

that opened after 4 minutes had an orifice greater than 15 mm in the anteroposterior plane. The mean time required for the initial dilatation was 65 seconds, while the mean time for the anus to reach maximum dilatation was 2 minutes, 11 seconds. The anus remained open once the sphincters dilated in 38% of the children, while the anus opened and closed intermittently in 62% of the subjects in which dilatation occurred. Anal dilatation of 20 mm or greater without the presence of stool in the rectal ampulla was unusual.

## FISSURES

Breaks in the skin/mucosal covering of the rectum, anus, and anal skin occur as a result of overstretching and frictional force exerted on the tissues (**see Figure 9-26**). This can occur after the passage of a hard stool or abusive traumatic penetration of the anus. Tiny superficial cracks in the anal verge or perianal skin often result from scratching with pinworms or with excoriation from acute diarrhea or diaper rash.

## LARGE TEARS

Large breaks in the skin extending into the anal canal or across the perineum are usually painful and can cause anal spasm. Tears often heal with scarring and leave a skin tag at the site of the trauma (**see Figure 9-26**). McCann et al. (1990)

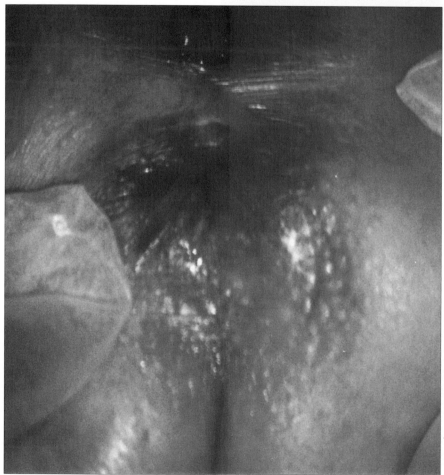

*Figure 9-23.* Abnormal anal exam, Category II, nonspecific findings. Chronic anal changes, especially from 9 to 1 o'clock where there is swelling and a breakdown of the mucosa, deep fissures, and erythema. This is secondary to the congenital anatomic abnormality—anterior displacement of the anus. Note the small perineum. This child was 12 months old and had been treated by her physician for anal fissures since 6 months of age. The problem was complicated by an older sibling who had genital warts and was sexually abused.

found anal skin tags **(see Figure 9-25)** or folds located anterior to the anal orifice in the midline equally in preschool, school-aged, and preadolescent children. They found no differences between the races; however, no tags were found in the males. Skin tags/folds posterior to the anus were not seen.

## Venous Congestion

Purple to blue discoloration around the anal margin corresponds to areas of venous congestion. The veins can extend as a ring around the whole anal circle or be limited to a segment. Venous congestion can be seen in the normal anus after excess traction, as from long periods in the knee-chest position. In the McCann et al. (1989) study, venous engorgement was seen in approximately three fourths of all the children who remained in the knee-chest position for 4 minutes or longer. Moderate to marked venous congestion at the outset of the examination was not seen.

Venous congestion is not specific for injury from abuse. McCann et al. (1989) found venous congestion present in 7% of the subjects initially, in 52% at the midpoint, and in 73% of the children by the end of the examination. No hemorrhoids were found in any of the children.

## Skin Changes

Paul reported that repeated acts of penetration will lead to changes in the anal verge skin **(see Figure 9-21).** Repeated friction and stretching of the fibers of the corrugator cutis and muscle result in thickening and smoothing away of the anal skin folds. The skin appears smooth, pink, and shiny, with a loss of normal fold pattern. The presence of these skin changes suggests chronicity of abuse.

Scars are evidence of earlier trauma. Paul states that the skin edges are pulled apart once the anal verge skin has split, leaving a triangular break in the continuity of the anal verge with the apex of the triangle pointing into the anal canal. The scar is often fan-shaped, radiating from the anal orifice, and appears as a pale thickened area distorting the normal folds. A skin tag is sometimes found, as well as linear scars. Healing is hampered by infection, passage of stools, or further abuse.

Smooth areas on or near the verge were observed in 26% of the children in the McCann et al. study (1989). These areas were always in the midline, at either the 6 or the 12 o'clock position. In 47% (8 of 17) of the children with this finding the smooth area was associated with a depression. Midline depressions without a smooth zone were detected anterior to the anus in 7 (41%) of the patients with this finding.

In that same study, perianal scars were found in 4 of the 240 children evaluated. Three of the lesions were located in the midline at the 12 o'clock position posterior to the rectum. The other one was at the 2 o'clock location and was observable by using the prone, knee-chest position. No fissures, abrasions, lacerations, or hematomas were found in any of the subjects. Perianal skin tags/folds and scars outside the midline were not seen. A prominent anal verge was also an unusual finding.

## Funnelling

Funnelling is a traditional sign of chronic anal sexual abuse, but its presence in children has been questioned. The appearance of funnelling or a hollowing-out of the perianal area is caused by loss of fat tissue or fat atrophy of the subcutaneous area. Although this is often associated with chronic anal sex, it has also been described in nonabused children.

## Hematoma and/or Bruising

Subcutaneous accumulations of old and new blood and bruising are strong indicators of trauma. It would be very unlikely for these to occur without a history to explain them. These injuries are not likely to be accidental.

## ANAL WARTS

Anal warts can occur as an isolated physical finding or in conjunction with other signs consistent with abuse, either anal or genital. Anogenital warts are frequently associated with human papillomavirus types 6 and 11 and less commonly with 16 and 18. DNA HPV typing should assist assessment when the question of nonvenereal transmission (e.g., from hand warts) is raised.

Anal warts in children under 2 years of age whose mother has a history of genital warts are most likely not the result of abuse. If no history of genital warts is elicited, the family should be evaluated for their presence. In children over 4 years of age with new genital warts, abuse should be considered and the child carefully interviewed by an experienced evaluator. Evaluation of genital warts is difficult in the nonverbal child. *See Chapter 15, Sexually Transmitted Diseases in Abused Children,* for further information on this topic.

## PIGMENTATION

McCann et al. (1990) found increased perianal pigmentation in 29.5% of nonabused children in their sample. The degree of pigmentation was minimal in 84%, moderate in 13.6%, and great in 2.2%. The mean radius of the pigmentation was 1.6 cm, with the maximum width being 4 cm. An analysis of variance revealed a significant difference between the races for the presence of increased pigmentation. Of the white children, 22% had this finding as compared to 53.3% of the black and 57.6% of the Hispanic children. The black children had the greatest incidence in the amount of perianal pigmentation, with 17.6% having a moderate to marked degree as compared to 5.1% for the Hispanic and only 2.5% of the white children.

## ANAL ASYMMETRY WHEN DILATED

McCann et al. (1989) in their study of nonabused children noted that the anal orifice had a symmetrical oval configuration in 89% of the children whose anus dilated open. In 9% of the subjects the anus was round in appearance, and in 3% it was irregular; 6 children had minimal asymmetry of their anal orifice as it opened and closed intermittently. Marked irregularity of the anal orifice during dilatation was unusual.

## ◆ NORMAL EXAMINATIONS IN SEXUALLY ABUSED CHILDREN

The physical examination is usually normal in children who have been sexually abused. Even with a confession of penetration by the perpetrator, the examination can be normal (Muram, 1989; Kerns & Ritter, 1992). Many types of sexual molestation do not involve penetration and will not leave physical findings. In addition, a significant number of rapes occur without ejaculation or damage to the hymen (Camps, 1968). The anal sphincter is pliant and, with care and lubrication, can easily allow passage of a penis or an object of comparable diameter without injury. The hymen is elastic, and penetration by a finger or penis, especially in an older child, may cause no injury or may only enlarge the hymenal opening.

Bays and Chadwick (1993) have summarized data from 21 studies of reported medical findings in children who were allegedly sexually abused. Normal examinations were reported in 26% to 73% of girls and 17% to 82% of boys. Diagnostic evidence (Category III or IV) of sexual abuse was found in 3% to 16% of the victims. Bays and Chadwick give several explanations for the wide range in percentages of positive and negative findings. Higher rates of physical findings occurred in earlier studies when only the most severe cases came to light. Criteria for what constitutes physical evidence of molestation have changed in the last 20 years as information from clinical studies on abused and nonabused children has been compiled and disseminated.

An absence of physical findings in sexually abused children can be explained in a number of ways. The sooner the examination occurs after the abusive event, the more likely it will reveal positive findings. In two studies comparing timing of examinations, 36% of children examined within 24 hours of a penetrating sexual assault had evidence of genital trauma, whereas 13% seen after 24 hours had positive findings (Rimza & Niggemann, 1982). Muram (1989) found irritation and inflammation of the genitalia in 21 of 31 child sexual abuse victims seen within 1 week of the assault, while no findings were noted in victims after a week or more.

Evidence of ejaculate is difficult to find if the child has washed, urinated, or defecated and if more than 72 hours has elapsed since the assault (Tipton, 1989; DeJong & Finkel, 1990; Paradise, 1990).

Injuries can heal rapidly. Hymenal healing occurs in 6 to 30 days and can be complete. Teixeira (1981) examined 500 patients for sexual abuse. He found single, partial hymenal tears healed as soon as 9 days after injury, while extensive tears took up to 24 days to heal. Finkel (1989) followed seven children with acute genital and anal trauma. Six children healed with no residual trauma in 7 to 13 days. Others have also reported complete healing of acute anal and genital injuries from sexual abuse (McCann, 1988; McCann et al., 1992).

At puberty, estrogen stimulates the hymen, causing thickening and proliferation, which can obscure injuries (McCann et al., 1992).

Groth and Burgess (1977) noted that 34% of rapists had erectile or ejaculatory dysfunction. The study was in adult women but may also apply to child molesters.

## ◆ PHYSICAL FINDINGS IN RAPE VICTIMS

Certain types and locations of hymenal injuries are often seen after abuse. McCann et al. (1990) observed that the hymenal membrane at its midline (6 o'clock position) attachment along the posterior rim of the introitus, during actual or attempted penetration, is the portion of the hymen most likely to be damaged. A narrowed (attenuated) hymen at this position is usually indicative of an injury. Mounds, projections, or notches on the edge of the hymen and the exposure of intravaginal ridges strengthen the possibility of abuse.

McCann et al. (1992) followed three girls with healing injuries resulting from an assault and found that a narrow hymenal rim at the point of injury persisted. The original injuries occurred along the posterior or lateral hymenal rim, between 5 and 9 o'clock. Teixeira (1981) examined 500 rape victims and found that the hymen ruptured most commonly at the 5 to 7 o'clock position. He noted that 310 of the victims had hymenal ruptures, 193 (62%) of which revealed tears in the 5 to 7 o'clock area. He noted that ectopic coitus, or penile impact without penetration, resulted in lesions of the fourchette and partial ruptures. Herman-Giddens and Frothingham (1987) generally concurred with the above study and found that attempted forced vaginal penetration generally resulted in hymenal tears and fissures between the 3 and 9 o'clock positions and may extend across the vestibule and fourchette.

## ◆ A CLASSIFICATION OF PHYSICAL FINDINGS IN SEXUAL ABUSE EXAMINATIONS

*The National Child Sexual Abuse Summit Meeting in 1985 (Tipton, 1989) concluded that some specific physical findings are strongly indicative of sexual abuse beyond reasonable doubt, as follows:*

1. Clear-cut tears, fresh or old; scars; significant distortion of the normal shape of the hymen and/or hymenal bruising.

2. Lacerations, scars, bruises, and healing abraded areas, often accompanied by neovascularization, of the posterior fourchette.

3. Anal dilation greater than 15 mm transverse diameter with gentle buttock traction with the child in knee-chest position. Large anal scars in the absence of a history that could explain the scars.

The authors have used the classification of physical findings in sexual abuse as listed in **Table 9-6**. The categories were suggested by Muram. We have expanded the classification and have placed several conditions Muram had in Category III into Category IV.

---

**Table 9-6. Classification of Sexual Abuse Physical Findings**

I. **Normal-appearing exam**
The majority (60% or more) of abused children fall into this category.
    Mounds
    Clefts
    Bands
    Septal remnants
    Urethral dilation (mild)

II. **Nonspecific findings of sexual abuse**
(often seen in children who have not been sexually abused)
    Condylomata (human papilloma virus, HPV)
    (in children under 2 years, may upgrade with a strong history or with supportive physical findings [hymenal tear, narrowing, etc.])
    Hymenal thickening or edema*
    Injection, erythema, vaginitis (nonspecific), areas of increased vascularity*
    Rounding of hymenal edges
    Labial adhesions
    (depending on history, could be Category III)
    Urethral dilation (moderate)
    Narrowing of hymen (greater than 2 mm)
    Enlargement of the hymenal opening (with no other findings)*
    Thickening of the perianal tissue
    Increased pigmentation
    Venous pooling
    (after prolonged knee-chest position)
    Funnelling, fat atrophy

III. **Specific (suspicious/highly suspicious) for sexual abuse**
    Hymenal and vaginal tears
    Hymenal scars (usually are retracted), mounted linear avascular areas

    Herpes II
    *Chlamydia trachomatis*†
    *Trichomonas vaginalis*
    Reflex anal dilation in absence of stool in antrum and greater than 20 mm
    Hymenal transections
    Hymenal narrowing, flattening (less than 2 mm)
    Hymenal attenuation (narrowing or flattening)
    Synechiae (lower pole, 3 to 9 o'clock; may be confused with bands of tissue extending from the vaginal wall caused by stretching with labial traction)
    Severe rounding of hymenal margin with loss of vascularity
    Perianal skin tags/folds outside the midline
    Anal scars outside the midline
    Marked irregularity of the anal orifice during dilation, persistence of a prominent anal verge
    Urethral dilation (severe)
    Pelvic inflammatory disease (PID)

IV. **Conclusive of sexual abuse**
(children under 12 years; older children may be sexually active)
    *Neisseria gonorrhoeae*†
    *Treponema pallidum* (syphilis)†
    Sperm, seminal fluid, acid phosphatase activity in discharge (must be very high if nonspecific assay, or prostatic specific)
    Pregnancy
    Human immunodeficiency virus (HIV)† (no history to explain)

*A nonspecific finding can become a specific finding when a child gives a clear history of recent sexual abuse, especially when describing pain.*
*†Nonneonatal.*

---

## ♦ CONDITIONS THAT CAN BE MISTAKEN FOR SEXUAL ABUSE

Bays and Jenny (1990) described a number of dermatologic, congenital, traumatic, and infectious physical findings that can be mistaken for sexual abuse (**Table 9-7**). The most common dermatologic condition confused with trauma from sexual assault is lichen sclerosis. It can present in various ways from mild irritation of the labia and vaginal mucosa to dramatic findings such as subepidermal hemorrhages of the genital or anal area involving the labia and vaginal mucosa and/or the anus.

| Table 9-7. Conditions That Can be Mistaken for Sexual Abuse |
| --- |
| Lichen sclerosis et atrophicus |
| Accidental straddle injuries |
| Accidental impaling injuries |
| Nonspecific vulvovaginitis and proctitis |
| Group A β-streptococcal vaginitis and proctitis |
| *Shigella* vaginitis |
| Diaper dermatitis |
| Foreign bodies |
| Lower extremity girdle paralysis as in myelomeningocele |
| Defects that cause chronic constipation, Hirschsprung disease, or anteriorly displaced anus |
| Chronic gastrointestinal disease, Crohn disease |
| Labial adhesions |
| Anal fissures |

A punch biopsy may be necessary to make the diagnosis. The diagnosis is usually suspected when a lighter, "halo" area is noted at the periphery of the reddened or hemorrhagic area.

Congenital hemangiomas, streptococcal infections, straddle injuries, and urethral caruncle or prolapse (Johnson, 1991) are other conditions that produce physical findings which can be confused with sexual abuse. We have seen three cases of *Shigella* vaginitis that had been reported as sexual abuse because the children presented with vaginal bleeding and severe vaginal mucosal edema.

Anal changes from Crohn disease, hemolytic uremic syndrome, postmortem anal dilation, neurogenic patulous anus, lichen sclerosis, and chronic constipation (Bays & Jenny, 1990) may also be mistaken for sexual abuse. Bays and Jenny warned that fissures and anal dilation can be particularly troublesome because they are found both in constipated and in sexually abused children. One study reported 6% to 26% of constipated children had anal fissures, and 15% to 18% had anal dilation. In that study, sexually abused children revealed a higher percentage with anal dilation (42%) and fissures (53%) (Hobbs & Wynne, 1989). In a comparable study of 171 children referred for gastrointestinal complaints, 8 (4.7%) revealed anal or perianal abnormalities. One of 30 children referred for constipation had an anal fissure. No child had anal dilation or distortion of the anal opening (Lazar & Muram, 1989). The authors suggest that perianal abnormalities should raise suspicions of possible sexual abuse and be investigated.

## ♦ QUESTIONS THAT ARE OFTEN ASKED

*Can a child be born without a hymen to explain the physical findings described?*

There is no documented case of an infant girl born without a hymen. In two studies (Jenny et al., 1987; Mor & Merlob, 1988) 26,199 newborn girls were examined; all had hymens.

*Can excessive masturbation or the use of tampons explain abnormal vaginal findings?*

Masturbation and tampons do not cause injury to the hymen or internal genital structures. There is no evidence that use of tampons causes trauma to the hymen (Dickinson, 1945; Cowell, 1981; Stewart, 1990). Masturbation in girls usually involves clitoral or labial stimulation and does not cause hymenal injury (Hobbs & Wynne, 1989; Tipton, 1989).

Labbe (1990) described 10 boys with urinary tract infections apparently caused by the boys injecting water into their own urethras while bathing. No genital injuries were described. However, similarly, no injuries were seen in 38 infants with neurogenic bladder whose parents or caretakers catheterized them every 4 to 6 hours during the day for a mean of 28 months (Joseph et al., 1989).

Children who masturbate excessively or insert foreign objects into body orifices usually show no genital or anal injuries. Hyman et al. (1990) examined 97 mentally retarded individuals between 11 months and 21 years old whose behaviors included excessive masturbation and insertion of foreign objects into various body orifices. None had evidence of genital or anal injury.

*Can a child contract a sexually transmitted disease by merely sharing the same bed, toilet seat, or towel with an infected individual?*

In general, as the title implies, sexually transmitted diseases are sexually transmitted *(see discussion of sexually transmitted diseases in this chapter).*

*Can horseback riding, gymnastics, or dancing cause permanent genital changes?*

Injuries can occur with physical activities. When such injuries involve the genitalia, the event is very dramatic and will be reported immediately. If a physician finds hymenal changes after a child has disclosed sexual abuse or during a routine examination, injury from one of these activities is not being investigated because it would not be a reasonable explanation for the changes.

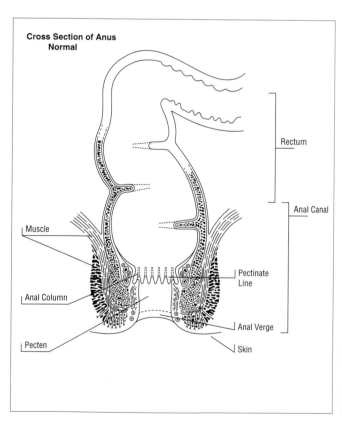

**Figure 9-24.** *Cross section of anus, normal.*

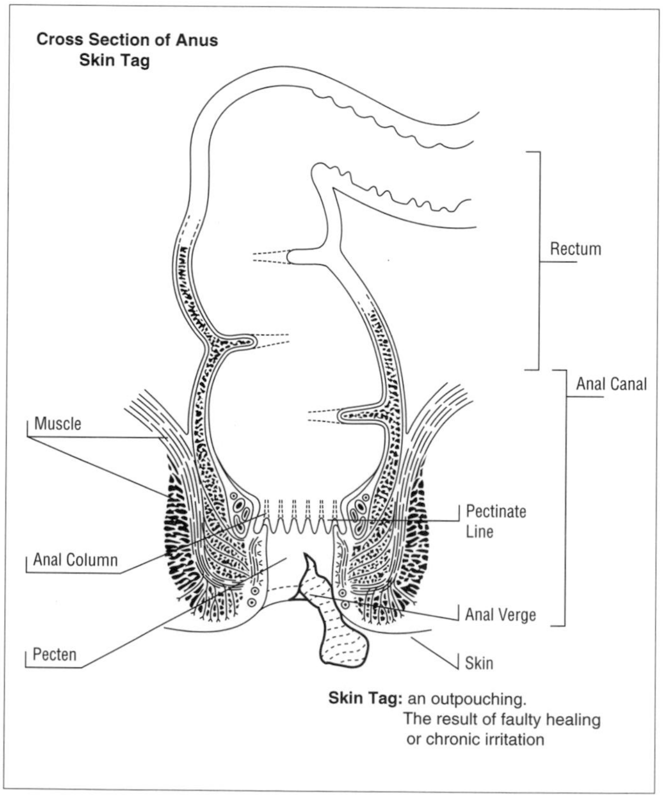

**Figure 9-25.** *Cross section of anus, skin tag.*

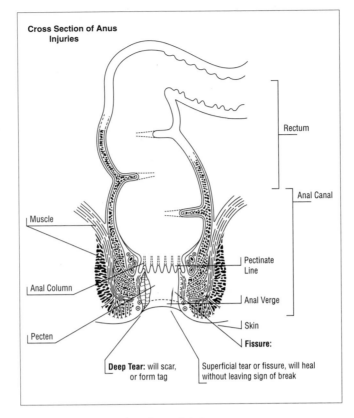

**Figure 9-26.** *Cross section of anus, injuries.*

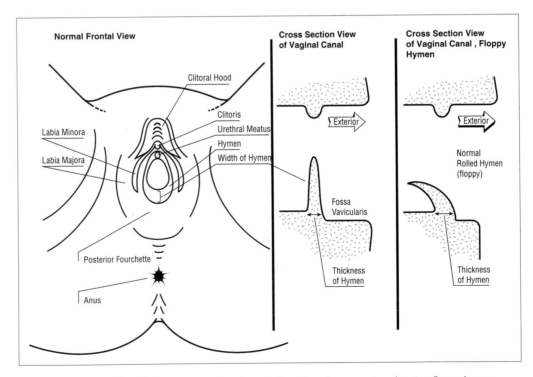

**Figure 9-27.** *Normal frontal view, cross section of vaginal canal, and cross section showing floppy hymen.*

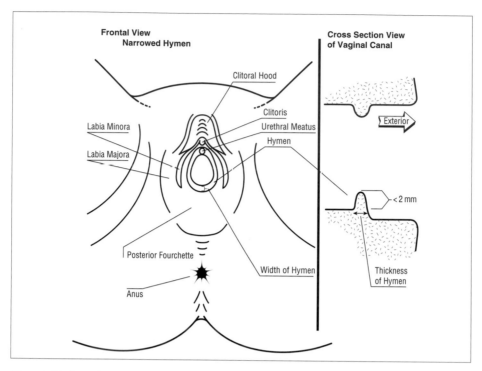

**Figure 9-28.** *Frontal view, narrowed hymen, and cross section of vaginal canal.*

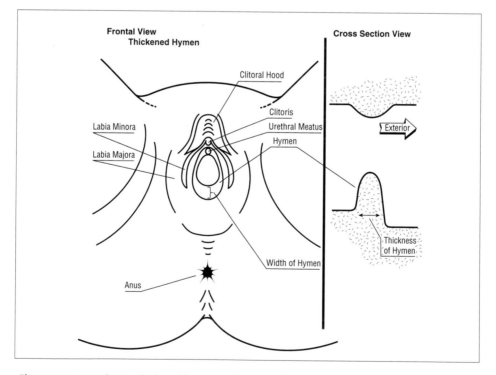

**Figure 9-29.** *Frontal view, thickened hymen, and cross section.*

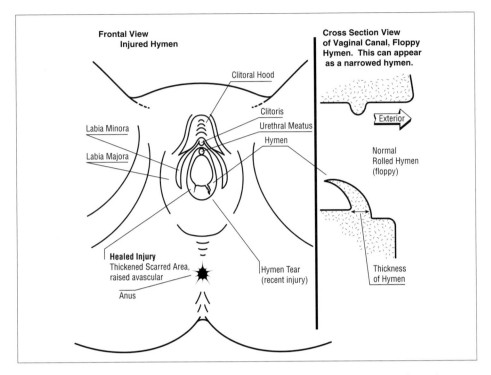

**Figure 9-30.** *Frontal view, injured hymen, and cross section of vaginal canal showing floppy hymen.*

## ♦BIBLIOGRAPHY

Bays, J, and Chadwick, D: Medical diagnosis of the sexually abused child, *Child Abuse Negl* 17:91-110, 1993.

Bays, J, and Jenny, C: Genital and anal conditions confused with child sexual abuse trauma, *Am J Dis Child* 144:1319-1322, 1990.

Berenson, AB, Heger, AH, Hayes, JM, Bailey, RK, and Emans, SJ: Appearance of the hymen in prepubertal girls, *Pediatrics* 89:387-394, 1992.

Bergeron C, Ferenczy, A, and Richart, R: Underwear: Contamination by human papillomaviruses, *Am J Obstet Gynecol* 162:25-29, 1990.

Bond GR, Dowd MD, Landsman I, and Rimsza M: Unintentional perineal injury in prepubescent girls: A multicenter, prospective report of 56 girls, *Pediatrics* 95:628-361, 1995.

Cantwell. 1983

Chadwick, DL, Berkowitz, CD, Kerns, DL, McCann, J, Reinhart, MA, and Strickland, SL: *Color Atlas of Child Sexual Abuse*, produced by the California Medical Association's Maternal, Perinatal and Child Care Subcommittee on Child Abuse, Year Book Medical Publishers, Inc, Chicago, 1989.

DeJong, AR, and Finkel, MA: Sexual abuse of children, *Curr Probl Pediatr* XX:490-567, 1990.

Enos, 1986

Finkel, MA: Anogenital trauma in sexually abused children, *Pediatrics* 84:317-322, 1989.

Fleming, KA, Venning, V, and Evans, M: DNA typing of genital warts and diagnosis of sexual abuse of children, *Lancet* 11:454, 1987.

Gabby, T, Winkleby, MA, Boyce, WT, Fisher, DL, Lancanster, A, Sensabaugh, GF, and Crim, D: Sexual abuse of children: The detection of semen on skin, *Am J Dis Child* 146:700-703, 1992.

Gardner, JJ: Descriptive study of genital variation in healthy, nonabused premenarchal girls, *J Pediatr* 120:251-257, 1992.

Graves, HCG, Sensabaugh, GF, and Blake, ET: Postcoital detection of a male-specific semen protein: Application to the investigation of rape, *N Engl J Med* 312:338, 1985.

Heger, A, and Emans, SJ: American Academy of Pediatrics: Introital diameter as the criterion for sexual abuse, *Pediatrics* 85:222-223, 1990.

Herman-Giddens, ME, and Frothingham, TE: Prepubertal female genitalia: Examination for evidence of sexual abuse, *Pediatrics* 80:203-208, 1987.

Herr, JC, Summers, TA, McGee, RS, Sutherland, WM, Sigman, M, and Evans, RJ: Characterization of a monoclonal antibody to a conserved epitope on human seminal vesicle-specific peptides: A novel probe/marker system for semen identification, *Biol Rep* 35:773, 1986.

Hobbs, CJ, and Wynne, JM: Sexual abuse of English boys and girls: The importance of anal examination, *Child Abuse Negl* 13:195-210, 1989.

Huffman, JW, Dewhurst, CJ, and Capraro, VJ: *The Gynecology of Childhood and Adolescence*, ed 2, WB Saunders Co, Philadelphia, 1981.

Hyman, SL, Fisher, W, Mercugliano, and Cataldo, MF: Children with self injurious behavior, *Pediatrics* 85:437-441, 1990.

Kellogg, ND, and Parra, JM: Linea vestibularis: A previously undescribed normal genital structure in female neonates, *Pediatrics* 87:926-929, 1991.

Kerns, DL, and Ritter, ML: Medical findings in child sexual abuse cases with perpetrator confessions, (Abstract) *Am J Dis Child* 146:494, 1992.

Kirby, LT: *Fingerprinting: An Introduction*, Stockton Press, New York, 1990.

McCann, J: Patterns of healing in cases of sexual abuse, Paper presented at symposium *Health Sciences Response to Child Maltreatment*, San Diego, CA, January, 1988.

McCann, J, Voris, J, and Simon, M: Genital injuries resulting from sexual abuse: A longitudinal study, *Pediatrics* 89:307-317, 1992.

McCann, J, Voris, J, Simon, M, and Wells, R: Perianal findings in prepubertal children selected for nonabuse: A descriptive study, *Child Abuse Negl* 13:179-193, 1989.

McCann, J, Voris, J, Simon, M, and Wells, R: Comparison of genital examination techniques in prepubertal girls, *Pediatrics* 85:182-187, 1990.

McCann, J, Wells, R, Simon, M, and Voris, J: Genital findings in prepubertal girls selected for nonabuse: A descriptive study, *Pediatrics* 86:428-439, 1990.

Monteleone, J, Brewer, J, Scalzo, A, Doerhoff, F, Munkel, W, Heaney, S, Bowen, K, Scherzinger, P, and LaRock, T: Urethral dilatation as a physical finding in sexual abuse (abstract). VII International Congress on Child Abuse and Neglect Book of Abstracts. FP106, 1988.

Muram, D: Anal and perianal abnormalities in prepubertal victims of sexual abuse, *Am J Obstet Gynecol* 161:278-281, 1989.

Muram, D: Child sexual abuse: Relationship between sexual acts and genital findings, *Child Abuse Negl* 13:211-216, 1989.

Neinstein, LS, Goldenring, J, and Carpenter, S: Nonsexual transmission of sexually transmitted diseases: An infrequent occurrence, *Pediatrics* 74:67-76, 1984.

O'Rahilly, R: *Anatomy: A Regional Study of Human Structure*, ed 5, WB Saunders Co, Philadelphia, 1986.

Pacheco, BP, Di Paola, G, Ribas, JM, Vighi, S, and Rueda, NG: Vulvar infection caused by human papilloma virus in children and adolescents without sexual contact, *Adolesc Pediatr Gynecol* 4:136-142, 1991.

Paradise, JE: Predictive accuracy and the diagnosis of sexual abuse: A big issue about a little tissue, *Child Abuse Negl* 13:169-176, 1989.

Paradise, JE: The medical evaluation of the sexually abused child, *Pediatr Clin North Am* 37:839-862, 1990.

Paul, DM: The medical examination in sexual offenses against children, *Med Sci Law* 17:251-258, 1977.

Pokorny, SF, and Kozinetz, CA: Configuration and other anatomic details of the prepubertal hymen, *Adolesc Pediatr Gynecol* 1:97-103, 1988.

Pokorny SF, Pokorny, WJ and Kramer, W: Acute genital injury in the prepubertal girl, *Am J Obstet Gynecol*, 166:1461-1466, 1992.

Steinhart, G, and Monteleone, JA: Unreported observation, 1990.

Teixeira, WRG: Hymenal colposcopic examination in sexual offenses, *Am J Forensic Med Pathol* 3:209-214, 1981.

Tipton, AC: Child sexual abuse: Physical examination techniques and interpretation of findings, *Adolesc Pediatr Gynecol* 2:10-25, 1989.

West R, Davies, A and Fenton, T; Accidental vulval injuries in childhood, *Br Med J*, 298:1002-1003, 1989.

White, S, Ingram, DL, and Lyna, PR: Vaginal introital diameter in the evaluation of sexual abuse, *Child Abuse Negl* 13:217-224, 1989.

Woodling, BA, and Heger, A: The use of the colposcope in the diagnosis of sexual abuse in the pediatric age group, *Child Abuse Negl* 10:111-114, 1986.

Wynne JM; Injuries to the genitalia in female children; *S Afr Med J*, 57:47-50, 1980.

# Sexual Abuse– The Interview

Vicki McNeese, M.S.

In recent years, child sexual abuse has captured the attention of professionals and the general public. This is largely due to the highly publicized stories of children sexually molested by the very adults entrusted with their care and well-being. Yet despite our increased awareness and understanding of the dynamics of child sexual abuse, it continues to be a difficult, if not painful, topic for many to contemplate and discuss. Recent attention focused on child sexual abuse clearly depicts the potentially significant effects on and vulnerability of the alleged victim, the perpetrator, and their respective families, as well as on evaluators charged with investigating such allegations. It has become increasingly important to develop stringent standards for the evaluation of sexual abuse allegations. Only through a comprehensive investigation of allegations, which includes objective, thorough, and well-documented interviews, can those involved best be protected.

In order to conduct objective, reliable, and child-sensitive interviews, professionals need an awareness and understanding of child development, the history and dynamics of sexual abuse, and a working knowledge of the continuing evolution of the evaluation process. Armed with this information, an evaluator can benefit from others' past experiences, positive and negative; assess potential pitfalls and risks to all those involved; and more confidently and comfortably address the challenging task at hand—the child interview.

## ♦History

In the late 1970s and early 1980s the growing battle against child sexual abuse, while not without opponents, seemed to be a safe and well-supported endeavor. However, as the momentum to identify and protect alleged victims of child sexual abuse grew, investigatory practices and disposition of such cases were increasingly called into question by critics. Hechler (1988) in *The Battle and the Backlash* described the mounting problems in the "child sexual abuse war." He identified clearly drawn lines between professionals regarding the prevalence of child sexual abuse, the credibility of children's statements, and the competence and objectivity of professionals who evaluate allegations of child sexual abuse.

## ♦Prevalence

The dramatic increase in reports of child sexual abuse in the past decade has caused professionals to ask if current statistics indicate an epidemic of child molestation or if greater public awareness and acceptance have resulted in increased reporting. Since the victims of child sexual abuse often delay reporting or may never disclose their victimization, the true incidence of child sexual abuse is difficult, if not impossible, to ascertain.

Results of a national study *(The National Study of the Incidence and Severity of Child Abuse and Neglect, 1981)* and a privately conducted survey *(Los Angeles Times Poll, 1985)* estimate that approximately one in four girls will be sexually victimized by age 18 (Finkelhor & Hotaling, 1984; Finkelhor, 1986; Finkelhor et al., 1990). Boys were initially considered to be less at risk for child sexual abuse; however, current epidemiological studies suggest that the incidence of sexual victimization of male children is notably higher than previously believed (Pescosolido, 1989). Childhood sexual abuse was reported by 16% of the males surveyed by the *Los Angeles Times* (1985). These findings, if extrapolated to the general population, suggest that one in six boys will experience sexual victimization. It has been proposed that victimization of boys may be comparable to that of girls, although, due to societal and gender expectations, males are less likely to report their victimization experiences. As a result, male victims are often not identified and thus do not receive appropriate intervention services.

As previously noted, there is considerable controversy and debate in the field of child sexual abuse regarding the accuracy of prevalence statistics. Many professionals contend that child sexual abuse continues to be underreported due to its nature of secrecy and lack of physical findings. On the other hand, critics of current practices cite significant problems in the investigatory process, particularly inadequate interviews conducted by overzealous and poorly trained evaluators, which leads to an overdiagnosis of child sexual abuse.

All professionals involved in evaluating allegations of child sexual abuse must attend to and objectively assess the criticism raised by colleagues. Rather than being viewed as forsaking the vigorous identification and protection of child victims of sexual abuse, honest consideration of criticisms can be used to ensure that evaluation practices are of the highest caliber. A comprehensive, well-documented evaluation by a competent evaluator will, in fact, serve to identify and protect a victimized child, as well as safeguard the rights of others involved. It should never be advocated that professionals, in our well-intended efforts to believe and protect a child, knowingly conduct a biased evaluation.

The evaluation of alleged victims of child sexual abuse is rapidly changing. Wherever possible, professionals responsible for assessing alleged victims and their families must be informed of recent findings in the disciplines of medical and mental health care as well as legal practice. Some clinicians responsible for a multiplicity of cases may feel ill-prepared to assess allegations of child sexual abuse. Even evaluators who feel confident in their knowledge of child development, as well as their ability to effectively communicate with children, are less confident in assessing the validity and credibility of a child's statement regarding sexual victimization. This is especially true if the alleged victim is a young child, developmentally delayed, and/or in any other way hindered in relating experiences and possible trauma.

Evaluators involved in interviewing children about child sexual abuse need to gather accurate information without suggesting particular responses to a child. A well-conducted interview should increase the likelihood that a child will be able to disclose any previous abusive experience and diminish the likelihood of obtaining false or inaccurate information. At the same time an objective, thorough, and well-documented interview will minimize the likelihood of erroneous conclusions.

It is critical that evaluators responsible for assessing allegations of sexual victimization of a child have knowledge and understanding specific to the field of child sexual abuse. Areas of particular concern include risk factors, the process of victimization, dynamics that may hinder a child's disclosure, and currently accepted techniques for evaluating alleged victims.

## ♦ RISK FACTORS

While any child is a potential victim of sexual abuse, Finkelhor (1986) has examined characteristics such as age, sex, ethnicity, and family relations to identify specific factors that may increase the risk for sexual victimization. His findings indicate that girls are at greater risk than boys. In general, children seem to be most vulnerable to sexual victimization during pre-adolescence, particularly between the ages of 8 and 12 years. Other risk factors cited include family disruptions; parental conflict, absence, or unavailability; and presence of a "nonbiological related father" (Finkelhor et al., 1990).

In recent years the literature concerning child sexual abuse has also started to examine and document the vulnerability of children when a sibling, cousin, or nonrelated child in the home is engaging in sexually reactive or abusive behaviors (Johnson, 1988). DeJong (1989) concluded that sexual interactions among siblings and cousins are common and that reported cases are usually abusive. Evaluators need to be aware of the potential risk to children who have unsupervised or minimally supervised contact with a child or adolescent who is sexually acting out. A history of sexual victimization in the parents' family of origin and/or a previous sexual abusive experience may also increase a child's risk for sexual victimization.

## ♦ VICTIMIZATION PROCESS AND DISCLOSURE INHIBITORS

Child sexual abuse should be viewed as a *process* rather than an isolated event. Most children who are abused recognize that something is wrong, but some lack the maturity to identify what that is or know how to respond to it (Fay et al., 1991). In assessing cases of possible sexual abuse, it is important that evaluators recognize and understand the process of victimization, including reasons children don't tell or delay disclosure of abuse. Findings reported by Berliner and Conte (1990) suggest that the victimization process involves three overlapping processes: sexualization of the relationship, justification of the sexual contact, and maintenance of the child's cooperation. Results of this study indicate that virtually all children who disclose a history of sexual abuse say they wish they would have told someone earlier.

One of the most common, compelling, and obvious reasons children often don't "tell" is fear (Smith, 1985). Child victims of sexual abuse not only fear physical repercussions, but also fear potential loss of home and/or the love and attention of a nonoffending parent. The offender is usually considerably larger and stronger than the child and wields overt or covert authority. From this perspective, even a vague threat of violence might be sufficient intimidation to leave a child feeling powerless and afraid (Tobin & Farley, 1990). In assessing suspected victims of abuse, recognition of the power differentiation between an offender and a child victim is a key consideration.

Victims of sexual abuse often feel ashamed or guilty and find few safe opportunities to disclose their victimization. Although shame is a powerful factor in maintaining a child's silence, ignorance of personal boundaries and appropriate physical contacts, especially in young children, also contribute to a child's silence or delayed disclosure. Often by the time a child recognizes the abusive nature of a trusted adult's behavior, the child is likely experiencing feelings of responsibility, shame, and/or isolation—feelings that further inhibit disclosure of victimization experiences. It should be noted that some offenders, rather than using threats, secure a child's compliance and silence through bribes and/or special privileges.

All too often a child's safety depends solely on his or her ability to report the sexually victimizing experience. A frustration for many professionals in the field of child sexual abuse is a child's denial of sexual abuse in the face of overwhelming physical and/or corroborating evidence.

Literature as well as clinical experience emphasizes that a child's disclosure of sexual abuse is a dynamic process. Sorensen and Snow (1991) explored this phenomenon and outlined a process with definable phases and characteristics. Their findings suggest that disclosure follows a progression that may include denial, tentative disclosure, active disclosure, recantation, and reaffirmation. These authors report that denial is a frequent response when a child is too frightened, threatened, or insecure to acknowledge his or her victimization experience. Conclusions of the study reveal that 72% of the children in confirmed cases of sexual abuse initially denied any history of abuse. In only 11% of the cases examined did children actively disclose when they were first questioned.

Recognition of a disclosure progression challenges the common assumption that children can immediately make a disclosure with questioning. These findings have far-reaching implications for investigative procedures and suggest that evaluation protocols which provide more than a single opportunity for disclosure are most likely to facilitate the collection of reliable and accurate information. While steps in the process of disclosure are identifiable and share common elements, it is important to recognize that the process for any individual child may be highly idiosyncratic.

## ♦ BEHAVIORAL INDICATORS

Children may manifest various behavioral changes in response to stress and/or trauma. The particular stress to which a child is reacting may be a divorce, death in the family, the family's relocations (which may necessitate multiple changes in the child's life), a significant illness or injury, physical maltreatment, and/or sexual victimization. Stress-related behaviors often observed in children include but are not limited to sleeping and eating disturbances, increased somatic complaints, regressed behaviors, anxiety and/or depression, changes in academic performance, and aggressive behaviors (Sgroi et al., 1983) (**Table 10-1**).

---

### Table 10-1. Nonspecific Stress-Related Behaviors Observed in Children and Adolescents

In assessing stress-related behaviors the abruptness of onset, severity, and chronicity are factors that should be carefully considered. Abrupt and severe behavioral changes may be particularly indicative of emotional distress and/or possible trauma.

1. Sleep disturbances (e.g., nightmares, night terrors, fear of the dark or sleeping alone, trouble falling asleep and/or frequently awakening during the night, or excessive sleeping).

2. Changes in eating behaviors (e.g., loss of or sudden increase in appetite with resulting weight loss or gain).

3. Regressive behaviors (child's behavior regresses to earlier developmental level, such as clinging and separation difficulties, thumbsucking, and/or diminished bladder and/or bowel control in a child who had been successfully toilet trained).

4. Hyperactivity/hypervigilance/insecure behaviors.

5. Excessive and/or inappropriate fears (e.g., fear of a particular or familiar place, person, or activity not previously noted).

6. Hostile, aggressive, or acting out behaviors/play.

7. Varied and repeated somatic complaints with no known physical etiology.

8. Change/decline in academic performance, school avoidance, poor peer relations.

9. Behaviors suggestive of or in response to a high level of anxiety and/or depression (e.g., excessive crying, expressed feelings of hopelessness, withdrawal from family and friends, diminished interest in previously anticipated activities, decline in personal appearance, suicidal ideation and/or gesture, and substance abuse).

10. Delinquent and/or runaway behaviors.

Research in the area of child sexual abuse (Finkelhor & Browne, 1985; Gomes-Schwartz et al., 1985; Conte & Schuerman, 1987) has consistently concluded that children who have a history of child sexual abuse exhibit more symptoms than children who have no known history of sexual victimization. However, recent studies indicate that there does not appear to be any significant difference in stress-related symptom presentation between child sexual abuse and other types of trauma that children experience (Beitchman et al., 1991). The presence of nonspecific stress-related behaviors is an important factor in the overall evaluation of a child, although evaluators must be cautious when interpreting children's behaviors. Evidence of stress-related behaviors should not be a primary determinant in the belief that a child has been abused. Similarly, the absence of such behavioral reactions should not lead a professional to conclude that a child has not been abused. While most children who have been sexually abused do display some nonspecific stress-related behaviors, other sexually victimized children exhibit no significant observable behavioral reactions. Stress-related behaviors in children should alert a professional to a child's feelings of distress and possible trauma, and should be assessed further. Sexually abused children may have an increased prevalence of certain traits, but these traits may also be found in children without histories of abuse.

*Specific behavioral reactions in children are often characteristic of that particular child's developmental level. The following outlines some abilities to be expected at specific levels:*

### Preschool Children

Preschool children demonstrate a variety of affective, cognitive, and behavioral symptoms in response to stress (Lusk & Waterman, 1986). Young children often respond to stress and/or trauma by exhibiting changes in eating and sleeping habits, chronic nightmares, regression, and an increase in fearful and clinging behaviors. Young children may also demonstrate changes in bowel and bladder control, with those who have been previously toilet trained beginning to wet and soil themselves. Preschool children may also demonstrate an increased activity level as well as aggressive behaviors in play activities and their interactions with others.

### School-aged Children

School-aged children may demonstrate various emotional, cognitive, and behavioral changes that can be observed by parents and/or school personnel. These children may display notable moodiness, behaviors indicating a high level of anxiety and/or depression, and diminished academic functioning (Gomes-Schwartz et al., 1985). These affective and behavioral reactions may be accompanied by varied and repeated somatic complaints with no known physical cause.

### Adolescents

Adolescents may come to the attention of mental health professionals in response to a crisis or an episode of acting out behavior such as a suicidal gesture, episodes of running away from home, or hostile, aggressive, and/or delinquent behaviors. Adolescents may also respond to personal and family stressors by withdrawing from family or friends, altering academic performance, or changing personal hygiene and appearance. It should be noted that due to the frequent delays in reporting incidents of child sexual abuse, adolescents may present with a history of chronic affective disturbances and behavioral problems. A comprehensive evaluation is indicated to fully assess the extent and origins of presenting problems.

Children may also come to the attention of professionals due to sexually reactive behaviors. While most stress-related behaviors are nonspecific for sexual abuse, Sgroi et al. (1988) have identified three sexually reactive behaviors likely to be seen in children who have been involved in direct or vicarious sexual experiences. Behaviors that have increased specificity for sexual abuse include excessive masturbation, sexual victimization of another child, and promiscuity. Developmentally inappropriate sexualized behaviors in children of all ages who have been sexually abused is one of the most consistent findings reported in the literature (Friedrich et al., 1986; Burns et al., 1988).

Children may also demonstrate sexualized behaviors that have not been identified as specific to sexual abuse but are suspicious for developmentally inappropriate sexual knowledge and/or experiences. If observed in a child or reported by a caregiver, such behaviors may warrant further evaluation.

*These behaviors include but are not limited to the following:*

— *Diminished personal boundaries, including indiscriminate kissing, hugging, and/or sexualized touching of other children or adults.*

— *Developmentally inappropriate "seductive" behavior to solicit attention, acceptance, and/or affection from significant others.*

— *Curiosity regarding genitalia or behavioral reactions to observed sexual material or situations that are atypical for that child's developmental level.*

— *Extreme reactions to bathing or toileting.*

— *Excessive fear or resistance to contact with the opposite sex.*

— *Strong resistance or refusal to participate in age-appropriate physical or social activities (i.e., physical education classes or sleeping over) where changing clothes or showering is involved.*

## DIFFERENTIATING NORMAL FROM ABNORMAL SEXUAL BEHAVIOR

Since it has been well-documented that children who have a history of child sexual victimization often act out sexually and/or engage in sexual activity with other individuals, it is important that evaluators involved in evaluating allegations of abuse have an understanding of normal sexual behaviors in children. While information regarding developmental norms for sexual behaviors in children is limited, Sgroi et al. (1988) and Friedrich et al. (1991) have presented a developmental context for sexual behaviors observed within different age ranges for children. Normative data regarding sexual behavior of children at different developmental stages can guide an evaluator in differentiating normal sexual behaviors from those indicative of sexual abuse experiences.

Children who have a history of trauma, including sexual victimization, may present with symptoms associated with a diagnosis of post-traumatic stress disorder (PTSD). While post-traumatic phenomena have long been recognized in the literature, PTSD has only recently been examined as a possible consequence of child sexual abuse. Although now recognized as occurring in children, little is known about the course of PTSD in childhood. McLeer et al. (1988) cite evidence of PTSD symptom clusters in sexually abused children, including reexperiencing phenomena, avoidance behaviors, and autonomic hyperarousal. A follow-up study (Deblinger et al., 1989) of children hospitalized with psychiatric disorders with a history of sexual abuse reported that sexually abused children suffered significantly more re-experiencing phenomena than physically abused or nonabused subjects. McLeer and colleagues caution that children who develop PTSD may not only suffer from the direct trauma of their abuse, but may also experience chronic symptoms that can interfere with a child's overall developmental progress.

## ◆ SCREENING AND REFERRAL PROCESS

Due to the complexity and the number of professionals who may be involved in evaluating alleged victims of child sexual abuse, it is necessary to organize initial screening and referral data. This can be accomplished using a standardized format *(see Telephone Referral/Screening Outline)*. The evaluators must exercise professional judgment when a request is received to interview an alleged victim of child sexual abuse, with an emphasis placed on meeting specific predetermined criteria before initiating any evaluation.

When it is determined that evaluation of an alleged victim of sexual abuse is appropriate, the standardized questionnaire can avoid duplicating services and facilitate communication among professionals. Similarly, when other action is indicated and/or referral to another agency is made, the information can be easily documented.

## Telephone Referral/Screening Outline

Date_____Taken by _____

**Patient Information:**

Caller_____Relationship to Child _____

Child's Name_____BD_____Age_____Sex:  M  F

Current Address_____Phone _____

Parent's Name _____

Living with:  Parents__  Mother__  Father__  Relative__  Foster Care__  Other__

Siblings (Names and Ages)_____

Current/Pending Legal Action:  Divorce  Y  N  Custody Visitation  Y  N

   Other_____

Developmental Level of Child: Age Appropriate_____Delayed _____

Behavioral Indicators:  Y  N  Sexual Acting Out_____Stress-Related _____

Describe_____

Physical Symptoms:  Y  N  Describe _____

**Referring Information:**

Referred by_____ Agency _____

Address_____Phone _____

Reason for Referral _____

_____

_____

Hot Line Call Made:  Y  N  When_____Reported by _____

Other Agencies Involved:  Y  N  Name, Address, Telephone _____

_____

Is Child Currently Protected?  Y  N

Alleged Perpetrator(s) Name_____Relationship _____

Male_____Female_____Adult_____Child_____(Age)_____(Other) _____

Disclosure: None_____Purposeful_____Accidental_____Describe _____

Child Disclosed to: Mother___Father___Other Family___Peer___Other___

Reported Incidence: Single  Multiple  Last incident _____

Previous Interview(s): Y N By: DFS_____(Date)_____Police_____

(Date)_____Other Professional_____(Date)_____

Results of Interview: Disclosed Sexual Abuse____Physical Abuse____Denied____

Previous P.E. Y N By:_____Date _____

Results of P.E. _____

Previous Allegations of Sexual Abuse: Y N When _____

Disposition of Those Allegations _____

Previous Sexual Abuse Evaluation: Y N Location_____Date _____

Is Child Currently in Counseling? Y N Provider _____

**Plan:**

Notified Caller to Make Hotline Report: Y N NA

Scheduled Appointment: Y N Interview_____P.E._____

Parent Consult_____Date_____

Referred Child to DFS___Police___Therapist___Attorney___Medical Services___

(Name)_____Other_____

Comments_____

_____

Additional Telephone Contacts: _____

_____

## ◆EVALUATION PROCESS

The following interview protocols reflect guidelines for the evaluation of sexual abuse of children proposed by the American Professional Society on the Abuse of Children (1990), the American Academy of Child and Adolescent Psychiatry (1988), and the American Academy of Pediatrics (1991).

## ◆CAREGIVER INTERVIEW

When abuse is suspected and it has been determined that a child will be interviewed, it is recommended that a minimum of one interview be conducted with the parent(s)/primary caregiver and/or other appropriate individual(s) in order to obtain applicable information in the following areas: family constellation and history, child's health history and current status, child's developmental level, behavioral indicators, psychosexual history including family's attitude and practices regarding privacy, nudity, sexual attitudes, and bath time and bedtime patterns, and allegations or suspicion of possible sexual abuse. Detailed information regarding the child's initial disclosure of the event is also obtained. This interview includes the parent or primary caregiver's interpretation of the child's statement and/or behavior regarding possible sexual abuse. It is recommended that this interview be conducted by the primary evaluator, prior to the initial child interview, and not with the child present. Information regarding sexual abuse allegations obtained from a caregiver in the presence of the child may contaminate any subsequent statements made by the child. A child may feel compelled to provide information to the evaluator that is consistent with the caregiver's statements. Statements made by caregivers should be documented specifically and in detail. Caregivers should be informed that information obtained may be shared with other professionals who are investigating allegations of abuse, as well as those making decisions regarding the appropriateness of legal action.

An information-gathering interview may be conducted with the alleged perpetrator, if he or she is a member of the child's immediate family (parent), when this is deemed appropriate. The purpose of this interview is to gather pertinent data regarding the child's level of functioning and behaviors, the family situation, and the alleged or suspected perpetrator's knowledge of current allegations. The alleged or suspected perpetrator, as well as other family members, may also be referred for further evaluation by an independent assessor.

If information gathered during a parent interview reveals a current pending divorce or custody dispute and the allegations of sexual abuse were first disclosed during legal proceedings, it may be advisable to refer some or all parties (parent[s] and child/children) to an evaluator with the capabilities and expertise to evaluate all family members. Appropriate referral information should be provided to the family as indicated.

## RELEASE OF INFORMATION

To facilitate review of all relevant information, parents are requested to sign release of information forms. This enables the evaluator to request information from other sources. Parents may also be requested to sign authorizations permitting the evaluation results to be shared with appropriate child protective, law enforcement, and/or treatment services.

Caregivers are informed that in the case of an open child abuse investigation, investigatory agencies (including child protective services, law enforcement agencies, and court officials) may have access to information gathered during an evaluation. They are also told that reports will be made as mandated by state law to child protective services. Information regarding evaluation procedures will be reviewed with parents at the initial interview.

## ASSESSMENT OF FAMILY DYNAMICS

In conducting the parent/caregiver interview the evaluator should carefully assess family dynamics and possible pathologies. It is important to identify stressors other than sexual abuse that may explain a child's statement or behaviors. Diagnostic information gathered at the time of the parent/caregiver interview is important, not only to the evaluation process, but also in the formulation of an appropriate treatment plan.

A behavior rating scale may also be used to gather specific information about the types and intensity of a child's problematic behaviors. The rating scale is completed by the child's parent(s) or primary caregiver.

The following is a sample of a parent/caregiver interview that organizes material gathered at the time of the initial contact with the parent or caregiver. This interview format may be modified to meet the needs of a particular agency and/or individual evaluator.

---

## Parent/Caregiver Interview Outline

Date: _____

Primary Evaluator: _____

Parent/Caregiver Interview (not to be conducted in presence of the child):

Person(s) Interviewed_____Relationship to Child _____

Family Constellation (Members in Household):

Adult _____Relationship to Child _____

Adult_____ Relationship to Child _____

Adult_____ Relationship to Child _____

Child_____ Relationship _____

Child_____ Relationship _____

Child_____ Relationship _____

Others_____ Relationship _____

Caretakers Outside of the Home _____

_____

_____

**Family History:**

Parents are:  Married_____Divorced_____Separated_____Single _____

If parents divorced or never married, does child have visitation with noncustodial parent? Y N   Visitation schedule _____

Date of last visit _____

Child lives with: Parents___Mother___Father___Foster Care___Other ___

Legal action pending: Y N  Divorce___Custody/Visitation_____

History of child sexual abuse in mother's family of origin:  Y N

If yes, victim_____Alleged perpetrator _____

History of child sexual abuse in father's family of origin:  Y N

If yes, victim_____ Alleged perpetrator _____

History of child sexual abuse of other siblings/children in household:  Y N

If yes, victim  _____

Alleged perpetrator  _____

Has child had unsupervised contact with any above named alleged perpetrators?  Y N
If yes, has child ever alleged child sexual abuse by person(s)?  Y  N
Identify/Describe_____

History of psychiatric illnesses in family:  Y  N _____

History of drug/alcohol abuse in family:  Y  N_____

History of domestic violence in family:  Y  N_____

History of previous child sexual abuse in family:  Y  N  _____

Physical abuse in family:  Y  N_____

Previous involvement of Child Protective Services:  Y  N   Date _____

Describe_____

Police involvement:  Y  N  Date_____Describe _____

Mother history of: Sexually transmitted disease_____Genital warts_____

I.V. drug use_____  HIV+ _____

Father history of: Sexually transmitted disease_____Genital warts_____

I.V. drug use_____ HIV+ _____

Has child been exposed to pornographic material?   Y  N   Describe_____

_____

**Background Information of Child:**

Birth history: Unremarkable_____Remarkable _____Describe_____

Developmental level: Age appropriate_____Delayed_____

Language development: Age appropriate_____Delayed_____

Toilet trained:  Y  N   Age: _____

Stress-related behaviors:  Y  N   Describe _____

Onset and length of behaviors:_____

School/Day care (Name):_____Grade _____

Academic performance: Average or above_____Below average_____

Special education services:  Y  N _____

History of chronic health problems:  Y  N _____

History of UTI/bladder infections:  Y  N   Date: _____

History of chronic constipation:  Y  N _____

History of genital injuries, surgeries, diagnostic procedures:  Y  N _____

Current medication:  Y  N _____

Past or current physical symptoms: _____

Present sleeping arrangements in household: _____

Family stressors during past year?_____

Has child disclosed history of child sexual abuse?  Y  N _____

Describe _____

_____

Child disclosed to: (Name) _____

Relationship_____Date _____

Disclosure: Purposeful_____Accidental_____Spontaneous_____

        Upon questioning_____ By whom_____

Has child displayed developmentally inappropriate sexual knowledge, sexualized behaviors, and/or excessive masturbation?  Y  N  Explain_____

_____

_____

_____

Alleged perpetrator(s) (Name):_____

Relationship:_____Location:_____

Last known contact (Date): _____

Does child have current contact with named individual?  Y  N

Describe_____

Hot line report made:  Y N  Date_____Reporter _____

Status of alleged perpetrator_____
Other agencies involved (*See Referral Form):*

Previous interview(s), P.E.(s), and results *(See Referral Form)*

_____

Does parent/caregiver believe child sexual abuse allegations?  Y  N

Uncertain_____

Reason: _____

**Collateral Information:**

Child reports others present at time of abuse:  Y  N

Describe_____

Others state they observed incident(s) of abuse:  Y  N

Describe_____

Release of information signed to obtain/release information to:

Name/Address:

> Private Pediatrician  Y  N  _____

> Hospital  Y  N_____

> Division of Family Services  Y  N_____

> Law enforcement  Y  N  _____

> Therapist  Y  N  _____

> Other  Y  N  _____

## ♦CHILD INTERVIEW GUIDELINES

The initial child interview is conducted after the caregiver interview has been completed. Ideally, a minimum of two interviews should be conducted with the child. A young child or a child identified as having special needs, such as developmental delay or language impairment, can require additional interviews. At some point in the evaluation process the child will be questioned directly about sexual abuse. However, repeated questioning of a child regarding sexual abuse, when the child is not reporting or denying abuse, is contraindicated.

It is preferable that one evaluator conduct both caregiver(s) and child interviews to foster continuity and consistency. Following collection of parent, child, and collateral information, impressions regarding the credibility and reliability of a child's statements, the probability that sexual victimization has occurred, and the presence of alternative explanations may be formulated. Based on all available information, conclusions and recommendations can be provided to caregivers and appropriate investigative authorities. The evaluator should attempt to reconcile the content of the interview with other information.

It is important to focus on and be sensitive to the child's needs at the time of the interview. Children quickly assess the interest, investment, and ease of the evaluator.

The evaluator must create a safe and private atmosphere that fosters rapport and trust, diminishes feelings of anxiety, and enables the child to talk openly. This includes securing child-sized furniture and arranging the surroundings in a way that is child-friendly. Availability of materials such as paper, pencils, and crayons is suggested to put the child at ease, facilitate nonverbal communication, and help the child clarify verbal statements. Adequate time should be allotted so that neither the evaluator nor the child feels rushed. The evaluator must be sensitive to the child's pace and emotional responses. If a child is hungry, tired, or needing a bathroom break, the outcome of the interview may be compromised.

It is important to make the evaluation as predictable as possible for the child. First, the evaluator should explain the purpose and format of the assessment, and address the child's expectations and/or fears. While appropriate reassurances can foster rapport and communication, the evaluator is cautioned not to make promises he or she will be unable to keep. Often a child will ask, "If I tell you, will you tell my Mom/Dad?" or "If I tell you, will you promise not to tell anyone?" The evaluator must be honest and supportive regarding the need to ensure the child's safety. An evaluator can respond to a child's concern by saying, "After we talk, I'll do everything I can to help keep you safe and tell you what I know will happen next." If a child feels betrayed by the evaluator's use of information obtained, it can potentially have negative effects on the child's well-being and on the outcome of the evaluation.

## The Developmentally Appropriate Interview

The interviewing approach and the language used by the evaluator should be developmentally appropriate and match the child's age and level of functioning. It is necessary to establish the terminology the child uses for people, things, body parts, and sexual behaviors. The evaluator should ask the child to define words that may be ambiguous before using them in the interview. Words such as "case" and "counselor" may not mean the same thing to a child as they do to the evaluator and should be clearly defined.

Given the importance of communication between the evaluator and child during the interview process, close attention should be given to the language exchange. The evaluator should use language sensitive to a child's developmental level. Language should be adapted to fit the child's vocabulary and kept consistent throughout the interview.

Using developmentally sensitive language is particularly important when interviewing young children. Saywitz (1990) advocates using several short questions, such as "Who was there?" or "Where was your mom?" rather than long complex questions. Questions that are direct and use short words, simple verbs, and single negatives are also more likely to be understood by a young child. Miscommunication is likely to occur when children are asked long and complex questions. This is particularly the case with young children who typically respond only to the part of the question they understand, disregarding other information contained in the questions. Likewise, young children are unable to recognize their partial understanding or confusion in order to ask for clarification. The use of developmentally sensitive techniques can contribute significantly to the evaluator's confidence that the child has a good understanding of the questions asked and has responded accordingly.

It is also helpful to clarify response options for the child before direct questioning. The child should know that he or she is not *required* to answer the question asked by the evaluator; the child has permission to refuse to answer. Explain to the child that saying "I don't want to talk about that now" in response to a direct question is preferable to giving inaccurate information or saying "I don't know" when he or she does in fact know. Also, if a child declines to respond to a specific inquiry, the evaluator may want to follow up with additional questions, such as "What do you think might happen if you talk about it?" This helps to clarify how the child is feeling and the source of any reluctance. Hopefully, more than one interview has been scheduled, so the evaluator will have the opportunity to return to sensitive questions that a child was unwilling to answer.

If following the initial interview with a child, the evaluator is uncertain of the child's cognitive functioning, has doubts about the child's level of language development, or suspects the presence of possibly severe emotional and/or psychiatric disturbance, further assessment by a mental health professional may be suggested as part of the evaluation. A psychological/psychiatric assessment is indicated in cases where the child's delayed development and/or disturbance could significantly interfere with the child's ability to participate in the evaluation. If the child was previously evaluated by a psychiatrist and/or psychologist, the evaluator should attempt to secure appropriate records before completing the sexual abuse evaluation.

As stated earlier, it is best to try to interview the child more than once. The following discussion outlines the stages of the process assuming that more than one interview is possible. If only one interview is feasible, the evaluator will need to be thorough and take sufficient time to obtain an accurate evaluation of the situation.

## INITIAL INTERVIEW WITH THE CHILD

At the initial interview the evaluator's primary tasks are to establish a safe and comfortable environment, develop rapport, and assess the developmental level of the child. Young children may be fearful and resistant to separating from their parent(s). While a parent may accompany the child to the initial meeting to assist in giving the child a sense of security, the evaluator should advise the parent(s) that sexual abuse allegations will not be discussed with the parent(s) present.

At the initial interview, in the context of acclimating the child to the evaluation process, the evaluator is advised to ask the child "Do you know why you are here today?" or "How come you are here today?" or "What did your (Mom, Dad, Grandma, etc.) tell you about coming here today?" If the child indicates that his or her intent is to discuss allegations of sexual abuse by saying "To tell what happened" or "To talk about what my (uncle, etc.) did," the evaluator should follow a child's lead by saying "Tell me about that." At that time, the evaluator should encourage a narrative statement from the child with minimal questioning. Follow-up inquiries to clarify a child's initial report can then be asked. However, if a child claims no understanding of the purpose of the appointment and appears reluctant to discuss it further, the evaluator should provide a simple explanation, identifying the interview as an opportunity for the child and evaluator to talk about the child's everyday experiences and anything that might be troubling the child.

At the first session the evaluator can begin assessing the child's overall development (cognitive, language, social and interpersonal, and emotional) and relevant skills through structured dialogue, informal tasks, and play activities. Concepts such as size, number, location, and time should be assessed. Observation and interaction with the child can yield an estimation of the child's level of functioning. The establishment of developmental landmarks can assist the evaluator to interpret information obtained during child interviews. If significant delays are detected in a child's intelligence and/or verbal skills, the interviewer must modify the interview to fit the child's particular level of development and special needs. This is critical for the information gathered to be considered valid.

*As part of developmental screening procedures, especially with young children, the evaluator can gather information by asking a child to:*

1. Provide basic personal identifying information (i.e., name, age, place of residence, members of household, school placement, and caretakers). Other pertinent questions may be asked to gather information regarding custodial care and relationships. Children may be asked to outline a typical day at their parent's/caregiver's house. This can give information regarding family practices, including bath and bedtime patterns.

2. State gender of self and others.

3. Identify and label general body parts.

4. Identify and label genitalia and functions of identified body parts.

Dolls (with or without anatomic detail) or simple standard boy and girl drawings may be used to aid and clarify a child's identification of general body parts and genitalia.

Unless a child is deemed to be at immediate risk or spontaneously reports allegations of sexual abuse, direct questioning regarding possible sexual abuse is not recommended during the initial interview.

## SUBSEQUENT INTERVIEWS WITH THE CHILD

The second (and subsequent) interview(s) begin with the evaluator reestablishing contact and rapport with the child. Conversation regarding the child's recent (since the first interview) family and school activities as well as play activities can put the child at ease. Reviewing activities and the content of the discussion of the initial interview can also help in reacclimating the child to the surroundings.

The primary purpose of the second and subsequent interviews is to directly question the child about any possible occurrence of sexual abuse. The evaluator uses open-ended questions that facilitate the child's disclosure rather than questions that suggest particular responses. Initially the evaluator should attempt to obtain a narrative response that involves only minimal nondirective questioning. The child should be encouraged to relate information regarding possible inappropriate touch in his or her own words. Later questioning can be directed from general open-ended questions to more focused and specific inquiries, as is appropriate for each child. For young and/or special needs children, it may be necessary and appropriate to ask more specific or directive questions (Faller, 1990). As questioning moves from general open-ended inquiries to more directive questions, the confidence level in a child's responses diminishes, although evaluators should be aware that information obtained from directive questions can be accurate and reliable.

One technique to note is the "cognitive interview," which is useful in interviewing some children by aiding their recall of reported experiences (Saywitz, 1992). This technique, developed by R. Edward Geiselman, is a guided memory search that has recently been modified for use with children. Modifications provide specific instructions to children regarding the demands of the interview task, as well as revisions of general retrieval aids. Saywitz (1992) reports that results from recent studies utilizing these techniques indicate improvement in the quality of useful information gained from latency age children without creating increased inaccuracy.

Upon completion of the evaluation, it is important to acknowledge a child's participation, cooperation, and assistance in providing information regarding his or her experiences. The evaluator can express understanding that the evaluation may have been challenging and stressful at times. The evaluator can be supportive by listening to and validating a child's feelings, although caution should be used not to suggest that a child should respond or feel a particular way. The child may be encouraged to ask the evaluator any questions, discuss any concerns or fears, or express current needs. As previously noted, one of the evaluator's responsibilities is to make the evaluation as predictable as possible for the child. Depending on information known to the evaluator, the child should be informed in age-appropriate language what is likely to happen next. A young child might be told, "We are done talking. You are going home with your mom now. Another man wants to talk to you about what you told me. He'll call your mom. Then you and your mom can go and see him at his office." If a child is referred for counseling, that may also be explained briefly. Lastly, the evaluator can help the child identify support people in his or her environment (i.e., "Who can you talk to if you have a question or feel worried, scared, etc.?"). It is also reassuring for the child to know that the evaluator can be available if a child wants to talk further.

The following interview format or a modified version may be helpful in guiding and documenting child interviews.

## Child Interview Outline

Child's name:_____Evaluator:_____

Date:_____Others present: _____

General identifying information obtained from child:

Name  Y  N  _____Age Y  N  _____Birthdate Y  N

Home address  Y  N  _____School placement  Y  N  _____

Identified members of household: _____

_____

Other: Caretakers/day care: _____

_____

**Developmental assessment (young children)**

Identification of:

Primary colors  Y  N    Letters/numbers  Y  N

Drawings: House  Y  N    Tree  Y  N    Person  Y  N    Other_____

Other measures:_____

_____

_____

Affect/mood: _____

Behavioral observations/activity level: _____

Information gathered during initial session (i.e., typical day): _____

_____

_____

**Subsequent Child Interview(s):**

Date:_____

*Assessment of Possible Sexual Abuse:*

Questioning presented to ascertain if child knows purpose of appointment on this date.

Do you know why you are here today? _____

Who brought (came with) you today?  If child gives name(s) only, attempt to establish relationship to child. _____

_____

Ascertain if named person told child to relate any specific information to evaluator on this date.

Did (named person) tell you to say anything to me today? If yes, what? _____

_____

Use of dolls (anatomically detailed or nonspecific) for identification and clarification of general body parts  Y  N    Genitalia  Y  N

Demonstrates knowledge of general body parts  Y  N    Method of parts labeled (pointing/verbally labeled)

Identifies private parts:  Male Y N  Female Y  N

Method of parts labeled (pointing/verbally labeled):

Labels male genitalia: Y  N_____

Demonstrates knowledge of function: _____

Labels female genitalia:  Y  N  _____

_____

Demonstrates knowledge of function: _____

Assessment of child's understanding of different kinds of touch.

Describe: _____ _____

_____

_____

Adequate understanding demonstrated:   Y  N

Questioning to address possible sexual victimization of child:

If the child discloses sexual victimization, the evaluator should attempt to obtain a narrative of the sexual abuse allegation.

Tell me about that (what happened). Continue to gather information with similar statements.

_____

_____

_____

_____

If the child gives a limited statement and/or is unable to give a narrative response, more direct questioning may be necessary to obtain additional identifying information and/or clarification.

If a statement of inappropriate touch is given, an attempt should be made to ascertain the following information: (If multiple perpetrators are identified, efforts should be made to gather information on a single individual or abusive experience at a time to avoid confusion.)

—Identification of alleged perpetrator(s)

—Relationship of alleged perpetrator(s) to child

—Sex and age of alleged perpetrator(s)

—Type(s) of inappropriate touch

—Time, location(s), frequency, and context of alleged abuse

—Presence or absence of element of secrecy

—Circumstances of initial disclosure, including person, time, location, and context

—Other children or adults directly or indirectly involved in present allegations of abuse

—Physical and/or behavioral response(s) of child at time of abuse (i.e., physical discomfort, actions taken, etc.)

—Any prior history or allegations of abuse

—Any attempts by adults to instruct child to give inaccurate information

—Dolls used in sexual abuse assessment for clarification of child's statements: Y N Anatomically detailed: Y N Nonspecific: Y N

## ANATOMICALLY DETAILED DOLLS

A word of caution should be added regarding the use of interview aids, such as anatomically detailed dolls and/or drawings. Although these may be useful for clarification and/or demonstration of a child's statement, the interpretation of a child's drawings or interactions with anatomically detailed dolls must be made cautiously. Information gathered from these techniques should be viewed as supplemental data, but never as conclusive evidence that sexual abuse has occurred. Doubt cast on the usefulness and reliability of the dolls was clearly illustrated by recent court decisions in California in which evidence obtained from use of anatomically detailed dolls was disallowed (*In re: Amber B. & Tella B., 191 Calif. 3rd 682, 1987*; *In re: Christine C & Michael C, Calif App. 3rd 676, 1987*). Critics alleged that anatomically detailed dolls are anatomically distorted and/or suggestive and lead normal nonabused children to engage in sexually explicit play that may be misinterpreted by evaluators as evidence of abuse. Others charge that the use of anatomically detailed dolls during interviews of suspected victims teaches children responses favored and reinforced by the interviewer (Wakefield & Underwager, 1988).

Current research findings support the usefulness of anatomically detailed dolls in evaluating child sexual abuse, but professionals are cautioned to know accepted practice and limitations in their use. Examination of 17 different sets of anatomically detailed dolls revealed that when extrapolated to adult human proportions, the sizes of genitalia and breasts of the dolls were not found to be exaggerated (Bays, 1990). Furthermore, Sivan et al. (1988) assessed interactions of nonabused children with anatomically detailed dolls and concluded that doll play of children with no reported history of sexual abuse is unlikely to be characterized by aggressive or explicit sexual activity. Likewise, Everson and Boat (1990) examined sexualized doll play among young children and found that anatomically detailed dolls are not overly suggestive to young, sexually naive children. They found the dolls useful in assessing a child's sexual knowledge and exposure to developmentally inappropriate sexual behaviors. These findings also were supported by a study conducted by White et al. (1986) who reported that sexually abused children exhibit more sexually specific behaviors than do children who have no known reported history of sexual abuse.

To address the criticism that the use of anatomically detailed dolls impacts a child's subsequent sexual behaviors, Boat and colleagues (unpublished) conducted follow-up interviews of 30 mothers whose children had been exposed to anatomical dolls. While some children were reported as demonstrating a heightened awareness of sexual body parts, none of the children were identified as displaying behaviors that might be misconstrued as indicating that sexual abuse had occurred (Everson & Boat, 1990). Similarly, Aman and Goodman (1987) had previously indicated that the use of anatomical dolls, in and of itself, does not lead to false reports of abuse, even under conditions of suggestive questioning.

As with any assessment instrument, the use of anatomically detailed dolls should be only one aspect of a comprehensive evaluation. It appears that, at the present time, anatomically detailed dolls may be most useful as a supportive tool in a comprehensive evaluation to assist young or linguistically impaired children to clarify and/or demonstrate alleged inappropriate sexual contact. With regard to their admissibility as evidence into court proceedings, Myers and White (1989) advise interviewers to be prepared to describe the specific use and reason for using the dolls in a particular case; to be familiar with the research on anatomically detailed dolls and be certain that accepted practice in the field was followed; and to know the limits in the use of anatomically detailed dolls and recognize them for what they are—an interview tool.

## DRAWINGS

As previously noted, drawings can be a useful interviewing aid. Drawing is a form of expression that is familiar even to young children. Often, through drawings, a child can communicate ideas and feelings to adults while achieving a sense of mastery and competence. The use of drawings may be especially helpful with young children, children who are hesitant, and/or those with immature verbal abilities.

For very young and/or highly traumatized children, drawings can provide a safe avenue for expression of both events and emotions (Burgess et al., 1981). A child may spontaneously depict an abusive experience that can be used to assist the child in disclosing a history of sexual victimization (**Figures 10-3 to 10-6**). Similarly, the evaluator can request that a child draw typical daily activities, family members, and/or interactions with significant others, which may illustrate areas in the child's life that warrant further evaluation. Drawings can also be used to clarify and validate a child's statement of sexual abuse (**Figure 10-2**). After a child completes a drawing, the evaluator should never assume understanding, but rather should ask the child to "Tell me about your picture." If the explanation is vague or incomplete, the evaluator can ask questions by beginning at the top of the figure(s) and progressively moving downward, asking "What is this?" or "Tell me about this part."

Clinical data in the literature suggest that sexually abused children are more likely to draw genitalia than those children who report no history of sexual victimization. Research findings on children 3 through 7 years of age reveal that young children with a history of sexual abuse are five to seven times more likely to draw genitalia than nonabused children (Hibbard et al., 1987; Hibbard & Hartman, 1990). However, it should be emphasized that although the presence of genitalia in a child's human figure drawing may be an indicator of possible sexual abuse, it is not conclusive. Likewise, the absence of genitalia does not exclude the possibility of sexual victimization (**Figures 10-4 and 10-7**).

## ♦ DOCUMENTATION

When an allegation of sexual abuse is assessed, the implications are profound for the child, alleged offender, and their respective families, as well as the evaluator. Accurate recording of information obtained is *critical*. It is common for court proceedings regarding sexual abuse allegations to take place months or even years after allegations were initially presented and evaluated. As a result, detailed written and/or taped documentation regarding evaluation procedures, including statements made by the child, caregiver, alleged offender, and collateral sources, is of utmost importance.

The ability of authorities to protect a child who is alleging sexual abuse frequently depends on the quality and comprehensiveness of the evaluator's records.

*Pertinent information to be noted each time a child is seen includes the following:*

1. Individual(s) who accompanied the child to evaluation sessions
2. Persons in the room at the time of the interview
3. The location of the interview
4. The date and time of day the interview took place
5. The length of the interview
6. The use of any interview tools

It is recommended that specific questions regarding possible sexual victimization as well as the exact responses (verbal and behavioral) made by a child are completely, accurately, and objectively documented. Myers (1991) has outlined factors in addition to interview questions and the content of a child's statement that have specific legal implications and should be carefully documented when obtained from a child or parent(s).

*He stresses the need to document factors that immediately surrounded the disclosure statement, including:*

1. The nature of the event(s) surrounding a child's disclosure
2. The lapse of time between the event(s) and the statement
3. The emotional condition of the child
4. The speech pattern displayed by the child (e.g., speech hurried)
5. The physical condition of the child at the time of the statement (e.g., injury and/or physical discomfort)
6. Spontaneity of child's statement
7. Child's statement in response to questions
8. Existence of first safe opportunity to make disclosure statement (e.g., child in prior custody of alleged offender with recent placement in safe setting).

As previously indicated, detailed documentation of all aspects of the evaluation, especially a child's statement, can have a significant impact on the protection of a child, as well as on the final disposition of the case. A primary responsibility of the evaluator is to accurately assess and document a child's competence to make a reliable statement. Factors surrounding a child's statement that should be documented include spontaneity in reporting an abuse experience, consistency of core details (over time and with prior statements), child's affective state, use of age-appropriate language and words to describe sexual contact(s), content of play behaviors or gestures that clarify or demonstrate a child's description of abuse, and evidence of developmentally inappropriate knowledge of sexual acts, anatomy, or vocabulary.

Myers (1991) also advises that information regarding a child's developmental competence and maturity, memory, and abilities to observe, communicate, and differentiate fact from fantasy should be noted in the record. Likewise, the evaluator should document any motive expressed by a child or adult to fabricate, deny, or postpone disclosure of sexual abuse. Drawings, handwritten statements, or other materials introduced by the child should be appropriately labeled and maintained as part of the permanent record.

### USE OF AUDIO AND VIDEOTAPING

Audio and videotaping of child interviews continues to be controversial and lacking apparent consensus among professionals. It is suggested that evaluators who utilize audio and videotaping closely follow accepted practice for taping, storage, and release of information. Myers (1992) presents an overview of the advantages, disadvantages, and legal implications of videotaping.

## ♦ALLEGATIONS OF SEXUAL ABUSE IN DIVORCE AND CHILD CUSTODY DISPUTES

Sexual abuse allegations that arise during divorce and child custody proceedings, as noted earlier, present particular challenges to the evaluator. Such allegations are often viewed with immediate skepticism. This may, in part, be due to general public opinion that in the context of a divorce and/or custody dispute a parent or child may be motivated to deliberately give false information in an attempt to secure a favored legal decision.

Professionals disagree on the true incidence of false allegations of sexual abuse that emerge during court litigation involving child custody and visitation rights. Green (1986) reported the incidence of false allegations in such cases as "strikingly high," failing to confirm sexual abuse allegations in 4 of 11 children he evaluated for suspected sexual abuse during child custody disputes. Citing "an emerging national hysteria regarding the problem of sexual abuse," Blush and Ross (1987) identified a pattern (SAID syndrome) believed to be specific to sexual abuse allegations in present and past divorce situations. The SAID syndrome (sexual allegations in divorce) is defined as a particular phenomenon that occurs when sexual abuse allegations develop within a pre- or post-divorce context and when a family unit has become dysfunctional as a result of the divorce process.

While allegations of sexual abuse in divorce and child custody disputes may be regarded by some with suspicion, research findings do not consistently support the assumption that false allegations of sexual abuse in separated and divorcing families are common. Results of a study by Thoennes and Tjaden (1990) do not support previous clinical conclusions that suggest a disproportionately higher incidence of false allegations in custody and visitation disputes. Their findings indicate that allegations of sexual abuse made at the time of litigation regarding custody and/or visitation are no more likely to be determined as false than are sexual abuse allegations in the general population.

In contrast to the dispute concerning false allegations, figures regarding the existence of sexual abuse allegations in families after separation or divorce do indeed indicate a higher incidence than in the general population (Corwin et al., 1987). Reasons cited for a higher incidence of allegations of sexual abuse in divorcing families include stress, familial dysfunction, and increased opportunities for sexual victimization due to parental separation or divorce. In addition, separation from the abuser may provide the first safe opportunity for a child to disclose that abuse has taken place. Corwin and associates suggest that separation weakens an abusive parent's ability to enforce secrecy, while increasing the willingness of the nonoffending parent to accept the disclosure and take protective action. It should also be noted that following a parental separation a child's risk for extrafamilial sexual abuse may be higher due to a change in caregivers, including the presence of a nonbiological parental figure in the home.

Allegations of sexual abuse made in the context of parental separation or divorce should not be readily dismissed due to situational factors, but rather given serious consideration and thoroughly evaluated. A complete evaluation of the parents, as well as the child, is indicated to ensure the child's safety and emotional well-being. Allegations of sexual abuse of a child by a parent indicate that a child is at emotional risk even when allegations are unsubstantiated (Bresee et al., 1986).

## ◆EVALUATION OF INFORMATION OBTAINED IN INTERVIEWS

The interview with the child is often denoted as the "cornerstone" of a sexual abuse evaluation. Upon completion, the evaluator must assess the reliability and credibility of a child's statement(s) to determine the degree of probability that sexual victimization has occurred.

The use of predetermined criteria to assess a child's statements and behavior in allegations of sexual abuse can assist in minimizing evaluator bias. The following characteristics of a child's statement and behavior are associated with true allegations of sexual abuse (Faller, 1990):

*Description and/or knowledge of sexual behavior:*
— description of specific sexual acts
— description of sexual acts from a child's viewpoint
— sexual knowledge beyond that expected for the child's developmental stage

*Emotional reaction of child to sexual abuse:*
— child's state of mind and affective responses at the time of disclosure
— child's recollection of feelings at the time of the abuse

*Details provided about the context of abusive situations:*
— identity and relationship of alleged offender
— sex and estimated age of alleged offender
— when and where abuse occurred
— what the victim and alleged offender were wearing
— what clothing was removed and by whom
— whereabouts of other family members
— how alleged offender induced child to be involved
— elements of secrecy or coercion
— other idiosyncratic details/events

*Note: Positive findings in the three major areas are not found routinely in every case of sexual victimization.*

Schetky (1988) has also proposed factors that enhance a child's credibility. She notes numerous characteristics, including (1) behavioral changes specific to sexual abuse and/or nonspecific stress-related changes; (2) the presence of sexual themes in a child's play and drawings; (3) progressive sexual activity over time; (4) secrecy; (5) delayed disclosure; (6) a description of psychological coercion; and (7) physical indicators.

In evaluating a child's statement for reliability and validity, close attention should be given to the child's language (words), ability to relate core events, and spontaneity. A child's interpretation and subsequent description of sexual victimization is dependent on the child's cognitive development, verbal abilities, and the extent of his or her life experiences.

Other factors that may corroborate a child's statement and should be considered include statements indicative of sexual victimization overheard by others, any eyewitness accounts, and the presence of multiple victims with consistent statements of sexual abuse (Myers, 1991).

## ◆ CONCLUSIONS

Evaluators are faced with the dilemma that there are few absolutes in the area of child sexual abuse. Exceptions include pregnancy in a child under 12 years of age or medical evidence of specific sexually transmitted disease in young children *(see Chapter 9, Physical Examination in Sexual Abuse)*. However, after careful consideration of all available information, an evaluator can render one of the following possible findings (Swan, 1989). Conclusions are based on degrees of probability that sexual abuse has occurred.

Reliable history of sexual abuse

Child gives clear, consistent statements of sexual abuse in age-appropriate language. There is no clear evidence of alternative explanations for a child's statement or behaviors, or motivation for a child or reporting adult to give false information. Corroborating factors may be present, including physical findings or behavioral indicators specific to sexual abuse.

Suspected sexual abuse

The presence of physical or behavioral indicators that are consistent with sexual abuse although child does not make a clear statement or denies sexual victimization.

Appropriate concern/insufficient information

A child may demonstrate stress-related behaviors or present vague statements of vulnerability. However, there is no statement or there is denial of inappropriate sexual contact, and supportive evidence is insufficient for findings.

No evidence of sexual abuse

Information indicates child or reporting adult made false statement. Presence of alternative explanation for child's statement and/or behaviors, or misinterpretation of initial statement or behavior of child by significant adults.

## ◆ RECOMMENDATIONS

Following evaluation of all available information and formulation of a conclusion, an interviewer may make recommendations regarding issues of protection, placement, custody and/or visitation, and the appropriateness of additional diagnostic or treatment services. The final deposition of cases regarding allegations of sexual abuse investigated by child protective services and/or law enforcement agencies is the responsibility of those agencies. However, conclusions and recommendations made by the evaluators may be valuable input in making placement and treatment decisions for children and their families.

*Figures 10-3, 10-4, 10-5, and 10-6 are a series of drawings by one child.*

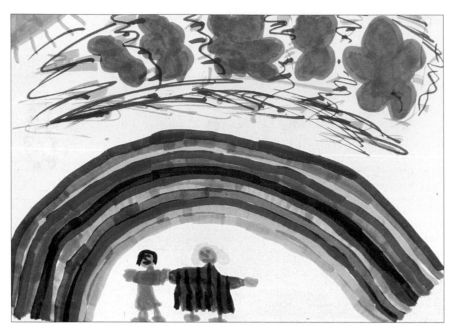

**Figure 10-1.** *A 9-year-old victim of sexual abuse drew a picture of herself, at right, with her therapist. A rainbow protects them from the turmoil and chaos shown above. Drawings by sexually abused children often depict some type of shield from environmental stressors.*

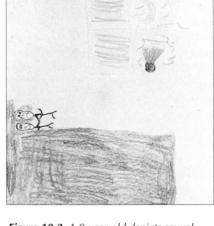

**Figure 10-2.** *A 9-year-old depicts sexual abuse by adult. Picture shows type of abuse, location and time of abuse, as well as emotional responses of child and offender.*

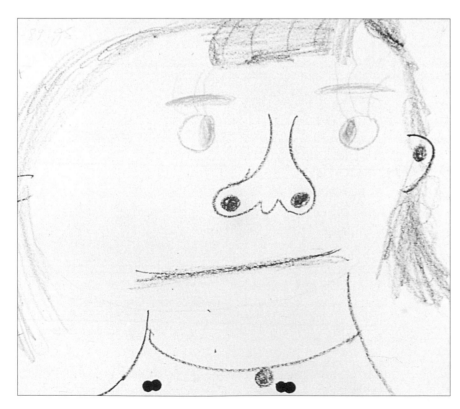

**Figure 10-3.** *A 4-year-old victim depicts abusive mother, above, and father (Figure 10-4).*

**Figure 10-4.** *Drawing by 4-year-old girl at initial interview when asked to draw a picture of her father. Presence of genitalia in drawing facilitated child's disclosure of sexual abuse.*

**Figure 10-5.** *Drawing by 4-year-old girl at initial interview when asked to draw a picture about her family. Child described fondling of her younger brother's genitalia at her father's instruction.*

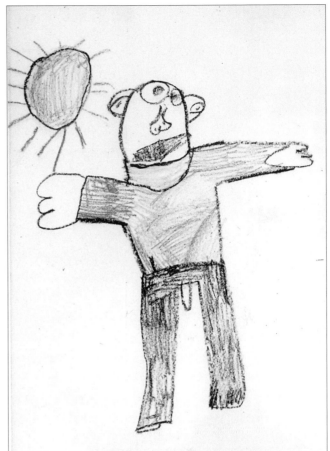

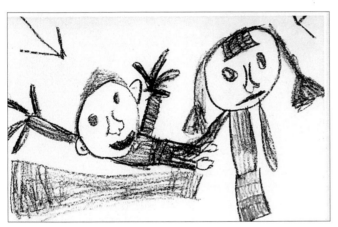

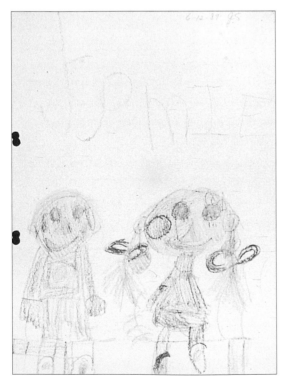

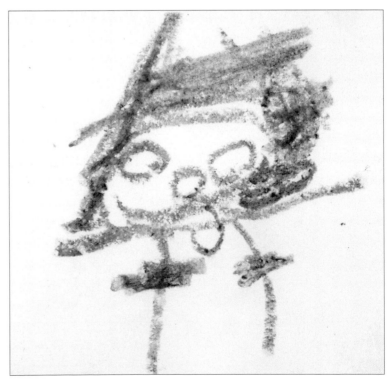

**Figure 10-6.** *A 4-year-old draws nurturing caregiver in foster home. There is a striking difference between this drawing and the previous ones.*

**Figure 10-7.** *Drawing of human figure with genitalia by 3-year-old boy.*

## ◆BIBLIOGRAPHY

Aman, C, and Goodman, G: Children's use of anatomically detailed dolls: An experimental study. Paper presented at the National Center on Child Abuse and Neglect's Symposium on Interviewing Children, Washington, DC, 1987.

Bays, J: Are the genitalia of anatomical dolls distorted? *Child Abuse Negl* 14:171-175, 1990.

Beitchman, J, Zucker, K, Hood, J, DaCosta, G, and Akman, D: A review of the short-term effects of child sexual abuse, *Child Abuse Negl* 15:537-556, 1991.

Berliner, L, and Conte, J: The process of victimization: the victim's perspective, *Child Abuse Negl* 14:29-40, 1990.

Blush, G, and Ross, K: Sexual allegations in divorce: The SAID syndrome, *Conciliation Court's Review* 25(1):1-11, 1987.

Boat, B, Everson, M, and Holland: Maternal perceptions of nonabused young children's exposure to anatomical dolls, (unpublished).

Bresee, P, Stearns, G, Bess, B, and Packer, L: Allegations of child sexual abuse in child custody disputes: A therapeutic assessment model, *Am J Orthopsychiatry* 56(4):560-569, 1986.

Burgess, A, McCausland, M, and Wolbert, W: Children's drawings as indicators of sexual trauma, *Perspect Psychiatr Care* 19(2):50-58, 1981.

Burns, N, Meyer-Williams, L, and Finkelhor, D: Victim impact. In *Nursery Crimes, Sexual Abuse in Day Care*, Sage Publications, Inc, Newbury Park, CA, 1988, pp. 114-123.

Conte, J, and Schuerman, J: Factors associated with an increased impact of child sex abuse, *Child Abuse Negl* 11:201-211, 1987.

Corwin, D, Berliner, L, Goodman, G, Goodwin, J, and White, S: Child sexual abuse and custody disputes: No easy answers, *J Interpersonal Violence* 2:91-105, 1987.

Deblinger, E, McLeer, S, Atkins, M, Ralphe, D, and Foa, E: Post-traumatic stress in sexually abused, physically abused and nonabused children, *Child Abuse Negl* 13:403-408, 1989.

DeJong, A: Sexual interactions among siblings and cousins: Experimentation or exploitation? *Child Abuse Negl* 13:271-279, 1989.

Everson, M, and Boat, B: Are anatomical dolls too suggestive? *The Advisor, Newsletter of the American Professional Society on the Abuse of Children* 3(2):6,14, 1990.

Everson, M, and Boat, B: Sexualized doll play among young children: Implications for the use of anatomical dolls in sexual abuse evaluations, *J Am Acad Child Adolescent Psychiatry* 29(5):736-742, 1990.

Faller, K: Criteria for judging the credibility of children's statements about their sexual abuse. Child Protective Investigative Team Training, UT Social Work/Office of Research and Public Service 1990.

Faller, K: Types of questions for children alleged to have been sexually abused, *The Advisor, Newsletter of the American Professional Society on the Abuse of Children* 3(2):3-5, 1990.

Fay, J, Adams, C, Flerchinger, BJ, Loontjens, L, Rittenhouse, P, and Stone, ME: *He Told Me Not to Tell*, King County Sexual Assault Resource Center, 1991.

Finkelhor, D: *A Sourcebook on Child Sexual Abuse*, Sage Publications, Inc, Beverly Hills, CA, 1986.

Finkelhor, D, and Browne, A: The traumatic impact of child sexual abuse: A conceptualization, *Am J Orthopsychiatry* 55(4):530-541, 1985.

Finkelhor, D, and Hotaling, G: Sexual abuse in the national incidence study of child abuse and neglect: An appraisal, *Child Abuse Negl* 8:23-33, 1984.

Finkelhor, D, Hotaling, G, Lewis, IA, and Smith, C: Sexual abuse in a national survey of adult men and women: Prevalence, characteristics, and risk factors, *Child Abuse Negl* 14:19-28, 1990.

Friedrich, W, Grambsch, P, Broughton, D, Kuiper, J, and Beilke, R: Normative sexual behavior in children, *Pediatrics* 88(3): 456-464, 1991.

Friedrich, W, Urquiza, A, and Beilke, R: Behavior problems in sexually abused young children, *J Pediatr Psychol* 11(1):47-57, 1986.

Gomes-Schwartz, B, Horowitz, J, and Sauzier, M: Severity of emotional distress among sexually abused preschool, school-age, and adolescent children, *Hosp Community Psychiatry* 36:503-508, 1985.

Green, A: True and false allegations of sexual abuse in child custody disputes, *J Am Acad Child Psychiatry* 25(4):449-456, 1986.

Guidelines for the clinical evaluation of child and adolescent sexual abuse: Position statement of The American Academy of Child and Adolescent Psychiatry, *J Am Acad Child Adolescent Psychiatry* 27:655-657, 1988.

Guidelines for the evaluation of sexual abuse of children. Committee on Child Abuse and Neglect: American Academy of Pediatrics, *Pediatrics* 87(2):254-260, 1991.

Guidelines for psychosocial evaluation of suspected sexual abuse in young children. Task Force chaired by Lucy Berliner, American Professional Society on the Abuse of Children, 1990.

Hechler, D: The battle for acceptance. In *The Battle and the Backlash, The Child Sexual Abuse War,* Lexington Books, Lexington, MA, 1988, pp. 1-12.

Hibbard, R, and Hartman, G: Genitalia in human figure drawings: Childrearing practices and child sexual abuse, *J Pediatr* 116(5):822-828, 1990.

Hibbard, R, Roghmann, K, and Hoekelman, R: Genitalia in children's drawings: An association with sexual abuse, *Pediatrics* 79(1):129-137, 1987.

Johnson, T: Child perpetrators: Children who molest other children: Preliminary findings, *Child Abuse Negl* 12:219-229, 1988.

*Los Angeles Times* poll, 1985.

Lusk, R, and Waterman, J: Effects of sexual abuse on children. In MacFarlane, K, and Waterman, J, eds: *Sexual Abuse of Young Children*, The Guilford Press, New York, 1986, pp. 101-118.

McLeer, S, Deblinger, E, Atkins, M, Foa, E, and Ralphe, D: Post-traumatic stress disorder in sexually abused children, *J Am Acad Child Adolescent Psychiatry* 27(5):650-654, 1988.

Myers, J: Legal implications of interviewing children. *In Legal Issues in Child Abuse and Neglect*, Sage Publication, Newbury Park, 1992, pp. 80-83.

Myers, J: Legal implications of interviewing sexually abused children. Presentation: The Seventh National Symposium on Child Sexual Abuse, Huntsville, AL, 1991.

Myers, J, and White, S: Dolls in court? *The Advisor, Newsletter of the American Professional Society on the Abuse of Children* 3(2):5-6, 1989.

National Center on Child Abuse and Neglect, US Department of Health and Human Services, Washington, DC, 1981.

Pescosolido, F: Sexual abuse of boys by males: Theoretical and treatment implications. In *Vulnerable Populations: Volume II*, Lexington Books, Lexington, MA, 1989, pp. 85-109.

Saywitz, K: Developmental considerations for forensic interviewing, *The Advisor, Newsletter of the American Professional Society on the Abuse of Children* 3(2):2,5,15, 1990.

Saywitz, K: Enhancing children's memory with the cognitive interview, *The Advisor, Newsletter of the American Professional Society on the Abuse of Children* 5(3):9-10, 1992.

Schetky, D: The clinical evaluation of child sexual abuse. In *Child Sexual Abuse, A Handbook for Health Care and Legal Professionals*, Brunner/Mazel, Inc, 1988, pp. 57-78.

Sgroi, S, Bunk, B, and Wabrek, C: Children's sexual behaviors and their relationships to sexual abuse. In *Vulnerable Populations: Volume I*, Lexington Books, Lexington, MA, 1988, pp. 1-13.

Sgroi, S, Porter, F, and Blick, L: *Validation of Child Sexual Abuse. Handbook of Clinical Intervention in Child Sexual Abuse*, Lexington Books, Lexington, MA, 1983, pp. 39-41.

Sivan, A, Schor, D, Koeppl, G, and Noble, L: Interaction of normal children with anatomical dolls, *Child Abuse Negl* 12:295-304, 1988.

Smith, S: Children's Story: *Sexually Molested Children in Criminal Court*, Launch Press, Walnut Creek, CA, 1985.

Sorensen, T, and Snow, B: How children tell: The process of disclosure in child sexual abuse, *Child Welfare* 70:3-15, 1991.

Swan, H: Presentation: Sexual abuse and the law, St. Charles County Family Stress Council, Inc, and Sexual Abuse Task Force, St. Charles, MO.

Thoennes, N, and Tjaden, P: The extent, nature, and validity of sexual abuse allegations in custody/visitation disputes, *Child Abuse Negl* 14:151-163, 1990.

Tobin, P, and Farley, S: *Keeping Kids Safe: A Child Sexual Abuse Prevention Manual*, Learning Publications, Inc., Holmes Beach, 1990.

Wakefield, H, and Underwager, R: *Accusations of Child Sexual Abuse*, Charles C Thomas, Publishers, Springfield, IL, 1988.

White, S, Strom, G, Santilli, G, and Halpin, B: Interviewing young sexual abuse victims with anatomically correct dolls, *Child Abuse Negl* 10:519-529, 1986.

# Developmental Aspects of the Young Child in Maltreatment Cases

Patricia M. Sullivan, Ph.D.

*Children who participate in the legal system as a result of child abuse and neglect have developmental characteristics and competencies that affect their abilities to recall and relate facts about an event and participate in the judicial process. Medical professionals evaluating children for possible abuse and neglect need to have a thorough working knowledge of impinging child development issues in order to make appropriate and uncontaminated referrals to law enforcement agencies and participate in legal proceedings. These include selected aspects of biological development, perception, memory, and attention that differ markedly between young children and adults.*

*Relevant aspects of cognitive, language, memory, and behavioral/emotional development of preschool and young children are presented that may impinge upon the young child's participation in legal proceedings. Conditions that may affect a young child's ability to relate events, including emotional trauma, inducements to keep secrets, and lying and coaching, are discussed. Particular attention is given to children's memory, the suggestibility of children's recollections, and the communicative competence of the questioner, which is necessary to elicit reliable information from children. Finally, children with disabilities are at increased risk to be victims of child maltreatment and disabilities often result from the child maltreatment. Results of an epidemiological research study on child maltreatment and disability conducted at the Boys Town National Research Hospital and funded by the National Center on Child Abuse and Neglect will be summarized, providing demographic information on maltreatment and perpetrator characteristics of children under 5 years of age with disabilities.*

"As long as little children suffer, there is no true justice in the world."

*—Isadora Duncan*

# ♦BIOLOGICAL DEVELOPMENT ISSUES

The ability to relate facts depends on several factors including the physical development of the brain, perception, and attention. These functions develop over time and affect information that is encoded and stored in memory. Memory for people, places, things, and events in our lives is a central part of knowing who we are as individuals (Drummey & Newcombe, 1995). Recent research in memory development has explored the relationships between memory tasks and neurological development. One's memory of infancy and early childhood is fragmentary at best, and memory for that developmental period is referred to as infantile amnesia (Newcombe & Fox, 1994). Although some individuals report some accurate memories from ages as early as 2 or 3 years, significant increases in the ability to remember childhood events occur by the ages of 5 or 6 years (Pillemer & White, 1989; Usher & Neisser, 1993). Information acquired before the age of 5 is forgotten more quickly and completely than information acquired later in life (Newcombe & Fox, 1994). Although poor recollection of childhood events cannot be explained as simply caused by developmental changes (Weltzler & Sweeney, 1986), understanding a child's capacity to relate events as they are remembered requires a cursory review of biological developmental issues related to myelination, perception, and attention.

## PHYSICAL DEVELOPMENT OF THE BRAIN

Although most myelination is completed by the time the child is 2 years of age, some myelin continues to develop until adolescence (Wedding et al., 1986). Growth rates are not uniform for all parts of the brain, and increased brain functioning occurs as myelination increases. The brains of young children permit them to accurately perceive events and communicate simple information about those events. Their brains are not mature enough to make complicated decisions and evaluations or to make inferences and draw conclusions about those occurrences. This occurs in adolescence. Preschool and school-aged children should not be expected to answer questions requiring them to make inferences or draw conclusions. They are developmentally incapable of doing so.

To be an effective witness, a child must be able to perceive the event accurately, which is primarily a function of the right hemisphere of the brain, and convey information about the perception, which is primarily a left hemisphere function (Perry & Wrightsman, 1991). The corpus callosum, or band of fibers that connects the right and left hemisphere and facilitates communication between the two, is not completely myelinated until 10 years of age (Wedding et al., 1986). However, there is communication between the hemispheres, to a limited degree, in children as young as 5 years of age.

## PERCEPTION

Children and adults are continuously bombarded by perceptual stimuli. The most basic perceptual processes involving the five senses (vision, hearing, smell, taste, and touch) function at an adult level even in infancy (Newman & Newman, 1995). However, several aspects of perception change with age (Perry & Wrightsman, 1991). As children mature, their perceptions become more selective and more purposeful, and they become more skillful at discerning the critical information from stimuli. Their perception becomes more selective as they learn to detect the increasingly subtle aspects of stimuli. As they mature, children also become increasingly more aware of the meaning of their perceptions. They also become more proficient at generalizing perceived meanings from one situation to another.

The ability to understand the distinction between appearance and reality is an aspect of perception that develops during the preschool years (Stott, 1990). Children can understand the difference between a friend dressed up as a policeman and an actual policeman around the age of 6 or 7 years (Stott, 1990). Before this age, children cannot think effectively about appearance and reality. To them, what they perceive the appearance to be is reality.

Young children can perceive events accurately if they pay attention to them. This applies to straightforward factual occurrences involving the five senses. However, young children have difficulty ordering and interpreting their perceptions. In interviewing very young children, it is helpful to ask them about their perceptual experiences in order to gain information about the possible abusive occurrence. For example, open-ended questions such as "Tell me what you saw, heard, smelled, tasted" or "What did it feel like?" often elicit a great deal of spontaneous information from a child less than 6 years of age and can provide valuable information about any physical and/or sexual maltreatment.

Young children should not be expected to answer questions that require them to identify relationships, recognize feelings, or attribute intentions. The ability to interpret perceptions at a reliable level does not occur until around 12 years of age (Newman & Newman, 1995). A concept of time is required to interpret and order perceptions. Children under the age of 8 generally have difficulty in understanding and reporting elapsed time and time of occurrence.

## ATTENTION

To perceive an event a child first and foremost must pay attention to the event. Children use their attending skills more effectively and systematically as they mature. The two basic components of attention are scanning and selectivity (Newman & Newman, 1995). Children younger than 5 years tend to scan downward and unsystematically and to stop scanning before they have obtained all the relevant information. They also attend to central, not peripheral, details. Thus, their testimony is limited by these attentional characteristics. Children under 5 years of age are also distracted by irrelevant details and may focus on them in relating the event. Between the ages of 5 and 7 years, children become more systematic and intentional in their attending.

Young children typically recall fewer details of events in their testimony because of their immature attention processes. However, even children as young as 3 or 4 years of age can attend to events happening around them if these events are straightforward and involve familiar people and places. They are quite capable of answering simply constructed questions asking what happened, who did it, and where it happened. Questions should address the central facts of the event rather than peripheral details.

## CONCLUSIONS

Medical professionals evaluating young children for suspected child abuse and neglect must phrase their questions to be congruent with the child's biological status and perception and attention capabilities. Young children can answer questions about their sensory experiences surrounding the event, and these open-ended questions often elicit corroborating factors about the abusive event. Questions regarding time frames ("When did this happen?"), the ordering and interpreting of events ("Did he touch you before you ate the ice cream?"), and attributions about the events ("Why would he touch you there?") should be avoided.

# ♦COGNITIVE DEVELOPMENT ISSUES

## DEFINITION OF INTELLIGENCE

The term *intelligence* refers to the whole class of cognitive behaviors that reflect a child's capacity to solve problems, adapt to new situations, think abstractly, and profit from experience (Neisser et al., 1996). Intelligence is an elastic concept that describes different kinds of behavior at different times in life. Therefore most theories of intelligence are developmental theories. The exact content of the abilities included in the concept of general intelligence is subject to great debate. Practically speaking, these abilities are defined by the subtests and items that appear on commonly accepted standardized tests of intelligence. The concept of intelligence is, thus, an invention that corresponds roughly to "cognitive capacity." At its best, it is only a description and not an entity. Currently, there are several different theories of intelligence, including analytic, creative, practical, and social (Neisser et al., 1996). Developmental and psychometric models of intelligence are considered in **Table 11-1.**

| Table 11-1. Classification of Intelligence | |
| --- | --- |
| **IQ Range** | **Classification** |
| 130+ | Very superior |
| 120–129 | Superior |
| 110–119 | High average |
| 90–109 | Average |
| 80–89 | Low average |
| 70–79 | Borderline |
| 69 & Below | Intellectually deficient |

*(Wechsler, 1991)*

An intelligence quotient (IQ) is a standardized score based on an individual's performance on an intelligence test. A given IQ corresponds to a percentile value, which, in turn, corresponds to a given raw score. Thus a given IQ for an individual means that he or she obtained a raw score, which, for a person in the standardization sample in the test, was of a given percentile value. In other words, it is the IQ associated with the percentile rank of the person in the standardization sample who obtained that particular raw score. All IQ scales have a mean defined at 100. The IQ scales of most intelligence tests define the standard deviation units as 15 IQ points.

Mental age (MA), like IQ, is only a test score representing performance obtained by a certain chronological age group. It is based on the old ratio IQ of MA/chronological age (CA) x 100. Children are often thought of in reference to their "mental age." While MA may serve as a baseline or reference point, such a conceptualization of MA must be employed with considerable caution. For example, a child who is 10 years old (CA) with an MA of 5 years, 2 months cannot do many things that average children can do who have both an MA and a CA of 5 years, 2 months. Conversely, there are probably a few things the 10-year-old child, because of his large size, age, and experience, can do that surpass the 5-year-old child, even though they have the same MA.

The diagnosis of mental retardation is based on capabilities (intelligence and adaptive skills in self-help, social, and motor domains), environments (home, work, school, and community), and functioning in terms of support available to the individual (American Association on Mental Retardation, 1992). Children who are mentally retarded are at increased risk to endure neglect, physical abuse, and sexual abuse. Mental retardation can also result from child abuse and neglect (Sullivan & Knutson, 1994). Given their special vulnerabilities for maltreatment, medical professionals should routinely screen children with mental retardation for abuse and neglect and screen abused and neglected children for the presence of disabilities. If the child has a mental disability, questions must be posed at a level commensurate with the child's cognitive developmental status.

## PERIODS OF INTELLECTUAL DEVELOPMENT

The premier developmental theorist in the ontogeny of children's intelligence is Jean Piaget, who has posited four developmental stages, which are summarized here.

### SENSORY-MOTOR

*(Birth to age 2 years).* The child passes through six stages, beginning with the exercise of simple reflexes and ending with the first sign of internal or symbolic

representations of actions. Language development occurs throughout the six stages. The child begins with simple reflexes, such as finger sucking or watching the hands, and proceeds through the endless repetition of actions, repeating procedures to make events occur again, trial-and-error behavior, goal-seeking behavior, and the beginnings of symbolic thought. If a child endures abuse or neglect during this phase of development, it is highly unlikely that he or she will have any recollection of it. In the absence of an eye witness or a confession, allegations of maltreatment are usually unfounded.

## PREOPERATIONAL PERIOD

*(Age 2 to 7 years).* During this developmental stage the child acquires language and symbolic functions. The child can search for hidden objects, perform delayed imitation, engage in symbolic play, and use language for social and communicative purposes. In general, thinking is flawed and not well organized. The child gains the ability to mentally represent an object. Pretend play and language are prevalent, and the child begins to distinguish between "for real" and "for pretend." The abilities to think symbolically and represent the world mentally predominate.

Two important limitations to preoperational thought are egocentrism and animism. Egocentrism is the inability to distinguish between one's own perspective and the perspective of someone else. Thus children are limited to answering questions about their own view or perspective of certain events rather than the perspective of others. Animism is the belief that inanimate objects have lifelike qualities and are capable of action. Children in this age range fail to distinguish the appropriate occasions for using human and nonhuman or animal perspectives. They may pretend to be an animal and attribute human characteristics to it.

Children begin to use primitive reasoning and want to know the answers to all sorts of questions, such as Why can't we hear the sun? or Why are rocks different sizes? They are very sure about their knowledge and understanding but unaware of how they know what they know.

The primary characteristic of preoperational thought is centration. Centration refers to focusing or centering of attention on one characteristic to the exclusion of all others. Examples include calling all vehicles a truck or thinking a penis is only for urination. Centration affects the child's ability to describe events or actions that they have experienced. Children in this developmental phase can answer questions about abusive experiences they may have endured. However, the interviewer must be highly skilled in communicating with children in this age range. A key rule of thumb is to ascertain what the child is saying vs. what an adult is saying the child is saying. Listening skills on the part of the adult conducting the interview are particularly important.

## CONCRETE OPERATIONS

*(Age 7 to 11 years).* During this stage of intellectual development the child develops conservation skills, and mental operations are applied to real (concrete) objects or events. The child can focus on height and width, whereas a preoperational child can focus on only one of these attributes at a time. The child can also classify or divide things into different sets or subsets and can consider their interrelationships.

The child understands that mental operations can be reversible and the concept of conservation, which is the idea that an amount stays the same regardless of how the container changes. A child who has mastered this developmental stage can understand that an erect and a flaccid penis are both a penis. A child who has not mastered this may think that a penis is only for urination and remains flaccid at all times. Thus this child may refer to semen as urine and not be aware that two distinct types of fluids may be emitted from a penis.

Children in this developmental stage have a host of ideas about the physical and natural world, but these ideas differ from those of adults. Adults need to listen and comprehend what children are saying and respond to them accordingly.

## FORMAL OPERATIONS

*(Age 11 years +)*. Children in this developmental stage are capable of thinking abstractly, formulating hypotheses, using deductive reasoning, and checking solutions. Thinking is no longer concrete and becomes increasingly more logical. The adolescent can conceive and reason about hypothetical possibilities. Thinking is more abstract, and the adolescent can conjure up make-believe situations, hypothetical possibilities, and purely abstract propositions about them.

There is much more individual variation in formal operational thought than Piaget originally hypothesized. Only about one in three young adolescents is a formal operational thinker, and many adults never become formal operational thinkers. There are cultural influences in the attainment of formal operations, and education in the logic of science and mathematics is an important cultural experience in this regard.

## APPLICATIONS TO THE INTERVIEW PROCESS

A child's credibility is directly affected by the questioner's knowledge of the norms of cognitive development and the content of the questions posed to the child (Saywitz et al., 1993). Information must be elicited from children in a manner that allows them to tell what they know. Problems occur when the question requires cognitive skills the child has not yet developed. The situation is compounded when the child attempts to answer the question without the necessary cognitive skills, and misinterpretations and misunderstandings result. One must always be cognizant of what the child is actually saying and avoid making projections and attributions of the content and meaning of the child's utterance that may not exist.

## TIME

Children do not learn to tell clock time until around 7 years of age and, even at this age, many have difficulties with calendar dates. Yet children are frequently asked time-related questions in interviews regarding the time and date of the incidents of maltreatment. It is often helpful with preschoolers to relate the time of occurrence to regularly occurring events in a given day, such as awakening, meal and snack times, and nap times. Holidays and the child's birthday may also be used as reference points. However, preschool children have difficulties indicating if an event occurred before or after another one. Developmentally, most children are able to do this around 8 or 9 years of age (Newman & Newman, 1995).

When asked the time something occurred, there is a risk that young children will try to answer even when they do not know how to tell time. This can ruin a child's credibility with an adult who is not familiar with the developmental nature of time concepts in young children. Saywitz and her colleagues (1991, 1993) have demonstrated that alternative forms of questioning, such as asking what type of clothing the child was wearing or what television program the child was watching at the time, and then inferring the season of year and time from the local television guide can elicit accurate time frames from young children.

Children can name the days of the week and the seasons around 8 years of age (Friedman, 1982; Newman & Newman, 1995). At this age, they can also describe when two events happened together (for example, the abuse occurred when I was visiting Aunt Martha) and can reason that if one was wearing a heavy coat, something probably happened in the winter (Saywitz et al., 1993). Although reporting events in chronological order is not developmentally expected until around 10 years of age (Brown, 1976), this does not affect the accuracy of the events reported (Saywitz et al., 1993). Thus children can accurately relate what happened to them of an abusive nature even though they cannot delineate the exact chronology of the events.

## QUANTITATIVE CONCEPTS

It is very difficult for preschool children to count events in time. Although they may be able to count from three to six or more objects, they are unable to count events in time (Geary, 1994). Thus, a child may be able to count to 10 but unable to indicate the number of times she was molested (Saywitz et al., 1993). This developmental fact can discredit a child's statements and confuse adults asking the questions. The following transcript involving the cross examination of a 10-year-old girl, with a diagnosed learning disability in mathematics, illustrates this point.

> *Defense Attorney:* Okay. Now, you say that you are the victim of, as you put it, sexual abuse. Is that right?
>
> *Child:* Yes.
>
> *Defense Attorney:* And how many times did you say that happened?
>
> *Child:* So many, I don't know.
>
> *Defense Attorney:* Like more than a hundred?
>
> *Child:* I don't know.
>
> *Defense Attorney:* You don't know, it could be more than a hundred?
>
> *Child:* Maybe.
>
> *Defense Attorney:* All the time your dad did that may be more than a hundred times?
>
> *Child:* Maybe.
>
> *Defense Attorney:* Could it be less than 10 times?
>
> *Child:* Maybe.
>
> *Defense Attorney:* Well, how may times did he sexually abuse you?
>
> *Child:* It happened so many times. I can't remember.

Questions about how many times something may have happened are often very confusing to young children and make them appear to be inconsistent in their accounts of maltreatment. In fact, these inconsistencies reflect on the interviewing skills of the adult and the child's lack of understanding of numerical concepts. The child being cross examined was abused on numerous occasions and could not identify a specific number of times the abuse had occurred. Her confusion was compounded by the fact that the abuse often happened multiple times during the same day or night. She was unable to distinguish these multiple events as discrete independent occurrences.

## MEASUREMENT

Numerical concepts for measuring time, distance, height, and weight are presented over the course of the elementary school years but not fully mastered until preadolescence (Geary, 1994). Asking young children questions that require numbers in time, distance, height, and weight can confuse the child and make the allegation seem inconsistent and the child incredible. Saywitz and her colleagues (1991) have described a method to address this difficulty wherein the child is asked to provide concrete bits of information that can enable the adult to reconstruct some of the physical characteristics of the person in question. Examples include asking the child if the person was old enough to drive a car, was tall enough to reach something from the top of the refrigerator, or what their hair color was. With preschool children, who tend to focus on only one salient feature of a person at a time, it is imperative to ask for clarifying information. Children in this age group may think that the tallest person in the room is also the oldest. Thus if the child tells you the person was old, it is important to ask: "How did you know he was old?" The child's answer of "He was tall" versus "He had white hair" provides valuable information for the interviewer.

### BODY PARTS

Children often do not know the proper names for body parts, although some are able to correctly name them. Knowledge of the names and functions of body parts should not be assumed. Some children have special names for body parts and these need to be ascertained early in the interview process. If a very young child uses sophisticated anatomical language in describing the sexual touch, the possibility of coaching by an adult should be considered. However, a verbally precocious child may simply be using the appropriate vocabulary. Also, many parents and preschool teachers present the proper anatomical names for penis and vagina to children who use them appropriately. It is helpful to pay close attention to and follow the child's lead in his or her use of language for body parts. One should never assume that the child knows the function of a given body part or that a child has been touched by a body part without an explanation from the child as to his or her meaning of the use of the term. Some children overgeneralize the term "rape" to mean being touched on the breasts. The use of drawings or dolls is helpful in assisting the child to demonstrate what he means. It is imperative that the interviewer guard against suggestibility in these situations by telling the child in a nondirective manner to "Show me where you were (raped or whatever word the child used)." Often very young children have different meanings for terms of human sexuality than adults, and one cannot infer the occurrence of maltreatment on the basis of verbalizations alone.

## ◆ LANGUAGE DEVELOPMENT ISSUES

### KEY CONCEPTS IN LANGUAGE DEVELOPMENT

Very young children are not sophisticated verbal communicators. Language develops slowly and dramatically during the first 7 years of life. Many fine points of language-related thinking continue to develop through adolescence. A listing of key language developmental milestones is presented in **Table 11-2**.

| Table 11-2. Milestones in Vocalization and Language Development | |
|---|---|
| **Age** | **Language Milestone** |
| 12 weeks | Markedly less crying than at 8 weeks; when talked to and nodded at, smiles, followed by squealing-gurgling sounds usually called cooing, that is, vowel-like in character and pitch-modulated; sustains cooing for 15-20 seconds. |
| 16 weeks | Responds to human sounds more definitely; turns head; eyes seem to search for speaker, occasionally some chuckling sounds. |
| 20 weeks | The vowel-like cooing sounds begin to be interspersed with more consonantal sound; acoustically, all vocalizations are very different from the sounds of the mature language of the environment. |
| 6 months | Cooing changing into babbling resembling one-syllable utterances; neither vowels nor consonants have very fixed recurrences; most common utterances sound somewhat like ma, mu, da, or di. |

**Table 11-2.** Milestones in Vocalization and Language Development—*Continued*

| Age | Language Milestone |
|---|---|
| 8 months | Reduplication (or more continuous repetition) becomes frequent; intonation patterns become distinct, utterances can signal emphasis and emotions. |
| 10 months | Vocalizations are mixed with sound play such as gurgling or bubble-blowing; appears to wish to imitate sounds, but the imitations are never quite successful; beginning to differentiate between words heard by making differential adjustment. |
| 12 months | Identical sound sequences are replicated with higher relative frequency of occurrence and words (mama or dada) are emerging; definite signs of understanding some words and simple commands ("Show me your eyes"). |
| 18 months than | Has a definite repertoire of words—more than 3 but fewer 50; still much babbling but now of several syllables with intricate intonation pattern; no attempt at communicating information and no frustration at not being understood; words may include items such as thank you and come here, but there is little ability to join any of the lexical items into spontaneous two-item phrases; understanding is progressing rapidly. |
| 24 months | Vocabulary of more than 50 items (some children seem to be able to name everything in environment); begins spontaneously to join vocabulary items into two-word phrases; all phrases appear to be own creations; definite increase in communicative behavior and interest in language. |
| 30 months | Fastest increase in vocabulary with many new additions every day, no babbling at all, utterances have communicative intent; frustrated if not understood by adults; utterances of at least two words; may have three or even five words; sentences and phrases have characteristic child grammar, that is, they are rarely verbatim repetitions of an adult utterance; intelligibility is not very good yet, though there is great variation among children, some seem to understand everything that is said to them. |
| 3 years | Vocabulary of some 1,999 words; about 80% of utterances are intelligent even to strangers; grammatical complexity of utterances is roughly that of colloquial adult language, although mistakes still occur. |
| 4 years | Language is well established; deviations from the adult norm tend to be more in style than in grammar. |
| 5 years | Language becomes more complete in structure and form; more abstract; up to 2,500 words; sentences have 7+words; asks many "how" and "why"questions. |
| 6 years | Language becomes increasingly symbolic; comprehends up to 6,000 words; some abstracting and categorizing; syntactical development. |
| 7 years | Begins to read and write; fluent language usage; understands cause and effect relationship. |

*Adapted from Bloom & Lahey, 1979; Newman & Newman, 1995.*

There is a critical period for speech and language acquisition between birth and 3 years of age. Children learn to understand and speak the language they hear spoken about them. Language is social and develops through communication between a child and his or her caretakers. Children who are victims of neglect and do not receive appropriate speech and language stimulation are at high risk to develop language-related learning problems that manifest themselves in poor academic achievement.

Speech and language are not synonymous. Speech refers to the acoustic articulatory code for oral language and includes the auditory sounds of speech and the movement of the articulators (larynx, pharynx, velum, tongue, teeth, lips, etc.) that make those sounds. Language is the symbolic code for representing ideas. It comprises various components or units, including vocabulary, syntax (grammar), semantics (meaning), pragmatics (the social use of language), and metalinguistic knowledge (the awareness of language and its uses).

Receptive language refers to what a child can understand or comprehend. Conversely, expressive language is what a child can communicate or state. During the early development of language there is a discrepancy between what a child understands and what a child can express. Thus young children are capable of understanding more language than they can produce. This is particularly the case with preoperational children.

Speaking ability depends on auditory or hearing ability. Thus one cannot judge thinking skills by speaking skills. Furthermore, one cannot assume understanding on the basis of speaking skills alone. It is possible to have good or intelligible speech and poor language skills, as in the case of some children with mental disabilities or traumatic brain injuries affecting language functioning. Conversely, it is also possible to have poor speech and good language skills, as in the case in many deaf and hard-of-hearing children and some children with cerebral palsy and dysarthria.

Language proficiency may be categorized as different (i.e., French, Spanish, or American Sign Language), delayed (i.e., behind in the attainment of language-related developmental milestones), or disordered (deviant in some aspect of language such as the formulation of words and sentences, the retrieval of words or phrases, or the comprehension of what is spoken). Before questioning a child, it is very important to ascertain his or her preferred mode of communication. If this is a language other than English, then a professional interpreter in the child's native language should be obtained to interpret the questions of the interviewer into the child's language, and the child's answers into the questioner's language. In some cases this means hiring a Spanish-speaking interpreter or one who is fluent in some form of sign language. Using a sibling or parent fluent in the child's preferred communication mode is not recommended in any situation because it contaminates the interview and may actually impede the child's disclosure, particularly in the case of a victim of intrafamilial abuse. With a deaf or hard-of-hearing child, it is important to identify the form of language used by the child, which may include oralism (speech and speech reading only), Cued Speech, American Sign Language, or one of the English-based sign language systems. Children with delayed or deviant language skills will most likely need to have questions formulated in simple grammatical constructions, such as the subject-verb-object format rather than complex grammatical constructions. For example, ask: "Who touched you?" Do not ask: "On the day you visited your grandfather's farm and wore your red dress, who touched you and where were you when it happened?"

Children may exhibit various speech and language disabilities, including articulation disorders, receptive language disorders, expressive language disorders, receptive and expressive language disorders, and stuttering. In interviewing these children, it is critical to use vocabulary and sentence structure within the child's comprehension level. A growing area of concern is the abuse of children with disabilities and the unique difficulties in obtaining evidence through appropriate interviewing techniques (Westcott, 1994, Sullivan et al., 1996). Research and development in this area may improve interviewing techniques with nondisabled children, particularly when they are highly reticent to disclose the maltreatment (Flin, 1995).

## AGE-APPROPRIATE QUESTIONS FOR CHILDREN

Child development specialists, including psychologists, social workers, and mental health therapists, are well aware of Piaget's (1965) dictum that children are not simply little adults. However, medical and legal professionals do not always demonstrate awareness of this in their questioning of children. When questioning children, it is imperative to be familiar with the child's developmental mastery of the various question forms in language development. Bloom and Lahey (1979) have derived norms of question comprehension in children's language development. These are presented in **Table 11-3**.

Some children older than 5 1/2 years chronologically may not have mastered comprehension of the various question types. This can result from language disabilities, learning disabilities, developmental disabilities, or hearing impairment. Questioning techniques used by lawyers and some physicians are generally designed for adults. Children must be addressed differently. Questions should be phrased at the child's cognitive and linguistic developmental level. Individuals who do not know how to talk to children will not obtain reliable information from them.

**Table 11-3.** Age-Appropriate Questions for Children

| Question Type | Age at Mastery |
| --- | --- |
| Yes-no | 2 years |
| What | 2 1/2 years |
| What do | 2 1/2 years |
| Where (place and directions) | 2 1/2 years |
| Who | 3 years |
| Whose | 3 years |
| Why | 3 years |
| How many | 3 1/2 years |
| How much | 4 years |
| How long (duration) | 4 years |
| How far | 4 1/2 years |
| How often | 5 years |
| How long (time) | 5 1/2 years |
| When | 5 1/2 years |

Children age 8 years and older can usually recount an experience in a straightforward manner and answer questions regarding it. Children younger than 8 years will have difficulty doing so. Most children with disabilities, irrespective of age, will have difficulties. This does not imply that their testimony is unreliable, but that it may appear so because of their speech and language, mental, learning, or hearing disabilities. These difficulties are overcome if the adult communicates with the child in a developmentally appropriate manner, including making sure the child understands the question posed by understanding how literally the child interprets and confidently answers the questions asked.

## UNDERSTANDING OF THE LEGAL PROCESS

Young children have a very limited understanding of the legal system, including the need for various people, their functions, or the rules by which people interact in the judicial process. Many 4- to 7-year-olds are not aware that the judge is in charge of the courtroom and assume that unknown persons in the jury are friends of the accused (Saywitz, 1990). Many similarly aged children misinterpret the adversarial process of the courtroom and fear they themselves may go to jail. Children in the 8- to 11-year-old range think that judges are capable of knowing if people are telling the truth. Children and youth do not become fully cognizant that courtroom proceedings are a part of the larger judicial process with roles for judges, attorneys, witnesses, juries, and themselves (Saywitz, 1990). The degree to which children understand the courtroom process significantly influences both the quantity and the quality of their verbalizations.

Saywitz (1994) recommends certain grammatical structures that should be both used and avoided when communicating with young children. She recommends using short sentences containing simple grammatical constructions (i.e., "Tell me what happened at Uncle Joe's house?") and avoiding long compound sentences with embedded clauses (i.e., "Now, Susie, is it not true, that on the day you say you were at your Uncle Joe's house, you were really at home?"). She also recommends that new topics be introduced (i.e., "Now, let's talk about your grandpa"). A similar technique has been used in courts in British Columbia wherein the attorney lists topics on a flip chart or writes them on the blackboard for the child and then asks open-ended questions about the topic (Harvey, 1995). Long compound sentences, multiword verbs (could not have been), passive voice ("Were you hit by him?"), double negatives ("Were you not told never to go there?"), and hypotheticals ("If you wanted it to stop, why didn't you just tell your mother?") are to be avoided with young children.

Adults sometimes use "Can you tell me" as a carrier phrase in questions they pose to children, for example, "Can you tell me how old you are?" or "Can you tell me what he did to you?" This is very confusing to the child because the answer to both of these questions is either "Yes" the child can tell you or "No" the child cannot tell you. The child may perceive that the adult is not sure whether he or she can answer the question and thereby unnecessary anxiety and apprehension develop within the child. It is best to directly say the child: "Tell me how old you are." "Tell me what happened to you." Children will not tell what they do not understand or know. If a child does not understand words in a given question, they will neither ask the adult the meaning of certain words nor inform him or her of their lack of understanding of the question. In these circumstances, young children generally attempt to answer the question, which may cause their answers to appear inconsistent when they have not fully understood the question. If a child is asked the same question repeatedly by an adult, he or she will often change the answer over time because they assume they are giving the wrong answer. Thus repeating the same question several times is not recommended and seriously contaminates the interview. To assist in these areas, Saywitz and her colleagues (1993) have recommended a series of instructions to young children prior to an interview. These include the following:

> *There may be some questions that you do not know the answers to. That's okay. Nobody can remember everything. If you don't know the answer to a question, then tell me "I don't know" but do not guess or make anything up. It is very important to tell me only what you really remember. Only what really happened. If you don't want to answer some of the questions, you don't have to. That's okay. Tell me "I don't want to answer that question." If you don't know what something I ask you means, tell me "I don't understand" or "I don't know that you mean." Tell me to say it in new words. I may ask you some questions more than one time. Sometimes I forget that I already asked you that question. You don't have to change your answer; just tell me what you remember the best you can.*

## ♦ CHILDREN AND LYING

Lying is a behavior that essentially everyone exhibits at some time in their lives. The essential elements of lying are an awareness of the falsity, an intention to deceive, and a preconceived goal or purpose for the deception (Ford et al., 1988). An awareness of the lie differentiates the liar from the misinformed and the deluded. A lie can be told in various modes, including exaggeration, pure fiction, or the combination, attribution, or addition of things or events to a factual occurrence. Lies are generally classified by their intent. Aggressive lies are told to cause harm to another person; defensive lies are told to escape punishment; and white, or altruistic, lies are told to benefit self or others.

Children's primary motivation in lying is to cover up for misdeeds (Bussey, 1992). If a child thought she might be in trouble for participating in a sexual incident with an adult, lying might be a strategy employed to avoid disclosure and thereby avoid punishment and displeasing adults. Children may also lie to comply with the demands of a significant person in their lives (Bussey, 1992). This can include a parent with whom the child is significantly aligned in a custody dispute or when a parent's own psychopathology involves insistence that the child was sexually abused. Children may also lie because of their own background or psychopathology (Quinn, 1988). Children with parents who model lying behavior for their children learn to lie from their parents. Children may also lie because of psychiatric illnesses that have symptoms which include lying, such as conduct disorder, oppositional disorder, and various personality disorders (Ford, 1995).

Research on detecting deception in children has focused on facial expression and voice quality to assist in detecting the lie (Quinn, 1988). Results have indicated that first graders cannot lie successfully (Feldman et al., 1979; Morency & Krauss, 1982; DePaulo et al., 1985); fourth and fifth graders are more proficient at lying and can fool peers, adult strangers, and parents (Allen & Atkinson, 1978; Morency & Krauss, 1982). Children become more adept at verbally hiding deceptions from ages 5 to 12 years (Braginsky, 1970). Children between the ages of 6 and 12 years become more proficient at using their faces to deceive (DePaulo & Rosenthal, 1979; Shennum & Bugental, 1982). It should be noted that children are less successful at deceiving when they have positive rather than negative feelings about the topic (Feldman & White, 1980).

A primary reason that children fail at lying is detection apprehension or the fear of being caught in the deception (Quinn, 1988). A child may experience a great deal of detection apprehension as a function of his or her belief in the parent's skill at detecting lies. Some parents can convince their children that they are highly skilled in detecting lying in the child. As a result, a parent who displays high amounts of suspicion even in the context of truthfulness will arouse fear and anxiety in a truthful child. This creates a difficult problem in detecting deception in children. Parents are usually aware that the severity of their punishment is a factor that influences whether children tell the truth or lie about their behavior in a given situation. Clarifying that the punishment for lying will be more severe than the transgression before questioning the child is highly effective in eliciting the truth (Ekman, 1986). However, if the child is exceedingly anxious in the face of a suspicious parent, it is almost impossible to differentiate between an innocent child's fear of being disbelieved and a lying child's detection apprehension (Ekman, 1986).

Children may also fail at deceiving others because of deception guilt or guilt about the act of lying (Quinn, 1988). Accordingly, a child experiences anxiety-arousing guilt because of the lie and seeks relief by admitting the lie even in the face of punishment. In fact, the punishment may alleviate the guilt surrounding the deception (Ekman, 1986). Deception guilt is a function of shared social values between the liar and the deceived. People feel less guilty about lying to those individuals they think are wrongdoers (Ekman, 1986; Quinn, 1988). Thus a child who feels attached to the noncustodial parent will feel guilty about making false sexual abuse allegations, whereas the child who feels emotionally alienated and aloof from the parent will not.

## CLINICAL ASSESSMENT OF CHILDREN'S LYING

The clinical assessment of children's lying addresses several specific evaluation issues (Quinn, 1988). First, one must ascertain whether or not the child has the developmental capacity to deceive. Very young children's statements may be untruths generated by their immature cognitive abilities with no intention to deceive. As a general guideline, children under the age of 6 years are unable to intentionally lie successfully (Quinn, 1988). If they do tell intentional lies, they are readily discernible by adults.

A second clinical question is whether or not the child or adolescent has a history of persistent lying. If so, then this baseline of previous lying influences the evaluation of the veracity of the child's current statement. Lying is a process and not a single event. If the child has a history of persistent lying, then the dynamics of that lying and the gain it affords the child must be determined.

Third, one must ascertain if the child has a psychiatric disorder that would alter reality testing or cause severe distortion, fantasy, or the use of defenses such as massive denial or dissociation. If this is the case, then one must ascertain if the child's presentation of a psychiatric or medical disorder is consistent with a well-recognized illness or syndrome.

With adolescents, one must ascertain whether or not the youth has a history of persistent lying. It also must be determined whether there are any psychosocial stressors that might promote lying, such as a divorce in the family, alcoholism or drug abuse in the family, or a history of family violence and/or abuse. It is most helpful to ascertain whether or not the youth is pursuing an objective such as custody with a particular parent or a change in visitation.

It is also essential to rule out whether an adult is lying for the child or distorting the child's communication. In addition, it is important to determine if previous assessments of the child contain interviewing errors resulting in incorrect assessment of the nature of the child's communication. Highly coercive and leading questions can lead to premature conclusions of abuse.

## DEVELOPMENTAL ASPECTS OF TRUTHFULNESS

In order to lie, one must have a knowledge of the truth because lying and truthfulness are inexorably entwined. Before the age of 5 years, children do not understand the concept of lying and therefore are not capable of telling a willful untruth with the intent to deceive another (Piaget, 1965; Feldman et al., 1979; DePaulo et al., 1985). After age 5 years, children begin to understand the concept of lying, but they tend to confuse and overgeneralize it. For example, they may equate lying with swearing or guessing. Around the age of 10 years children can judge lies by their intent and the damage or benefit they may cause (Piaget, 1965). Thereafter, children may intentionally lie.

Anna Freud (1965) and Piaget (1965) have described lying as a normal part of a child's development with distinct phases that evolve as the child grows. This lying is developmental and not pathological. As the child matures, three types of lying occur. Very young children, from 3 to 5 years of age, tell innocent lies that are largely determined by wishful thinking. An example is: "I met Michelangelo" (the Ninja Turtle). From 6 to 8 years, the child may tell fantasy lies about things wished to be true. In the later states of development, 8 years and older, children lie to gain material things, escape punishment, protect themselves from feared authority, or enhance their images to others.

Although Piaget's developmentally related definitions of lying have generally been confirmed in studies of the changes in children's understanding of lying (Peterson et al., 1983; DePaulo et al., 1985), recent theorists view lying as a normal developmental variant that occurs in the process of learning to tell the truth (Leekam, 1992; Ford, 1995). Accordingly, lying is part of a process wherein the child develops autonomy from the parent, thereby facilitating the development of both ego and superego functions. In telling falsehoods the child is able to separate himself or herself autonomously from the parent and establish a distinct and individual identity (Ford, 1995). In addition, the process of learning how to lie is developmentally influenced by how the child learns about the morality of lying (Bussey, 1992), child-rearing styles (Stouthamer-Loeber, 1986), exposure to truthfulness or deception in others (Ford, 1995), and the social impression the child wants to convey in others (Saarni & von Salisch, 1993). Thus learning how and when to be truthful and deceitful are developmental tasks.

Most children speak the truth as they understand it, if speaking the truth is defined for them and the obligation to tell the truth is impressed on them (Whitcomb, 1992). Children are not more likely to lie than adults. Research suggests there is little reason to differentiate children from adults in relation to their propensity to lie on the witness stand (Whitcomb, 1992). Telling the truth does not necessarily result from understanding the difference between a truth and a lie, and comprehending the oath does not guarantee honesty (Goodman, 1988; Gordon & Follmer, 1994). When speaking truthfully is defined for young children and the importance of doing so is impressed on them, most children will tell the truth as they understand it (Perry & Wrightsman, 1991).

## CHILDREN'S PLAY AND FANTASIES

Play and fantasies are the serious business of childhood, according to Piaget. Play parallels the development of language and, accordingly, has its egocentric aspects in which children play next to one another without interaction (parallel play) and slowly progress toward associative interaction, which culminates developmentally in cooperative interaction in rule-governed games. All children engage in reality play, in which they manipulate objects for their intended purpose, such as putting sand in a dump truck or playing with dolls. Object fantasy is most popular with 2- and 3-year-olds and entails the attribution of an entirely new identity to the object, such as designating the truck as a rocket ship and the doll as an airplane. Person fantasy involves the portrayal of characters and occurs in children from 3 to 5 years of age, usually decreasing after 6 years of age.

The dramatic play of children reflects their cognitive development, the social issues with which they are grappling, and the environmental stimuli with which they come in contact, including television, books, and the actions of others around them (Singer, 1995). Preoperational children depend on actual experiences to produce images of fantasy, that is, they fantasize about what they have actually experienced (DeYoung, 1986). The fantasies of preoperational children reflect wishful thinking and are tied to the pleasure principle. Thus they are hedonistic in nature. In fantasy, the child obtains what he or she does not have, removes sources of irritation, goes where he or she cannot go, and solves problems with positive and rewarding results. Accordingly, the child's fantasies stress mastery and competence, and the child is a hero and a problem solver, not a victim.

Research has indicated that television does not enhance a child's fantasy or imagination (Singer & Singer, 1990; Van der Voort & Valkenburg, 1994). In fact, children who watch a great deal of television have less imagination than children who do not. In addition, heavy television viewers also have less expressiveness in language and a greater tendency toward aggression and uncooperativeness than children who do not watch a good deal of television (Singer et al., 1984). Thus exposure to television does not increase a child's creativity or imagination.

Given what we know about the effects of television viewing on children and the nature of children's fantasies, they are not a likely source of false allegations of child sexual abuse. Fantasy lies occur in children in response to intolerable realities in which they regress and engage in infantile forms of wishful thinking in order to cope with an exceedingly distressing world (DeYoung, 1986; Ford, 1995).

## Factors Affecting a Child's Ability to Relate Events
### Traumatic Events

Traumatic events, such as exposure to violence or abuse, have effects on the memory abilities of both children and adults. The stress related to trauma can interfere with the accurate memory of the details of the trauma. Pynoos and Nadar (1989) investigated the effects of a sniper attack on the memories of children and found that those who were close to the sniper attack minimized their exposure to the gunfire during their recall of the event. In contrast, children who were far from the gunfire tended to maximize their exposure to it in their recall of the incident. In their free recall, the children reported intended and planned actions to protect themselves and others as if they had carried them out.

Other research has indicated that high anxiety at the time of trauma is associated with interference in the memory of the event, but low and moderate anxiety are not (Perry & Wrightsman, 1991). Intense stress may create a state of hyperarousal within the individual that causes high levels of anxiety which impede memory functioning. One possible response to high stress is to focus only on major details and to ignore minor or peripheral details. For example, when raped at knife point, the victim may remember little about the facial features of the attacker but may have vivid memories of the weapon and sexual assault itself. However, the effects of anxiety and stress on the memory process are not simple or easily explained. The results of several studies involving memories of medical procedures and the space shuttle disaster have indicated that high levels of stress at the time of the remembered event are associated with detail in recall and resistance to suggestion (Batterman-Faunce & Goodman, 1993).

Central features of highly emotional events are retained in memory for long periods of time but peripheral details are not as readily encoded or retained (Christiansson, 1992). Ceci and Bruck (1993) maintain that stress has a debilitating effect on memory. However, in studies addressing children's memory for stressful events, results have indicated that core features of stressful events are retained well in memory (Goodman et al., 1991) and stressful memories are associated with both greater recall and resistance to suggestion (Warren-Leubecker, 1991; Steward, 1992). Some children may remember stressful events more accurately than others, and individual differences in children's memory skills may account for these differences (Ornstein et al., 1993; Goodman et al., 1994). More research is needed to identify these differences.

### Incentives/Coercion to Keep Secrets

Incentives to keep secrets may induce a child not to tell about a particular event and thereby impact a child's account of events. These incentives can take several forms. A common one is physical threats against the child and/or her loved ones or family. Tangible rewards may be offered to the child if she keeps the secret. The child may be told that the perpetrator will get in trouble if the child discloses the secret, which may lead to disruption of the family unit that is the child's main source of support. The child may be told that she will get in trouble if she discloses the secret or that no one will believe or understand her if she tells. These inducements can cause a young child to omit important information in giving an account of an event or to not provide any information about the event at all.

The process by which children come to make reports of sexual abuse has been addressed in both theory (Summit, 1983) and research (Sauzier, 1989; Sorensen & Snow, 1991; Goodman et al., 1992; Campis et al., 1993). In the sexual abuse accommodation syndrome, Summit (1983) posits that children go through a series of stages in disclosing their sexual abuse, including secrecy, helplessness, entrapment, disclosure, and retraction. There is some frequently cited empirical support for these stages. Sorensen and Snow (1991) examined a sample of 116 treated cases of child sexual abuse and found accidental disclosures for a majority of the children; denial of the abuse at some time by 75% of the children; and recantation of the disclosure by 22% of the children. However, other data indicate that children readily report their victimization and the disclosure varies as a function of age (Campis et al., 1993), with preschool children making accidental disclosures in 75% of cases and older children overwhelmingly making deliberate ones. This is in contrast to previous research, which found that over half of preschoolers made deliberate disclosures of their victimization (Mian et al., 1986). Goodman and her colleagues (1992) reported that almost half (42%) of the children in their study reported their sexual victimization within 48 hours of its occurrence. In contrast, Sauzier (1989) reported that only 24% of children told about the abuse within 1 week and 39% did not disclose but were brought to the attention of authorities through accidental disclosures. Furthermore, the likelihood of disclosure was not related to threats by the offender. Even in the presence of aggressive threats for disclosure, children were equally likely to immediately or never disclose the sexual abuse. Other research has indicated that two thirds of children disclosed sexual abuse even despite being physically threatened by the perpetrator (Gray, 1993).

Thus, a number of children either accidentally or deliberately disclose sexual abuse and a number delay their disclosures for long periods of time (Ceci & Bruck, 1995). Currently, there are no identified empirical parameters to differentially distinguish between these two groups of children.

## COACHING

Despite lack of evidence (Bussey et al., 1994), many people believe that it is easy to coach young children to lie. False recantations were found to be a greater problem than false allegations (Everson & Boat, 1989) in a study of 1,249 Child Protective Service (CPS) referrals in North Carolina. In a review of research on false allegations, the American Prosecutor Research Institute (1989) found false allegation rates to range from 3% to 8% with most false allegations made by adults rather than children. Among many mental health professionals, it is common practice to ask very young children what is happening in their families because they are a very good source of uncensored and truthful information. As a rule of thumb, it is informative to ask the child what the parent (both father and mother) told him to tell the interviewer as well as what not to tell. These questions need to be open ended and simply constructed: What did your mother tell you to tell me? What did she tell you not to tell me?

Situations commonly associated with coaching and false allegations of child sexual abuse have been identified (Faller, 1991). These include post-traumatic stress disorder or serious psychiatric disorder in the adult; a symbiotically disturbed mother-child relationship; certain ongoing custody and visitation disputes; and a professional committed prematurely to the truth of the allegation. These situations underscore the necessity of evaluating all parties making allegations of childhood sexual abuse. Some adults have unresolved trauma from their own victimization and over-identify with the child. This over-involvement often manifests itself in the parent's preoccupation with the child's abuse and becomes apparent when the adult is clearly influencing the child in making the allegations. In other cases the parent may possess a serious psychiatric disorder (i.e., psychoses, personality disorder, or Munchausen Syndrome by Proxy). In these cases the disclosure is initiated by the parent and the allegations are presented from a perspective of genuine concern. The reports of molestation become increasingly embellished, and the parent may keep and provide copious notes on the molestation and minute anecdotes and documentation of the child's behavior. The child's statement, if present, lacks detail and emotional consistency and is often very similar to the parent's. In some cases the parent's psychopathology contributes significantly to a highly unhealthy parent/child dyad. The child becomes "parentified" or is used to meet the unmet parental needs causing significant self-other boundary disturbances within the parent/child dyad. The child depends on the parent and, threatened with the loss of parental love, adheres to the delusional misinterpretation of events. Faller (1991) also describes professional bias wherein a physician, psychologist, social worker, or mental health therapist prematurely commits to the allegation of sexual abuse and over-values, misinterprets, or distorts available data. These professionals may unwittingly contribute to the perpetuation of false allegations by interviewing the child repeatedly about the allegations or seeing the child for numerous therapy sessions in which the allegations are discussed repeatedly.

### INTERVIEWER REINFORCEMENT

Goodman (1988) investigated the effects of interviewer reinforcement on children's accuracy. Interviewer reinforcement has no effect on children's accuracy for children aged 5 years and older. However, 3- and 4-year-old children are more accurate when the interviewer provides reinforcement. This study was conducted because interviewers were criticized for being too nice to children and bribing them to say the things they wanted. The implications for the physician interviewing children are obvious: a cold physician will receive less accurate reports from very young children, and interviews during which the child receives some type of reinforcement are not invalidated or contaminated by the reinforcement. However, one must ensure that the child does not perceive that the content of his or her utterances should be changed to obtain specific reinforcement. Rather, giving the child a reward for being brave and discussing things that happened to him or her does not contaminate the interview if it is provided after the completion of the interview.

## ♦ CHILDREN'S MEMORY

Memory is not a unitary construct, and, accordingly, there are different types of memory that must be addressed separately. These include the memory process, recognition memory, free recall, episodic memory, and script memory. These constructs exemplify current psychological approaches in conceptualizing the memory process (Ceci & Bruck, 1995).

The primary phases of the *memory process* are attention, encoding, storage, and retrieval (Baddeley, 1990). Very briefly, these entail attending to the stimulus event through one or more of the five senses (Baddeley, 1990), encoding or registering the memory trace within the memory system (Baddeley, 1990), storing the memory trace in either short- or long-term memory (Brainerd et al., 1990), and retrieving the stored memories (Baddeley, 1990). However, several cognitive and social factors influence the retrieval of stored memories that may either enhance recall or decrease the accuracy of retrieved memories (Ceci & Bruck, 1995).

Memory is a central component to most cognitive activity, and current theorists support Piaget and Inhelder in not separating it conceptually from cognition itself. Children's ability to remember things is linked to their knowledge and understanding of what they are trying to remember (Newcombe et al., 1995), and children acquire strategies for enhancing their memory (i.e., rehearsal, chunking, and mnemonics) as they gain experience in academic settings.

### TYPES OF MEMORY

*Recognition memory* is required when the child is asked to recognize the presence or absence of something. Children as young as age 4 or 5 years do as well as older children on recognition tasks involving picture or face recognition (Saywitz, 1987). One published account in the literature details a 3-year-old recognizing an assailant in a photo line up (Jones & Krugman, 1986). Recognition memory is essentially a matching process, and both adults and children find it easier than recall memory tasks (Cole & Loftus, 1987). Preschool children can recognize previously experienced locations as well as older children and adults (Sivan, 1991).

*Free recall* involves recounting information or events from the past. Preschool children tend to do quite poorly on this when compared to older children and adults. Free recall is the most complex form of memory in that it requires that previously observed and coded events be retrieved from memory storage with few, if any prompts. The narrative provided in response to open-ended questions such as "Tell me what happened" is the most accurate form of memory report (Dent & Stephenson, 1979). This has been a consistent and robust finding in the memory research literature (Saywitz & Goodman, 1996). However, this form of memory is age-related, and young children find it difficult to describe events in free-recall situations (Whitcomb, 1992). Children's recollections under free recall contain less information, but the information given is accurate (Saywitz & Goodman, 1996). Young children have a less complex view of the world than adults and, accordingly, provide less information to open-ended questions. They also assume that adults know the answers to the questions they ask them. Thus children give only bits of information to questions posed because they assume the adult is fully aware of the incident in question. Furthermore, because of this assumption, children's disclosures typically are incremental and include partial disclosure of a given event over time. Thus, although a preschooler's total amount of information about a given event does not change over time, he recalls different information each time he recalls an event (Fivush & Shukat, 1995). These factors can make preschoolers appear inconsistent in their recall of events because preschoolers often rely on external cues from adults to guide their recall and specific questions and cues are needed to elicit specific details of memory (Fivush & Shukat, 1995). Studies have indicated that these cues tend to enhance accuracy among preschool children (Pipe et al., 1993).

*Episodic memory* refers to those memories of specific details about times, dates, and locations. Episodic memory requires the understanding of abstract concepts, such as time, duration, sequence, and succession. School-aged children can make accurate judgments about time, but younger children cannot (Geary, 1994). Preschool children are tied to regular behavioral routines such as bedtime, bathtime, breakfast, etc. in order to anchor events in time. A child's episodic memory of an abusive event encompasses episodes or experiences that include specific times, dates, locations, and events. School-aged children can make accurate judgments about time, whereas younger children cannot. Young children have problems recalling the correct order of events, although they do not have problems recalling the events themselves. The episodic memories of preschool children are significantly poorer than those of older children and adults (Sivan, 1991).

*Script memory* describes the recall of a past event in a free manner. The child is required to report details that are personally relevant rather than specifics, which are demanded by an interview. Children as young as 35 months of age have been found to accurately relate some events occurring from 1 month to over a year previously. With young children, repeated exposure to a given event brings about a more elaborate script memory. Thus children who are molested in routine settings, such as during bath or at bedtime, have script memories of the events that can be elicited in interviews. Preschool children develop scripts to organize the elements and memories of events into categories that enhance recall: participants, setting, actions, conversations/affect, and consequences (Stein & Glenn, 1978; Nelson & Hudson, 1988). These scripts can be elicited by asking the child simple, basic questions such as "Who was there?" "Where were you?" "What did he do to you?"

"What did he say?" "How did you feel?" and "What happened?"

When allowed to relate a tale in his or her own words, the preschool child does not create a false picture. When prompted, preschool children add relevant and true details to what has occurred. Their cognitive limitations related to the knowledge of time and sequence render a child's version of the story qualitatively different from that of an adult. However, children can produce elaborate and exact recollections under these conditions (Fivush & Shukat, 1995; Saywitz, 1995).

## MEMORY PROCESSES

*Encoding* is the first phase of the memory process and is the mechanism by which a trace of an experience is coded or registered within the memory system (Ceci & Bruck, 1995). The information encoded is limited by the attention of the child to the events in the episode. Obviously, all events in a given episode cannot be remembered, and selectivity of attention to relevant elements determines what is registered through the senses into memory store. Selectivity of attention is determined by prior knowledge of events, the interest value of the events, and stress level of the child at the time of encoding (Perry & Wrightsman, 1991). Thus a child may not remember the shirt or hair color of the person who abused him but he can remember that the individual smelled like cigarette smoke and had a missing tooth. Young children typically remember central rather than peripheral details and events that are repeated over time.

*Storage*, the second phase of the memory system, is the process by which encoded events enter a short-term or long-term memory store where they are preserved either temporarily or permanently. Several factors, including the passage of time, re-experiencing the event, and intervening experiences, can influence the stored memories (Ceci & Bruck, 1995). Memories can be strengthened or weakened depending on the number of times they are recalled and the length of time in storage. During the storage process itself, expectancies, knowledge, and experiences surrounding the event can affect the content of the memory trace (Ceci & Bruck, 1995). Retrieval processes access information from these stored representations. The retrieval task varies as a function of the questioning stimulus, that is recognition tasks such as "Was it a tall or short man?" or "Is this the man?" or free recall such as "Tell me what happened to you at the farm."

Saywitz and her colleagues (1991) investigated different types of recall in children for their memories of a medical examination involving genital touch. The memories of 5- and 7-year-old girls were evaluated after a physical evaluation in which one group received a vaginal and anal examination and the other group did not receive the sexual evaluation. Memories were elicited through free recall, anatomically correct dolls, and direct questions. The anal and vaginal touches were unreported in the free recall and the doll conditions. The sexual touch was reported only when the children were asked directly to talk about it. Children are socialized not to talk to strangers about sexual matters and will do so only with permission. The direct questioning provided this permission. This suggests that interviewers should use direct questions when interviewing young children about sexual issues. False reports of vaginal and anal touch from the children in the nongenital condition were virtually nonexistent in the free recall, dolls, and direct questioning conditions. With the genital touch group, the doll questioning condition did not elicit additional reports of vaginal or anal touch. For the genital touch group, 5- and 7-year-olds performed at the same level in free recall. In free recall, 5-year-olds were more likely to reveal the genital touch. It would appear that younger children are more likely to reveal genital touch than older children when asked simply to recall the events in an open-ended manner. Direct questioning and the use of dolls elicited the most information from girls who had been touched on the genitals. An intriguing finding is an 8% false-report rate of genital touch among the children who did not experience this during the physical examination. Some children in the study were more vulnerable to false report than others.

In a replication of this research with a sample of 2- and 3-year-olds, a high number of false reports were found (Bruck et al., 1995). Younger children seem to succumb to suggestive questioning more readily than older children (Goodman & Aman, 1991) and may require a supportive context within the interview situation to resist providing suggestive misinformation (Goodman et al., 1991). Suggestions in this regard include the following: keep questions short, grammatical constructions simple, and vocabulary familiar; do not pressure or coerce the child during questioning; remain nonjudgmental both verbally and nonverbally during the interview and do not reinforce the child for providing specific content; and when a "yes-no" question is posed, follow it with "How do you know that?" or "What makes you think so?"

Memory abilities, including the encoding, storage, and retrieval of events, are not static or invariant, and vary, at any age, depending on the type of event experienced and information to be remembered, the conditions surrounding the elicitation of the memory during the interview, the strength of the memory, the language used in the interview, and post-event influences (Saywitz & Goodman, 1996).

## ◆ SUGGESTIBILITY

Suggestibility can affect children's memory. Unrelenting questioning or telling the child repeatedly that something has occurred can influence the child to give false information. Children are most likely to do this when they are asked the same questions repeatedly over multiple interviews with a long time delay between the events and the questioning (Ceci & Bruck, 1993). However, there are individual variations in suggestibility and some children are highly resistant to false suggestions (Ceci & Bruck, 1993).

There are conflicting research results concerning the suggestibility of children's recollections. Some research indicates that young children are as immune to suggestion as older children (Saywitz et al., 1991), and other studies conclude that young children are more suggestible than older children (Ceci & Bruck, 1993). This discrepancy in research results may reflect the fact that several factors interact with age to influence suggestibility (Loftus & Ceci, 1991). Nevertheless, preschool children seem to be more suggestible than school-aged children and adults (Ceci & Bruck, 1995; Saywitz & Goodman, 1996). Suggestibility is not a stable factor and is influenced by the interaction of variables within the child, the environment, and significant individuals within the child's environment.

### SUGGESTIVE QUESTIONING

The first such factor is strongly suggestive questioning such as "I bet your Daddy touched your pee pee, isn't that right?" Such questions greatly increase the chances of an inaccurate response. The same is true for asking the same question on multiple occasions throughout the interview. Children want very much to please adults. They may concur with a highly leading question because they want to please the adult asking it, or they may change a response to a repeated question because they assume they have not given the adult the correct answer.

### MEMORY STRENGTH

Another factor influencing suggestibility is the strength of the memory in question. Memory can be weakened by the passage of time, the level of interest in the events at the time of occurrence and their understanding, and the imposition of misleading information. Memory strength is enhanced by the personal significance of the event. Even in children, strong memories are very resistant to change.

However, they are more likely to be suggestible about peripheral or poorly retained information than about salient and memorable information (Saywitz & Goodman, 1996). Thus a young child would not be suggestible to abusive genital contact (a highly salient and memorable experience) but might be to peripheral details such as the hair or eye color of the assailant.

## INTERVIEWER STATUS

Children are more likely to be suggestible if the questioner represents high status or power, such as a parent, teacher, physician, therapist, or police officer. Parents often unwittingly set the stage for suggestibility by bringing the child to the high-status professional with the instruction "Tell Dr. Jones everything that Mr. Smith did to you on your private parts."

## QUESTIONING CONTEXT

Children are influenced by leading questions if they are pressured to supply more details, questioned repeatedly, questioned under intimidating circumstances, or instilled with a negative stereotype about a person when questioned about him or her (Ceci & Bruck, 1993, 1995). Very young children have made inaccurate statements to policemen when asked free recall questions within an accusatory context (Tobey & Goodman, 1992). The free recall statements of preschool children can be distorted if they are asked misleading questions that are repeated and are within a negative context about a given individual (Clarke-Stewart et al., 1989; Leichtman & Ceci, 1995). Thus if preschoolers are interviewed repeatedly with false suggestions in an accusatory context, false information is likely to be present in the narrative of their free recall of events (Saywitz & Goodman, 1996). Conversely, sexually abused preschoolers are vulnerable to repeated suggestions that they were not sexually victimized, which can result in false recantations.

## STATE OF KNOWLEDGE ON SUGGESTIBILITY

Medical professionals who interview young children need to have a cursory knowledge of the current state of scientific knowledge regarding the reliability and suggestibility of children's testimony. *It is briefly summarized as follows:*

1. Reliable age differences have been identified in suggestibility, with preschool children being more suggestible than school-aged children, adolescents, and adults (Ceci & Bruck, 1995; Saywitz & Goodman, 1996).

2. No current evidence supports the confirmation of sexual abuse on the basis of very young children's play or interaction with anatomically correct dolls (Berry & Skinner, 1993; Ceci & Bruck, 1995). These dolls can be suggestive (Ceci & Bruck, 1995); there are no uniform standards for conducting interviews with the dolls (American Psychological Association, 1992); and sexualized play with the dolls does not reliably differentiate between abused and nonabused children (Realmuto et al.,1990; Cohn, 1991; Kenyon-Jump et al.,1991; Realmuto & Wescoe, 1992). However, the dolls can be useful adjuncts to assist children and youth in communicating abusive experiences in the presence of speech and/or language delays, differences or disabilities, emotional concerns, or difficulty in verbally discussing sexual topics (American Psychological Association, 1991). However, a verbal or language-based disclosure should be made before the dolls are introduced into the interview.

3. Highly suggestive interviewing techniques (i.e., multiple interviews, suggestive questioning, repeated questioning, and demanding interviewers) can cause inaccuracies in the reports of young children, including central and salient events in the report (Ceci & Bruck, 1995).

4. Suggestibility effects tend to occur most often in young children after repeated questioning in multiple interviews over time (Saywitz & Goodman, 1996). Suggestibility effects are best viewed on a continuum ranging from mild effects

on the recall of peripheral details of the event to prolonged and repeated interviews eliciting horrifying content of child murders or satanic or ritualistic abuse. Ritualistic and satanic child sexual abuse is a low baserate phenomenon (Kelley, 1995; Bottoms et al., 1996) and there is no evidence for a large satanic conspiracy of child abusers preying on children across the United States (Lanning, 1991).

5. There is no syndrome or constellation of behavioral manifestations that result from child sexual abuse (Kendall-Tackett et al., 1993). Both abused and nonabused children can exhibit similar behavioral difficulties (i.e., aggression, withdrawal, bedwetting, sexual acting out, masturbation). Thus the occurrence of sexual abuse cannot be inferred by the presence of one of these behavioral difficulties. Indeed, approximately one-third of child sexual abuse victims do not exhibit symptoms of psychological distress or behavior problems (Kendall-Tackett et al., 1993).

6. There is nothing in the scientific literature indicating that a child who is resistive to a medical examination for child sexual abuse has been a victim of sexual abuse. Available research suggests that most children do not have negative perceptions about the physical examination and that previous negative medical experiences play a determining role in how the child interprets the experience (Lazebnik et al., 1994).

## STRENGTHS IN CHILDREN'S MEMORY

An examination of suggestibility issues in children's memory is not complete without also addressing the strengths in children's memory skills. Research has demonstrated that children can be highly resistive to interviewer biases (Ceci & Bruck, 1995). Furthermore, some inconsistencies in the recall of events are a normal occurrence in both children and adults, and, given the selectivity of memory itself, no one can realistically be expected to recall all details of a given event accurately and consistently. Thus some inconsistencies in the recall of details cannot be used to discredit the narratives of children. Nothing in the scientific literature suggests that an incorrect memory resulting from suggestibility in one aspect of a child's narrative generalizes to the entire narrative of the child (Ceci & Bruck, 1995). This is a very important distinction. Even though suggestibility effects can be strong, they are not always large in magnitude and do not necessarily permeate the entire interview.

## SUGGESTIONS FOR AVOIDING SUGGESTIBILITY

1. Keep the number of interviews to a minimum. Consider an interview to encompass all conversations between a child and an adult about the alleged sexual event.

2. Use simple grammatical constructions and familiar vocabulary in questioning young children. Ask questions that are appropriate to the child's developmental question comprehension level **(Table 11-3).** Do not ask leading questions, which suggest answers to the child.

3. Avoid acquiring a confirmatory bias before interviewing the child. Avoid making an alliance with an adult initiating the allegation before examining the child. Keep a nonbiased attitude and be open to other explanations for the alleged sexual event, behavioral manifestations, and previous verbalizations of the child throughout the interview.

4. If you anticipate that the results of your interview will be used for forensic purposes, preserve it electronically in some manner.

5. Avoid inculcating a negative stereotype about the alleged perpetrator with the child during the interview. Be patient with the child and nonjudgmental about the sexual events, the child, and the alleged perpetrator.

6. Try not to repeat questions or use close-ended yes/no questions in the

interview. Do not praise the child for providing specific content or answers, and do not pressure or coerce the child to discuss sexual issues.

## ♦ VULNERABILITY OF CHILDREN WITH DISABILITIES

### MEDICAL AND PSYCHOLOGICAL NEEDS OF CHILDREN ENTERING FOSTER CARE

A comprehensive study of children taken into foster care completed by the University of Chicago School of Medicine found an overwhelming majority in need of medical and psychological intervention (Hochstadt et al., 1987). Physical evaluations found only 13% (out of 200) of the children to be normal. Physical problems included growth problems (height, weight, and head circumference); dermatologic, ophthalmologic, neuromuscular, cardiovascular, dental, and pulmonary abnormalities; fetal alcohol syndrome (FAS); congenital anomalies; ear infections; and pregnancy. Psychological evaluations found 56% of the children over 3 years of age in need of psychological treatment, 52% of the children under 3 years of age in need of infant stimulation due to developmental delays, and 2% in need of psychiatric residential treatment. These findings are consistent with previous research indicating that abused and neglected children have significant cognitive, developmental, and emotional deficits (Elmer & Gregg, 1967; Fitch et al., 1976; Applebaum, 1977; Kline, 1977; Koski & Ingram, 1977).

Hochstadt and colleagues (1987) concluded that at the time of placement, most foster children have had inadequate physical and emotional nourishment and poor medical and psychological care. This tragedy is often compounded by lack of medical and psychological care after foster placement. Parental neglect is replaced, as it were, by community neglect. As a result of this research, the authors recommended that medical and psychological screening be completed on all children entering foster care; treatment be provided for children needing these services; centralized medical and psychosocial records be developed that follow the child throughout the system; case management be ongoing; and support for foster parents be given in obtaining these services.

### RISK FOR MALTREATMENT

Children with disabilities are presumed to increase the level of stress among parents and, thereby, be at risk for abuse (Blacher, 1984; Krents et al., 1987) or be at risk by the very nature of their disability (Friedrich & Boriskin, 1978; Cole, 1986; Watson, 1995). It has been argued that mentally retarded children are at risk because ordinary standards of care are inadequate for them (Schilling & Schinke, 1984) and they may be less protected by the incest taboo than children of normal intelligence (Neutra et al., 1977). Many children with disabilities exhibit behavioral characteristics such as tantrums, aggressiveness, and noncompliance that impact negatively on parents and caregivers, increasing the risk for abuse (Solomons, 1979). Perceptions of high rates of physical and sexual abuse have been reported for children who are blind (Zadnik, 1973; Elonen & Swarensteyn, 1975), chronically ill (Glaser & Bentovim, 1979), schizophrenic (Green, 1968), and multihandicapped (Ammerman et al., 1989). Various disabilities, including mental retardation (Sangrund et al., 1974), cerebral palsy (Jaudes & Diamond, 1985), developmental delays (Augoustinos, 1987), speech and language disabilities (Fox et al., 1988; Law & Conway, 1992), and multiple personality disorders (Putnam et al., 1986) have been attributed to abuse and neglect. Finally, research with juveniles condemned to death in the United States indicates that they possess multiple disabilities and were severely physically and sexually abused by their families before their crimes (Lewis et al., 1988).

## RELATIONSHIP BETWEEN CHILD ABUSE AND NEGLECT AND DISABILITIES

Children with disabilities represent a significant number of children in the United States, but little attention has been afforded this population in the field of child maltreatment. The *Child Abuse and Prevention, Adoption, and Family Services Act of 1988* (PL 100-294) mandated the study of the incidence of child maltreatment among children with disabilities. In response, research was undertaken to determine the prevalence of maltreatment among children with disabilities and to identify risk factors for maltreatment (Sullivan & Knutson, 1994). Archival data were collected on a random sample of 3,001 abused subjects and 880 nonabused subjects identified by merging the patient data base of Boys Town National Research Hospital (BTNRH) with two social service and five law enforcement data bases within the state of Nebraska. Both social service and law enforcement records were used to determine the rate of intra- and extrafamilial child maltreatment among children referred for evaluation and treatment at a pediatric hospital.

Demographic and descriptive information was collected on the children through a system of medical and victim record review. The following information was collected from hospital, social service, and law enforcement files on each child in this study: age, gender, disability type, severity of disability, schooling, hair color, attractiveness, race, presence of multiple disabilities, agency source, site of abuse, type of abuse, perpetrator characteristics, age when abused, severity of abuse, and duration of abuse.

### TYPE OF MALTREATMENT

The vast majority of children in the sample were victims of neglect, followed by physical abuse and then sexual abuse. The types of maltreatment endured by the children studied are listed in **Table 11-4** in descending order of magnitude.

### AGE AT MALTREATMENT

Children with disabilities are maltreated at very young ages. About half (53%) of the maltreatment was reported before the child was 5 years of age.

### TYPE OF DISABILITY

Among children identified as maltreated from social service and police agencies, 73% were found to have some type of disability in contrast to 32% of the nonabused children. The identified disabilities, in descending order of magnitude for the abused and nonabused groups, are given in **Table 11-5**.

### SITE OF ABUSE

*The vast majority of children with disabilities*

**Table 11-4.** Type and Prevalence of Maltreatment

| Maltreatment Type | Percent (%) of Study Sample |
|---|---|
| Neglect | 74 |
| Physical | 52 |
| Sexual | 31 |
| Emotional | 27 |
| Multiple types of abuse | 54 |

*Findings included the following:*

Nearly three fourths (74%) of the maltreated children endured some form of neglect. Thus, for both children with and without disabilities, *neglect is the most prevalent form of maltreatment* followed by physical abuse and sexual abuse.

Approximately half of them experienced physical abuse.

Slightly less than a third (27%) of the children had records of emotional abuse.

A little over half of the children studied (54%) endured multiple forms of maltreatment.

*Children who experienced either emotional (94%) or physical (83%) abuse almost always experienced additional forms of maltreatment.*

Nearly two of every three sexually abused children (67%) and neglected children (64%) also endured other forms of maltreatment.

| Table 11-5. Prevalence of Disabilities | | |
|---|---|---|
| | **Percent (%)** | |
| **Disability** | **Abused** | **Nonabused** |
| Behavior disorders | 37.8 | 0.9 |
| None | 27.4 | 67.6 |
| Speech/language | 8.7 | 8.4 |
| Mental retardation | 6.2 | 1.3 |
| Hearing impairment | 6.1 | 7.5 |
| Learning disability | 5.7 | 2.6 |
| Other disability* | 4.1 | 6.7 |
| Health impairments† | 2.4 | 4.0 |
| Attention deficit disorder (with no conduct disorder) | 1.6 | 0.8 |

*Includes visual impairments, cleft palate, cerebral palsy, orthopedic impairments, autism, and neurological impairments.

†Includes chronic allergies, asthma, middle ear and lung problems, epilepsy, Crohn's disease, sickle cell anemia, muscular dystrophy, Reyes syndrome, Tay Sachs disease, juvenile rheumatoid arthritis, heart problems, and diabetes.

*(88%) are abused in their own homes.*

Of those abused outside of their home, one third (4%) were abused in the perpetrator's home, while only 1% were abused in school.

Other less frequent sites of abuse include foster homes, public restrooms, public transportation vehicles, hospitals, juvenile detention centers, bus stops, car washes, and public shopping malls.

## PERPETRATORS

Children with disabilities tend to be maltreated by individuals they know and trust. The overwhelming majority of perpetrators are parents of disabled children. Parents account for 95% of neglect perpetrators, 76% of physical abuse perpetrators, and 39% of sexual abuse perpetrators.

The majority of the *remaining* physical abuse and neglect was perpetrated by extended and other family members, such as grandparents, adoptive step- or foster parents, or siblings, spouses, uncles, aunts, and cousins.

Half of sexually abused children with disabilities were abused by family members, while the other half were abused by people outside their family. *In most cases (92.4%) of the sexual abuse, perpetrators were known to the child victim.* Only 7% were strangers.

Men perpetrated 82% of the sexual abuse of children with disabilities.

Women perpetrated almost 70% of neglect, 51% of physical abuse, and 18% of sexual abuse of children with disabilities.

Prevention programs for children with disabilities need to take these perpetrator characteristics into account in the development of program content and target groups.

## CHILDREN WITH DISABILITIES ARE RISK FACTORS

1.8 times more likely to be neglected by family members than children without disabilities.

1.6 times more likely to be physically abused than children without disabilities.

2.2 times more likely to be sexually abused than children without disabilities.

*Children with behavior disorders and mental retardation* are at increased risk for all forms of maltreatment.

## IMPLICATIONS

This epidemiological research indicated that 15% of children referred to a national pediatric hospital had verified records of child maltreatment in social service and/or police records. This suggests that the rate of referral of maltreated children to medical facilities is quite high. Child maltreatment is a significant public health issue and should be an integral part of primary care, particularly for infants, toddlers, and preschoolers less than 5 years of age. Health care professionals must be aware of the increased incidence of maltreatment among children referred to them for care and treatment and should screen for histories of maltreatment and be alert for signs and symptoms of abuse and neglect. Given the high percentage of children with disabilities among maltreated children, health care professionals also need to routinely screen for disabilities so this information can be available to law enforcement and social service personnel in the conduct of child maltreatment investigations. Medical personnel need to play a key role in the identification and treatment of maltreated children with disabilities.

> **Child abuse can be considered the most potent and damaging influence on the development of children and consequently on the increasing incidence of serious social problems (Brown University Child and Adolescent Behavior Letter, 1993).**

## ◆ BIBLIOGRAPHY

Allen, VL, and Atkinson, ML: Encoding of nonverbal behavior by high-achieving and low-achieving children, *J Educ Psychol* 70:298-305, 1978.

American Association on Mental Retardation: *Mental Retardation: Definition, Classification, and System of Support*, ed 9, American Association on Mental Retardation, Washington, DC, (1992).

American Psychological Association (APA): Statement issued by the APA counsel of representatives, Feb 8, 1991.

Ammerman, RT, Van Hasselt, VB, Hersen, M, McGonigle, JJ, Lebetsky, MH: Abuse and neglect in psychiatrically hospitalized multihandicapped children, *Child Abuse Negl* 13(3):335-343, 1989.

Applebaum, A: Developmental retardation of infants as a concomitant of physical child abuse, *J Abnorm Child Psychol* 5:417-423, 1977.

Augoustinos, M: Developmental effects of child abuse: Recent findings, *Child Abuse Negl* 11:15-27, 1987.

Baddeley, AD: *Human memory: Theory and practice*, Allyn & Bacon, Boston, 1990.

Bala, N: Children, psychiatrists and the courts: Understanding the ambivalence of the legal profession. Part 1—General principles, *Can J Psychiatr* 39:526-539, 1994.

Batterman-Faunce, JM, and Goodman, GS: Effects of context on the accuracy of suggestibility of child witnesses. In GS Goodman and BL Bottoms, eds: *Child Victims, Child Witnesses*, Guilford, New York, 1993, pp. 301-330.

Berry, K, and Skinner, LG: Anatomically detailed dolls and the evaluations of child sexual abuse allegations: Psychometric considerations, *Law Hum Behav* 17:399-422, 1993.

Blacher, J: Attachment and severely handicapped children: Implications for intervention. *J Dev Behav Pediatr* 5(4):178-183, 1984.

Bloom, L, and Lahey, M: *Language Development and Language Disorders,* John Wiley Publishers, New York, 1979.

Bottoms, BL, Shaver, PR, and Goodman, GS: An analysis of ritualistic and religion-related child abuse allegations, *Law Hum Behav* 20(1):1-34, 1996.

Braginsky, DD: Machiavellian and manipulative interpersonal behavior in children, *J Exp Soc Psychol* 6:77-89, 1970.

Brainerd, CJ, Reyna, VF, Howe, ML, and Kingman, J: The development of forgetting and reminiscence, *Monog Soc Res Child Dev* 55(3-4): Serial No. 222, 1990.

Brown, A: The construction of temporal succession by the preoperational child. In A Pick, ed: *Minnesota Symposium on Child Development*, vol 10, University of Minnesota Press, Minneapolis, 1976, pp. 28-83.

Bruck, M, Ceci, SJ, Francouer, E, and Renick, A: Anatomically detailed dolls do not facilitate preschoolers' reports of a pediatric examination involving genital touching, *J Exp Psychol: Appl* 1(2):95-109, 1995.

Burton, K, and Myers, WC: Child sexual abuse and forensic psychiatry: Evolving and controversial issues, *Bull Am Acad Psychiatry Law* 20(4):439-453, 1992.

Bussey, K: Lying and truthfulness: Children's definitions, standards and evaluative reactions, *Child Dev* 63:129-137, 1992.

Bussey, K, Lee, K, and Grimbeek, E: Lies and secrets: Implications for children's reporting of sexual abuse. In GS Goodman and BL Bottoms, eds: *Child Victims, Child Witnesses*, Guilford, New York, 1993, pp. 147-168.

Campis, LB, Hebden-Curtis, J, and DeMaso, DR: Developmental differences in detection and disclosure of sexual abuse. *J Am Acad Child Adolescent Psychiatry* 32(5):920-924, 1993.

Ceci, SJ, and Bruck, M: *Jeopardy in the Courtroom: A Scientific Analysis of Children's Testimony*, American Psychological Association, Washington, DC, 1995.

Ceci, SJ, and Bruck, M: Suggestibility of the child witness: A historical review and synthesis, *Psychol Bull* 113(3):403-439, 1993.

Ceci, SJ, Leichtman, MD, and Putnick, M, eds: *Cognitive and Social Factors in Early Deceptions*, Lawrence Erlbaum Associates, Hillsdale, NJ, 1992.

Ceci, SJ, Toglia, MP, and Ross, DF, eds: *Children's Eyewitness Memory*, Springer-Verlag, New York, 1987.

Christiansson, SA: Emotional stress and eyewitness memory: A critical review, *Psychol Bull* 12:284-309, 1992.

Clarke-Stewart, A, Thompson, L, and Lepore, S: Manipulating children's interpretations through interrogation. In GS Goodman (Chair): *Can Children Provide Accurate Testimony?* Symposium presented at the Society for Research in Child Development Meetings, Kansas City, MO.

Cohn, DS: Anatomical doll play of preschoolers referred for sexual abuse and those not referred, *Child Abuse Negl* 15:455-466, 1991.

Cole, CB and Loftus, EF: The memory of children. In SJ Ceci, MP Toglia, and DF Ross, eds: *Children's Eyewitness Memory*, Springer-Verlag, New York, 1987, pp. 178-208.

Cole, SS: Facing the challenges of sexual abuse in persons with disabilities, *Sexuality Disability* 7(3-4):71-87, 1986.

Dent, H, and Stephenson, G: An experimental study of the effectiveness of different techniques of questioning child witnesses, *Br J Soc Clin Psychol* 18:41-51, 1979.

DePaulo, BM, and Rosenthal, R: Telling lies, *J Personality Soc Psychol* 37:1713-1722, 1979.

DePaulo, BM, Stone, JI, and Lassiter, GD: Deceiving and detecting deceit. In BR Schlenker, ed: *Self and Identity: Presentations of Self in Social Life*, McGraw-Hill, New York, 1985, pp. 323-370.

DeYoung, M: A conceptual model for judging the truthfulness of a young child's allegations of sexual abuse, *Am J Orthopsychiatry* 56(4):550-559, 1986.

Drummey, A, and Newcombe, N: Remembering versus knowing the past: Children's explicit and implicit memories for pictures, *J Child Psychol* 59:549-565, 1995.

Ekman, P: *Telling Lies*, Berkeley Books, New York, 1986.

Elmer, E, and Gregg, CS: Developmental characteristics of abused children, *Pediatrics* 40:596-602, 1967.

Elonen, AS, and Swarensteyn, SV: Sexual trauma in young blind children, *A New Outlook for the Blind* 69:440-442, 1975.

Everson, M, and Boat, B: False allegations of sexual abuse by children and adolescents, *J Am Acad Child Adolescent Psychiatry* 28(2):230-235, 1989.

Faller, KC: Possible explanations for child sexual abuse allegations in divorce, *Am J Orthopsychiatry* 6:86-91, 1991.

Feldman, RS, Jenkins, L, and Popoola, O: Detection of deception in adults and children via facial expressions, *Child Dev* 50:350-355, 1979.

Feldman, RS, and White, JB: Detecting deception in children, *J Communication* 30:121-139, 1980.

Fitch, MJ, Cadol, RV, Goldson, E, Wendell, T, Swartz, D, and Jackson, E: Cognitive development of abuse and failure to thrive children, *J Pediatr* 1:25-31, 1976.

Fivush, R, and Shukat, J: What young children recall: Issues of content, consistency, and coherence. In M Zaragoza, JR Graham, GCN Hall, R Hirschman, and YS Ben-Porath, eds: *Memory and Testimony in the Child Witness*, Sage, Thousand Oaks, CA, 1995, pp. 5-23.

Flin, R: Hearing and testing children's evidence. In G Goodman and B Bottoms, eds: *Child Victims, Child Witnesses*, Guilford, New York, 1993, pp. 279-299.

Ford, C: *Lies! Lies!! Lies!!!: The Psychology of Deceit*, American Psychiatric Press, Inc., Washington, DC, 1995.

Ford, CV, King, BH, and Hollender, MH: Lies and liars: Psychiatric aspects of prevarication, *Am J Psychiatry* 145:554-562, 1988.

Fox, L, Long, SH, and Langlois, A: Patterns of language comprehension deficit in abused and neglected children, *J Speech Hearing Disorders* 53:239-244, 1988.

Freud, A: *Normality and Pathology in Childhood: Aspects of Development*, International Universities Press, New York, 1965.

Friedman, W: *The Developmental Psychology of Time*, Academic Press, New York, 1982.

Friedrich, WN, and Boriskin, JA: Primary prevention of child abuse: Focus on the special child, *Hosp Community Psychiatry* 29(4):248-256, 1978.

Geary, DC: *Children's Mathematical Development: Research and Practical Applications*, American Psychological Association, Washington, DC, 1994.

Glaser, D, and Bentovim, A: Abuse and risk to handicapped and chronically ill children, *Child Abuse Negl* 3:565-575, 1979.

Goodman, G: Summaries of research and children's lying, *Am Prosecutor's Res Institute* 2(1): January, 1988.

Goodman, GS, and Aman, CJ: Children's use of anatomically detailed dolls to recount an event, *Child Dev* 61:1859-1871, 1991.

Goodman, GS, Batterman-Faunce, JM, Quas, JA, Riddlesberger, MM, and Kuhn, J: Optimizing children's testimony: Research and social policy issues concerning allegations of child sexual abuse. In D Cicchetti and S Toth, eds: *Child Abuse, Child Development, and Social Policy*, Ablex, Norwood, NJ, 1994, pp. 139-166.

Goodman, GS, Bottoms, BL, Schwartz-Kenney, B, and Rudy, L: Children's memory for a stressful event: Improving children's reports, *J Narrative Life History* 1:69-99, 1991.

Goodman, GS, Hirschman, J, Hepps, D, and Rudy, L: Children's memory for stressful events, *Merrill-Palmer Q* 37:109-158, 1991.

Goodman, GS, Pyle-Taub, EP, Jones, DPH, England, P, Port, LK, Rudy, L, and Prado, L: The effects of criminal court testimony on child sexual assault victims, *Monographs of the Society for Research in Child Development* 57: Serial No. 229, pp. 1-163, 1992.

Gordon, BN, and Follmer, A: Developmental issues in judging the credibility of children's testimony, *J Clin Child Psychol* 23(3):283-294, 1994.

Gordon, BN, Jens, KG, Hollings, R, and Watson, TE: Developmental issues in judging the credibility of children's testimony, *J Clin Child Psychol* 23(3):239-244, 1994.

Gray, E: *Unequal Justice: The Prosecution of Child Sexual Abuse*, MacMillan, New York, 1993.

Green, A: Self destruction in physically abused schizophrenic children: Report of cases, *Arch Gen Psychiatry* 19:171-197, 1968.

Harvey, W: Preparing children for court. In D Peters, ed: *The Child Witness: Cognitive, Social and Legal Issues*, Kluwer, Deventer, 1995.

Hochstadt, NJ, Jaudes, PK, Zimo, DA, and Schachter, J: The medical and psychosocial needs of children entering foster care, *Child Abuse Negl* 11:53-62, 1987.

Illinois Child Witness Project, State's Attorneys Appellate Prosecutor: *Under 10... And in the Witness Chair*, Chicago, 1990.

Jaudes, PK, and Diamond, LD: The handicapped child and child abuse, *Child Abuse Negl* 9:341-347, 1985.

Jones, DPH, and Krugman, R: Can a three year old bear witness to her sexual assault and attempted murder? *Child Abuse Negl* 10(2):253-258, 1986.

Kelley, SJ: Ritualistic abuse of children. In J Briere, L Berliner, JA Bulkley, C Jenny, and T Reid, eds: *The APSAC Handbook on Child Maltreatment*, Thousand Oaks, CA, 1996, pp. 90-99.

Kendall-Tackett, KA, Williams, LM, and Finkelhor, D: Impact of sexual abuse on children: A review and synthesis of recent empirical studies, *Psychol Bull* 113:164-180, 1993.

Kenyon-Jump, R, Burnette, M, and Robertson, M: Comparison of behaviors of suspected sexually abused and nonsexually abused preschool children using anatomical dolls, *J Psychopath Behav Assess* 13:225-240, 1991.

Kline, DF: Educational and psychological problems of abused children, *Child Abuse Negl* 1:301-307, 1977.

Koski, MA, and Ingram, EM: Child abuse and neglect: Effects on the Bayley Scale, *J Abnormal Child Psychol* 5:79-91, 1977.

Krents, E, Schulman, V, and Brenner, S: Child abuse and the disabled child: Prospectus for parents, *Volta Rev* 89(5):78-95, 1987.

Lanning, K: Ritual abuse: A law enforcement view or perspective, *Child Abuse Negl* 15:171-173, 1991.

Law, J, and Conway, J: Effect of abuse and neglect on the development of children's speech and language, *Dev Med Child Neurol* 34:943-948, 1992.

Lazebnik, R, Zimet, GD, Ebert, J, Anglin, TM, Williams, P, Bunch, DL, and Krowchuk, DP: How children perceive the medical evaluation for suspected sexual abuse, *Child Abuse Negl* 18(9):739-745, 1994.

Leekam, SR: Believing and deceiving: Steps to becoming a good liar. In SJ Ceci, MD Leichtman, and ME Putnick, eds: *Cognitive and Social Factors in Early Deception*, Erlbaum, Hillsdale, NJ, 1992, pp. 47-62.

Leichtman, M, and Ceci, SJ: Effects of stereotypes and suggestions on preschoolers' reports, *Dev Psychol* 31:568-578, 1995.

McIlwraith, RD, and Schallow, JR: Television viewing and styles of children's fantasy, *Imagination Cognition Personality* 2(4):323-331, 1983.

Mian, M, Wehrspann, W, Klajner-Diamond, H, LeBaron, D, and Winder, C: Review of 125 children six years of age and under who were sexually abused, *Child Abuse Negl* 10:223-229, 1986.

Morency, NL, and Krauss, RM: The nonverbal encoding and decoding of affect in first and fifth graders. In RS Feldman, ed: *Development of Nonverbal Behavioral Skills,* Springer-Verlag, New York, 1982, pp. 181-199.

Neisser, U, Boodoo, G, Bouchard, TJ, Boykin, AW, Brody, N, Ceci, SJ, Halpern, DF, Loehlin, JC, Perloff, R, Sternberg, RJ, and Urbina, S: Intelligence: Knowns and unknowns, *Am Psychol* 51(2):77-101, 1996.

Nelson, K, and Hudson, J: Scripts and memory: Functional relationships in development. In F Weinert and M Perlmutter, eds: *Memory Development: Universal Changes and Individual Differences*, Lawrence Erlbaum, Hillsdale, NJ, 1988, pp. 221-242.

Neutra, R, Levy, J, and Parker, D: Cultural expectations versus reality in Navajo seizure patterns and sick roles, *Culture, Medicine Psychiatry* 1:225-275, 1977.

Newcombe, N, Drummey-Bullock, A, and Lie, E: Children's memory for early experience, *J Exp Psychol* 59:337-342, 1995.

Newcombe, N, and Fox, N: Infantile amnesia: Through a glass darkly, *Child Dev* 65:31-40, 1994.

Newman, BM, and Newman, PR: *Development Through Life: A Psychosocial Approach,* Brookes Cole Publishing Co., Pacific Grove, CA, 1995.

Ornstein, P, Baker-Ward, L, Gordon, B, and Merritt, R: Children's memory for medical procedures. In N Stein (Chair): *Children's Memory for Emotional Events.* Symposium presented at the Society for Research in Child Development Meetings, New Orleans, LA, 1993.

Perry, NW, and Wrightsman, LS: *The Child Witness: Legal Issues and Dilemmas*, Sage Publications, Newbury Park, CA, 1991.

Peterson, CC, Peterson, JL, and Seeto, D: Developmental changes in ideas in lying, *Child Dev* 54:1529-1535, 1983.

Piaget, J: *The Moral Judgment of the Child* (Translated by M Gabain), Free Press, New York, 1965.

Pillemer, DB, and White, SH: Childhood events recalled by children and adults. In HW Reese, ed: *Advances in Child Development and Behavior*, Academic Press, New York, 1989, pp. 297-340.

Pipe, ME, Gee, S, and Wilson, C: Cues, props, and context: Do they facilitate children's reports? In GS Goodman and GL Bottoms, eds: *Child Victims, Child Witnesses*, Guilford, New York, 1993, pp. 25-45.

Putnam, FW, Guroff, JJ, Silberman, EK, Barban, L, and Post, RM: The clinical phenomenology of multiple personality disorders: Review of 100 recent cases, *J Clin Psychiatry* 47(6):285-293, 1986.

Pynoos, RS, and Nadar, K: Children's memory and proximity to violence, *J Am Acad Child Adolescent Psychiatry* 28:236-241, 1989.

Quinn, KM: Children and deception. In R Rogers, ed: *Clinical Assessment of Malingering and Deception*, Guilford Press, New York, 1988.

Realmuto, G, Jensen, J, and Wescoe, S: Specificity and sensitivity of sexually anatomically correct dolls in substantiating abuse: A pilot study, *J Am Acad Child Adolescent Psychiatry* 29:743-746, 1990.

Realmuto, G, and Wescoe, S: Agreement among professionals about a child's sexual abuse status: Interviews with sexually anatomically correct dolls as indicators of abuse, *Child Abuse Negl* 16:719-725, 1992.

Saarni, C, and von Salisch, M: The socialization of emotional dissemblance, in lying and deception in everyday life. In M Lewis and C Saarni, eds: *Lies! Lies!! Lies!!!* Guilford, New York, 1993, pp. 106-125.

Sangrund, A, Gaines, RW, and Green, AH: Child abuse and mental retardation: A problem of cause and effect, *Am J Ment Defic* 79(3):327-330, 1974.

Sauzier, M: Disclosure of child sexual abuse: For better or for worse, *Treatment Victims Sexual Abuse* 12:455-469, 1989.

Saywitz, K: Children's testimony: Age-related patterns of memory errors. In Ceci, SJ, Toglia, MP, and Ross, DF, eds: *Children's Eyewitness Memory*, Springer-Verlag, New York, 1987.

Saywitz, K: Children's knowledge of legal terminology, *Law Hum Behavior* 14(6): 523-535, 1990.

Saywitz, K: Questioning child witnesses, *Violence Update* 4(7):3-10, 1994.

Saywitz, K: Improving children's testimony: The question, the answer, and the environment. In MS Zaragoza, JR Graham, GCN Hall, R Hirschman, and YS Ben-Porath, eds: *Memory and Testimony in the Child Witness*, Sage, Thousand Oaks, CA, 1995, pp. 113-140.

Saywitz, K, and Goodman, G: Interviewing children in and out of court: Current research and practice implications. In Briere, J, Berliner, L, Bulkley, J, Jenny, C, and Reid, T, eds: *The APSAC Handbook on Child Maltreatment*, Sage, Thousand Oaks, CA, 1996, pp. 297-318.

Saywitz, KJ, Goodman, GS, Nicholas, E, and Moan, SF: Children's memories of a physical examination involving genital touch: Implications for reports of child sexual abuse, *J Consult Clin Psychol* 59(5):682-691, 1991.

Saywitz, KJ, Nathanson, R, and Snyder, LS: Credibility of child witnesses: The role of communicative competence, *Topics Language Dis* 13(4):59-78, 1993.

Schilling, RF, and Schinke, SP: Maltreatment and mental retardation. In JM Bern, ed: *Perspectives and Progress in Mental Retardation*, University Park Press, Baltimore, 1984, pp. 11-22.

Shennum, WA, and Bugental, DB: The development of control over affective expression in nonverbal behavior. In RS Feldman, ed: *Development of Nonverbal Behavior in Children,* Springer-Verlag, New York, 1982, pp. 101-121.

Singer, DG, and Singer, JL: *The House of Make-Believe: Children's Play and the Developing Imagination*, State University of New York Press, Albany, NY, 1990.

Singer, JL: *Imaginative Play in Childhood: Precursor of Subjective Thought, Daydreaming, and Adult Pretending Games*, State University of New York Press, Albany, NY, 1995.

Singer, JL, Singer, DG, and Rapaczynski, W: Children's imagination as predicted by family patterns and television viewing: A longitudinal study, *Genetic Psychol Monogr* 110(1):43-69, 1984.

Singer, JL, Singer, DG, and Sherrod, LR: A factor analytical study of preschoolers' play behavior, *Acad Psychol Bull* 2(2):143-156, 1980.

Sivan, AB: Preschool child development: Implications for investigations of child abuse allegations, *Child Abuse Negl* 16(2):485-493, 1991.

Solomons, G: Child abuse and developmental disabilities, *Dev Med Child Neuro* 21:101-105, 1979.

Sorensen, T, and Snow, B: How children tell: The process of disclosure in child sexual abuse, *Child Welfare League of America* 70:3-15, 1991.

Stein, N, and Glenn, C: The role of temporal organization in story comprehension, University of Illinois, Center for Study of Reading, Urbana, IL, 1978, Tech Rep. No. 71.

Steward, M: Preliminary findings from the University of California, Davis, Child Memory Study, *APSAC Advisor* 5:11-13, 1992.

Stott, F: Children as sources of information for adults. In Illinois Child Witness Project, State's Attorneys Appellate Prosecutor: *Under 10...And in the Witness Chair*, Chicago, 1990.

Stouthamer-Loeber, M: Lying as problem behavior in children: A review, *Clin Psychol Rev* 6:267-289, 1986.

Sullivan, PM, Brookhouser, PE, and Scanlan, JM: Maltreatment of deaf and hard of hearing children. In P Hindley and N Kitson, eds: *Mental Health and Deafness.* Whurr Publications, London, 1996.

Sullivan, PM, and Knutson, JF: *The Relationship Between Child Abuse and Practice Neglect and Disabilities: Implications for Research and Practice,* National Center on Child Abuse and Neglect Clearinghouse, Washington, DC, 1994.

Summit, RC: The child sexual abuse accommodation syndrome, *Child Abuse Negl* 7:177-193, 1983.

Terr, L: Childhood traumas: An outline and overview, *Am J Psychiatry* 148:10-20, 1991.

Tobey, A, and Goodman, GS: Children's eyewitness memory: Effects of participation and forensic context, *Child Abuse Negl* 16:779-796, 1992.

Usher, A, and Neisser, U: Childhood amnesia and the beginnings of memory for four early life events, *J Exp Psychol General* 122(2):155-165, 1993.

Van der Voort, TH, and Valkenburg, PM: Television's impact on fantasy play: A review of the research, *Dev Rev* 14(1):227-251, 1994.

Warren-Leubecker, A: Commentary: Development of event memories or event reports. In J Doris, ed: *The Suggestibility of Children's Recollections,* American Psychological Association, Washington, DC, 1991, pp. 24-26.

Watson, JF: Talking about the best kept secret: Sexual abuse and children with disabilities, *Exceptional Parents* 14(6):15-20, 1985.

Wechsler, D: *Manual for the Wechsler Intelligence Scale for Children—III.* The Psychological Corporation, Harcourt-Brace-Jovanovich, Inc., New York, 1991.

Wedding, D, Horton, AM, and Webster, J: *The Neuropsychology Handbook: Behavioral and clinical perspectives,* Springer, New York, 1986.

Weltzler, SE, and Sweeney, JA: Childhood amnesia: An empirical demonstration. In DC Rudin, ed: *Autobiographical Memory,* Cambridge University Press, London, 1986, pp. 191-201.

Westcott, H: The memorandum of good practice and children with disabilities, *J Law Practice* 3:21-32, 1994.

Whitcomb, D: *When the Victim is a Child,* ed 2, National Institute of Justice: Issues and Practices, Washington, DC, 1992.

Zadnik, D: Social and medical aspects of the battered child with vision impairment, *New Outlook for Blind,* 67(6):241-250, 1973.

# ART THERAPY

COLETTE M. RICKERT, LPCC, A.T.R.-BC

Art therapy was established as a human service profession in the United States in 1969 when the American Art Therapy Association was formed. Although many attempts have been made through the years to concisely define art therapy, the intricate blending of the creative process and clinical insights needed to access, diagnose, and treat make this difficult.

Two primary philosophies have existed in the profession. One approach takes the stand that art, by its very nature, is healing and the role of the art therapist is to promote the use of art to facilitate healing. The other approach holds to the belief that doing art is a good beginning, but the role of the art therapist is to companion the client and serve as an assistant in the healing process. This latter philosophy has moved to the forefront during the past few years, and much is being done to create a more clinically compatible profession.

*The American Art Therapy Association 1996 defines art therapy as follows:*

> Art therapy is a human service profession that utilizes art media, images, the creative art process, and patient/client responses to the created products as reflections of an individual's development, abilities, personality, interests, concerns, and conflicts. Art therapy practice is based on knowledge of human development and psychological theories which are implemented in the full spectrum of models of assessment and treatment including educational, psychodynamic, cognitive, transpersonal, and other therapeutic means of reconciling emotional conflicts, fostering self-awareness, developing social skills, managing behavior, solving problems, reducing anxiety, aiding reality orientation, and increasing self-esteem.

## ◆ EDUCATIONAL REQUIREMENTS FOR ART THERAPISTS

Art therapists are required to complete a master's degree in art therapy and have between 600 and 1000 hours of supervised practicum experience. After meeting these requirements, the art therapist can apply for registration. A registered art therapist (A.T.R.) is then eligible to take a written certification examination. After successfully passing this, the therapist is qualified as a board-certified art therapist (A.T.R.-BC). This credentialing is maintained by continuing education credits.

## ◆ MEMBERSHIP

Approximately 4,750 professionals and students are currently members of the American Art Therapy Association. Bi-annual reports are published to illustrate national and international distributions of art therapists. **Figure 12-1** reflects the geographical distribution of art therapists according to the 1994-1995 Membership Survey Report.

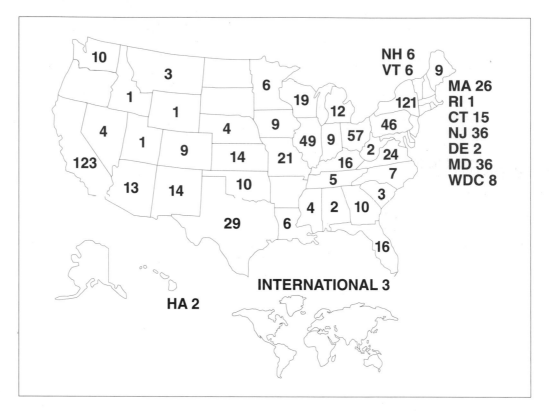

**Figure 12-1.** *American Art Therapy Association U.S. National Membership. (From Art Therapy: Journal of the American Art Therapy Association, vol 13, #2, 1996.)*

## ◆LICENSING OF ART THERAPISTS

Art therapists in each state are exploring options for licensing, while national efforts are made with other organizations and governmental agencies to find the most effective way to achieve licensing. Art therapists are affected by various efforts to change the ways health care is being made available. Governmental, insurance, and licensing issues are evolving as regulatory decisions are explored. New Mexico has had licensing for art therapists since 1993, and Kentucky has just adopted licensing standards. Texas recognizes art therapists as a separate specialty. Art therapists in other states may be eligible for licensing as a counselor based on state requirements.

## ◆HISTORY OF ART THERAPY

The field of art therapy evolved from the shared insights of professionals in three main occupations: fine and creative arts, education, and mental health. The people in these fields learned that certain individuals could be reached, could be productive, and could get better when art became a part of their activities.

Artists and writers find that the act of creating art gives them access to their innermost selves. This could be seen as either self-destructive or healing. Artists are often portrayed as people living on the edge of madness, people who cannot function in the "real world" because they are consumed by their art. Vincent Van Gogh certainly represents this stereotyped image—a man so lost in his art and pain that he had to be hospitalized and still succeeded in harming himself. Tennessee Williams, Ernest Hemingway, and many others have struggled with maintaining balance between their art and functioning in real life.

History is also full of people who have used the arts to achieve great successes and solve seemingly impossible dilemmas. Diagnosed as manic-depressive, Winston Churchill struggled with his ups and downs. First, he turned to landscaping his country estate. When he had exhausted those projects, he dreamed about a Muse who brought him brushes and paints and suggested that he might find them useful. In an article about the importance of the arts, he wrote that stress is not reduced by trying to avoid a subject, but is managed and reduced by doing something else. "Change," he said, "is the Master Key." He credited his ability to survive the turmoil and channel the passions that Hitler evoked in him to his use of the arts, painting in particular. Other artists who have certainly paved new paths for mankind by surrendering to their creative process include Pablo Picasso, Norman Rockwell, Robin Williams, and Maya Angelou.

Educators have long struggled with how to teach students effectively. Teaching techniques have mixed success rates, with some students learning no matter what, others benefitting greatly from a teacher's efforts, and some students, despite the best efforts of those around them, unwilling or unable to learn. Yet, it is often this most difficult group of students who respond best to the arts. The student who spends most of his or her time visiting the principal's office, suspended, truant, or in special educational programs for behaviorally challenging students often responds positively to classes or teachers employing or allowing art as part of his or her expression.

In the past when hospitalizations for mentally ill persons were more primitive with regard to understanding what people needed, often those charged with managing clients became frustrated. Mostly by accident and in response to the need to keep these people occupied, workers discovered that patients who drew would sometimes spontaneously stabilize and, in time, recover. Walt Whitman cared for a brother who was mentally unstable and allowed him to use art materials to draw and paint. It was his belief that this was a kinder and more productive healing technique for his brother than any others he knew. As Whitman aged, he explored options for his brother's care should Whitman die before his brother. His belief in the arts led him to an English doctor who was willing to consider the possibility that healing for the mentally ill might require treatments that allowed them to be considered as creative, spiritual beings in pain rather than creatures to be feared. Freud believed in the importance of dreams, which are nothing more than pictures created while sleeping. Jung believed that art was the key that opened the door not only to our unconscious, but also to the collective unconscious of all of mankind. Those who work with children, the ill, and those in pain know that words are not enough.

Today most art therapists see art therapy as an intricate blend of the creative process and clinical interventions. Just as walking can be beneficial and therapeutic, so too can art activities. But walking, by itself, is not therapy. When a person is injured or recovering from an illness or surgery, walking alone will not provide the cure. It may be part of the recovery process but must be under the guidance of a trained professional (doctor, nurse, physical therapist) who will companion that person to the point of recovery. Accessing, diagnosing, and treating an individual using art requires training, education, and experience in how to blend the creative process and clinical theories so that healing and resolution can occur.

At this point, art therapists function in many settings and work with many populations. Art therapy is based on creativity, and where and with whom it is used are limited only by our imaginations. With thoughtfulness and coordination of efforts and needs, it can be applied in most settings and with most populations.

*According to the American Art Therapy Association, 1996:*

> The art therapist treats a variety of populations in diverse settings, including but not limited to, the emotionally disturbed, the physically disabled, the elderly, the developmentally delayed, both inpatient and outpatient, community mental health centers, family service agencies, rehabilitation centers, medical hospitals, corrections institutions, developmental centers, educational institutions, private practice, and other facilities.

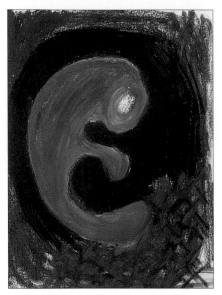

**Figure 12-2.** *This client stated, "The fires hurt the baby. She feels the fires."* *It represents a prenatal memory.*

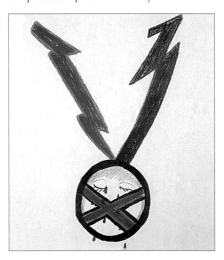

**Figure 12-3.** *This picture was drawn in response to a structured activity asking participants to make a drawing showing why art therapy has been helpful for them. The client said that the red and orange X across the mouth came from her mother's messages to "shut up" and "quit complaining." The mother is shown as the red and orange lightning bolt at the top left of the picture. The brown and black X across the mouth came from her father's message to "never speak to me unless you have something decent to say." He is represented as the black and brown lightning bolt at the top right of the picture.*

# ◆ VERBAL VERSUS NONVERBAL COMMUNICATION

Some experts estimate that 65% to 93% of our communication is done through nonverbal means. Art can tap into our nonverbal communication needs and help facilitate a deeper level of relating both with ourselves and with others.

*Georgia O'Keefe said,*

> I have just been trying to express myself — I just have to say things, you know — Words and I — are not good friends at all except with some people — when I am close to them and I can feel as well as hear their response — I have to say it some way [and so I paint].

The human mind functions much like a computer, and, like a computer, it needs programming. Whereas a computer might operate with a specially designed data entry system, the human mind is programmed with language. An individual gradually learns the language used in the environment and gains access to the mental aspect of personality. As language skills increase, verbalization increases and mental processing skills mature.

There are some basic drawbacks to relying on words to communicate experiences. First, any language has only so many words to describe the world and our experiences in it. For example, English contains about 96 words to describe feelings. What words can adequately describe the experience of a person who survives a plane crash, or the experience of a person who has been told that his child was killed in a plane crash? Second, we only have access to the words we already know. If a child goes through an experience that she does not have adequate words to describe, she will only be able to intellectually think of the event with the words she knows at that point in time. If the child is mistreated in utero or as an infant, no words are available to think about that event. This, however, does not mean that the experience is not recorded. Instead of being linguistically recorded in the mind, the computer, or the mental aspect of the child, it is recorded in the emotional, physical, and creative aspects (**Figure 12-2**). Third, abusers often threaten to further harm or kill the child or a pet or another loved one if the child ever tells what happened. In many cases, the ability to put on paper what occurred seems to bypass the inner fears and injunctions not to tell and allows maltreated children to "tell" in another, safer way. Often the pictures by these children reflect some kind of "don't tell" message or handicapping condition that makes it impossible for them to convey the information verbally (**Figure 12-3**). For example, the mouth might be missing from the picture.

It is vital to provide all children with alternative methods of expressing themselves, not only to give them options so that they can "tell," but also so that they can more fully connect with the world around them and learn balance through better integration of their mental, emotional, physical, and creative aspects.

# ◆ ASPECTS CHART

The mental, emotional, physical, and inspirational aspects of an individual help create a more complete picture of that person. When these aspects are working well together, integration is present. When they are not working well together, disintegration is seen. When people are hurt and the wound is not healed, they move through life in an off-balanced, nondirected way because they are not cohesively connected internally to themselves with respect to mind, heart, body, and spirit.

People with effective inner connections to these aspects can work in a balanced, self-directed way because they are internally cohesive—they are integrated. The Greeks called this being in "timeless time," a term that refers to the experience of being so absorbed in an activity that you forget all sense of time. Integrated individuals have an inherent joy in what is being done and a general lack of stress. The task may be difficult, but the unity within the individual allows him or her to proceed in a controlled, focused, integrated way.

When the four aspects of an individual are considered for assessment, diagnosis, and treatment, a more complete profile can be formulated regarding the actual needs and problems of that individual. Just as a teacher might provide a pretest assessment for the class or a doctor might order a diagnostic test, exploring these four aspects of an individual in visible form creates an opportunity for an art therapist and a client to better see what is actually needed—not what the individual thinks he needs based only on mental perceptions. **Figure 12-4** is a shape used to invite individuals to explore themselves from a more holistic point of view.

When individuals have been subjected to abuse, its impact will be reflected in their aspects chart. They will not be able to function in an integrated way because some aspect or aspects of themselves have been injured so that they cannot move forward in a focused, balanced, cohesive way. The aspects of themselves that they are not allowed to use are blocked off or not developed **(Figures 12-5 and 12-6).**

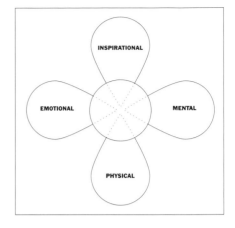

*Figure 12-4.* Aspects chart.

*Figure 12-5.* This aspects chart was created by a child, age 12, who has been subjected to emotional abuse due to isolating, rejecting, and overpressuring during visits to a noncustodial parent. Although no overt sexual activities are known, age-inappropriate bathing activities occurred and covert sexual activities have abounded within the home. Note the lack of body-specific features in the physical areas, with colors surrounding the form. Although the mental aspect appears ordered with bricks neatly in place, the window could be broken. This child often dissociates during visits and reports experiencing a see-through barrier. In her words, In the top part of my chart (creative), I drew a plant with buds on it. To me that symbolizes my creative self really growing and full. I feel that at the present time I am trying to work more with that section and make it as big as the other parts have been. In the past I think that it has been smaller than some of the other parts, but now I think it is equal. In the right part of my chart (mental) I drew a clear window, with a brick wall around it. I think that that section is very strong and also very clear. Sometimes my mental side can be "out of it" (i.e., she dissociates) but it seems to always stay clear. In the bottom part of my chart (physical) I drew an outline of a human body with many colors. I think that I am starting to show how great I am on the inside as well as the outside. In the left part of my chart (emotions) I drew a heart with half of the background green and the other half blue. The heart symbolizes that I am starting to be able to show my emotions, but yet they aren't as sad and dreary as they have been in the past. The green and blue is to symbolize how much I love the earth and how happy I feel outside and on the earth. In the center part of my chart (integration) I drew scribbles, but I used all the colors that I used in the loops and I made them flow in a nice even circle that started in the center and worked its way out. I feel that this symbolizes all of them working together and making me "even."

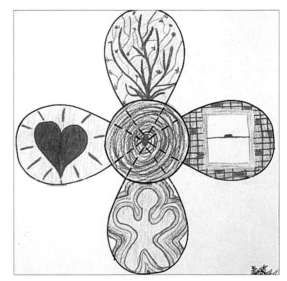

*Figure 12-6.* This aspects chart was created by a woman during a deep depression. At the time of the drawing, she was aware of growing up in a home filled with physical violence, high degrees of emotional and verbal abuse, and general neglect. She was not aware of having been sexually abused until she began having recurring nightmares approximately 2 years later that eventually led her to uncovering abuse memories. Note that the physical area at the bottom is drawn with lines that appear fluid and blood-like. All of the areas contain circles that interrupt their areas. Boundary problems pervaded her home situation. Rectal intrusions were a regular part of her upbringing and "interrupted" her personal spaces and development.

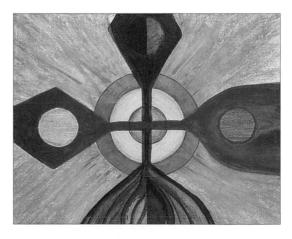

251

## ◆ STAGES OF CHILD DEVELOPMENT AND ART

Children progress through specific developmental stages as they move toward adulthood: learning to trust, becoming an individual, belonging to a group, thinking, identifying with their gender, and developing values. In the same way children must progress through developmental stages with regard to artistic expression. **Table 12-1** is a basic outline of these stages.

| Table 12-1. Developmental Stages of Children Related to Their Art | |
| --- | --- |
| *Age and Stage* | *Characteristics* |
| 2 to 4 years—Scribbling | Twenty basic scribbles (see **Figure 12-7**) form the building blocks of art. Generally disordered in approach with controlled, repeated motions, and employing naming, which marks a change from kinesthetic to imaginative thinking. Human figures are not common. |
| 4 to 7 years—Preschematic | Find relationship between drawing, thinking, & environment. Use various symbols in search of a definite concept. For human figures, use circular motion for head, longitudinal for legs and arms. |
| 7 to 9 years—Schematic | Have a definite concept of man and environment; show self-assurance through repeated forms, schemes, symbols; represent the thing itself, with experiences represented as deviances from that scheme; use geometric lines. For human figures, reproduce definite concept of figure. |
| 9 to 11 years—Drawing realism | Removed from geometric lines and from baseline expression; first conscious approach toward decoration. For human figures, attention paid to clothes, emphasizing differences between male and female; more stiffness and emphasis on details; tend to be more realistic. |
| 12 to 14 years—Pseudo-naturalistic | Drawings reflect critical awareness of own shortcomings in art, can become shorthand notations; can focus on selected parts of environment; tend not to engage in spontaneous art activity; for some, focus on details such as wrinkles or folds; project nonliteral, personal meaning onto objects and events. For human figures, closer to correct proportions with greater awareness of joints and body actions; facial expressions vary; cartooning; person can be represented by less than complete figure; sexual characteristics overemphasized. |
| 14 to 17 years—Adolescent | Without further instruction, drawings tend to resemble those done at age 12; conscious development of artistic abilities; subjective interpretation to drawings; visually minded may derive pleasure from details such as light and shade; longer attention span with mastery of all art materials; control over purposeful expression. For human figures, some attempt at naturalistic depiction, with awareness of proportion, action, and detail; exaggeration of detail for emphasis; imaginative use of figure for satire. |
| *(Based on Lowenfeld and Brittain, 1987, Plate 26, pp. 474-479.)* | |

| Scribble 1 | , ⌐ | Dot | Scribble 2 | │ | Single vertical line |
|---|---|---|---|---|---|
| Scribble 3 | — | Single horizontal line | Scribble 4 | ╲ ╱ | Single diagonal line |
| Scribble 5 | ⌒ | Single curved line | Scribble 6 | ⋀⋀⋀⋀ | Multiple vertical line |
| Scribble 7 | ≊ | Multiple horizontal line | Scribble 8 | ⫽ ⫽ | Multiple diagonal line |
| Scribble 9 | ⌒ | Multiple curved line | Scribble 10 | ∿ | Roving open line |
| Scribble 11 | ⌁ | Roving enclosing line | Scribble 12 | ∿∿∿ | Zigzag or waving line |
| Scribble 13 | ℓ | Single loop line | Scribble 14 | ℓℓℓ | Multiple loop line |
| Scribble 15 | ◎ | Spiral line | Scribble 16 | ⬤ | Multiple-line overlaid circle |
| Scribble 17 | ⬭ | Multiple-line circumference circle | Scribble 18 | ⬭⬭⬭ | Circular line spread out |
| Scribble 19 | ⬭ | Single crossed circle | Scribble 20 | ◯ | Imperfect circle |

**Figure 12-7.** *The basic scribbles. (From Kellogg, R: Analyzing Children's Art, Mayfield Publishing Co., Palo Alto, CA, 1970. Copyright© 1969, 1970 by Rhoda Kellogg. Reprinted by permission of the publisher.)*

Maltreatment affects creative development as well as other aspects of the child's well-being, making it difficult to move through the stages correctly. Often children become stuck at the stage where the abuse predominantly occurred, or they regress consistently to that age when they try to make representational art. Creative development for the well-treated child flows from stage to stage, always moving toward a more complete and mature expression of the self (**Figure 12-8**). Because art accesses their nonverbal communication areas, when victims of maltreatment try to create, they create from what they see, who they are, and where they have been, which is founded on a baseline of injury rather than good health. Children who are not mistreated and can explore their mental, emotional, physical, and inspirational aspects without fear learn to integrate themselves internally and then integrate with their external world. Children who have to disintegrate themselves to survive cannot explore integration because they must use their energy to brace, dissociate, protect, and defend themselves. These efforts to survive are reflected in their art.

♦ **ART MATERIALS**

Caretakers of children and professionals who interact with children, although not art therapists, can have available various art materials so that a child can easily access them. It is natural for children to want to explore and play with art materials, and this helps to create an environment that allows them to express themselves, even when words may not be known or permitted. Art activities not only foster integration of the individual, but also allow children to express the many complicated experiences they go through on their way to adulthood.

Each person develops his or her own way of thinking, speaking, walking, and dressing, and these individual characteristics eventually come to be the way we know that person. The same is true of a child's creative expressions. When permitted, each child will develop a nonverbal symbolic system of expression. His or her dreams, feelings, thoughts, and experiences will be expressed in his or her own personal style. Over time, caretakers and professionals can learn to understand and communicate

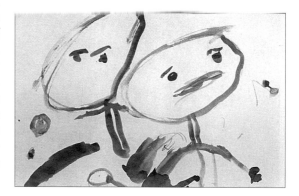

**Figure 12-8a.** *"Mommy and Daddy" painted by a 4-year-old child who had just left the scribbling stage.*

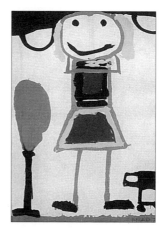

**Figure 12-8b.** *"I am Standing in My Back Yard," painted by a 6 1/2-year-old girl. Note the developing signs of the child's awareness of the relationship between objects and color. She has painted herself as much larger than the tree, showing the egocentrism at this stage of development.*

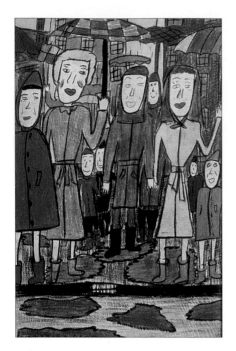

*Figure 12-8c.* *"Standing in the Rain," drawn by an 11-year-old girl. Color, use of space, and wealth of detail combine to give an aesthetically pleasing whole. The artist's growing visual awareness is coupled with her directness and freshness. (From Lowenfeld, V, and Brittain, WL: Creative and Mental Growth, ed. 7, Macmillan Publishing Co., Inc., New York, 1982.)*

with a child on his or her creative level in much the same way that we learn to communicate with a child verbally. If children do not feel "spied on" or criticized, they continue to express themselves in their academic, personal, and creative efforts. Caretakers who observe the drawings and creations with sensitivity to the child's feelings will find a way of "hearing" what the child is saying. If a problem exists or is developing, the caretaker who has learned to listen to the child's creative voice will hear and see what is happening. If they expect children to communicate with them at this very deep and personal level, it is crucial that caretakers and professionals resist the urge to define themselves as responsible by exerting control over children. It is much more effective to focus on providing a safe, structured, and protective environment within which children can grow and evolve their own ability to control themselves. The freedom to explore oneself is too often a luxury not afforded to children. Instead they are forced to use their creative energies to construct defenses against forces that are bigger and stronger than them physically, psychologically, mentally, and emotionally. This kind of environment does not allow for creative and honest exploration or development.

**Table 12-2** lists various art materials that can be made readily available for children to use. It is important to provide materials appropriate for children's ages, interests, and ability levels.

| Table 12-2. Art Materials | |
| --- | --- |
| Paper—all shapes, sizes, types | Traditional 8½ × 11 or 11 × 14 sheets |
| Old wallpaper books | Used wrapping paper |
| Tissue from inside shoe boxes | "Stuff"—anything that is interesting to touch or see |
| Pencils | Clay |
| Shoulder pads | Pens |
| Popsicle sticks | Construction paper |
| Colored pencils | Small tree branches |
| Flour and water | Crayons |
| Pipe cleaners | Food coloring |
| Cray Pas | Stickers |
| Pastels | Beans |
| Markers | Beads |
| Oil crayons | Nuts and bolts |
| Plastic crayons | Tape of all sizes and shapes |
| Water pencils | Old holiday cards |
| Water crayons | Magazines and catalogs |
| Water colors | Paper towel or toilet paper rolls |
| Tempera paints | Styrofoam boards (from food packages) |
| Finger paints | Rubberbands |
| Brushes | Scissors |
| Newspapers | Buttons |
| Boxes | Glues of all colors and styles |
| Fabrics | Thread and yarn |
| Plasticine | Scrap fabrics |

| Table 12-3. Trends and Indicators Related to Abuse Found in Children's Art |
|---|

This list is based on Dr. Spring's conclusions after studying 8,000 drawings and completing her empirical research in 1988.

- Contain noticeable use of disembodied eyes (adults) and wedges (adults and children)

- Display extremes in both color and content; may be more intense, may be avoided

- Exhibit an overall fragmented, separated, and confused quality showing degrees of incongruity

- Lean more toward abstraction than realism or representation (adults); fantasy and stories (children)

- Expose more angular properties in the compositions, but also include many circles that are not eye shaped

- Style tends to be inconsistent, fluctuating from passive to aggressive use of materials and forms

- Express intense feelings that focus on rage and sadness, depression and confusion, helplessness and inescapability, threat and fear, as well as lack of control

- Show an absence of the future and an enjoyment of life, as well as an inability to solve problems

- Reveal a confusion about life, suicidal ideation, detachment, and an inability to concentrate or understand their emotional state, which is expressed verbally as an inadequacy in attempting to solve problems

- Have an explosive and/or scattered quality

- Reveal fragmented bodies, disembodied eyes and genitalia, stick figures, and other forms that suggest regression to an earlier developmental stage

- Victims tend to direct their drawings toward the past and feelings about their traumatic experiences whether remembered or not; children focus on uncomfortable relationships

- Victims consistently use red or black or combined red and black in the same drawing in varying degrees and patterns. They use yellowish green colors less than nonvictims but use yellow at about the same frequency

*Repetitive symbolic forms chosen by victims include the following:*

1. Circles: circular pattern of crisis cycle, depression, obsessive thinking, circular behavior, "can't break the chain," and addictions

2. Chains: trapped, helpless, chained to abuse (adults)

3. Chains with penises or female genitalia: chained to sexuality, sex, and sexual abuse (adults)

4. Floating or detached objects: dissociation

5. Yellow sun with wedge rays: "it is threatening to hope"; hope disguised with magical thinking

6. Encapsulation and compartmentalization: withdrawal, isolation, protection, and addictions

7. Concentric circles: depression and suicidal ideation

8. Ears, no mouth: heard, cannot tell

9. Closed eyes: "don't see," "don't tell"

*(Spring, 1993, pp.54,55.)*

## ♦ SYMBOLIC INDICATORS OF POTENTIAL ABUSE

Although every individual has a personal style of creative expression, no matter how primitive or practiced they may be, certain symbols seem to reappear in the creations of individuals who have been maltreated. However, even if a person's artwork does incorporate these symbols repeatedly, it does not necessarily mean that the person has been abused.

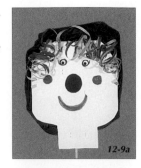

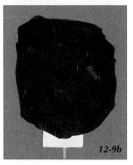

***Figure 12-9a,b.*** *Front and back of mask on a stick. This mask is of a brother the client considered "two-faced."*

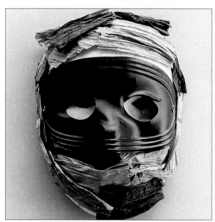

***Figure 12-10.*** *Mask of brother who never spoke to the client.*

Symbolic communication is subjective. It is vital that caretakers and professionals remember that indicators of abuse are exactly that—indicators. Abuse cannot be determined on the basis of one picture, not even many pictures. Symbolic language must be looked at in the context of the individual's overall life, circumstances, and intent.

Dr. Spring's research with known adult survivors of abuse found that the trends and symbols obtained in **Table 12-3** occur more frequently than in the artwork of people not identified as victims of abuse. I also see these in the artwork of adults abused as children. Many of these indicators also appear in the artwork of abused children. The understanding of symbolic communication is not intended to intrude on people and their art. Art therapists are trained to evaluate art and yet must continually receive both supervision and education to maintain their objectivity in regard to their clients' artwork. It is with somber and serious warnings to view children's artwork as a whole and as an expression of their entire self that these possible indicators are presented.

## ♦ THE ROLE OF ART THERAPISTS IN THE LEGAL SYSTEM

The art therapy profession is playing a greater role in the assessment, diagnosis, and treatment of child abuse. With this expanded role, art therapists are now being called into court cases to provide expert testimony. Because of the demands placed on witnesses and the role of art in this process, careful study and in-depth preparation are required. Publications are available for review before testifying.

## ♦ SUMMARY

Art therapy is a human service profession that focuses on the process involved in healing. Each time a person creates a work of art, he or she moves a piece of himself or herself outside for the world to see. The individual is looking at the inner self and seeing a reflection of their true self in the artwork. Art therapy can benefit almost anyone if the person is willing to more fully express inner feelings and thoughts.

An art therapist can and should be consulted when a child's or an adult's drawings consistently and significantly deviate from developmental norms. Issues that may be resistant to traditional therapy or those that are too difficult to talk about can be quite responsive to art therapy. Art therapy bypasses the criticism of technique and focuses on helping the client move toward integration by helping him or her express how they experience themselves, others, and events in a more complete way.

The rest of this chapter will present case studies showing how, through art therapy, abused individuals were able to communicate about their abuse. These studies also illustrate the thoughts and feelings of persons who have experienced abuse or neglect.

### CASE STUDY 1

This client attended group therapy sessions for a number of years and spoke very rarely in the group. When asked specifically if she preferred to discontinue therapy or be moved to another group, she stated that she wanted to stay. Eventually an art activity was suggested that she responded to with noticeable interest. When asked to make an object that would represent her siblings, she created these masks (**Figures 12-9 and 12-10**). Her therapeutic journey became more fluid after these masks were done. She was raised in a family where children were never to speak unless spoken to first by an adult. She was supposed to sit still and not move whenever she was at home, and if she did express herself or move, her brothers verbally assaulted her. She was isolated from other children and rejected and ignored by other members of her family. She cannot recall if she was physically or sexually assaulted.

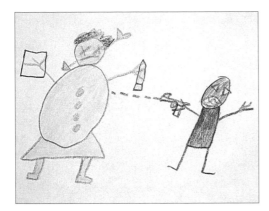

**Figure 12-11.** *The client drew what he wishes he could do—kill his teacher.*

## CASE STUDY 2

This child was first brought to therapy because of behavioral problems at school. He appeared to have attention-deficit hyperactivity disorder with moderate indications of a learning disability in the area of reading comprehension. After initial resistance to coming to therapy, when he said "There's nothing wrong with me. It's everybody else!" he became comfortable in the therapy setting and began doing art activities that were a blend of topics suggested by the therapist for assessment and diagnostic purposes (for example, **Figure 12-11**) and spontaneous drawings he created based on the things that seemed to be worrying him at that time. During the process of treatment, a prior sexual assault was depicted (**Figure 12-12**). The mother had known about it and proper authorities had been involved, so everyone thought that the experience had been resolved and the child was simply a "behavior problem" at school. During treatment he received medication for depression and difficulty paying attention at school. After therapy, moving to a new house in a different neighborhood, and beginning a different school, he was no longer considered a behavior problem. He adjusted well (**Figure 12-13**), and medications were reduced significantly.

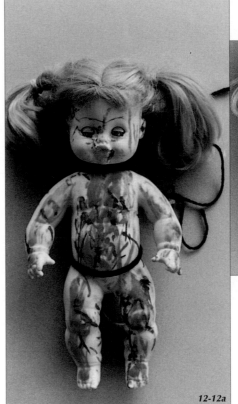

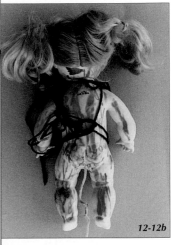

**Figure 12-12a,b.** *Spontaneous creation of an abused child wherein he replicated the rectal sexual abuse that he had experienced. The experience was confirmed by his mother. At the time of the abuse, counseling had been sought and all of the proper steps had been taken so that the issue seemed resolved.*

12-12a  12-12b

## CASE STUDY 3

This young adult male murdered his father. Therapeutically this case is of note because his artwork had been saved by his mother from the time he was very young, so that samples exist from most of the stages of his life. Legally it is of interest because it explores the impact of sexual abuse, post-traumatic stress disorder, and dissociative states in relation to a crime where the client admitted killing his father and was able to verbally address, during the trial, his experience as a child and a man.

The art was first reviewed without the therapist being aware of the criminal case, the events connected with the case, or the person's prior history. Yet the art is filled with commonly seen indicators of possible abuse. The symbolic language the client developed and expressed in art shows probable sexual abuse by sodomy. The abuser seems to be male and the creator of the art seemed to have nonspecific tensions with a female, probably his mother. Indicators of possible abuse that exist throughout his artwork include the following:

- Partial rather than whole figures (**Figure 12-14a**)

- Phallic symbols exaggerated beyond common levels of developmental sexual concerns (**Figure 12-14b**)

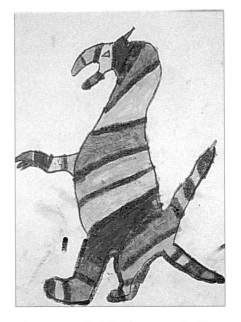

**Figure 12-13.** *Final drawing presented to his therapist as a going-away present, indicating that he was done with counseling. He stated that the therapist "no longer needed to know his private business" and that he did not need to come to therapy any more. This final picture shows a full-figured and colorful character, depicting the client when he chose to leave therapy—having set boundaries, full-figured, and richly colored.*

257

- Secret or "hidden" pictures (many were drawn on the back of another picture) **(Figure 12-14c)**

- Indicators of disintegration **(Figure 12-14d,e)**

**Figure 12-14a.** Indications of abuse. Partial figures rather than whole.

**Figure 12-14b.** Phallic depiction of house.

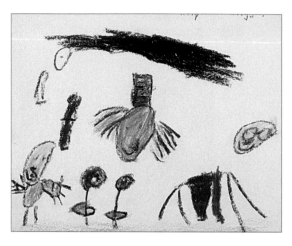

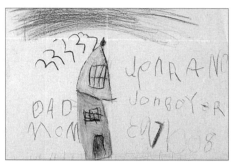

**Figure 12-14d.** Here the client is showing himself as the dog between a man with a blue shirt and a huge pair of red pants; there is a spider coming up from the ground that is also threatening him.

**Figure 12-14c.** "Hidden" pictures—one drawn on the back of another.

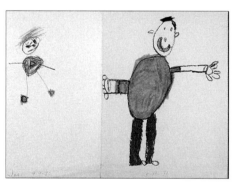

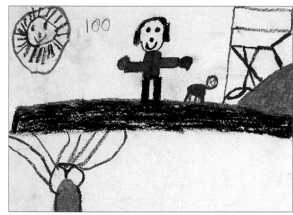

**Figure 12-14e.** This picture is an example of disintegration. The client is "telling" his story at a young age. The abuse by sodomy and enemas done by his father with a turkey baster are depicted here as a dark man with a phallically projected gun, wedged lamps, a space ship that he wants to take him away, and a turkey hovering over him.

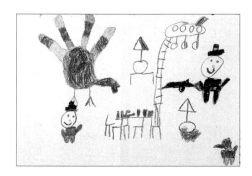

**Figure 12-15a.** *Drawing to show something the client's father would like. Note the anal shape of the buckeye.*

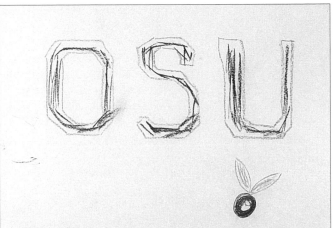

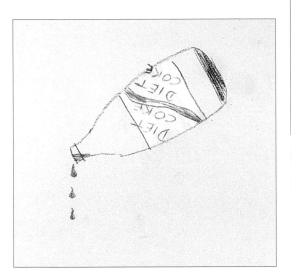

**Figure 12-15b.** *Drawing to show something the client's mother would not like—blood dripping out of a Coke bottle.*

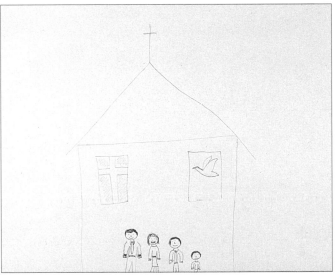

**Figure 12-15c.** *Drawing of what everyone saw when they looked at this family—proper, church-going people.*

**Figure 12-15d.** *Drawing of what went on when his mother was gone. His mother is outside the house, ready to return. His father is downstairs playing with his brother and the client (as a child) is hiding up in his closet.*

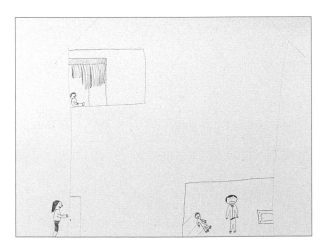

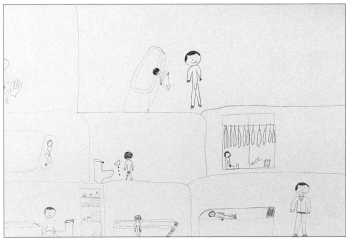

**Figure 12-15e.** *After the client had killed his father, this picture was drawn in response to the art therapist's request to describe what happened to him while he was growing up. He drew and described these scenes. He told of being sodomized, hiding near his mother's bed to be safe, hiding in the closet to be safe, bleeding from rectal intrusions, fearing his father, and keeping silent, never telling about these events.*

As the client went from drawing to drawing, he verbally and nonverbally depicted the abuse he had experienced. When the assessment was complete, it became apparent that the client had "told" his story at a much earlier time in his life. The sodomy and the enemas administered by his father using a turkey baster can be seen in a number of the pictures. Of particular interest is the similarity of the art in **Figure 12-16, a and b,** which were done many years apart. The positioning of the shovel in his father's hand is paralleled, and these pictures essentially tell the same story.

**Figure 12-16a,b.** *Parallel pictures drawn many years apart.*

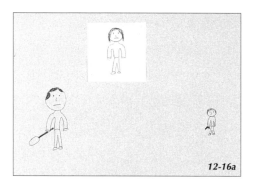

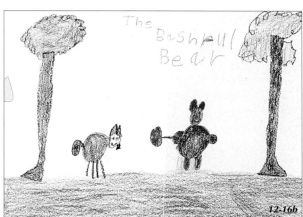

**Figure 12-17a.** *Hopeful aspects are seen in these two pictures. The client is small and everyone is basically drawn the same.*

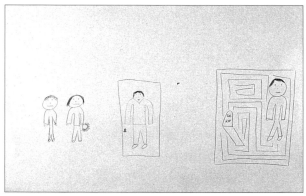

**Figure 12-17b.** *He draws himself as still encapsulated, but bigger. Dad (in the maze) is not as rigid and not as large. Mom and her husband are matched in color and are shown as different from the others.*

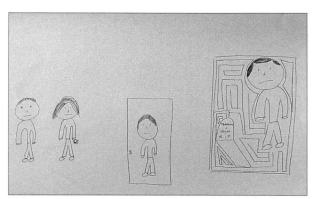

## CASE STUDY 4

This client grew up in a house with a violent and sexually abusive mother. Many times during therapy, she was completely unable to speak, aware that she was unable to speak, and frustrated with this condition. A person of extremely high intelligence, she was deeply distressed with her inability to understand why she drew seemingly inexplicable pictures of violence, enemas, sexual trauma, and cruelty **(Figures 12-18 to 12-23).**

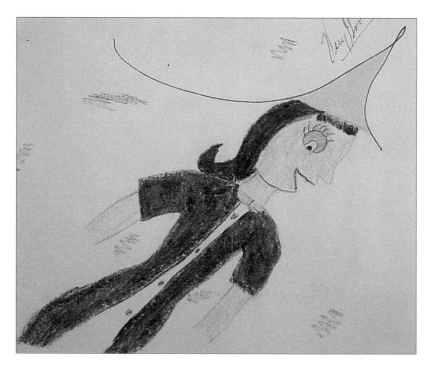

***Figure 12-18.*** *Picture created during elementary school years.*

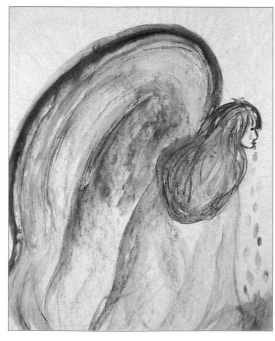

***Figure 12-19.*** *After continued and repeated physical and sexual abuse, the client became aware of the presence of an angel who would watch over her. This painting reflects the client's sense of the angel weeping about what this woman was experiencing as a child. It was done 4 years before the client had any conscious memories of having been sexually assaulted.*

**Figure 12-20a.** *The drawings in a and b depict a lack of boundaries or protective images; transparencies; X's; and distorted or missing body parts. They were done 5 years apart and reflect abuse memories the client is still trying to sort out. Shows the client at the age of 5 years.*

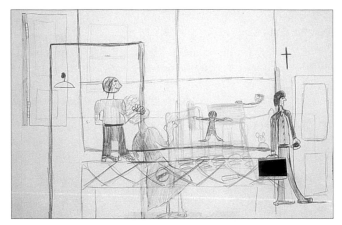

**Figure 12-20b.** *Shows the client at about the age of 1 year.*

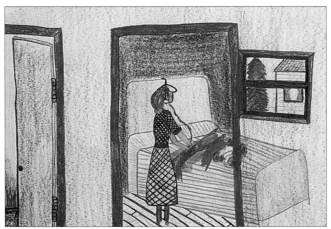

**Figure 12-21a-c.** *These three drawings reflect the client's relationship with her mother and the abusive behaviors she experienced that led to her eventual dissociation at the age of 4 years. The client saw herself as having an evil companion who would deal with the mother while the client went to sleep crying.*

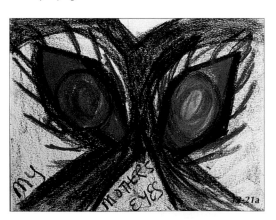

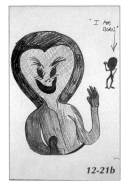

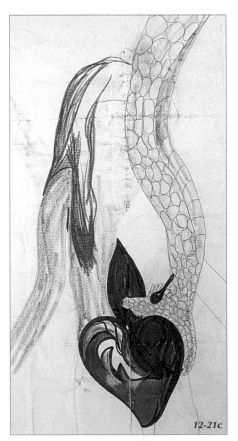

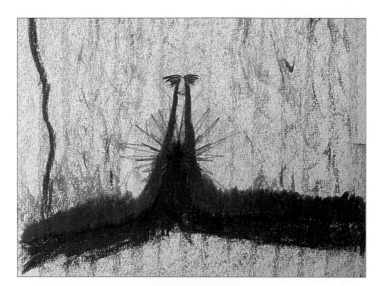

***Figure 12-22.*** *Shows client feeling sad and locked in behind a glass wall as a child.*

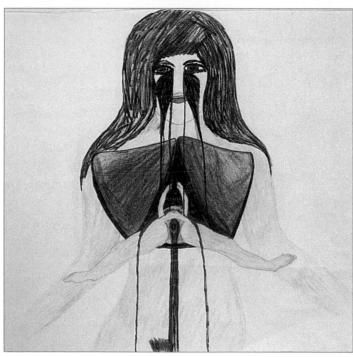

***Figure 12-23.*** *This drawing is an integration and awareness picture. It was done during a time when the client was first aware that she had been sexually assaulted both vaginally and rectally by her mother. She depicts her "child self" being taken into her own heart to love and protect. Although the tears of the woman flow down on the "child self," the client expressed an awareness that these were cleansing tears and that, in time, she was certain that the wounds would be washed clean.*

## ◆ BIBLIOGRAPHY

Adamson, E (in association with Timlin, J): *Art as Healing*, Nicholas-Hays, Inc., York Beach, ME, 1984.

American Art Therapy Association: *Art Therapist: Model Job Description*, American Art Therapy Association, Mundelein, IL, 1987.

American Art Therapy Association: *Education Standards for Programs Providing Art Therapy Education*, effective April 30, 1994, American Art Therapy Association, Inc., Mundelein, IL, March 1996.

American Art Therapy Association: *Information and Membership*, American Art Therapy Association, Inc., Mundelein, IL, April, 1996.

Anderson, FE: *Art for All the Children: A Creative Sourcebook for the Impaired Child*, Charles C Thomas, Publisher, Springfield, IL, 1978.

Andrews, LV: *Crystal Woman: The Sisters of the Dreamtimes*, Warner Books, Inc., New York, 1987.

Andrews, LV: *Flight of the Seventh Moon: The Teaching of the Shields*, Harper & Row, Publishers, New York, 1985a.

Andrews, LV: *Jaguar Woman and The Wisdom of the Butterfly Tree*, Harper & Row, Publishers, San Francisco, 1985b.

Andrews, LV: *Medicine Woman*, Harper Paperbacks, New York, 1991.

Andrews, LV: *Shakkai: Woman of the Sacred Garden*, HarperCollins Publishers, New York, 1992.

Andrews, LV: *Star Woman: We Are Made From Stars and to the Stars We Must Return* (illustrations by David Tamura), Warner Books, Inc., New York, 1986.

Andrews, LV: *Teachings Around the Sacred Wheel: Finding the Soul of the Dreamtime*, Harper San Francisco, San Francisco, 1990a.

Andrews, LV: *Windhorse Woman: A Marriage of Spirit*, Warner Books, Inc., New York, 1990b.

Andrews, LV: *The Woman of Wyrrd: The Arousal of the Inner Fire*, HarperCollins Publishers, New York, 1990c.

Arnheim, R: *Art and Visual Perception: A Psychology of the Creative Eye* (the new version), University of California Press, Berkeley, CA, 1974.

Art Therapy Credentials Board: *Certification Examination in Art Therapy: Bulletin of Information*, Art Therapy Credentials Board, Inc., Mundelein, IL.

Babin, A: Safer substitutes in art (appendix), *Art Therapy* 11(4):274, 1994.

*Beautiful dreamers*, videotape, copyrighted 1990, released 1992, Hemdale Pictures Corporation, Los Angeles, CA.

Chamberlain, DB: *Consciousness at Birth: A Review of the Empirical Evidence*, Chamberlain Communications, San Diego, 1983.

Cohen-Liebman, MS: The art therapist as expert witness in child sexual abuse litigation, *Art Therapy* 11(4):260-265, 1994.

Dalley, T, ed: *Art as Therapy: An Introduction to the Use of Art as a Therapeutic Technique*, Tavistock Publications, London, 1984.

Drachnik, C: The tongue as a graphic symbol of sexual abuse, *Art Therapy* 11(1):58-61, 1994.

Emerson, W: *Infant and Child Birth Re-facilitation*, Human Potential Resources, California and Institute for Holistic Education, Surrey, England, 1984.

Feder, E, and Feder, B: *The Expressive Arts Therapies: Art, Music and Dance as Psychotherapy*, Prentice-Hall, Inc., Englewood Cliffs, NJ, 1981.

Field, J: *On Not Being Able to Paint*, J.P. Tarcher, Inc., Los Angeles, 1957.

Freud, S: In Strachey, J, ed: *New Introductory Lectures on Psychoanalysis, Part II: Dreams*, vol. XV, Hogarth Press, London, 1963.

Furth, GM: *The Secret World of Drawings: Healing Through Art*, Sigo Press, Boston, 1988.

Gardner, H: *Artful Scribbles: The Significance of Children's Drawings*, Basic Books, Inc., Publishers, New York, 1980.

Good, D, and Sly-Linton, K: Art therapy licensure update, *Art Therapy* 12(2):100, 1995.

Good, DA: 1993 Distinguished Service Award, *Art Therapy* 11(1):12, 1994.

Gussak, D: Governmental Affairs Committee chairperson: Personal communication, July 15, 1996.

Hagood, MM: Diagnosis or dilemma: Drawings of sexually abused children, *Art Therapy* 11(1):37-42, 1994.

Jung, CG, and von Franz, M-L, Henderson, JL, Jacobi, J, Jaffe, A: *Man and His Symbols*, Doubleday & Co., Inc., Garden City, NJ, 1983.

Junge, MB: The formation of the American Art Therapy Association, special 25th anniversary section, *Art Therapy* 11(3):175-179, 1994.

Kaufman, B, and Wohl, A: *Casualties of Childhood: A Developmental Perspective on Sexual Abuse Using Projective Drawings*, Brunner/Mazel, Publishers, New York, 1992.

Kellogg, R: *Analyzing Children's Art*, Mayfield Publishing Co., Palo Alto, CA, 1970.

Kellogg, R: *Children's Drawings/Children's Minds*, Avon, New York, 1979.

Klaus, MH, and Klaus, PH: *The Amazing Newborn*, Addison-Wesley Publishing Co., Inc., Reading, MA, 1985.

Klepsch, M, and Logie, L: *Children Draw and Tell: An Introduction to the Projective Uses of Children's Human Figure Drawings*, Brunner/Mazel, Publishers, New York, 1982.

Kramer, E: *Art as Therapy with Children*, Schocken Books, New York, 1971.

Landgarten, HB: *Clinical Art Therapy: A Comprehensive Guide*, Brunner/Mazel, Publishers, New York, 1981.

Levick, MF: *They Could Not Talk and So They Drew: Children's Styles of Coping and Thinking*, Charles C Thomas, Publisher, Springfield, IL, 1983.

Levick, MF, Safran, DS, and Levine, AJ: Art therapists as expert witnesses: A judge delivers a precedent-setting decision, *The Arts in Psychotherapy* 17:49-53, 1990.

Liebman, M, ed: *Art Therapy with Offenders*, Jessica Kingsley Publishers, London, 1994.

Lisle, L: *Portrait of an Artist: A Biography of Georgia O'Keeffe*, University of New Mexico, Albuquerque, NM, 1986.

Lowenfeld, V, and Brittain, WL: *Creative and Mental Growth*, ed 7, Macmillan Publishing Co., Inc., New York, 1987.

Malchiodi, C: *Breaking the Silence: Art Therapy with Children from Violent Homes*, Brunner/Mazel, Publishers, New York, 1990.

Neumann, E: *Art and the Creative Unconscious: Four Essays* (translated from the German by Ralph Manheim), Bollinger Series LXI, Princeton University Press, Princeton, NJ, 1974.

Orleman, J: Looking in—looking out: An artist's journey through childhood sexual abuse, *Art Therapy* 11(1):62, 1994.

Painting as a pastime, Churchill Reader, Whittlelsey House, 1950; quoted in Jacoby, S: *Asylum, Connoisseur*, pp. 176-180, November, 1987.

Pearson, SL, Walker, KK, Martinek-Smith, M, Knapp, NM, Weaver, KA: American Art Therapy Association, Inc.: The Results of the 1994-1995 Membership Survey, *Art Therapy* 13(2):121-125, 1996.

Prinzhorn, H: *Artistry of the Mentally Ill* (translated by Eric von Brockdorff from the second German edition), Springer-Verlag New York, Inc., New York, 1972.

Rankin, A: Tree drawings and trauma indicators: A comparison of past research with current findings from the Diagnostic Drawing Series, *Art Therapy* 11(2):127-130, 1994.

Rubin, JA: *Child Art Therapy: Understanding and Helping Children Grow Through Art*, Van Nostrand Reinhold Co., New York, 1978.

Spring, D: *Shattered Images: Phenomenological Language of Sexual Trauma*, Magnolia Street Publishers, Chicago, 1993.

Stewart, J, and D'Angelo, G: *Together: Communicating Interpersonally*, Addison-Wesley Publishing Co., Reading, MA, 1980.

Storm, H: *Seven Arrows*, Ballantine Books, New York, 1973.

Terr, L: *Too Scared to Cry: Psychic Trauma in Childhood*, Basic Books, New York, 1990.

Towne, T, Edelstein, L, Brancheau, D, Anand, SA, Council, T, Leonard, A, Lombardo, D: Governmental affairs, *AATA Newsletter* 28(4), 1995.

Uhlin, DM: *Art for Exceptional Children*, ed 2, Wm. C. Brown Publishers, Dubuque, IA, 1982.

Ulman, E, Kramer, E, Kwiatkowska, HY: *Art Therapy in the United States*, Craftsbury Common, VT, 1978.

Vernon, PE, ed: *Creativity: Selected Readings*, Penguin Education, Harmondsworth, Middlesex, England, 1973.

Verny, TR, ed: *Pre- and Perinatal Psychology: An Introduction*, Human Sciences Press, Inc., New York, 1987.

Wadeson, H: *Art Psychotherapy*, Wiley Series on Personality Processes, a Wiley-Interscience Publication, John Wiley & Sons, New York, 1980.

Waller, CS: Art therapy with adult female incest survivors, *Art Therapy* 9(3):135-138, 1992.

Wirtz, G: Essential legal issues for art therapists in private practice, *Art Therapy* 11(4):293, 1994.

Wohl, A, and Kaufman, B: *Silent Screams and Hidden Cries: An Interpretation of Artwork by Children from Violent Homes*, Brunner/Mazel, Publishers, New York, 1985.

# MULTIPLE PERSONALITY DISORDER

BARBARA Y. WHITMAN, PH.D.
PASQUALE J. ACCARDO, M.D.

Sheryl, a 12-year-old seventh grader, was referred to a multidisciplinary clinic for evaluation of continuing learning problems that had become more problematic after she entered a departmentalized learning situation with multiple teachers. She was noted to be behind in reading, had severe spelling and other sequential processing difficulties, and displayed attentional and reading comprehension problems. She was described as chronically withdrawn, asocial, and moody, and her parents would frequently find her sitting in the family room and staring for hours, particularly when upset. It was also reported that she exhibited occasional flashes of rage. However, it was noted that she seemed to display episodes of brilliance and talent. She occasionally wrote sophisticated and spellbinding poetry and sometimes produced astonishingly talented artwork. She could not explain what enabled her to perform so brilliantly or prevented her from regularly producing work of this caliber.

Although socially withdrawn and inept most of the time, it appeared that if Sheryl wanted to reach a goal she would single-mindedly pursue it. For example, she managed to get herself elected class president, and she succeeded at track and field events. She was described by both of her physician parents as a misfit in the family, unable to relate to or get along with her three highly successful siblings. After extensive psychoeducational and psychological testing, she was diagnosed as having a neurologically based specific learning disability, a dysthymic disorder, and an overanxious disorder of childhood. Appropriate therapies were recommended.

Sheryl made an emergency return to the clinic when she was a senior in high school.

She was talking of suicide, and her parents wanted additional evaluation. During this emergency visit, it was reported that psychotherapy had never been pursued because her parents felt her behavioral problems were related to stubbornness; they did not believe a child could be "depressed." This episode of suicidal ideation was actually her second. Her first episode had occurred 2 years previously, and Sheryl had been referred to her pastor for counseling. This second episode concluded with an immediate referral to a psychiatrist for medication and therapy.

The following September Sheryl enrolled as a freshman at a local private college. Within 6 weeks she was exhibiting major vegetative symptoms, so noticeable that college personnel contacted Sheryl's therapist. She was hospitalized for 4 weeks. After the first week she was allowed to leave the hospital during the day to attend classes. After being admitted to the hospital there was an instant stabilization of mood, occurring within 48 hours. During hospitalization it was noted that she had a shallow level of understanding of the need to explore how she got there, how to cope when leaving, and a generally oppositional demeanor toward any subject other than how she could "get out of here." After discharge she exhibited no engagement or effort during her weekly therapy sessions, a marked alteration in her demeanor. Before she left college for winter break, she reported being afraid to go home because "she didn't want the voices to start again."

After she returned from the school break, the subject of voices was vigorously pursued during therapy. Simultaneously, reports from a consulting psychiatrist noted that she was presenting an "entirely different" young

lady to him than was reported as being presented to the primary therapist. Confrontation of these discrepancies with Sheryl ultimately led to discussions of incidents such as memory loss, articles appearing that she didn't remember buying, and people telling her she had a good time at a movie she didn't remember attending. Ultimately the therapist invited the source of the "voices" to emerge. To date, 33 personalities have been identified. Etiology appears to have been chronic and sadistic sexual abuse from age 3 to age 10 by her maternal grandfather. Both Sheryl and her family indicated that "she was his special grandchild" and they further emphatically reported that "she was devastated when he died." She has, as yet, not divulged the facts of the abuse to her family.

Sheryl typifies the difficulty of diagnosing multiple personality disorder (MPD) in children. For her, there was never any indication or even an index of suspicion of any sort of abuse, which is the major etiologic factor for this disorder. Her "host" personality is indeed "learning disabled," although several of her other personalities are artisans. She was so scared of the "voices" that she never divulged their presence until moving to her college dorm. This move so greatly altered her external environment that she was unable to continue to function and hospitalization was required. Even with this episode, it was not until she was going home for a month and would be unable to see her therapist that she "let it slip" that she heard voices. Her age of presentation of this symptom, combined with her history, was compatible with a schizophrenic process. However, enough contradictory data were present that shortly thereafter, the MPD diagnosis was confirmed.

## ◆ DEFINITION

Multiple personality disorder (MPD) can be a devastating and refractory psychiatric disorder, the origins of which lie in the pre-latency period of childhood (Braun & Sachs, 1985; Frischholz, 1985; Kluft, 1985a; Putnam et al., 1986; Baldwin, 1990; Hornstein & Tyson, 1991). Since more than 90% of all cases are directly attributable to severe abuse in early childhood (Greaves, 1980; Boor, 1982; Braun & Sachs, 1985), current theories interpret MPD as one form of childhood post-traumatic stress disorder (Spiegel, 1984, 1986; Putnam, 1985).

MPD is characterized by the existence within an individual of two or more distinct personalities or personality states. In classic cases each personality is fully integrated, having his or her own unique memories, behavior patterns, and social relationships; in others there may be some sharing of memories and commonalities of behavior. When the personality is dominant, it determines the host individual's behavior (DSM-III-R, 1987). Transition from one personality to another is usually sudden (within seconds to minutes) and is most often precipitated by stress, reflecting a complex psychophysiologic process termed dissociation.

### PREDISPOSING FACTORS

Two predisposing factors for MPD are currently recognized: (1) exposure to severe and overwhelming trauma, particularly during childhood, such as frequent and inconsistent alternating abuse and love, and (2) an innate and probably genetically determined psychophysiologic tendency to dissociate. Both factors—exposure and genetic tendency—are necessary; neither factor alone is sufficient to produce the disorder (Braun, 1984).

## ◆ EPIDEMIOLOGY AND HISTORY

Determining the incidence and prevalence of MPD has been hampered by two difficulties: (1) diagnosing the disorder and (2) dealing with the sociopolitical and professional context in which diagnoses are conceptualized. A brief understanding of the history of this disorder in psychiatric thinking is needed to understand the current state of knowledge regarding incidence and prevalence.

MPD is not a new psychiatric entity. Recognizable case histories of MPD in both adults and children were reported as early as 1817 (Taylor & Martin, 1944; Alvaredo, 1989). In the last major pre-Freudian psychology textbook, cases of MPD were given extensive coverage (James, 1890). The disorder was then lost in psychiatric controversy for a number of years and has only recently resurfaced as a "legitimate" psychiatric entity (Putnam, 1991a). Since 1980 a number of investigators have begun to clarify the epidemiology and consequences of this disorder.

In the earliest reports, MPD was described as the splitting of the total consciousness into complementary parts that coexist and mutually ignore each other, yet can share objects between or among themselves. The primary self often needs to invent "hallucinations" to mask and hide from itself the strange incidents and incongruous deeds of the secondary personalities. Each personality, nevertheless, has a conscious unity, continuous memory, habits, a name, and a sense of its own identity. This phenomenon was considered rare, associated with hysterical anesthesia, and discussed in conjunction with hypnotism, spiritualism, and the question of the location of the seat of the soul.

Although trauma similar to what might produce amnesia was considered a possible precipitating factor, the explanatory model used was post-hypnotic suggestion. Descriptions of the dissociative process were subjected to conflicting theoretical interpretations by Janet and Freud (Alexander & Selesnick, 1968). Unfortunately, the recommended use of a planchette to facilitate communication with these alter egos tended to link the entire MPD phenomenon with the interpretation of Charcot's hystero-epilepsy as a product of suggestion, if not fraud (Freud, 1948; Owen, 1971). Because of these linkages, Freud's theory of psychic repression prevailed over Janet's theory of dissociation (Masson, 1984) as the accepted description of unconscious functioning, resulting in a 60-year hiatus (circa 1920-1980) in the study of dissociative disorders. At the same time that interest in dissociation as a psychic concept was declining, Bleuler introduced the diagnostic entity "schizophrenia," which misinterpreted disorders of thought accompanied by hallucination as a psychic schism or two personalities. Subsequently, many MPD patients were misdiagnosed as schizophrenic (Rosenbaum, 1980).

Accurate statistical evaluation of MPD also relates to its etiologic relationship with severe abuse. Only recently have we recognized the widespread incidence of child abuse and child sexual abuse.

> In 1980 in the brief section of the *Comprehensive Textbook of Psychiatry* dealing with incest, the only epidemiological comment is a reference to a 1955 paper estimating that incest affects one family out of a million in North America. This estimate was low by four orders of magnitude...Child abuse underwent a 10,000 fold shift in prevalence in a very short time, and was transformed from a vanishingly rare curiosity to a major public health problem (Ross, 1991).

A parallel shift in the epidemiologic estimates of MPD is only now beginning to follow the earlier shift in its major etiologic determinant. Current prevalence estimates range from a very conservative 0.5% of the general population to a high of 10%. A recent prevalence study in the city of Winnipeg, Manitoba, Canada, yielded a 1% population prevalence rate (Ross et al., 1990); there is no reason to think American rates are substantially different. In a referred population (individuals who have come for counseling and been referred to psychologists and psychiatrists), prevalence rates may reach 25%.

## ♦ ETIOLOGY AND PATHOPHYSIOLOGY

MPD is most often associated with maltreatment beginning in early childhood and frequently extending through adolescence. The abuse, which can be sexual, physical, emotional, or often some combination of these, is usually "unprovoked" and often exhibits "marked deviance." "Unprovoked" implies that the abuse is not excessive discipline in response to child misbehavior; rather, it is purposefully imposed, takes unusually severe forms, and often exhibits both bizarre form and sadistic ambience. The extreme end of this abuse spectrum is exemplified by satanic cult practices, which can include witnessed child sacrifice (Young, 1988). Finally, the abuse is usually inflicted by the parent or another primary caregiver.

The last two decades have forced the recognition of the reality that the sexual abuse of children is common. Simultaneously, mental health professionals have acquired a new and deeper understanding of the psychological impact of traumatic events. This knowledge is both derived from and focused by the post-traumatic stress disorders resulting from the Vietnam combat experience. Research has yielded better understandings of the nature of trauma and the trauma response mechanisms that define these disorders. Research has also highlighted the potential for long-term sequelae after traumatic events, particularly when appropriate psychological intervention is unavailable. Such knowledge has contributed to the evolution of procedures such as routine "crisis debriefing" and supportive therapy following major traumatic events, for example, earthquakes, hurricanes, riots, and other natural or man-made disasters.

While much of the progress in this area evolved from post-trauma work with adults, children have not escaped attention. Events such as The Chauchilla bus incident, firearm tragedies in schools, and similar events where children were the primary targeted victims have all broadened our understanding of both the immediate impact and the long-term sequelae of such trauma in children. While emotional health cannot be guaranteed through immediate and competent intervention, emotional devastation and long-term illness are inevitable when intervention is lacking. The prevalence of severe child abuse and child sexual abuse as well as the increased knowledge regarding the long-term consequences of such trauma allow the recognition and identification of MPD as the most severe form of post-trauma consequence.

## DISSOCIATION

Since physical escape from abuse or trauma is often impossible for the victims, the only form of escape is psychological via dissociation. Dissociation is a psychological separation from the current feeling or cognitive state. In MPD the dissociation is so complete that a discontinuity of "self" and "memory" results. In this situation, escape by dissociation, while psychologically creative, is also a psychologically devastating solution to an inescapable evil. The solution is creative in that the child maintains his or her love for the perpetrator in one personality, the memory of the painful experience and feelings in another, and frequently the angry and aggressive emotions and behaviors in yet another. Unfortunately, once that route of defense has been chosen, external stimuli unrelated to the original stress can precipitate dissociative episodes and the creation of additional personalities.

Not all victims of severe child abuse or child sexual abuse dissociate. Many authors note that some forms of dissociation are normal developmentally (Putnam, 1991b). Even among a severely abused population, not all dissociation leads to MPD; many children and adults dissociate emotionally as a coping strategy. This dissociation, however, is limited to the emotional sphere with no loss of continuity of self or memory. Thus many victims will describe severe abuse in great detail, with no apparent demonstration of affect. They often note companion depersonalization and out-of-body phenomena such as "there was a spot on the wall where I routinely went and watched as he raped me." For these victims, therapy involves a reintegration of the emotions and the experiences along with a working through of the feelings.

The ongoing puzzle of MPD is that the dissociation is so complete that the multiple personalities can continue to coexist. Each personality is either unaware of the others or there is an internal system of personalities who are aware of each other, but who operate outside the conscious awareness of the host personality. Frequently one or several of these personalities will emerge, engage in behavior not compatible with the host personality, and then retreat, leaving the host personality "holding the bag." Thus the prevailing personality, unaware of the existence of the others, must often manage the consequences of another personality's actions, such as meeting the demands of the promises made by these other selves. All the while the host personality remains unclear as to why he or she does not remember either the interactions described or the periods of time during which they occurred. People with MPD become masters at covering up these perceived deficiencies. Their lives are a constant balancing and disguising act for what each personality perceives as its "terrible memory," if not its "craziness," which must be kept secret from other people.

## ◆DIFFERENTIAL DIAGNOSIS

Despite clear-cut and readily identifiable risk factors, the diagnosis of MPD in high-risk pediatric populations remains the exception rather than the rule. In addition to the factors already discussed, underdiagnosis is also due, in part, to the nature of the disorder itself.

### DIAGNOSTIC CRITERIA

*There are two diagnostic criteria for MPD:*

1. The existence within an individual of two or more distinct personalities or personality states, each with its own relatively enduring pattern of perceiving, relating to, and thinking about the self and the environment.

2. The recurrent assumption of full control of the person's behavior by at least two of these personalities.

These criteria are deceptively straightforward. Conceptually, confirming the diagnosis of MPD, particularly in children, is complex, as illustrated by the reported 6.8-year average interval between the first mental health contact and an accurate diagnosis made in adults (Putnam et al., 1984). Studies also indicate that the MPD child receives an average of 2.7 other psychiatric diagnoses before an accurate diagnosis of MPD is made (Hornstein & Putnam, 1992).

What is it about this disorder that makes diagnosis so difficult? Unlike the diagnosis of depression, where a clearly defined symptom list can be used to make systematic inquiry for critical findings, MPD presents the examiner with multiple personalities who frequently are not consciously aware of one another. Since dissociative processes occur, by definition, out of consciousness, one cannot merely ask "Do you dissociate?" In the majority of MPD adults, unless an episode of dissociation is witnessed and recognized, diagnostic data must be pursued through more indirect approaches.

Diagnosing childhood MPD is doubly difficult. The presenting plethora of affective symptoms, post-traumatic indicators, conduct disorders, hallucinatory signs, attention discrepancies, and school difficulties parallels the presentation of dissociative disorders in adults. The investigation of these symptoms in children, however, is more often performed through physical or developmental channels rather than psychiatric services. Thus many MPD children are referred to neurological services for possible seizure disorders presenting as "staring episodes," or to developmental clinics for evaluation of inconsistent attention and learning problems. Even when a child psychiatric evaluation is obtained, a number of developmental factors make it difficult to determine if a given child's dissociative behavior is normal or pathological. Even when clearly pathological, some personalities can be nonverbal or preverbal. These personalities can exhibit marked acting out that is diagnostic, but they still could be unable to understand or respond to diagnostically useful questions.

For the diagnosis of children the data collection must start from the diagnostic red flag of possible abuse, and the examiner must obtain information from both the child and the caregivers. A family history of MPD represents a significant and heavily weighted risk factor. To the extent that such a history is present, the clinical task is more to rule out MPD rather than to rule it in. The diagnostic process precisely parallels that of adult MPD but seeks signs that are exhibited within the child's developmental sphere of action (**Table 13-1**).

| Table 13-1. Differences Between Adult and Child Dissociation | |
| --- | --- |
| **Adult** | **Child** |
| *Forgetfulness and Amnesia* | |
| Inexplainable and bothersome forgetfulness leading to a sense of always being on edge and needing to constantly conceal and check their behavior | Amnesia for recent events such as abuse, schoolwork, tantrums, rage attacks |
| Unexplained periods of lost time (both minutes and days) sometimes viewed by patient as "walking blackouts," but unrelated to alcohol use | Perplexing forgetfulness such as time lost or tardiness with an inability to remember where they just were |
| *and/or* | |
| Waking up and not knowing how they got where they were or what they were doing in the recent past | |
| The appearance of items of clothing, jewelry, books, or other personal goods in their possession that they cannot recall buying (or, conversely, the unexplained disappearance of such items) | The appearance of items of clothing, toys or school supplies that they have not been given by parents and cannot recall buying (or the unexplained disappearance of such items) |
| Long periods of lost time such as several childhood years in succession | Adolescent MPDs may report this same phenomenon |
| Flashbacks or broken threads of memory | Adolescent MPDs may report this same phenomenon |
| *Forgetfulness Reflected in Interpersonal Relations* | |
| People calling them other names and seeming to know them while they do not recognize these people | Confusion regarding the names of teachers or peers |
| *and /or* | |
| People telling them things they have done or said that they can't remember and the lack of memory is not explained by the use of drugs or alcohol | Denial of behavior witnessed by others—often accompanied by a fierce sense of injustice if punished or confronted for lying |
| A childhood reputation for being called a liar that remains puzzling to the host personality | Apparent inability to learn from experience such as discipline or punishment |
| *Affective Symptoms* | |
| Unexplained severe mood swings | Severe periodic depression, sometimes including suicidal gestures but with no clear precipitating factor |

## Table 13-1. Differences Between Adult and Child Dissociation–*Continued*

| Adult | Child |
|---|---|
| *Multiple Psychiatric Diagnoses* | |
| *Behavior Symptoms* | |
| Dichotomous behavior states and/or impulsive and dangerous risk taking as reported by friends | Subtle alternating personality changes such as a basically shy child exhibiting depressed, angry, seductive, or regressive episodes |
| | Extreme regressive episodes followed by amnesia such as thumbsucking in a pre-teen or sudden dramatic yet transient loss of language or motor skills |
| An awareness of sometimes being unable to control their own behavior | Frequent angry outbursts without apparent provocation and frequently with extreme physical strength |
| Marked differences in handwriting from time to time | Dramatic fluctuations in conduct and performance (especially in abilities relating to school work, games, and music) |
| | Continuously changing preferences in food, clothing, and social relationships |
| *Somatic Symptoms* | |
| A history of many somatic complaints unexplained by a physical disorder or other psychiatric entities (e.g., panic disorder) | Physical complaints and injuries of vague origin, sometimes clearly self-inflicted |
| *Daydreaming, Sleepwalking, Depersonalization* | |
| Frequent troublesome "dreamlike" states, including sleepwalking | Excessive daydreaming, sleepwalking, and trancelike and spacey behavior, including concentration and attentional difficulties, not seizure disorder based |
| *Auditory "Hallucinations" and Imaginary Companions* | |
| Occurrence of voices that argue in their heads but are not psychotic in character—that is, voices from inside (other personalities) perhaps speaking of "we" or "us" | Hallucinated voices, either friendly or unfriendly, often attributed to an imaginary companion |
| History of imaginary companion beyond age 6 years | Imaginary companion still real to a child 6 years or older |

## ◆CLINICAL PRESENTATION

MPD is depicted in the popular media as a flamboyant, rare female disorder. The cinematic presentations of *The Three Faces of Eve* (Thigpen & Checkley, 1957) and *Sybil* (Schreiber, 1973) compellingly depict the complexity, devastation, and totality of this disorder. MPD, however, is neither rare nor, in most affected individuals, flamboyant (Kluft, 1985b, 1991). Unlike most psychiatric disorders, where the presenting problem usually indicates a specific differential diagnostic decision tree, the chief complaint in MPD rarely suggests an MPD diagnosis. The most frequently described presentation of MPD is depression in the host personality (Putnam, 1989). A typical MPD history will be vague and unclear. There are many "I can't remember for sure" answers or clever and subtle redefining of the questions by the MPD patient through oblique or tangential responses aimed at covering up half-realized memory gaps. Facts stated at one time may be "forgotten" or denied by another personality at another time. A useful diagnostic clue is presented when the therapist begins to wonder who is more forgetful—the professional or the patient. When this occurs, it should raise the question of need for a major reorganization of the presenting data to account for this "forgetfulness." That perspective should lead to consideration of MPD in the differential diagnosis, particularly in the presence of a previous history of abuse.

Clinical diagnosis of MPD in both children and adults requires a different perceptual filter for the "third ear"; the usual clues and cues regarding truthfulness or defensiveness can be missing. A host personality asked about diagnostic behaviors could truthfully deny their presence because that personality can be completely unaware of events that were engaged in by another of the subject's personalities. The clinician's usual "lie detection" parameters such as eye gaze, body posture, nervous gestures, and defensive voice tones are of little use for the simple reason that the particular personality is not "lying." This phenomenon is of special importance to professionals investigating the possibility of multigenerational child sexual abuse. We will illustrate the diagnostic process from the perspective of diagnosing an adult. As complex as this process is, it must be remembered that this complexity is magnified in children because of their developmental level and language developmental issues.

### TWO-LEVEL INVESTIGATION

Once adult MPD is suspected, confirmation requires a two-level diagnostic investigation. Since independent external validation of continuity and discontinuities of psychological functioning and behavioral contrasts is frequently sought from friends or relatives, a conclusive diagnosis will usually need to evolve over several sessions and involve sources of information other than the patient.

### FIRST LEVEL

During the first level of investigation, adult victims of child abuse are questioned about the presence of extreme, unexplainable, and bothersome forgetfulness that causes them to have a sense of always being on edge and needing to constantly conceal and check their behavior.

*Other areas to be investigated are as follows:*

1. Flashbacks or broken threads of memory

2. Unexplained periods of lost time, both minutes and days, sometimes viewed by the patient as "walking blackouts," but unrelated to alcohol use

3. Waking up and not knowing how they got where they were or what they were doing in the recent past

4. People they do not know frequently calling them by other names and seeming to know them

5. A childhood reputation for being a "liar" that remains puzzling to the host personality

6. The appearance of items of clothing, jewelry, books, or other personal goods in their possession that they cannot recall buying or, conversely, the unexplained disappearance of such items

7. Frequent and troublesome "dreamlike" states, including sleepwalking

8. Marked differences in handwriting from time to time

## SECOND LEVEL

When several of these symptoms have been documented, the clinician can then probe more deeply for the presence of second-level diagnostic markers: the occurrence of voices (other personalities) that argue in their heads but that are not psychotic in character; an awareness of sometimes being unable to control their own behavior; long periods of lost time such as several childhood years in succession; and unexplained severe mood swings and dichotomous behavior states (such as impulsive and dangerous risk-taking alternating with cautious or phobic states) as reported to them by friends.

When a diagnosis of MPD becomes almost certain and other personalities have not yet spontaneously revealed themselves, a direct invitation for them to come forward can be proffered. Thus the diagnosis proceeds from a suspicion to an investigation of possible external signs that, in turn, point the way to internal signs. Such signs sometimes are confirmed by the patient and lead to external validation of suspicions and finally to the appearance of alternate personalities.

## ◆IS MPD REAL?

Despite substantial corroborative research the persistent, overriding question surrounding MPD continues to be "Is it real?" This has remained unchanged for most of the professional community over the past century. As Putnam (1991a) notes, "The data supporting the validity of this diagnosis are quite robust, particularly when compared with some better-accepted disorders . . . . [There seems to be an] extra burden of proof on MPD that is not demanded of other psychiatric disorders." Recognition and acceptance of this disorder have been slow. For many, MPD is deemed an iatrogenic product of hypnotic suggestion recently termed false memory syndrome, hysteria or malingering, or a variant of other personality disorders. External validation of the abuse and of the functional status of many MPD victims provides clear evidence that this disorder is real and extraordinarily debilitating to those affected. In many case reports the therapist makes no use of hypnotism nor have the patients ever been subjected to hypnotism. Clearly then, the recognition of childhood MPD has lagged even further behind in acceptance than has adult MPD.

## ◆PROGNOSIS

When these abused children are appropriately identified and adequately treated, outcomes and prognoses are positive (Fagan & McMahan, 1984; Kluft, 1986). When, however, children with MPD remain undiagnosed and untreated until adulthood, the therapeutic course is protracted, stormy, and prognostically uncertain. In contrast to many other psychiatric disorders, the etiologic factors of this disorder along with the psychological efficacy and cost effectiveness of early identification and treatment can be documented (Kluft, 1986).

The past decade has seen a reemergence in the study of this disorder and the stark realization that unless this disorder is recognized and treated at the point of its inception, early childhood, a public health problem of epidemic proportions can be created, potentially impacting succeeding generations.

Multiple personality disorder is currently recognized as a creative psychophysiologic defensive response to a specific set of inescapable and uncontrollable experiences occurring within a circumscribed developmental time frame. Effective treatment requires an understanding of the developmental antecedents and the initial adaption to cope with the overwhelming trauma while it is occurring. More importantly, both effective treatment and primary prevention require that professionals identify MPD in its incubation phase, those childhood years following identified abuse incidents.

## ISSUES

Despite recent advances in the understanding of MPD and an increased ability to diagnose it in both children and adults, there remains resistance among professionals working with abused populations to screen for this disorder (Kluft, 1985c). One reason rests in an appropriate concern that an MPD diagnosis might invalidate an abused child's testimony; such a diagnosis should be considered prima facie evidence of abuse rather than negating the testimony. Thus the real answer to this objection lies in public and judicial education through pediatric and other professional advocacy.

More importantly, however, ignoring the possibility of this disorder in high-risk populations constitutes nothing less than continuing abuse of the child. One glimpse of the pain of these children, and that of those adults who have never been diagnosed or treated, can stun and momentarily immobilize the most sophisticated and experienced therapist. To recognize the energy it requires for any MPD victim to negotiate even one ordinary day is to gain a new understanding of coping and resilience. It is imperative that professionals working with abused children be able to recognize, diagnose, and obtain appropriate treatment for MPD. It should be routine that all such child victims receive therapy from a professional knowledgeable about MPD.

## FORENSIC QUAGMIRE

MPD presents us with several forensic issues that are, as yet, unresolved. From the point of view of the person with MPD as a victim, recent court rulings have suggested that when one personality is seductive, promiscuous, and cooperative in getting into a compromising situation and another personality then emerges to stop, then continued forceful sexual interaction with this latter declining personality constitutes rape. This decision suggests that the person with MPD may be incapable of fully informed consent.

The more difficult ethical and legal conundrum occurs when one or more personalities has perpetrated abuse or murder. Incarceration or long-term institutionalization for these offenses accompanied by treatment for the "insanity or incompetency" may yield an integrated person who no longer has MPD. Does one then release this person, or does the person remain in care or custody based on the actions of a "person" who no longer exists? These and a number of other legal issues are just beginning to emerge as the diagnosis of MPD is more often a factor in litigation procedures.

MPD challenges our most basic beliefs and assumptions concerning the workings of the mind and leaves us with questions we are currently ill equipped to answer. Perhaps this gestalt also contributed to its loss of stature in the psychiatric literature for a number of years: What we don't see doesn't haunt us. Current evidence regarding the prevalence and destructiveness of this disorder strips us of the luxury of this blindness.

## ♦BIBLIOGRAPHY

Alexander, FG, and Selesnick, ST: *The History of Psychiatry: An Evaluation of Psychiatric Thought and Practice from Prehistoric Times to the Present*, New American Library, New York, 1968, p. 223.

Alvaredo, C: Dissociation and state-specific psychophysiology during the nineteenth century, *Dissociation* 2:160-168, 1989.

Baldwin, L: Child abuse as an antecedent of multiple personality disorder, *Am J Occup Ther* 44:978-983, 1990.

Boor, M: The multiple personality epidemic: Additional cases and inferences regarding diagnosis, etiology, dynamics and treatment, *J Nerv Ment Dis* 2(170):302-304, 1982.

Braun, B: Towards a theory of multiple personality and other dissociative phenomena. In B Braun, ed: Symposium on multiple personality, *Psychiatr Clin North Am* 171-194, 1984.

Braun, B, and Sachs, R: The development of multiple personality disorder: Predisposing, precipitating, and perpetuating factors. In R Kluft, ed: *Childhood Antecedents of Multiple Personality*, American Psychiatric Press, Inc, Washington, DC, 1985, pp. 37-64.

*Diagnostic and Statistical Manual of Mental Disorders*, ed 3, revised, American Psychiatric Association, Washington, DC, 1987, pp. 269-277.

Fagan, J, and McMahan, P: Incipient multiple personality in children: Four cases, *J Nerv Ment Dis* 172:26-36, 1984.

Freud, S: *Hypnotism and Suggestion*, Collected Papers, Hogarth Press, London, 1948, pp. 16-22.

Frischholz, EJ: The relationship among dissociation, hypnosis, and child abuse in the development of multiple personality disorder. In R Kluft, ed: *Childhood Antecedents of Multiple Personality*, American Psychiatric Press, Inc, Washington, DC, 1985, pp. 99-126.

Greaves, GB: Multiple personality: 165 years after Mary Reynolds, *J Nerv Ment Dis* 164:385-393, 1980.

Hornstein, N, and Putnam, F: Clinical phenomenology of child and adolescent dissociative disorders, *J Am Acad Child Adolescent Psychiatry* 31:6, 1077-1085, 1992.

Hornstein, N, and Tyson, S: Inpatient treatment of children with multiple personality/dissociative disorders and their families, *Psychiatr Clin North Am* 14(3):631-648, 1991.

James, W: *Principles of Psychology*, Henry Holt, New York, 1890, 2 volumes.

Kluft, R: Childhood multiple personality: Predictors, clinical findings, and treatment results. In R Kluft, ed: *Childhood Antecedents of Multiple Personality*, American Psychiatric Press, Inc, Washington, DC, 1985a.

Kluft, R: The natural history of multiple personality disorder. In R Kluft, ed: *Childhood Antecedents of Multiple Personality*, American Psychiatric Press, Inc, Washington, DC, 1985b, pp. 197-238.

Kluft, R: Introduction: Multiple personality disorder in the 1980s. In R Kluft, ed: *Childhood Antecedents of Multiple Personality*, American Psychiatric Press, Inc, Washington, DC, 1985c, pp. viii-xiv.

Kluft, R: Treating children who have multiple personality disorder. In B Braun, ed: *Treatment of Multiple Personality Disorder,* American Psychiatric Press, Inc, Washington, DC, 1986, pp. 79-105.

Kluft, R: Clinical presentations of multiple personality disorder, *Psychiatr Clin North Am* 14(3):605-629, 1991.

Masson, JM: *The Assault on Truth: Freud's Suppression of the Seduction Theory,* Farrer, Strauss and Giroux, New York, 1984.

Owen, A: *Hysteria, Hypnosis and Healing: The Work of JM Charcot,* Garrett Publications, New York, 1971.

Putnam, F: Dissociation as a response to extreme trauma. In R Kluft, ed: *Childhood Antecedents of Multiple Personality,* American Psychiatric Press, Inc, Washington, DC, 1985, pp. 65-97.

Putnam, F: *Diagnosis and Treatment of Multiple Personality Disorder,* Guilford Press, New York, 1989.

Putnam, F: Recent research on multiple personality disorder, *Psychiatr Clin North Am* 14(3):489-502, 1991a.

Putnam, F: Dissociative disorders in children and adolescents, *Psychiatr Clin North Am* 14(3):519-531, 1991b.

Putnam, F, Guroff, J, Silberman, E, Barban, L, and Post, R: The clinical phenomenology of multiple personality disorder: Review of 100 recent cases, *J Clin Psychiatry* 47:285-293, 1986.

Putnam, FW, Lowenstein, RJ, and Silberman, EK: Multiple personality disorder in a hospital setting, *J Clin Psychiatry* 45:172-175, 1984.

Reagor, P, Kasten, J, and Morelli, N: A checklist for screening dissociative disorders in children and adolescents, *Dissociation* 5(1):4-19, 1992.

Rosenbaum, M: The role of the term schizophrenia in the decline of diagnoses of multiple personality, *Arch Gen Psychiatry* 37:1383-1385, 1980.

Ross, C: Twelve cognitive errors about multiple personality disorder, *Am J Psychother* 348-356, 1990.

Ross, C: Epidemiology of multiple personality disorder and dissociation, *Psychiatr Clin North Am* 14(3):503-517, 1991.

Ross, C, Joshi, S, and Currie, R: Dissociative experiences in the general population, *Am J Psychiatry* 147:1547-1552, 1990.

Schreiber, FR: *Sybil,* Regnery, Chicago, 1973.

Spiegel, D: Multiple personality as a post-traumatic stress disorder. In B Braun, ed: Symposium on multiple personality, *Psychiatr Clin North Am* 101-110, 1984.

Spiegel, D: Dissociation, double binds, and posttraumatic stress in multiple personality disorder. In B Braun, ed: *Treatment of Multiple Personality Disorder,* American Psychiatric Press, Inc, Washington, DC, 1986, pp. 61-78.

Taylor, W, and Martin, M: Multiple personality, *J Abnorm Psychol* 39:281-300, 1944.

Thigpen, C, and Checkley, H: *The Three Faces of Eve,* McGraw-Hill, New York, 1957.

Tyson, G: Childhood MPD/dissociative identity disorder: Applying and extending current diagnostic checklists, *Dissociation* 5(1):20-27, 1992.

Young, W: Issues in the treatment of cult abuse victims. Proceedings of the Fifth International Conference on Multiple Personality/Dissociative States, Chicago, 1988.

# Psychopathology and the Role of the Child Psychiatrist

Stuart L. Kaplan, M.D.
Thomas F. Weeston, M.D.

As a physician who specializes in the treatment of child mental illness, the child psychiatrist working as a member of a child maltreatment team is primarily concerned with identifying and treating psychopathology. Thus this chapter will focus, in part, on the psychopathology of abused children. In addition, we will consider the causes of abuse related to its prevalence in some psychopathological groups to illustrate associations between abuse and psychopathology. In exploring these relationships some of the psychopathological disorders associated with child abuse will be discussed. Our focus will be on post-traumatic stress disorder, because it seems to represent a paradigm of the relationship between child abuse and psychopathology, and multiple personality disorder, because of the controversy surrounding this reported association. Psychobiological responses of the organism to overwhelming stress and pharmacological management of posttraumatic stress disorder will also be covered. The value of the child psychiatrist as a member of the child maltreatment team can be seen in all these areas.

## ◆ General Considerations of Psychopathology and Child Maltreatment

Psychopathology, for most American mental health professionals, is defined by the *Diagnostic and Statistical Manual (DSM-IV)* of the American Psychiatric Association (1994). Conferring a psychiatric diagnosis or labeling a child or adolescent as having a psychiatric disorder can be stigmatizing to the victim and add to his or her burden of painful feelings associated with maltreatment. Among the advantages of using a categorical diagnostic system like the DSM-IV is its organization of a wide array of clinical data. The meaningfulness and validity of the diagnostic categories are susceptible to empirical confirmation (family studies, follow-up studies, treatment outcome studies, and other epidemiological investigations), but the categorical approach helps in choosing appropriate treatment.

The criteria for post-traumatic stress disorder (PTSD) are listed in **Table 14-1**. As with most diagnoses in the DSM-IV, the criteria are clearly defined, allow for inter-rater reliability, and do not presuppose a particular theoretical orientation.

---

**Table14-1. Diagnostic Criteria for Post-Traumatic Stress Disorder**

A. The person has been exposed to a traumatic event in which both of the following were present:

1. The person experienced, witnessed, or was confronted with an event or events that involved actual or threatened death or serious injury, or a threat to the physical integrity of self or others.
2. The person's response involved intense fear, helplessness, or horror. **Note:** In children, this may be expressed instead by disorganized or agitated behavior.

---

**Table14-1. Diagnostic Criteria for Post-Traumatic Stress Disorder— *Continued***

B. The traumatic event is persistently re-experienced in one (or more) of the following ways:

1. Recurrent and intrusive distressing recollections of the event, including images, thoughts, or perceptions. **Note:** In young children, repetitive play may occur in which themes or aspects of the trauma are expressed.
2. Recurrent distressing dreams of the event. **Note:** In children, there may be frightening dreams without recognizable content.
3. Acting or feeling as if the traumatic event were recurring (includes a sense of reliving the experience, illusions, hallucinations, and dissociative flashback episodes, including those that occur on awakening or when intoxicated). **Note:** In young children, trauma-specific reenactment may occur.
4. Intense psychological distress at exposure to internal or external cues that symbolize or resemble an aspect of the traumatic event.
5. Physiological reactivity on exposure to internal or external cues that symbolize or resemble an aspect of the traumatic event.

C. Persistent avoidance of stimuli associated with the trauma and numbing of general responsiveness (not present before the trauma), as indicated by three (or more) of the following:

1. Efforts to avoid thoughts, feelings, or conversations associated with the trauma.
2. Efforts to avoid activities, places, or people that arouse recollections of the trauma.
3. Inability to recall an important aspect of the trauma.
4. Markedly diminished interest or participation in significant activities.
5. Feeling of detachment or estrangement from others.
6. Restricted range of affect (e.g., unable to have loving feelings).
7. Sense of a foreshortened future (e.g., does not expect to have a career, marriage, children, or a normal life span).

D. Persistent symptoms of increased arousal (not present before the trauma), as indicated by two (or more) of the following:

1. Difficulty falling or staying asleep.
2. Irritability or outbursts of anger.
3. Difficulty concentrating.
4. Hypervigilance.
5. Exaggerated startle response.

E. Duration of the disturbance (symptoms in criteria **B**, **C**, and **D**) is more than 1 month.

F. The disturbance causes clinically significant distress or impairment in social, occupational, or other important areas of functioning.

Specify as:
**Acute:** If duration of symptoms is less than 3 months.
**Chronic:** If duration of symptoms is 3 months or more.
Specify as:
**With Delayed Onset:** If onset of symptoms is at least 6 months after the stressor.

Determining the effects of child maltreatment on psychopathology is complicated by the dimension of time. As the child develops, symptoms may vary and disorders express themselves differently at different developmental stages. For example, preschool children do not seem depressed or guilt ridden after an episode of sexual abuse, but during adolescence they may become guilt-ridden over the same abusive preschool episode. The passage of time between the abuse and the evaluation can also be important. Immediate or short-term effects often differ from longer term consequences.

## ♦ CAUSES OF CHILD MALTREATMENT

The correlations of incidence, prevalence, and demographic variables can lead to important hypotheses. A striking aspect of the epidemiology of child maltreatment is its strong association with various psychopathological disorders.

To appreciate the breadth of this association, we will briefly review the incidence and prevalence of the various forms of child maltreatment among the general population. Because of state maltreatment reporting requirements, incidence figures for abuse and neglect are more widely reported than prevalence figures. The incidence of physical abuse is estimated to be 4.9 per 1000 children, and the incidence of physical neglect is estimated at 8.1 per 1000 children (Knutson, 1995). Green (1993) has summarized contemporary studies of the rates of sexual abuse in the general population, stating that the incidence of sexual abuse is estimated to be 155,900 children per year or 2.5/1000 children per year. A survey of female college students reported a prevalence of sex abuse in females of 20% and a prevalence of sex abuse in male college students of 10%. Females are sexually abused more often than males at a ratio of 2.5:1 (Green, 1993). The incidence of sexual abuse is universally believed to be much higher than reported. Because the most frequently studied sex abuse cases are those that have been reported to departments of social services, generalizations applied to sex abuse cases that are not reported to departments of social service may be inaccurate. In addition, incidence and prevalence figures for physical abuse, sexual abuse, and neglect vary, depending on definitions, sampling method, and wording of the instruments used.

Although child maltreatment occurs at every level of society, it appears to be more frequent among the poor. Children in families earning $15,000 or less are 4 times more likely to be physically abused or sexually abused and 12 times more likely to be physically neglected than children in families with more favorable economic circumstances (Knutson, 1995).

## ♦ EXAMPLES OF RELATIONSHIPS BETWEEN MALTREATMENT AND SPECIFIC PSYCHOPATHOLOGICAL DISORDERS

### SOMATIZATION DISORDER

In somatization disorder patients have a large number of physical complaints without any physical basis for them. It is strongly associated with a childhood history of having been abused. Somatization disorder has also been termed Briquet's syndrome or hysteria (Guze, 1975). Criteria for the diagnosis of Briquet's syndrome include a minimum of 25 physical complaints in at least nine body systems (Feighner et al., 1972). Pribor (1993) found a prevalence rate for any abuse as a child or adult of 92.2% and a prevalence of sexual abuse as a child or adult of 80.4% in a sample of 51 adult female outpatient clinic attendees who met the criteria for Briquet's syndrome. There was no comparison sample. The extraordinary high rate of abuse in Briquet's syndrome illustrates a problem in associating abuse with psychiatric illness. Because patients with somatization disorder or Briquet's syndrome are understood as having a tendency to complain, it is difficult to know if their willingness to acknowledge having been sexually abused reflects an underlying interest in complaining that characterizes their illness, or if their having been sexually abused is related etiologically to their having many physical complaints.

### EATING DISORDERS

Several reports have suggested a strong association between eating disorders and sexual and physical abuse (Smolak, 1990; Stuart et al., 1990). In the study by

Folsmo et al. (1993), information is given about the prevalence of self-reported sexual abuse in samples of psychiatrically hospitalized women with and without eating disorders such as anorexia nervosa and bulimia. Sixty-nine percent (N=70) of those with eating disorders and 80% (N=39) of those without an eating disorder reported a history of sexual abuse. Fifty-one percent of those with eating disorders who had been victimized sexually had also been physically abused, and 56% of those without eating disorders who had been victimized sexually had also been physically abused. There were no significant differences in the prevalence of sexual or physical abuse rates between the two populations. The unusually high prevalence rates for self-reported maltreatment may be explained in part by the investigators having used the self-report inventory *Sexual Life Events Questionnaire,* which includes "requests or invitations to engage in sexual activity" as part of its definition of sexual abuse. The study also illustrates the importance of controlling for psychiatric illness in assessing a relationship between abuse and specific psychiatric disorders because the rates of maltreatment in psychiatric hospitalized female patients seem to be very high regardless of the disorder.

## BORDERLINE PERSONALITY DISORDER

Borderline personality disorder (BPD) is often associated with both sexual and physical abuse (**see Table 14-2 for diagnostic criteria for borderline personality disorder**). The validity of borderline personality disorder remains controversial among psychiatric epidemiologists, but many clinicians find this diagnosis useful in classifying certain patients who do not fit other diagnostic categories. However, borderline personality disorder is a personality disorder and personality disorders are rarely diagnosed in children and adolescents. By convention, personality disorder diagnoses are not made before the age of 18 years based on a presumption that the personality is still developing up to that age. Some influential theoreticians, however, believe that the diagnosis of borderline personality disorder can be made during childhood and adolescence.

Goldman et al. (1992), using modified diagnostic criteria for children based on the adult DSM-III-R (third edition, revised version), found 44 children who met the criteria for the diagnosis of borderline personality disorder. They compared the prevalence of abuse in this sample (N=44) with the prevalence of abuse in a general child psychiatric outpatient sample (N=100). The prevalence in the first sample was 38.6%, and the prevalence in the child psychiatric outpatient sample was 9%. There was significantly more abuse among the individuals in the borderline sample than in the child psychiatric outpatient sample (P<0.001). Because abuse is more common in girls than boys, Goldman et al. (1992) believed that the low prevalence of abuse in both samples might result from the high proportion of males in both samples (2:1 males to females).

## *CONDUCT DISORDER*

As Dorothy Otnow Lewis has noted (1992), even animals who have pain inflicted on them react with anger, and presumably humans are no different in this regard. There is considerable evidence that physically abused youngsters are more aggressive than nonabused children (Widom, 1989). In addition to becoming more aggressive, physically abused children are often hypervigilant and prone to misinterpret stimuli in a paranoid fashion, responding as if harm were intended or as if they were being cheated or taken advantage of. Lewis has documented the high prevalence of abuse in very selected aggressive clinical populations such as death row inmates (Lewis et al., 1986) and incarcerated adolescent boys (Lewis et al., 1982). There is a high percentage of physical abuse in these selected samples, along with a high prevalence of central nervous system damage and social deprivation. Lewis (1992) notes that not all physically abused children have conduct disorders or become criminals. It seems to take a combination of central nervous system disabilities, psychosocial disadvantages, and physical abuse to lead to violent behavior.

---

**Table14-2. Diagnostic Criteria for Borderline Personality Disorder**

A pervasive pattern of instability of interpersonal relationships, self-image, and affects, and marked impulsivity beginning by early adulthood and present in a variety of contexts, as indicated by five (or more) of the following:

1. Frantic efforts to avoid real or imagined abandonment. **Note:** Do not include suicidal or self-mutilating behavior covered in criterion 5.

2. A pattern of unstable and intense interpersonal relationships characterized by alternating between extremes of idealization and devaluation.

3. Identity disturbance: markedly and persistently unstable self-image or sense of self.

4. Impulsivity in at least two areas that are potentially self-damaging (e.g., spending, sex, substance abuse, reckless driving, binge eating). **Note:** Do not include suicidal or self-mutilating behavior covered in criterion 5.

5. Recurrent suicidal behavior, gestures, or threats, or self-mutilating behavior.

6. Affective instability due to a marked reactivity of mood (e.g., intense episodic dysphoria, irritability, or anxiety usually lasting a few hours and only rarely more than a few days).

7. Chronic feelings of emptiness.

8. Inappropriate, intense anger or difficulty controlling anger (e.g., frequent displays of temper, constant anger, recurrent physical fights).

9. Transient, stress-related paranoid ideation or severe dissociative symptoms.

---

## ◆ AN EPIDEMIOLOGICALLY BASED STUDY OF THE RELATIONSHIP BETWEEN PSYCHOPATHOLOGY AND ABUSE

Searching for relationships between categories of abuse and categories of psychopathology can be problematic because of the lack of precision of diagnostic criteria for many of the categories, variations in defining the different forms of abuse, absence of blindness of the raters, and selection of samples from disturbed populations rather than from general epidemiologically selected populations, among other factors. Ascertainment bias is a critical methodological flaw in the studies we have described that purport to show a significant prevalence of abuse in various diagnostic categories. It can be expected that psychiatrically disturbed people in treatment—a setting in which self-disclosure is highly valued—will acknowledge maltreatment experiences more often than would general population samples. This may inflate the relationship between maltreatment and psychiatric disorders in treatment settings relative to the general population.

Mullen et al. (1993) designed a study that deals directly with the problem of ascertainment bias by selecting subjects from a community sample using epidemiological sampling techniques rather than studying subjects who are already identified as ill and are seeking help. These authors conducted a survey of 2250 women in New Zealand and then interviewed a subsample of 298 women who reported sexual abuse and a subsample of 716 women who did not report sexual abuse. The interviews took between 1 and 5 hours and employed the *General Health Questionnaire,* the *Present State Examination,* and measure of the relationship between the adult respondent and the respondent's parent—the *Parent*

*Bonding Instrument.* Sexual abuse was stratified by severity. The sexually abused women had significantly more psychopathological conditions than the nonsexually abused women. The severity of the sexual abuse was related to the severity of the adult psychopathology. Those with genital contact or penetration during childhood had significantly more psychopathological conditions as adults. Genital contact or penetration significantly predicted the presence of eating disorders, tendency to be suicidal, and psychiatric hospitalization. A sexual abuse history that did not involve genital contact did not significantly predict adult psychopathological conditions. For sexual abuse other than penetration, family functioning played a significant role. In cases of noncontact sexual abuse in well-functioning families there was no difference in psychopathological conditions between the abused groups and the control sample. In noncontact sex abuse cases in poorly functioning families the children developed psychopathological conditions more often than in poorly functioning families without sex abuse. The exception to this was severe sexual abuse involving penetration, which led to psychopathological conditions independent of family functioning. Those who were sexually abused and developed psychopathological conditions engaged in help-seeking behaviors for their conditions more often than those who were not sexually abused and developed problems. This higher rate of help seeking among the sexually abused mentally ill may explain in part the high prevalence of psychiatric patients with histories of abuse in various treatment settings.

---

### Table14-3. Diagnostic Criteria for Acute Stress Disorder

A. The person has been exposed to a traumatic event in which both of the following were present:

1. The person experienced, witnessed, or was confronted with an event or events that involved actual or threatened death or serious injury, or a threat to the physical integrity of self or others.

2. The person's response involved intense fear, helplessness, or horror.

B. Either while experiencing or after experiencing the distressing event, the individual has three (or more) of the following dissociative symptoms:

1. A subjective sense of numbing, detachment, or absence of emotional responsiveness.

2. A reduction of awareness or his or her surroundings (e.g.,"being in a daze").

3. Derealization.

4. Depersonalization.

5. Dissociative amnesia (i.e., inability to recall an important aspect of the trauma).

C. The traumatic event is persistently re-experienced in at least one of the following ways: recurrent images, thoughts, dreams, illusions, flashback episodes, or a sense of reliving the experience; or distress on exposure to reminders of the traumatic event.

D. Marked avoidance of stimuli that arouse recollections of the trauma (e.g., thoughts, feelings, conversations, activities, places, or people).

E. Marked symptoms of anxiety or increased arousal (e.g., difficulty sleeping, irritability, poor concentration, hypervigilance, exaggerated startle response, or motor restlessness).

> **Table14-3. Diagnostic Criteria for Acute Stress Disorder — *Continued***
>
> **F.** The disturbance causes clinically significant distress or impairment in social, occupational, or other important areas of functioning or impairs the individual's ability to pursue some necessary task, such as obtaining necessary assistance or mobilizing personal resources by telling family members about the traumatic experience.
>
> **G.** The disturbance lasts for a minimum of 2 days and a maximum of 4 weeks and occurs within 4 weeks of the traumatic event.
>
> **H.** The disturbance is not due to the direct physiological effects of a substance (e.g., a drug of abuse, a medication) or a general medical condition, is not better accounted for by *brief psychotic disorder,* and is not merely an exacerbation of a preexisting Axis I or Axis II disorder.

## ♦ POST-TRAUMATIC STRESS DISORDER—A PARADIGM

The notion of psychic trauma in childhood leading to emotional distress in childhood and continuing on into adulthood has intrigued psychotherapists and formed the basis for much of the popular imagination about psychological illness and its treatment. This view of mental illness is often found in movies and the theater. That new stressful events can have psychological consequences received clinical support in World War I with the observation that combatants with "shell shock" seemed to have been stressed beyond the limits of their psychological endurance by the horrors of combat and developed conversion reactions in what was understood to be an unconscious effort to avoid further risk of combat. Similar phenomena were observed during World War II. Several civilian disasters provided an opportunity for clinical investigators to document the human ravages of unexpected life-threatening events on the lives of the survivors. During the Vietnam War the phenomena of flashbacks and other psychological sequelae were well known. The concept of post-traumatic stress disorder began to be accepted as a psychological response to an overwhelming real threat to life. In addition to the criteria for post-traumatic stress disorder in DSM-IV (**see Table 14-1**), the disorder is also often characterized by psychic numbing or lack of emotional response to the surrounding environment and possible loss of memory for the event. Many of these additional criteria are contained in the DSM-IV criteria for acute stress disorder (**see Table 14-3**). The symptoms of acute stress disorder cannot last more than 4 weeks to meet the DSM-IV criteria. Although it is important to understand shorter term psychological responses to stress, the long-term consequences of exposure have been of greater concern to psychopathologists. Are these responses transient or do they change the way the personality develops, leading to truncation and deformation?

Lenore Terr (1979) strongly suggests that severe stress has major consequences for future personality development. Terr (1993a) studied 26 children who had been kidnapped from a school bus. The children were placed in vans in which they were driven in total blackness for 11 hours and then were buried under gravel and rock for 17 hours in a truck trailer. Terr (1993a) noted that 100% of the children suffered from post-traumatic stress disorder.

*From this and other clinical experiences with single-event external traumas, Terr observed many characteristics of children who have been the victims of a single episode of an overwhelming trauma (Terr, 1991):*

1.  Victims tend to revisualize the event, "seeing" it over and over again. The experience can come to them during times of relaxation and boredom. The events occur in play repeatedly, but there is no element of pleasure or joy in the repetition.

2. The experience is associated with specific fears directly related to the distressing event.

3. The events appear to be incorporated into the developing personality and to be repeated out of the awareness of the victim. For example, adult occupation choices may be made in an unconscious effort to "play out" or repeat a childhood trauma.

4. The victims of a single external traumatic event experience changed attitudes about life and their future. Their sense of the future may be foreshortened, and they may embody the attitude "one day at a time," reflecting their feeling that the future is so uncertain that no predictions can be made about it. Because the single external event was highly improbable, their sense that anything can happen and no certainties can be entertained leads them to lack confidence about the future of the world and their future in particular.

Children older than 3 years who have been victimized by a single external event almost always remember the event with great clarity. Terr notes that they blame themselves for failing to avoid the event by imagining "omens" or clues that might have served as warnings of the event to come. These self-blaming victims believe that had they heeded these unrealistic omens, they would have avoided the events.

Pynoos et al. (1987) investigated a group of students who came under attack by a sniper while attending school. He noted the high percentage of post-traumatic stress disorder in the students after the attack and reported distortions in time and space by the victims. Those who were close to the sniper tended to see themselves as having been far from the sniper and those who were far from the sniper tended to see themselves as having been closer to the attack than they were.

Clinicians tend to diagnose abused children as having post-traumatic stress disorder. An excessive willingness to label children who have been abused with this diagnosis even if the children do not meet criteria can obscure other important diagnostic considerations.

To illustrate an unwarranted extension of the criteria of post-traumatic stress disorder to sexually abused children as well to suggest the modest percentage of abused children who actually meet the criteria for such a diagnosis, Deblinger et al. (1989) performed a chart review study comparing the prevalence of post-traumatic stress disorder in (1) sexually abused children, (2) physically abused but not sexually abused children, and (3) nonabused psychiatric inpatient children. Before the chart review, clinicians caring for the children had only found three cases of post-traumatic stress disorder. Deblinger et al. (1989) counted as part of the re-experiencing phenomena of post-traumatic stress disorder the sexualized behavior of the sexually abused children. Although sexualized behavior (such as public masturbation, sexually predatory behavior toward young children, sexual talk, and sexual play) is an important aspect found in sexually abused children, it may or may not be a form of the re-experiencing phenomena of post-traumatic stress disorder. The sexualized behavior of the sexual abuse victim can result from excessive sexual stimulation or be a learned behavior that has led to interpersonal rewards of attention or affection from adults. Even with this broadened definition of the re-experiencing phenomena, Deblinger et al. found that only 20.7% of the sexually abused children met criteria for post-traumatic stress disorder, compared with 10.3% of the nonabused children. Thus clinicians should not automatically attribute the diagnosis of post-traumatic stress disorder to abused children despite the appalling stress they have endured.

In a more recent study, McLeer et al. (1994) found a 42.3% prevalence rate of post-traumatic stress disorder in 26 sexually abused girls referred from a sexual abuse crisis center and rape counseling center to an outpatient psychiatry clinic, compared to an 8.7% rate in nonsexually abused girls enrolled for treatment in an outpatient child psychiatry clinic. The fact that the sexually abused girls were referred from a sexual abuse crisis center and a rape center suggests that their sexual abuse was recent. All of the sexual abuse was classified as severe. Because of these facts, the high percentage who received a diagnosis of post-traumatic stress disorder is probably reasonable. Of interest in this study was the high prevalence of attention-deficit/hyperactivity disorder (ADHD) (46%) in the sexually abused group; 23.1% of the sample had both post-traumatic stress disorder and attention-deficit/hyperactivity disorder. The authors speculate that attention-deficit/hyperactivity disorder may have made the victims more vulnerable to the development of post-traumatic stress disorder or, alternatively, that the symptoms of attention-deficit/hyperactivity disorder may be a behavioral consequence of the sexual abuse (McLeer et al., 1994).

Terr (1991) believes that the psychological consequences of having been a victim of a single external event differs from the consequences of having been a victim of recurrent trauma, which often occurs in physical or sexual abuse. The psychological responses to a single external event (Terr's type I trauma) were discussed earlier. The latter ("type II") traumas, according to Terr, are characterized by substantial amounts of psychic numbing and poor or incomplete recollection of the event. Nonconsenting victims who are repeatedly abused sexually by an adult family member may tend to dissociate or to think of something else during the abusive act itself, something like the response of an adult undergoing a painful dental procedure. This repeated effort to enter a trance-like state during the abusive act may lead to forgetting or dissociating from the abusive act. This creates fertile psychological ground for the development of multiple personality disorder (Terr, 1991) (see also Chapter 13).

## ♦ MULTIPLE PERSONALITY DISORDER—A CULTURE-BOUND SYNDROME?

Many cultures have culturally determined specific symptoms for displaying distress and seeking help. The Hmong of Laos have episodes of agitation in which they experience their genitalia disappearing (Westermeyer, 1989). The phenomenon of multiple personality disorder (MPD) may be a culture-bound syndrome of our culture. The DSM-IV notes that anorexia nervosa and dissociative identity disorder (another term for MPD) may be culture-bound syndromes of industrialized cultures (APA, 1994). MPD may develop when sexually abused children repress the memory of the event. Indeed, a high proportion of patients who have MPD report sexual abuse as children, with Ross et al. finding that 95.1% of 102 adults with MPD reported having been abused (Ross et al., 1991).

The mechanism that leads from sexual abuse to MPD, it is posited, is a "splitting off" of the abuse from consciousness by the development of another personality out of conscious awareness. Thus, it is hypothesized, the traumatic memory of the abuse is avoided. This leads to the development of two or more personalities occupying the same body. Often the personalities are not aware of each others' existence. Therapists who are interested in this phenomenon often employ unusual interventions to discover the existence of additional personalities and often infer their existence based on limited clinical data (Piper, 1994; Seltzer, 1994; McHugh & Putnam, 1995).

Support for a cultural interpretation of MPD is found in the recent dramatic increase in the number of reported cases of MPD. Ross (1991) reports that only 8 cases of MPD were reported between 1960 and 1970, but 843 cases were published between 1986 and 1990. The number of personalities that patients with MPD report has increased dramatically (Mersky, 1992). In earlier decades, patients reported up to 3 personalities, but recently reports of 40 personalities are not unusual in a patient with MPD.

These findings do not suggest that patients who present with MPD are not psychologically disturbed or that they are merely malingering. Evidence suggests that patients with MPD are disturbed. The *Minnesota Multiphasic Personality Inventory (MMPI),* an exceptionally well-validated measure of psychological disturbance, shows these patients to be quite disturbed on many dimensions of personality unrelated to their MPD. Regarding psychotherapy for MPD, the clinician should be sensitive to the possibility that focusing on the various personalities of the patient with MPD might unwittingly encourage the development of even more personalities. Attention to the despair and misery of these patients rather than their bizarre presentation may be more constructive for them (North et al., 1993; McHugh & Putnam, 1995).

The issues raised by MPD are closely related to those of false memory or repressed memory syndromes. In these syndromes, adults (usually in their 20s or 30s) consult a therapist for difficulties in life. The therapist who believes in the theory that many people have been sexually abused but have repressed the memory searches for clinical evidence in the patient's material that the patient has been sexually abused but has repressed the memory. The patient is encouraged to remember the inferred abuse episode. With guidance from the therapist the patient may recall such an episode. Often, upon such recollection, the patient is strongly advised to cease communicating with his or her family. Many such patients have filed legal suits against their families for child abuse. In the United States these families have banded together to form the False Memory Syndrome Association to advocate against therapists they believe unscrupulously impose false memories onto patients who in fact were never abused. Loftus (1993) has made it clear that in some individuals who are particularly suggestible, it is remarkably easy to implant memories of events that have never occurred. This phenomenon can lead to criminal confessions of sexual and satanic ritual abuse by alleged perpetrators. The alleged perpetrators can also be deeply convinced that they have committed these acts when they are entirely innocent of them (Loftus, 1993; Garry & Loftus, 1994).

These controversies have raised anew questions concerning the empirical basis for repression, the validity of memory in childhood, the validity of adult memories of childhood, and the legal interpretation of testimony about child abuse. The meaning of the repressed memory syndrome remains controversial, with vigorous opponents and adherents. Most who have been sexually abused during childhood do not forget or repress the experience, but some do. Those who evaluate such situations are well advised to be skeptical but open to the possibility that the patient's claim is valid. It is particularly important to avoid foisting the idea of unremembered sexual abuse on a patient based solely on clinical inference from clinical interview material. Such a possibility must always be confirmed by externally valid sources of information.

## ♦PSYCHIATRIC CHARACTERISTICS OF MALTREATING PARENTS

Few studies have addressed the psychopathological condition of maltreating parents. The topic is clinically relevant because if the parent has a treatable psychopathological disorder, the maltreatment situation may be helped with mental health or psychiatric intervention. Alcoholism (Sirles et al., 1989), depression (Kaplan et al., 1983), and personality traits such as rigidity and unhappiness (Milner & Wimberly, 1980) seem to distinguish abusive parents from control groups. Famularo et al. (1992) compared 54 mothers of maltreated children to 37 mothers whose children were receiving treatment at a children's hospital but had not been abused. Both the experimental and control groups received a structured psychiatric interview. The two samples were well controlled for socioeconomic status. Examining for current diagnoses, the group of abusive mothers had more mood disorders, more alcoholism, and more personality disorders, and they were more likely to have post-traumatic stress disorder than the control group. The data suggest that these disorders are significantly more prevalent in abusive samples than in nonabusive samples. A systematic effort to identify psychopathological conditions in abusive parents is a necessary aspect of the family treatment of the abused child.

## ◆Causality in Child Abuse Research

The relationship between abuse and psychopathology and the relationship between parental psychopathology and the probability of abusing both presuppose a linear, univariate view of causality, meaning that one variable causes another, e.g., sexual abuse causes eating disorders. This oversimplification distorts reality greatly because several variables generally interact together over time to lead to specific pathological behaviors, such as child abuse or mental illness. Social class, culture, genetics, temperament, early childhood experience, current family interaction, and life stress all interact to determine individual behavior. Theories to explain this process have been termed "ecological" (Belsky, 1980) or "transactional" (Cicchetti & Rizley, 1981) models. These comprehensive theories are important, in part, because they consider the role of the child in the development of the abusive behavior without blaming the child for the event. Instead the child and the child's behavior are simply additional variables that interact in complex ways with all of the other variables that finally culminate in the abusive act. The child and the child's predispositions, behavior, and history may be regarded as risk factors that increase or decrease the probability of an abusive act.

One child characteristic that is strongly linked to the probability of abuse is age, with younger children more likely to be abused than older children. Younger children spend more time with their parents and are less able to defend themselves from abuse by leaving the situation or notifying authorities. Younger children are also more seriously injured than older children who have been abused.

Other variables that may increase the child's vulnerability to abuse are mental retardation, physical handicap, prematurity, high-pitched crying, and oppositionality. Ammerman (1991) offers an excellent review of this area.

## ◆Developmental Psychopathology

The DSM system may be too blunt an instrument to record the subtle changes in personality and affect that could be the residue of the maltreatment experience. Several important scholars believe that child maltreatment distorts development in profound ways that may not manifest themselves in the categorical diagnoses assessed by the DSM-IV, but that nevertheless have significance for individual development. For example, the low self-esteem often found in adult survivors of sexual abuse by itself would not merit a DSM diagnosis because it does not meet the criteria for the diagnosis of dysthymic disorder (chronic depression or neurotic depression). However, the low self-esteem could have devastating consequences for the well-being of the sexual abuse survivor.

Although children and others in the maltreatment situation must be assessed for psychopathological conditions during the evaluation of the abusive episode, the psychopathological model is limited in its understanding of abuse. Most abused children do not have diagnosable psychopathological conditions, but many are profoundly affected both in current functioning and in subsequent development. Study of the developmental processes related to abuse offers considerable promise for enhancing our understanding of the impact of abuse and lends sensitivity to treatment and research efforts.

Earlier it was stated that children sexually abused at a young age may reflect on the experience during adolescence and respond to the earlier experience with depression not experienced previously. Similarly, the excessive sexualized behavior often encountered in younger children and the predatory sexual behavior they may display after abuse contrast markedly with the inhibited attitude toward sexuality often found in sexually abused adolescents. Finkelhor (1995) cites Shirk (1988) as having coined the apt phrase "developmental symptom substitution." The child's interpretation of the abusive event varies depending on the level of cognitive and emotional development. Also, this perspective emphasizes areas known to have a particular salience for children, such as the quality of a young child's attachment to the mother and an older child's peer relationships, school behavior, and academic performance. These areas are adversely affected by abuse and neglect but may not enter directly into a DSM-IV criterion-based assessment of psychopathological conditions.

Cicchetti and Toth (1995) describe several psychotherapeutic interventions based on developmental psychopathological principles and provide a compelling case that a developmental psychopathological perspective may lead to better intervention efforts.

## ◆NEUROCHEMICAL AND NEUROHORMONAL RESPONSES TO STRESS

The major central nervous system neurotransmitters are dopamine (DA), norepinephrine and epinephrine (NE/E), and serotonin (5HT) (**Figure 14-1**). These are the most widely studied of more than 30 neurotransmitters. These transmitters are diffusely distributed throughout the brain, network dynamically and physically, and are intimately coordinated in an interdependent feedback system. They influence and are influenced by neurohormonal activity, especially corticotropin-releasing factor (CRF). Recent information concerning the dynamic relationships of these neurotransmitters comes from the study of human temperament (Cloninger, 1987). Serotonin is thought to be a more primitive, earlier ontogenic system that mainly inhibits behavior or sends a "stop" signal in the presence of threats. Dopamine is a behavioral activator, providing a "go" signal that motivates the organism into exploratory behavior and attention to novelty. Norepinephrine functions to increase learning, stabilize behavior in the face of anticipated reward, and promote social bonding. It functions as a "maintain" signal for learning, which shapes and affects the salience of future cues. Together with "persistence," these four domains constitute constraints on how we see and interpret the continuous flow of experiential data. The intimate control of these neurotransmitters over the processing of experience plays a central role in the sequelae of maltreatment.

Few studies have examined these neurotransmitter systems in abused children. Some researchers (DeBellis et al., 1994) have found that sexually abused girls excrete significantly higher urinary levels of norepinephrine and epinephrine, dopamine and their metabolites than do control subjects. Another study (Glavin et al., 1991) discovered low activity levels of dopamine-beta hydroxylase (see **Figure 14-1; this is the rate-limiting enzyme for conversion of phenylalanine and tyrosine to norepinephrine**) in psychiatrically hospitalized boys with

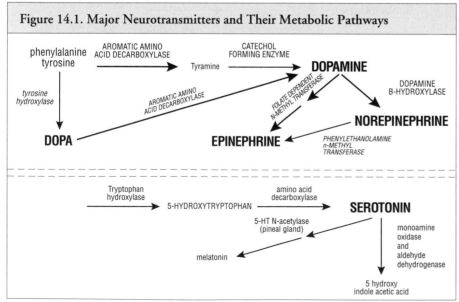

**Figure 14.1. Major Neurotransmitters and Their Metabolic Pathways**

*Figure 14-1*. *Major neurotransmitters and their metabolic pathways.*

conduct disorder and histories of abuse or neglect. Such studies suggest the potential for identifying biochemical correlates of abuse, but more study is needed.

## NEURAL SUBSYSTEMS AND STRESS

The endogenous opiates (endorphins, enkephalins, and dynorphins) control pain responses within the central nervous system, an effect that can be reversed with naloxone (Pittman et al., 1990). The highest concentration of endorphin receptors and enkephalins is in the amygdala, an area especially significant for aggression and channeling of drives toward the appropriate extrapersonal objects (Trimble, 1981). These agents have significant control over autonomic, endocrine, and behavioral responses to stress (Watson et al., 1988). They modulate the stress response by reducing the response rate of neurons in the locus coeruleus (LC) (Brenner et al., 1993). High levels of stress have been associated with an opiate-withdrawal-like state in animals and the development of "stress-induced analgesia" in those with post-traumatic stress disorder (Akil et al., 1984). A phenomenon referred to as stress-induced analgesia (SIA) has been noted in studies of veterans during exposure to visual material associated with combat experiences (van der Kolk et al., 1989). There may be a connection between this biological, opioid-mediated analgesia and the psychological need to re-experience trauma in that the activation of opioid receptors can produce a calming effect (van der Kolk et al., 1989). This is consistent with data associating opioids with a role in producing dissociative phenomena.

Corticotropin-releasing factor is a neuropeptide that acts as a mediator between the behavioral and physiological effects of stress. This mechanism is central to the stress and arousal experiences involved in post-traumatic stress responses. Corticotropin-releasing factor also has an activating role in behavior and helps coordinate behavioral responses to stress (Mcnazaghi et al., 1993). It can, therefore, act not only on the hormonal responses via the anterior pituitary but also exert effects that coordinate responses to stress at multiple levels. For instance, noradrenergic and serotonergic systems activated by stress are subsequently restrained by glucocorticoids, and it seems that corticosteroids exercise both "suppressive and permissive functions" in an attempt to prevent damage to the organism by overactive stress responses (McEwen et al., 1993; Munck et al., 1994).

Post-traumatic stress syndrome also seems to have distinct neurophysiological and neuroendocrinological aspects when compared to other psychiatric illnesses. These may allow its separation from phenotypically similar diagnoses, such as anxiety disorder, depression, and personality disorders. Twenty-four-hour urine assays of norepinephrine and epinephrine, dopamine, and cortisol have differentiated normal individuals from those with post-traumatic stress syndrome. While responses to exogenous steroids appear to be enhanced in post-traumatic stress syndrome patients, these same responses are blunted in many depressed patients (see dexamethasone suppression test; Yehuda et al., 1993).

Stress-response homeostasis includes a significant genetic contribution but is also affected by experience. The times of maximum exposure and risk are in early development (birth through adolescence), when we experience greater biological dependency as well as physiological and psychological immaturity. Thus we are more vulnerable to maladaptive stress responses when the assault takes place earlier in life.

Neuroendocrine responses are necessary for normal development and psychosexual growth. Dysregulation of this system may cause disturbances of growth, psychiatric illness, endocrine/metabolic disorders, and vulnerability to disease not only during childhood but also into adulthood (Statakis et al., 1995). Fluctuations in the functioning of the hypothalamic-pituitary-adrenal (HPA) axis have been demonstrated in sexually abused girls (DeBellis et al., 1994).

Psychogenic dwarfism and nonorganic failure to thrive are interruptions in normal growth that are believed to be mediated by a poor infant-caregiver relationship. The effects may operate through interruptions in normal hypothalamic-pituitary-growth hormone axis activity. Sustained, but not acute, stress is correlated with reduced levels of growth hormone resulting from the effects of corticotropin-releasing hormone activity (Chrousos et al., 1992). In a study of sexually abused boys, a significantly elevated ratio of growth hormone response to clonidine vs levo-dopamine (l-dopa) was discovered in the abused sample when compared to a control group (Jensen et al., 1991), suggesting a noradrenergic/corticotropin-releasing hormone interaction in the regulation of growth hormone. In addition, thyroid function can be inhibited by stress indirectly through the inhibition of thyroid-stimulating hormone (TSH) and thyroid-releasing hormone (TRH) by hypothalamic somatostatin and by corticosteroid inhibition of conversion of thyroxine (T4) to triiodothyronine (T3) (Yehuda et al., 1993).

## ◆ PHARMACOLOGICAL TREATMENT OF POST-TRAUMATIC STRESS DISORDER

The pharmacological treatment of post-traumatic stress disorder in children and adolescents is complicated by the relative lack of data for this age range in comparison to adults. Because pharmacological treatments for adults often serve as models for treatment in children, we will briefly review the treatment of post-traumatic stress disorder in adults.

The hyperarousal that follows sexual victimization is a symptom of post-traumatic stress disorder that may be amenable to pharmacological intervention. Hyperarousal symptoms include elevated heart rate and elevated 24-hour urinary excretion of catecholamines, both suggesting a high sympathetic tone (Orr, 1990). Agents that offer promise include clonidine, tricyclic antidepressants (TCAs), monoamine oxidase inhibitors (MAOIs), beta-blockers, lithium, benzodiazepines, carbamazapine, and propranolol (van der Kolk, 1983; Kolb et al., 1984).

Kolb et al. (1984), in assessing medications that affect the adrenergic nervous system in adults, found decreases in startle response, explosiveness, intrusive reexperiencing, and nightmares using both propranolol (120 to 180 mg/day) and clonidine (0.2 to 0.4 mg/day). Other studies in adults have shown the need for much higher doses of propranolol before such a response can be obtained, but these doses are often prohibited by side effects. Famularo et al. (1988, 1993) found propranolol in doses of 2.5 mg/kg per day to be effective in reducing hyperarousal and hypervigilance in children with acute post-traumatic stress disorder.

Benzodiazepines are classified as anxiolytics, affecting the central nervous system gamma aminobutyric acid (GABA) receptors by altering chloride conductance into the cell. As a class, they improve sleep and reduce nightmares as well as reduce anxiety. Their profile also includes tolerance and dependence potential as well as interference with learning, making long-term use of concern. Proper management must take into account the properties of distribution and elimination half-life (e.g., short distribution half-life associated with euphoria and higher dependency potential; short elimination half-life associated with withdrawal anxiety and rebound symptoms), prior addictive behavior, hepatic functioning (e.g., lorazepam, oxazepam, and temezapam are safest in hepatic dysfunction), and drug-drug interactions (e.g., increased toxicity when combined with agents known to inhibit hepatic enzyme systems).

Tricyclic antidepressants (2 to 5 mg/kg per day in divided doses) and monoamine oxidase inhibitors also have direct effects on adrenergic neurotransmission. The persistent arousal associated with the post-traumatic state is often accompanied by depression and anger, factors also to be considered in the choice of medication. The central role of corticotropin-releasing factor over adrenergic responsiveness under stress suggests a future role for corticotropin-releasing factor antagonists in pharmacological research (Sutherland et al., 1994).

Each class of drugs has significant potential toxicity in children, ranging from cardiac arrhythmias with tricyclic antidepressants to hypertensive crisis with monoamine oxidase inhibitors. Children present unique pharmacokinetic and pharmacodynamic considerations that must be considered when prescribing these medications. The child psychiatrist can offer a valuable consulting role in their use.

The finding of low levels of 5-HT metabolites in the CSF of those who exhibit violence, impulsivity, and suicidal behavior suggests that serotonin may provide an inhibitory aspect to behavior (Braun et al., 1990). Serotonin also facilitates nonassociative and avoidance learning, while animal models show increasing CSF levels of 5-HT when the animals successfully adapt to stress (Joseph et al., 1983). In a randomized double-blind comparison of placebo with fluoxetine, van der Kolk et al. (1994) found improvement in arousal, numbing symptoms, and depression (22 women, 42 men; 31 veterans, 33 non-veterans; 5-week, double-blind, randomized design; placebo vs fluoxetine). Researchers found that those with post-traumatic stress disorder symptoms had a more positive response to selective serotonin-reuptake inhibitor when they also demonstrated decreased platelet 3H-paroxetine binding (Fichtner et al., 1994). Another selective serotonin-reuptake inhibitor, sertraline, was studied in comorbid post-traumatic stress disorder–alcohol dependence and provided significant improvement, although these results are limited by lack of controls, open design, and a small number of subjects (Brady et al., 1995).

In a 1994 review of pharmacological treatments for post-traumatic stress disorder in adults, Sutherland et al. (1994), reviewing six controlled, double-blind studies, noted (1) conflicting effects of phenelzine to reduce intrusive symptoms; (2) the usefulness of desipramine to reduce intrusive and depressive symptoms without a change in anxiety, but only if there was concurrent major depression; (3) minor resolution of intrusive symptoms and anxiety with amitriptyline; and (4) improvement of depressive, anxious, and intrusive symptoms with fluoxetine. Several studies required considerable time (8 weeks or more) to separate placebo from actual drug effects, suggesting that medication trials should be given adequate periods of time before being discontinued.

In adults there is significant evidence that tricyclic antidepressants, monoamine oxidase inhibitors, and selective serotonin-reuptake inhibitors are useful in the treatment of the intrusive, depressive, and numbing symptoms of post-traumatic stress disorder. Mood stabilizers (lithium, CBZ, VPA) have less support but have proved effective in select populations where hyperarousal, irritability, aggression, and hostility are prominent. Alpha-2-agonists (e.g., clonidine, guanfacine) are believed to be useful for similar patterns of hyperarousal. In all age ranges, neuroleptics should be reserved for psychotic symptoms such as auditory hallucinations. Buspirone may be helpful for exaggerated startle responses; it has been used in a small trial where improvement occurred in seven of eight adult patients (Duffy et al., 1994).

In children the currently most studied agents include clonidine, benzodiazepines, and tricyclic antidepressants (Botteron et al., 1993), with a lesser emphasis on beta-blockers such as propranolol. Thus psychopharmacology may be a helpful adjunct in the treatment of children with post-traumatic stress syndrome.

## ◆ THE CHILD MALTREATMENT TEAM

The professionals forming the child abuse team share overlapping roles with child psychiatrists; all are committed to securing the safety of endangered children, promoting circumstances that will provide for maltreated children's future development, and treating families with whom they have contact with respect and empathy. Child psychiatrists may share a number of competencies with other mental health professionals on the team, including the skills to interview maltreated children and their parents, collaborate with outside agencies such as law enforcement agencies, and collaborate with disciplines other than their own. Yet each discipline brings special expertise and makes a unique contribution, strengthening the overall functioning of the team. Most child psychiatrists bring to the team a knowledge of individual psychodynamics, an understanding of child development, and an advanced skill level in various forms of psychotherapy. Arguably, the critical contributions that contemporary child psychiatrists can make to the team is an understanding of the assessment of psychopathology and the use of psychotropic medication.

## ◆ BIBLIOGRAPHY

Akil, H, Watson, SJ, Young, E, Lewis, ME, Khachaturian, H, and Walker, JM: Endogenous opioids: Biology and function, *Ann Rev Neurosci* 7:223-255, 1984.

American Psychiatric Association: *Diagnostic and Statistical Manual of Mental Disorders,* ed 4, American Psychiatric Association, Washington, DC, 1994.

Ammerman, RT: The role of the child in physical abuse: A reappraisal, *Violence and Victims* 6(2):87-100, 1991.

Belsky, J: Child maltreatment: An ecological integration, *Am Psychologist* 35:320-335, 1980.

Botteron, K, and Geller, B: Disorders, symptoms, and their pharmacology. In JS Werry, and MG Aman, eds: *Practitioners Guide to Psychoactive Drugs for Children and Adolescents,* Plenum Medical Book Company, New York, 1993.

Brady, KT, Sonne, SC, Roberts, JM: Sertraline treatment of comorbid posttraumatic stress disorder and alcohol dependence, *J Clin Psychiat* 56(11):502-505, 1995.

Braun, P, Greenberg, D, Dasberg, H, et al.: Core symptoms of posttraumatic stress disorder unimproved by alprazolam treatment, *J Clin Psychiat* 15:236-238, 1990.

Brenner, JD, Davis, M, Southwick, SM, et al.: Neurobiology of posttraumatic stress disorder. In JM Oldham, MB Riba, and A Tasman, eds: *Review of Psychiatry,* APA Press, Washington, DC, 1993, pp. 183-205.

Cicchetti, D, and Rizley, R: Developmental perspectives on the etiology, intergenerational transmission, and sequelae of child maltreatment, *New Directions Child Dev* 11:31-55, 1981.

Chrousos, GP, and Gold, PW: The concepts of stress system disorders: Overview of behavioral and physical homeostasis, *JAMA* 267:1244-1252, 1992.

Cicchetti, D, and Toth, SL: A developmental psychopathology perspective on child abuse and neglect, *J Am Acad Child Adolesc Psychiat* 34:5:541-545, 1995.

Cloninger, CR, and Gilligan, SB: Neurogenetic mechanisms of learning: A phylogenetic perspective, *J Psychiat Res* 21(4):457-472, 1987.

Debillis, MD, Chrousos, GP, Dorn, LD, Burke, L, Helmers, K, Kling, MA,Trickeet, PK, and Putnam, FW: Hypothalamic-pituitary-adrenal dysregulation in sexually abused girls, *J Clin Endocrinol Metab* 78:249-255, 1994.

Deblinger, E, McLeer, SV, Atkins, MS, Ralphe, D, and Foa, E: Post-traumatic stress in sexually abused physically abused and non-abused children, *Child Abuse Negl* 13:403-408, 1989.

Famularo R, Kinscherff, R, and Fenton, T: Psychiatric diagnoses of abusive mothers: A preliminary report, *J Nerv Ment Dis* 180(10):658-661, 1992.

Famularo R, Kinscherff, R, and Fenton, T: Propranolol treatment of childhood post-traumatic stress disorder, acute type, *Am J Dis Child* 142:1244-1247, 1988.

Feighner, JP, Robins, E, Guze, SB, Woodruff, RA, Winokur, G, and Munoz, R: Diagnostic criteria for use in psychiatric research, *Arch Gen Psychiat* 26:57-63, 1972.

Finkelhor D: The victimization of children: A developmental perspective, *Am J Orthopsychiat* 65(2):77-193, 1995.

Folsmo, V, Krahn, D, Nairn, K, Gold, L, Demitrack, MA, and Silk, KR: The impact of sexual and physical abuse on eating disorders and psychiatric symptoms: A comparison of eating disorders and psychiatric inpatients, *Int J Eating Dis* 13:249-257, 1993.

Glavin, M, Shekhar, A, Simon, J, et al.: Low dopamine-beta hydroxylase: A biological sequelae of abuse and neglect? *Psychiat Res* 39:1-11, 1991.

Garry, M, and Loftus, EF: Pseudomemories without hypnosis, *Int J Clin Exp Hypnosis* 42(4):363-378, 1994.

Goldman, SJ, D'Angelo, EJ, DeMaso, DR, and Mezzacappa, E: Physical and sexual abuse histories among children with borderline personality disorder, *Am J Psychiat* 149:1723-1726, 1992.

Green, AG: Child sexual abuse: Immediate and long-term effects and intervention, *J Am Acad Child Adolesc Psychiat* 32(5):890-902, 1993.

Guze, SB: The validity and significance of the clinical diagnosis of hysteria (Briquet's syndrome), *Am J Psychiat* 132(2):138-141, 1975.

Jensen, JB, Pease, JJ, Ten Bensel, R, and Garfinkel, BD: Growth hormone response patterns in sexually or physically abused boys, *J Am Acad Child Adolesc Psychiat* 30:784-790, 1991.

Joseph, MH, and Kennett, GA: Corticosteroid response to stress depends upon increased tryptophan availability, *Psychopharmacology* 79:79-81, 1983.

Kaplan, SJ, Pelcovitz, D, and Salzinger, S: Psychopathology of parents of abused and neglected children, *J Am Acad Child Psychiat* 22:238-244, 1983.

Knutson, JF: Psychological characteristics of maltreated children: Putative risk factors and consequences, *Annu Rev Psychol* 46:401-31, 1995.

Kolb, LC, Burris, BC, and Griffiths, S: Propranolol and clonidine in the treatment of post traumatic stress disorders of war. In BA van der Kolk, ed: *Post Traumatic Stress Disorder: Psychological and Biological Sequelae,* APA Press, Washington, DC, 1984.

Lewis, DO: From abuse to violence: psychophysiological consequences of maltreatment, *J Am Acad Child Adolesc Psychiat* 31(3):383-391, 1992.

Lewis, D, Pincus, JH, Feldman, M, Jackson, L, and Bard, B: Psychiatric, neurological and psychoeducational characteristics of 15 death row inmates in the United States, *Am J Psychiat* 143:838-845, 1986.

Lewis, D, Pincus, JH, Shanok, S, and Glaser, G: Psychomotor epilepsy and violence in a group of incarcerated adolescent boys, *Am J Psychiat* 139:882-887, 1982.

Loftus, EF: The reality of repressed memories, *Am Psychol* 48(5):518-537, 1993.

McEwen, BS, Sakai, RR, and Spender, RL: Adrenal steroid effects on the brain: versatile hormones with good and bad effects. In J Schullkin, ed: *Hormonally Induced Changes in Mind and Brain,* Academic Press, Washington, DC, 1993, pp. 157-189.

McHugh, PR, and Putman, F: Debate forum resolved: Multiple personality disorder is an individually and socially created artifact, *J Am Acad Child Adolesc Psychiat* 34(7):957-963 1995.

McLeer, SV, Callaghan, M, Henry, D, and Wallen, J: Psychiatric disorders in sexually abused children, *J Am Acad Child Adolesc Psychiat* 33(3):313-319, 1994.

Menazagh, F, Heinrichs, SC, Pich, EM, Weiss, F, and Koob, GF: The role of limbic and hypothalamic corticotropin-releasing factor in behavioral responses to stress, *NY Acad Sci* 697:142-154, 1993.

Mersky, H: Multiple personality disorder and false memory syndrome, *Br J Psychiat* 166:281-283, 1992.

Milner, JS, and Wimberly, RC: Prediction and explanation of child abuse, *J Clin Psychol* 36:875-884, 1980.

Mullen, PE, Martin, JL, Anderson, JC, Romans, SE, and Herbison, GP: Childhood sexual abuse and mental health in adult life, *Br J Psychiat* 163:721-732, 1993.

North, C.A., Ryall, J.E., Ricci, D.A., Wetzel, R.D.: *Multiple Personalities, Multiple Disorders: Psychiatric Classification and Media Influence.* Oxford University Press, New York, 1993.

Orr, SP: Psychophysiological studies of PTSD. In E Giller, ed: *Biological Assessment and Treatment of PTSD,* APA Press, Washington, DC, 1990.

Piper A: Multiple personality disorder, *Br J Psychiat* 164:600-612, 1994.

Pittman, PK, van der Kolk, BA, Orr, SP, et al.: Naloxone-reversible analgesic response to combat-related stimuli in posttraumatic stress disorder, *Arch Gen Psychiat* 47:541-544, 1990.

Pribor, EF, Yutzy, SH, Dean, JT, and Wetzel, RD: Briquet's Syndrome, dissociation and abuse, *Am J Psychiat* 150(10):1507-1511, 1993.

Pynoos, R, Frederick, C, Nader, K, et al.: Life threat and post-traumatic stress in school age children, *Arch Gen Psychiat* 44:1057-1063, 1987.

Ross, CA, Miller, SD, Bjornson, L, Reagor, P, Fraser, GA, and Anderson, G: Abuse histories in 102 cases of multiple personality disorder, *Can J Psychiat* 36:97-101, 1991.

Seltzer, A: Multiple personality: A psychiatric misadventure, *Can J Psychiat* 39:442-445, 1994.

Shirk, SR: The interpersonal legacy of physical abuse of children. In MD Struas, ed: *Abuse and Victimization Across the Life Span,* John Hopkins University Press, Baltimore, 1988, pp.57-81.

Sirles, EA, Smith, JA, and Kusama, H: Psychiatric status of intrafamilial child sexual abuse victims, *J Am Acad Child Adolesc Psychiat* 28:225-229, 1989.

Smolak, L, Levine, MP, and Sullins, E: Are child sexual experiences related to eating-disordered attitudes and behavior in a college sample? *Int J Eating Dis* 9(2):167-178, 1990.

Stratakis, CA, Gold, PW, and Chrousos, GP: Neuroendocrinology of stress: Implications for growth and development, *Horm Res* 43:162-167, 1995.

Stuart, GW, Laraia, MT, Ballenger, JC, and Lydiard, RB: Early family experiences of women with bulimia and depression, *Arch Psychiat Nurs* 4(1):43-52, 1990.

Sutherland, SM, and Davidson, JRT: Pharmacotherapy for post-traumatic stress disorder, *Psychiat Clin North Am* 17:2:409-423, 1994.

Terr, L: Childhood traumas: an outline and overview, *Am J Psychiat* 148(1):10-20, 1991.

Terr, L: Children of Chowchilla, *Psychoanal Study Child* 34:547-623, 1979.

Trimble, MR: *Neuropsychiatry,* John Wiley & Sons, Chichester, 1981.

van der Kolk, BA: Psychopharmacological issues in posttraumatic stress disorder, *Hosp Commun Psychiat* 34:683-691, 1983.

van der Kolk, BA, Dreyfuss, D, Michaels, M, Shera, D, Berkowitz, R, Fisler, R, and Saxe, G: Fluoxetine in posttraumatic stress disorder, *J Clin Psychiat* 55(12):517-522, 1994.

van der Kolk, BA, Greenberg, MS, Orr, SP, and Pittman, RK: Endogenous opioids, stress induced analgesia, and posttraumatic stress disorder, *Psychopharmacol Bull* 25(3):417-421, 1989.

Westermeyer, J: A case of koro in a refugee family: Association with depression and folie a deux, *J Clin Psychiat* 50(5):181-183,1989.

Widom, CS: The cycle of violence, *Science* 244:160-166, 1989.

Yehuda, R, Giller Jr, EL, and Mason, JW: Psychoneuroendocrine assessment of posttraumatic stress disorder: Current progress and new directions, *Prog Neuro-Psychopharmacol Biol Psychiat* 17:541-550, 1993.

# Sexually Transmitted Diseases in Abused Children

Allan D. Friedman, M.D., M.P.H.

*A 2-year-old girl was admitted to the emergency room for dysuria and a purulent bloody vaginal discharge. A vaginal smear was covered with polymorphonuclear leukocytes, many having gram-negative diplococci intracellularly. The vaginal mucosa was edematous and erythematous, with copious purulent discharge.*

*The hospital called Social Services and notified the Division of Family Services, via the hot line, of suspected sexual abuse.*

*The following day the vaginal cultures were reported positive for Neisseria gonorrhoeae and Chlamydia trachomatis. The child was taken into protective custody and placed in a foster home.*

*Because the child was preverbal, examiners could obtain no history. The mother and stepfather denied any possibility of sexual abuse. They postulated that the child had acquired the infection from either a towel or bedding, since she slept between the parents and shared a towel with them. The stepfather and a 12-year-old sibling tested positive for gonorrhea. The mother was negative. The sibling also denied abusing the child. The perpetrator was not discovered and the case went unresolved. The child was returned to the parents. She was seen again at 4 years of age with another gonococcal infection. At that time she was acting out sexually and disclosed that her brother had abused her. The sibling tested positive for gonorrhea.*

Sexually transmitted diseases (STDs) are one of a few objective measures of sexual abuse in preadolescents (McIntyre, 1986). Until proven otherwise, an STD in a preadolescent means sexual abuse (Felman & Nikitas, 1983; Finkel, 1983). The spectrum of STDs that children acquire mimics that seen in adults. Therefore the practitioner must become familiar with the signs and symptoms of these infections, know how to properly establish the etiologic agent in these diseases, and know how to effectively treat the patient.

A thorough evaluation, including oral, rectal, and genital sites, is important if sexual abuse is suspected. The main infections for which children who are suspected victims of sexual abuse should be evaluated include gonorrhea, *Chlamydia*, syphilis, genital warts (human papillomavirus [HPV]), herpes simplex, *Trichomonas*, and human immunodeficiency virus (HIV). **Not all children with an STD infection will be symptomatic; therefore cultures should be obtained in all suspected cases of sexual abuse (De Jong, 1986).** Fifty percent of gonococcal infections in sexually abused children are asymptomatic. Thirty percent of these infections have been found in locations not reported by the children to have been involved in the abuse.

**Table 15-1** lists the screening studies for sexually transmitted diseases, recommended by the Centers for Disease Control and Prevention (CDC), in children suspected to be victims of sexual abuse. Ideally, all these studies should be obtained, although cost may dictate a more conservative approach.

*General guidelines for the evaluation of children who are believed to be sexually abused include the following:*

1. The interview and examination of children suspected to be sexually abused require special skills. Institutions providing health care for children should have a team of individuals who are trained to evaluate these children. If such a team is available, involve it in the workup.

2. For legal reasons, make certain all samples and cultures are labeled and logged carefully at all places where they are processed. Have them personally transported from the clinic or emergency room to the laboratory so as to ensure chain of custody.

3. If the child is believed to be sexually abused, contact Social Services immediately. Report the case via the hot line if it involves a caretaker or to the police sex crimes unit if it does not involve a caretaker. In the latter case, getting permission of the Division of Family Services or the parent is advisable before contacting the police. Do not discharge the child without first making sure he or she is going to a safe environment.

4. The majority of children (60% to 70%) have no physical findings of abuse. Do not let a negative examination influence your impression of sexual abuse or your decision to involve Social Services.

5. Do not begin therapy in symptomatic children before obtaining all appropriate samples. Therapy may be necessary in specific incidences before the organism and antibiotic sensitivities are known.

   Prophylactic antibiotics are not usually necessary in asymptomatic children suspected to be victims of sexual abuse. The infection rate is low in children, and prophylactic antibiotics are unlikely to prevent an infection. In addition, the risk of STD complications is low in children, and the risk of pelvic inflammatory disease and peritonitis is very low in prepubertal children.

6. Use an experienced reference laboratory. On occasion, inexperienced laboratories have mistaken nonsexually transmitted gonorrhea organisms for *Neisseria gonorrhoeae*. Also, some laboratories that primarily deal with adults

have used rapid diagnostic tests such as that for monoclonal antibodies in direct immunofluorescent stains or the enzyme-linked immunoassay test for *Chlamydia trachomatis* in children. These tests are neither sensitive nor specific enough and have too many false positives to be used in medical-legal cases. Too much is at stake to make these kinds of errors.

---

**Table 15-1. Summary of Suggested Laboratory Tests for Sexual Abuse**

**AIDS and Hepatitis B**
Test for HIV infection and hepatitis B if the perpetrator is in the high-risk group (drug user, homosexual, prostitute, multiple sex partners) for these infections or is known to be seropositive for these conditions. Some believe that with the high incidence of these infections in the population, all sexually abused children should be screened for these conditions. Perform follow-up test in 3 to 6 months.

*Neisseria gonorrhoeae*
Obtain rectal, throat, vaginal/urethral cultures.

In males, checking the first 10 ml of freshly voided urine for white blood cells can be an effective screening procedure. Obtain blood, joint fluid, and conjunctival cultures if clinically indicated.

*Chlamydia trachomatis*
Obtain vulvovaginal, urethral, rectal, pharyngeal cultures.

*Gardnerella vaginalis*
Wet preparation of vaginal secretions for clue cells and amine odor with 10% KOH solution.

*Herpes simplex*
Obtain lesion culture or vulva/cervix culture, if no lesions are present.

**Human papillomavirus**
Confirm clinical examination with biopsy and histological exam. Acetic acid (10%) solution can aid in detecting subclinical cases.

*Treponema pallidum,* **syphilis**
Perform VDRL, with follow-up test at 6 to 12 weeks.

*Trichomonas vaginalis*
Examine urine for organisms and culture vaginal secretions.

*In cases of acute assault, obtain follow-up cultures after 2 weeks and repeat serology testing after 6 weeks. Perform a pregnancy test in pubertal children, and repeat this test in 2 weeks in cases of acute assault.*

---

## ♦GONORRHEA

Gonorrhea is caused by the gram-negative intracellular diplococcal organism *Neisseria gonorrhoeae*. The organism is fragile and will not grow without proper culturing procedures. Although precise numbers are difficult to find, it has been estimated that between 3% and 26% of sexually abused children are infected with gonorrhea (Frau & Alexander, 1985). In the author's institution the incidence is about 1% in sexually abused children. The infection occurs only in humans. In the United States the infection is reported in about 1 million patients of all ages each year, but the actual number of cases is probably significantly greater (Friedman, 1987).

## CLINICAL PRESENTATION

Gonorrhea may be asymptomatic or may present as urethritis, cervicitis, vulvovaginitis, proctitis, conjunctivitis, pharyngitis, epididymitis, bartholinitis, or pelvic inflammatory disease (American Academy of Pediatrics, 1988).

In prepubertal females, gonococcal infections most frequently present as vulvovaginitis and urethritis. In postpubertal girls the presentation is usually cervicitis or pelvic inflammatory disease. In males the primary site of infection is the urethra, but urethritis is infrequent in prepubertal males. Bacteremic spread can result in arthritis, dermatitis, perihepatitis, meningitis, or endocarditis (American Academy of Pediatrics, 1988).

Incubation periods for gonorrhea vary with the infection site. Urethritis in males can occur as early as 2 to 5 days after infection. In females, symptoms may not occur until 2 weeks after exposure or later (Parish & Gschnait, 1989). This longer incubation period increases the risk of unknowingly spreading the infection to sexual partners.

Symptoms in females include vaginal discharge, frequency of micturition, dysuria, backache, lower abdominal pain, pelvic pain, and rectal discharge and bleeding. Local complications include skenitis. In males, uncomplicated gonorrhea presents as purulent urethral discharge with dysuria. Frequency may also be a symptom. The urethral discharge is often yellow or yellowish green, and the external urethral meatus may be swollen and red. Untreated, a posterior urethral infection may occur, which may result in pain, burning, urgency, and frequency with a few drops of blood at the end of micturition. Ultimately this can lead to prostatitis, epididymitis, vesiculitis, and cystitis.

Less common symptoms of gonorrhea result from the involvement of the rectal mucosa, the pharynx, and the conjunctiva. Symptoms of anorectal gonorrhea may be mild and cause anal pruritus, a mucopurulent discharge, and scant rectal bleeding. If severe, gonorrhea can cause an acute proctitis that presents as rectal pain, tenesmus, and constipation. The mucosa is often red, friable, edematous, and mucopurulent. Most anorectal infections are symptomatic.

Pharyngeal gonorrhea is usually symptomatic. Common findings are fever, sore throat, and cervical adenopathy.

After the neonatal period, gonococcal conjunctivitis is uncommon. It results from direct contamination of the eye, often from fomites or fingers (Parish & Gschnait, 1989).

Children appear to be more susceptible to gonococcal infection than adults. The vaginal mucosa in prepubertal girls is thin with an alkaline pH and a poor glycogen content, making vulvovaginitis more likely. The discharge may be profuse. The vulva may be swollen, red, and sore (Parish & Gschnait, 1989).

## LABORATORY DIAGNOSIS

Culture of the gonococcal organism is necessary to confirm the clinical diagnosis of gonococcal disease. In males, swabs from the urethra should be obtained for Gram stain and culture. In females, when possible, cervical and urethral specimens should be obtained. Because sexual abuse may involve other orifices, swabs should also be obtained from the anus and pharynx. The specimen should be directly plated onto appropriate media and placed in an optimal environment for growth. Modified Thayer-Martin media are commonly used and are effective in preventing overgrowth of other organisms and facilitating the growth of most *N. gonorrhoeae*.

Positive cultures for *N. gonorrhoeae* should be confirmed by a reference laboratory. As stated earlier, nonpathogenic *Neisseria* organisms can be mistaken for *N. gonorrhoeae*. Nonculture techniques for diagnosing gonorrhea are not appropriate in children because they lack the requisite sensitivity and specificity.

## THERAPY

Current recommendations for the treatment of gonorrhea are based on the following considerations: the spread of infections due to organisms resistant to older therapies, the strong association of gonorrhea with chlamydial infections, the risk of serious complications of untreated gonorrhea or chlamydial infection, and the lack of accurate, fast, inexpensive diagnostic tests for chlamydial infection. In addition, sexually abused children may also have pharyngeal and anal infections. Infections at these sites are less susceptible to traditional therapies.

Children less than 45 kg body weight who have gonococcal vulvovaginitis, cervicitis, urethritis, pharyngitis, or proctitis should receive 125 mg intramuscularly of ceftriaxone once. If the patient is unable to tolerate ceftriaxone therapy, he or she can receive 40 mg/kg of spectinomycin intramuscularly once (not effective for pharyngeal infection). Children 45 kg or greater should follow the adult regimen, which is 250 mg of ceftriaxone intramuscularly once or, if the patient cannot tolerate ceftriaxone, 2 gm of spectinomycin intramuscularly once. **Table 15-2** summarizes treatment of STDs in children. Other acceptable regimens include oral cefuroxime axetil with probenecid (1 gm of each); cefixime, 400 mg orally once; cefotaxime, 1 gm intramuscularly, and ceftizoxime, 500 mg intramuscularly, once.

In patients proven to have infection not resistant to penicillin, 3 gm of amoxicillin may be given orally with 1 gm of probenecid. All patients 8 years of age and older should also receive doxycycline, 100 mg orally, twice daily for 7 days.

---

**Table 15-2. Treatment of STDs in Children***

*Chlamydia trachomatis*
Erythromycin base 40-50 mg/kg/day $\times$ 7 days po *or* sulfisoxazole 120-150 mg/kg/day $\times$ 14 days po *or* tetracycline 500 mg q6h $\times$ 7 days po (> 8 yr old) *or* doxycyline 100 mg bid $\times$ 7 days po (> 8 yr old)

*Gardnerella vaginalis*
Metronidazole 15 mg/kg/day $\times$ 7 days po *or* clindamycin 300 mg bid $\times$ 7 days po (older children)

**Herpes simplex**
Acyclovir oral 200 mg 5 times daily for 10 days (older children); topical (5%) 5 times daily $\times$ 7 days

**Human papillomavirus**
Podophyllin (10%-20%), apply for 2-4 hours, then wash off

*Neisseria gonorrhoeae*
< 45 kg body weight: ceftriaxone 125 mg IM $\times$ 1 *or* spectinomycin 40 mg/kg IM $\times$ 1 (may fail to eradicate pharyngeal disease); $\geq$ 45 kg body weight: ceftriaxone 250 mg IM $\times$ 1 *or* spectinomycin 2 gm IM $\times$ 1

*Treponema pallidum*
Penicillin G (benzathine) 50 $\times$ 10 U/kg (up to 2.4 $\times$ 10 U) IM $\times$ 1 (early disease) *or* penicillin G (benzathine) 2.4 $\times$ 10 U IM q week $\times$ 3 (> 1 yr duration of disease) *or* penicillin G (aqueous crystalline) 20 $\times$ 10-30 $\times$ 10 U/kg/day (up to 2-4 $\times$ 10 U q 4 hr) IV $\times$ 10-14 days (CNS disease)

*Trichomonas vaginalis*
Metronidazole 15 mg/kg/day $\times$ 7-12 days po *or* metronidazole 2 gm po $\times$ 1 (adolescents) *or* metronidazole 500 mg po bid $\times$ 7 days (adolescents)

*\* Alternative treatment may exist.*

---

With disseminated disease, children weighing less than 45 kg should receive 50 mg/kg per day of ceftriaxone (maximum of 1 gm/day) for 7 days for bacteremia or arthritis, and 10 to 14 days of therapy for meningitis (maximum of 2 gm/day). After treatment is completed, cultures should be obtained to ensure that therapy was effective (Centers for Disease Control, 1989).

# ♦ CHLAMYDIAL INFECTIONS

*Chlamydia trachomatis* is the most common cause of sexually transmitted disease and is believed to account for as many as 3 million new infections each year (Holmes, 1981). As many as 20,000 adolescent females become sterile from their chlamydial infection each year (Schachter et al., 1975). Whenever a child has a chlamydial infection in the vagina or rectum, abuse must be considered. The infection reportedly can be contracted at birth; however, it is not known how long the infection can be carried asymptomatically and therefore at what age neonatal infection need no longer be considered (Ingram et al., 1986).

## CLINICAL PRESENTATION

The most common clinical presentation of chlamydial infection in females is cervicitis. However, asymptomatic infections are common. If the patient is symptomatic, a mucopurulent discharge is present initially. A purulent yellow discharge on a cervical swab introduced into the cervical canal indicates leukorrhea. Urethritis may also occur in female patients, often in association with cervicitis.

Symptoms often include dysuria and increased frequency of micturition (Stamm et al., 1980). In teenage and adult female patients, salpingitis may result from chlamydial infection and may lead to infertility. Symptoms of salpingitis, such as mild to moderate abdominal pain, may be absent. Other complications of chlamydial infection include perihepatitis, which often presents with acute, right upper quadrant abdominal pain, and endometritis (Muller-Schoop et al., 1978).

In males, urethritis is the most common symptomatic presentation of chlamydial infection, which is believed to be the most common cause of nongonococcal urethritis. Discharge, when present, is mucoid or mucopurulent. Symptoms develop 1 to 3 weeks after infection. Untreated, these patients may progress to epididymitis and infertility. Simultaneous infection with both *N. gonorrhoeae* and *C. trachomatis* may result in a recurrence of symptoms after appropriate gonococcal therapy due to the longer incubation time for the chlamydial infection. Proctitis and Reiter's syndrome may also occur as a result of chlamydial infection (Holmes et al., 1975).

## LABORATORY DIAGNOSIS

Both serological and cell culture methods are available for the diagnosis of chlamydial infection. Serologic methods, however, are of limited value because of the high prevalence of chlamydial antibodies in the population. Cultures are highly specific, but the sensitivity depends on obtaining an adequate specimen. Appropriate cultures are obtained by vigorously swabbing the site so that cells attach to the swab. Either cotton wool or calcium alginate-tipped swabs can be used to collect the specimen (Schachter et al., 1979).

Using chlamydial antigen detection tests to evaluate suspected sexual abuse in children has been largely unsuccessful. Both false positive and false negative results have been reported. Because of the profound implications for both the victim and the accused, accurate diagnosis is essential. Therefore adequate cultures must be obtained (Fuster & Neinstein, 1987; Hammerschlag et al., 1988).

## THERAPY

Children 8 years of age or older can be treated according to the adult regimen. Treatment is doxycycline, 100 mg orally, twice daily for 7 days, or tetracycline,

500 mg orally, four times a day for 7 days. Alternative therapy for simple cervicitis or urethritis is azithromycin, 1 gm orally, once. Younger children or children who are unable to take the tetracyclines can receive erythromycin base in a dose of 40 to 50 mg/kg per day, by mouth, four times a day for 7 days or erythromycin ethylsuccinate, 40 to 50 mg/kg per day orally, four times a day for 7 days. Children unable to tolerate erythromycin receive sulfisoxazole or amoxicillin, although few clinical data are available regarding the efficacy of the alternative regimens (Centers for Disease Control, 1989).

## ◆BACTERIAL VAGINOSIS

Previously called nonspecific vaginitis, bacterial vaginosis is a result of overgrowth of *Gardnerella vaginalis* and anaerobes. This condition is thought to affect children infrequently, as the organisms prefer an estrogenic vagina; nevertheless, the organism can occasionally be recovered from prepubertal girls. Although the organism can be recovered from the male urethra, it is not clear what role male colonization with the organism has in female infection or if there is a symptomatic condition associated with this infection in males (Spagna & Prior, 1985; Bartley et al., 1987).

The organism is more prevalent in sexually active adolescent males and females. It is also more common in sexually abused children than in controls. Although the organism is not pathognomonic for sexual abuse, its presence should raise suspicion about possible sexual abuse.

### CLINICAL PRESENTATION

Adults with bacterial vaginosis may be asymptomatic. The classic symptoms are a foul-smelling, fishy vaginal odor that in postpubertal females may increase with menses and after intercourse (Spagna & Prior, 1985). The patient may have a discharge that is thin, gray, and homogeneous. The pH of the discharge is greater than 4.5, and the fishy odor becomes obvious after mixing KOH with the discharge.

Children may be asymptomatic. Symptoms may include pruritus and the classic discharge described for adults. Occasionally the discharge is more white than gray (Parish & Gschnait, 1989).

### LABORATORY DIAGNOSIS

The presence of a discharge with a foul, fishy smell on adding 10% KOH is helpful in making the diagnosis of bacterial vaginosis. Further evidence of infection is the presence of clue cells on Gram stain or Papanicolaou stain. Usually few white blood cells are found (Parish & Gschnait, 1989). Culture of the discharge or of a vaginal swab for *G. vaginalis* is of controversial value because, at least in postpubertal females, the organism may be present as nonpathogenic flora (Spagna & Prior, 1985). Nevertheless, its presence in children should always raise concern about possible sexual abuse.

### THERAPY

The treatment of *G. vaginalis* is 15 mg/kg per day of metronidazole given orally in three divided doses for 7 days. In older children and adults the infection can be treated with 500 mg orally twice a day for 7 days. Patients unable to take metronidazole can be treated with clindamycin 300 mg by mouth twice a day for 7 days (Centers for Disease Control, 1989).

## ◆SYPHILIS

In children, syphilis is almost always sexually transmitted. The causative organism is *Treponema pallidum*, a spirochetal organism with an incubation period of about 3 weeks. In children, syphilis undergoes a primary and a secondary stage. In adults a tertiary stage can also occur. In one series, about 6% of sexually abused children were infected with *T. pallidum* (Frau & Alexander, 1985). In the author's institution, however, the incidence of syphilis in postnatal sexually abused children has been essentially zero. This is consistent with other centers. A survey of 80 physicians showed that only 25 children had syphilis in a population of 49,000 sexually abused children. All these tested children were infected with other sexually transmitted diseases. Though the incidence of syphilis is believed to be low in these children, with the recent rise in syphilis in the adult population it is prudent to screen all children who have been sexually abused.

## CLINICAL PRESENTATION

Primary syphilis presents with a macule that evolves into a papule. The surface of the lesion then erodes with a sharply defined border. The lesion contains serous material. Usually only one primary lesion develops. This chancre is painless and is associated with nonsuppurative regional lymphadenopathy. It heals without therapy in 3 to 8 weeks.

The second stage occurs about 6 to 8 weeks after the chancre appears. A nonpruritic rash may develop that is maculopapular and generalized and involves the palms and soles.

Mucosal lesions, called mucous patches, and enlarged nontender lymph nodes may also be present. Skin lesions contain the organism and are a source of spread of the infection (Chapel, 1980). Less commonly, alopecia, periostitis, hepatomegaly, and acute glomerulonephritis may occur (Crissey & Denenholz, 1984).

## LABORATORY DIAGNOSIS

Spirochetes can be identified by dark-field microscopic examination of specimens taken from moist areas. False negative results are common. Reliable nontreponemal tests for syphilis include the Venereal Disease Reference Laboratory (VDRL) slide test, the rapid reagin (RPR) card test, and the automated reagin test (ART). These tests are convenient rapid screens that are useful in indicating disease activity. False-positive nontreponemal tests can occur in patients with connective tissue disease, tuberculosis, and endocarditis. False negatives occur in early primary syphilis and in late disease.

Specific treponemal tests should be performed to confirm results. These tests include the fluorescent treponemal antibody absorption (FTA-ABS) test, the microhemagglutination test (MHA-TP), and the immobilization test (TPI). FTA-ABS and MHA-TP remain positive for life even after successful treatment. The TPI is rarely used today.

## THERAPY

The recommended treatment for early acquired syphilis, which includes primary, secondary, and latent disease of less than 1 year's duration, is penicillin G (benzathine), intramuscularly, 50,000 units/kg, but not to exceed 2.4 million units. If patients are allergic to penicillin, they can receive tetracycline, 2 gm/day, by mouth, divided into four doses for at least 15 days. If the child is 8 years or younger, treatment may be either hospitalization and desensitization of the child to penicillin or the use of erythromycin for 15 days with good follow-up, since erythromycin is not believed to be as effective as penicillin or tetracycline (Centers for Disease Control, 1989).

## ◆ HERPES SIMPLEX

Approximately 10% of the adult population has symptomatic genital herpes (Friedman, 1987). Although herpes simplex type 2 is more commonly associated with genital infection, type 1 can also be found. After the neonatal period the presence of herpes lesions, especially in the genital region, strongly suggests sexual abuse.

Fomite transmission of the disease is unlikely. Transmission requires direct contact of live virus with a mucous membrane or an abraded skin area of the person becoming infected.

Other viruses and bacteria that cause lesions in the genital area of children can resemble herpes simplex. Viral cultures should, therefore, be obtained from all suspect lesions.

## CLINICAL PRESENTATION

Symptoms of herpes simplex vary from mild to severe. Soreness, itching, and dysuria along with inguinal or femoral lymphadenopathy are common. Systemic symptoms such as headache and fever may also occur. Female patients with primary herpes may experience erosive cervicitis and vaginal discharge. Males may have urethritis with dysuria. There may be little or no discharge. Lesions, if present, start as vesicles or vesiculopustules and are often found on the shaft of the penis or the vulva. These lesions ulcerate and are painful. Healing begins during the second week and is complete by the end of the third week. Recurrent infections are milder. Contact with lesions spreads the disease, but infection may be present without obvious lesions (Friedman, 1987).

## LABORATORY DIAGNOSIS

Lesions can be scraped and stained with Giemsa or Papanicolaou stains for multinucleated giant cells. This test is highly suggestive but not diagnostic, as other herpes viruses may also stain positively. A more specific test is immunofluorescent staining against herpes simplex antigen. Both tests require a good specimen from an unroofed lesion. Diagnostic confirmation is by viral culture for herpes simplex. Cultures are positive in 40 to 72 hours.

## THERAPY

Acyclovir is effective in treating primary herpes infections. The drug is available in topical, oral, and intravenous forms. Topical therapy can be applied six times a day for 7 days. Oral therapy (200 mg capsules) given five times a day for 7 to 10 days is available for older children.

For serious infection, intravenous therapy is available (Nelson, 1989). Recurrences of genital herpes infection are common. Although usually symptomatic, recurrences can be asymptomatic. In patients with frequent recurrences, the long-term administration of oral acyclovir can decrease the frequency of infection as long as the patient continues to take the medicine.

## ♦HUMAN PAPILLOMAVIRUS

Condyloma acuminatum is an infection caused by human papillomavirus (HPV). The incidence of these infections reportedly has increased more than 450% since 1954. Most patients are between 15 and 29 years of age, but infections have been reported in children and, when present, must lead to a suspicion of sexual abuse (Norins et al., 1984). Neonates, however, may acquire the infection while passing through the birth canal. Condyloma infection in the first 2 years of life is likely the result of contact during delivery, although sexual abuse is still a possibility. Since these children are preverbal, if there are no other physical or historical findings consistent with sexual abuse, it must be assumed the infection is not due to sexual abuse. Other members of the family should be examined for possible lesions, even if they are asymptomatic.

The incubation period for HPV is 3 to 20 months. Among the consequences of infection in children are the concerns about the oncogenicity of certain strains of the virus (HPV-16, HPV-18) and the possibility of transmission (Schachner & Hankin, 1985). Spread is by direct contact with the lesions.

## CLINICAL PRESENTATION

Genital and anorectal lesions are flesh colored, focal, and verrucous tumors. Lesions on the cervix are flat and wart-like. These lesions may be missed by the naked eye but can show up in colposcopy. In males the lesions are typically skin colored, slightly pink, or white verrucous papules. They may be solitary lesions or confluent, forming the typical cauliflower appearance. They may appear anywhere along the penile shaft or on the glans. Anal and perianal lesions also may occur. Lesions in both sexes range from small and painless to large, ulcerated lesions that are secondarily infected. These lesions may be pruritic and burn.

Infection can be subclinical. An application of acetic acid (10%) turns nonapparent lesions white. The solution should be allowed to remain in contact with the suspected area for 5 to 10 minutes before determining that this test is negative for HPV lesions. The solution is painful when applied to mucous membranes. Care must be taken when deciding to use it on children.

## LABORATORY DIAGNOSIS

Histological examination is diagnostic. Characteristic findings include acanthosis, papillomatosis, and parakeratosis of the epithelial projections. Koilocytotic cells are visible in the upper stratum malpighii.

## THERAPY

Condyloma acuminatum is treated topically. Infected areas should be kept cool and dry. Podophyllin, 10% to 20%, should be administered and then washed off after about 2 to 4 hours. Alternative therapies include trichloroacetic acid, electrocautery, and cryotherapy. Human lymphoblastoid interferon has also been used successfully (Centers for Disease Control, 1989).

## ◆ TRICHOMONIASIS

*Trichomonas vaginalis* is the protozoon responsible for trichomoniasis. It is uncommon in prepubescent patients and can be transmitted both sexually and nonsexually. In adults the prevalence varies from 5% to 75%, depending on the population studied (White et al., 1983).

## CLINICAL PRESENTATION

*T. vaginalis* infection is often asymptomatic. Infected females are more likely to be symptomatic than males. Erythema and edema of the external genitalia are often present. A frothy, gray discharge may occur. The patient may have vaginitis along with symptoms of cervicitis and punctate hemorrhages (White et al., 1983). Untreated, the infection may progress to prostatitis and salpingitis.

## LABORATORY DIAGNOSIS

The parasite is a motile protozoan that can be seen under microscopy. A specimen of vaginal discharge should be placed on a wet mount slide preparation with a drop of saline solution. The swimming motion of the organism is visible. Alternative means of identification are culture and Papanicolaou smear. Because the wet mount test for diagnosing *T. vaginalis* infections has been shown to miss 40% of those proven by culture, in children suspected to be infected with *T. vaginalis*, cultures and wet mount should be done.

## THERAPY

The drug of choice is oral metronidazole, 15 mg/kg/day, divided into three doses, for 7 to 10 days. In older children and adults, 2 gm of metronidazole may be given once or 500 mg twice a day for 7 days.

## ◆ ACQUIRED IMMUNODEFICIENCY SYNDROME (AIDS)

The human immunodeficiency virus (HIV) is the causative agent of AIDS. Fortunately, few reported cases of AIDS have been attributable to sexual abuse. The risk of transmitting the disease during sexual contact is well-documented, however, and the consequence of infection can be devastating.

HIV is particularly tropic for CD4 (T-helper) lymphocytes and macrophages. Humans are the only reservoir of HIV. The incubation period for this infection is variable, and infection acquired in adolescence may not result in clinical disease until adulthood.

### CLINICAL PRESENTATION

The spectrum of disease caused by HIV infection ranges from asymptomatic to full-blown, devastating, opportunistic infection in a severely debilitated, immunocompromised host. Common clinical findings include lymphadenopathy, hepatosplenomegaly, parotitis, recurrent diarrhea, failure to thrive, progressive neurological disease, recurrent invasive bacterial infections and opportunistic infections, malignancies, and lymphoid interstitial pneumonia. Opportunistic organisms commonly occurring in children with HIV infection include *Pneumocystis carinii, Candida, Mycobacterium, Avium-intracellularae*, and *Cryptosporidium*.

### LABORATORY DIAGNOSIS

HIV infection can be detected by serological testing. Enzyme-linked immunosorbent assays (ELISA) with confirmatory Western blot and immunofluorescent antibody testing are used. Serological tests may not become positive for months after infection has occurred, so retesting is indicated. Because symptoms resulting from infection may be delayed months to years, children suspected of sexual abuse should be evaluated for HIV infection along with the other infections. If the perpetrator is known, he or she should be tested for HIV infection. The victim should also be tested for baseline HIV status and retested at least one more time, 3 to 6 months later, during which period most infected people develop antibodies.

### THERAPY

Currently, HIV infection has no cure. Drugs reported to have a beneficial effect on the progression of the disease include azidothymidine (AZT), also called zidovudine; dideoxyinosine (ddI); and dideoxycytidine (ddC). Management also involves the treatment and prevention of secondary infections (Centers for Disease Control, 1989).

## ◆ MOLLUSCUM CONTAGIOSUM

While molluscum contagiosum is often sexually transmitted in adults, in children it is easily spread by casual contact. Without a reliable history of sexual abuse, molluscum in children should be considered nonsexually transmitted. When genital lesions are present in children, a careful history usually reveals that the lesions began on other parts of the body.

## ◆ MISCELLANEOUS INFECTIONS

Many other infections can be spread through sexual contact but have a relatively low incidence in the United States.

Although examiners do not routinely screen for them, chancroid (*Hemophilus ducreyi*), lymphogranuloma venereum (*C. trachomatis,* LGV serovars), viral hepatitis (mostly hepatitis B), and ectoparasites (pediculosis pubis, scabies) are other diseases that should be considered in abused children.

## ♦ SUMMARY

While not all of the illnesses discussed in this chapter are exclusively transmitted sexually, in most cases it would be inappropriate to assume nonsexual transmission before doing a full evaluation of the child. Many of these infections can be asymptomatic. A child suspected of being sexually abused requires a full workup to identify both symptomatic and asymptomatic infections. **Table 15-2** summarizes treatment for the infections discussed in this chapter.

When evaluating children for sexually transmitted diseases, the practitioner should keep in mind that it is common for more than one disease to be transmitted at the same time. It is therefore essential to do a comprehensive evaluation. The presence of one infection makes the presence of another more, not less, likely.

## ♦ BIBLIOGRAPHY

American Academy of Pediatrics, Committee on Infectious Diseases: *Report of the Committee on Infectious Diseases*, Elk Grove Village, IL, 1988, pp. 193-203.

Bartley, DL, Morgan, L, et al: *Gardnerella vaginalis* in prepubertal girls, *Am J Dis Child* 141:1014-1017, 1987.

Centers for Disease Control: *1989 Sexually Transmitted Diseases Treatment Guidelines,* US Department of Health and Human Services, 1989, pp. 21-26.

Chapel, TA: The signs and symptoms of secondary syphilis, *Sex Transm Dis* 7:161-164, 1980.

Crissey, JT, and Denenholz, DA: Syphilis, *Clin Dermatol* 2:1-166, 1984.

DeJong, AR: Sexually transmitted diseases in sexually abused children, *Sex Transm Dis* 13:123-126, 1986.

Feigin, R, and Cherry, J: *Textbook of Pediatric Infectious Diseases*, ed 3, WB Saunders Co, Philadelphia, 1992.

Felman, YM, and Nikitas, JA: Sexually transmitted diseases and child sexual abuse, Part 1, *NY State J Med* 83:341-343, 1983.

Finkel, KC: *Recognition and Assessment of the Sexually Abused Child*, Ontario Medical Association, Toronto, 1983.

Frau, LM, and Alexander, ER: Public health implications of sexually transmitted diseases in pediatric practice, *Pediatr Infect Dis* 4:453-467, 1985.

Friedman, AD: *Handbook of Pediatric Infectious Diseases*, Ishiyaku EuroAmerica Inc, St. Louis, 1987, pp. 109-111.

Fuster, CD, and Neinstein, LS: *Vaginal Chlamydia trachomatis* prevalence in sexually abused prepubertal girls, *Pediatrics* 79:235-238, 1987.

Hammerschlag, M, and Rawstron, S: Sexually transmitted diseases. In S Krugman, S Katz, A Gershon, and C Wilfert, eds: *Infectious Diseases of Children*, ed 9, Mosby-Year Book, St. Louis, 1992, pp. 419-456.

Hammerschlag, MR, Rettig, PJ, and Shields, ME: False positive results with the rise of chlamydial antigen detection tests in the evaluation of suspected sexual abuse in children, *Pediatr Infect Dis* 7:11-12, 1988.

Holmes, KK: The chlamydia epidemic, *JAMA* 245:428-435, 1981.

Holmes, KK, Handsfield, HH, Wang, SP, et al: Etiology of non-gonococcal urethritis, *N Engl J Med* 292:1109-1205, 1975.

Ingram, DL, White, ST, Occhiuti, AR, et al: Childhood vaginal infections: Association of *Chlamydia trachomatis* with sexual contact, *Pediatr Infect Dis* 5:226-229, 1986.

McIntyre, L: Sexual abuse and sexually transmitted diseases in children, *CMAJ* 134:1272-1273, 1986.

Muller-Schoop, JW, Wang, SP, Munzinger, J, et al: *C. trachomatis* as a possible cause of peritonitis and perihepatitis in young women, *Br Med J* 1:1022-1024, 1978.

Nelson, JD: *Pocketbook of Pediatric Antimicrobial Therapy*, ed 8, The Williams & Wilkins Co, Baltimore, 1989, p. 36.

Norins, AL, et al: Genital warts and sexual abuse, *J Am Acad Dermatol* 11:529-530, 1984.

Parish, LC, and Gschnait, F: *Sexually Transmitted Diseases, A Guide for Clinicians*, Springer-Verlag, New York, 1989, pp. 59-76.

Schachner, L, and Hankin, DE: Assessing child abuse in childhood condyloma acuminatum, *J Am Acad Dermatol* 12:157-160, 1985.

Schachter, J, Cles, L, Ray, R, et al: Failure of serology in diagnosing chlamydial infections of the female genital tract, *J Clin Microbiol* 10:647-649, 1979.

Schachter, J, Hanna, L, Hill, EC, et al: Are chlamydial infections the most prevalent venereal disease? *JAMA* 231:1252-1255, 1975.

Spagna, VA, and Prior, RB: *Sexually Transmitted Diseases, A Clinical Syndrome Approach*, Marcel Dekker, Inc, New York, 1985, pp. 147-152.

Stamm, WE, Wagner, KF, Amsel, R, et al: Causes of the acute urethral syndrome in women, *N Engl J Med* 303:409-415, 1980.

White, ST, Loda, FA, Ingnam, DL, et al: Sexually transmitted diseases in sexually abused children, *Pediatrics* 72:16-21, 1983.

# Poisoning

Kevin Coulter, M.D.
Anthony J. Scalzo, M.D., F.A.A.P., A.C.M.T.

*A 13-month-old boy was seen in the emergency room because of convulsions. The mother and boyfriend both smelled of alcohol, and social services was notified.*

*The child was found to have a blood glucose level of 15 mg/100 ml; the etiology of the convulsion was determined to be hypoglycemia, with alcohol-induced hypoglycemia suspected. A blood alcohol level was obtained and the child reported to the Division of Family Services via the abuse hot line for suspected abuse, specifically alcohol poisoning. The blood alcohol level was determined to be significantly elevated. The mother initially denied any possibility of the child ingesting alcohol but later acknowledged that the boyfriend had convinced her to give the child vodka to "help him sleep."*

Poisoning is one of the most common medical emergencies faced by health practitioners caring for children. It accounts for numerous emergency room visits and is a significant cause of pediatric morbidity and mortality. The Centers for Disease Control in 1986 reported 4,740 unintentional poisoning deaths. Of these deaths, 93 were children under 5 years, 24 were between 5 and 9 years, and 249 were adolescents (Olsen & Banner, 1991). A review of calls to 63 poison control centers participating in a national data collection program during 1987 disclosed 1.2 million ingestion cases. In this study, 60% of the ingestion cases involved children under the age of 5 years, 22 children died, and 107,844 had symptoms of poisoning. In another study the median age of the victims, 2 years, was similar to that in physical abuse, and indeed, evidence of coincident battering was present in 20% of the children (Dine, 1982). The most common agents used were found to be salt (eight cases), water (six cases), tranquilizers (six cases), and barbiturates (five cases). Unusual causes are sometimes seen. In one case report, of a 21-month-old child, a baby-sitter used hydrochloric acid (Gotschlich & Beltran, 1995). In his landmark discussion of the battered child syndrome in 1962, Kempe was the first to propose poisoning as part of the spectrum of injury in child abuse. As he stated, "In an occasional case the parent, or parent-substitute, may also have assaulted the child by administering an overdose of a drug or by exposing the child to natural gas or other toxic substances" (Kempe et al., 1962).

Poisoning as it relates to child abuse can occur in two major contexts: as an intentional act or as the result of neglect. Each has its own implications and complexities. Over the past 30 years, intentional poisoning has remained an uncommon form of reported child abuse. Yet cases continue to be identified (Dees & Dees, 1993). Similarities in the epidemiology of abuse and poisoning point to two overlapping and possibly frequently related problems. Both of these "environmental dangers" are commonly seen in children under 5 years of age and in social settings marked by similar stresses. Marital discord, unemployment, parental psychiatric disturbances, inadequate housing, and geographic mobility are common factors in both child abuse and poisoning. The similarities are not surprising when considering the relationship between neglect and the child with repeated ingestions. While many pediatric ingestions may represent a failure to provide adequate protection in chaotic, stress-burdened homes (acts of omission), health practitioners must remember that some ingestions, the exact proportion being unknown, result from intentional poisoning (acts of commission) (Kresel & Lovejoy, 1981).

## ♦ INTENTIONAL POISONING

Since Kempe first suggested that poisoning could be nonaccidental, scattered reports of this type of abuse have appeared in the literature. The intentional poisoning of children seems to occur by two general mechanisms: the acute assault of a child by forced ingestion or aspiration of a drug or other substance as a method of discipline. Case reports of these types of abuse in the literature include the forced ingestion of water through a garden hose in a 4-year-old boy who developed hyponatremic seizures (Mortimer, 1980) and homicidal pepper aspiration (Cohle et al., 1988).

### CHARACTERISTICS OF THE PERPETRATOR

Cases of abuse are usually perpetrated by an individual with poor impulse control, a low tolerance for a child's upsetting behavior, and a tendency to act out violently against the child using a poison. While some of these cases undoubtedly represent a deranged individual attempting to directly harm a child, other cases can be viewed as a spectrum of parental dysfunction in attempting to cope with the stresses of caring for children. In a 2-year prospective study looking at cases of Munchausen Syndrome by Proxy, intentional poisoning and nonaccidental suffocation, it was found that on 85% of the occasions the perpetrator was the child's mother

(McClure et al., 1996). At one end of the spectrum are the young parents distressed by their fussy, colicky infant. They may try at times, with the direction of their physician, to sedate their infant with an antihistamine or paregoric. Usually this does not prove to be injurious. There is the danger that the parents will continuously increase the dose to accomplish sedation without awareness of the potential ill effects that can be associated with these agents. In addition, with highly stressed, impulsive parents the situation may escalate to physical abuse, often by shaking, or possibly to chemical abuse with doses of potent sedatives such as alcohol or narcotics. At the far end of this spectrum are adults or older children who intentionally introduce children to the effects of illicit drugs. A recent survey was conducted of adolescent females in a drug treatment program who had been babysitters. Nine girls (11%) stated they had blown marijuana smoke into the faces or mouths of the children being cared for in an attempt to make them "high" (Schwartz et al., 1986). In a far more malicious setting, pedophiles may attempt to chemically sedate children before molesting them.

## Munchausen Syndrome by Proxy

A mechanism for intentional poisoning that occurs only rarely is Munchausen Syndrome by Proxy (MSBP). Briefly, this syndrome is defined as an illness in a child that is simulated or produced by a parent, usually the mother. The illness is frequently dramatic and results in repeated visits to physicians, leading to multiple diagnostic and therapeutic procedures. The perpetrator of this medical hoax denies any knowledge of the cause of the illness. Physical signs of illness usually promptly resolve when the child is separated from the perpetrator. In cases of MSBP where disease is actually produced, surreptitious poisoning of the child is a common mechanism. In a review of published cases of MSBP (Rosenberg, 1987), seven of the eight most common presentations of MSBP were poisoning (**Table 16-1**); the lone common presentation not involving poisoning was fever. In the majority of cases where actual illness was produced, including that produced by poisoning, the abuse continued after the child was admitted to the hospital. The placement of intravenous lines or gastrostomy tubes while in the hospital in some cases afforded other routes of poisoning (Saulsbury et al., 1984).

*For a more complete review of MSBP, refer to Chapter 17.*

| **Table 16-1. Munchausen Syndrome by Proxy** |
|---|
| *Presentations Produced by Poisoning* |
| Bleeding |
| Seizures |
| CNS depression |
| Apnea |
| Diarrhea |
| Vomiting |
| Fever |

## Neglect

While all childhood poisonings represent some degree of lack of proper supervision, it can be difficult to decide when a poisoning has resulted from true neglect. In an important study on the epidemiology of caustic ingestions, no difference was found in the number of safety hazards or safety precautions between homes where the ingestions occurred and control homes (Sobel, 1970). Similar factors appear in studies of homes of children who have experienced multiple ingestions. Sobel's and other studies consistently show that the common denominator in homes with accidental ingestions is not neglect but significant family stress. Marital conflicts, mental or physical illness, transiency, and other factors combined with poor coping mechanisms for stress seem to set the stage for poisonings. The resultant poisoning brings to the attention of the health care provider the child whose basic needs are unmet. The child may appear dirty, malnourished, and lack immunizations. There may be a delay in seeking medical care for the ingestion because the child is left unattended for long periods of time or the parents have been in a prolonged alcohol- or drug-induced stupor. When neglect is suspected, child protective services must be contacted to save the child from further harm (Fischler, 1983).

As noted, neglect may be a factor in some poisonings involving families with parental drug and alcohol abuse. As the extent and variety of drug use have proliferated over the latter portion of this century, the risk of ingestion of these drugs by children has similarly increased. Case reports of phencyclidine ingestion began to appear in the 1970s. Poisonings were presumed to have occurred from passive inhalation in a smoke-filled car. Younger children especially may be at increased risk of passive exposure to the smoke of crack cocaine because of their decreased mobility, although this remains an unproven theory. Accidental ingestion of PCP crystals left from a party was cited in one report (Schwartz & Einhorn, 1986). Benzodiazepines, opiates, and methamphetamines have been detected in children poisoned in drug-abusing environments (Bays, 1990).

## ILLICIT DRUG USE

The danger to a child living in the presence of illicit drug use includes not only the prenatal effects of drug exposure and the increased risks of neglect and physical abuse postnatally (Leventhal et al., 1989), but also the risk of the child actually ingesting an illicit drug. Close proximity to recreational drugs can result in the poisoning of a child through four possible routes: passive inhalation, accidental ingestion of drugs left around the home, accepting drugs from an older child or other nonparent adult, or deliberate poisoning (Schwartz et al., 1986).

The phrase "morning after syndrome" was first used to describe children poisoned by ethanol after sampling alcohol left out in the home, frequently from a party the night before. Typically these children came to the emergency room obviously intoxicated and then progressed to seizures and coma secondary to alcohol-induced hypoglycemia (Tolis, 1965).

### COCAINE INTOXICATION

As the epidemic of cocaine use has spread, reports of cocaine intoxication in young children have appeared. Apnea and seizures have been reported in infants exposed to cocaine in breast milk (Chasnoff et al., 1987) and in a breast-fed infant whose mother placed topical cocaine on her painful nipples (Chaney, 1988). Much of the epidemic of cocaine use has been fueled by the ready availability of the relatively cheap form of freebase cocaine referred to as "crack," which is easily vaporized by heat and then smoked. Passive inhalation of these cocaine vapors was the presumed route of ingestion of four children who were seen at Harlem Hospital, two of whom had seizures and two of whom were lethargic. Toxicological screens of the urine identified the presence of cocaine in all four children (Bateman & Heagerty, 1989). One of these children, who also presented with burns of uncertain etiology, also had an opiate found in the urine. In this case, deliberate poisoning seems a more likely mechanism. Oral ingestion of cocaine was believed to have caused seizures reported in four children under 3 years old who were unexpectedly found to have cocaine on routine urine toxicologic screening (Ernst & Sanders, 1989). On further evaluation by social services, all the children were found to have been in the company of cocaine-abusing adults. One infant, a 4-month-old, was believed to have been intentionally fed cocaine in an attempt to quiet her.

In addition to the ingestion of cocaine, the chemicals used in the conversion of cocaine hydrochloric acid to freebase cocaine ("crack") can be a serious hazard. A 20-month-old child who sustained severe caustic esophageal burns requiring gastrostomy feedings and central hyperalimentation has been reported. The injury occurred after the ingestion of a lye solution, which was used in making freebase cocaine. The lye had been left in her home following a party. This child's urine was also positive for cocaine metabolites (Kharasch et al., 1990).

Children who have clinical evidence of acute cocaine poisoning are likely to be only a small portion of all children who actively or passively ingest cocaine. This was demonstrated in a survey of children between 2 weeks and 5 years of age presenting to the emergency room at Boston City Hospital (Kharasch et al., 1991). In those children who did not have life-threatening emergencies or any history suggestive of cocaine exposure, the urine was screened for cocaine metabolites. Of 250 children whose urine was collected before discharge from the emergency room, six (2.4%) tested positive for cocaine. All of the children testing positive were younger than 2 years of age, and four of the six were less than 1 year old. Only one of these children was being breast-fed at the time of the study.

Regardless of the mechanism by which cocaine gains access to children's bodies, it seems clear that children in close proximity to this drug are at significant risk. They may not show obvious clinical signs of exposure, but can be at risk of behavioral, intellectual, and physical damage from repeated exposure. Although it may be difficult to determine the mechanism of ingestion in any given case of a child poisoned by an illicit drug, child protective services should be routinely involved in evaluating the home situation. Whether it is the purposeful intoxication of children by parents or babysitters (Schwartz et al., 1986) or an accidental ingestion, one must presume the child is a victim of abuse or neglect and act accordingly.

## ♦ MANAGEMENT

### HISTORY

In most incidents involving accidental poisoning the ingestion is either witnessed or is discovered soon after ingestion. The child still has the container in hand, with the pills or solution in the mouth or nearby. Usually little has been ingested and the child has no symptoms, or very mild, transient symptoms. Death is an uncommon occurrence following accidental ingestion. Accidental poisoning can also occur in homes that have not been child-proofed, for example, at a friend's or relative's home where there are no children.

The child who has been poisoned by intent or neglect presents with a confusing or misleading history. *One of four presentations commonly occurs (Meadow, 1989):*

1.  A parent brings the child to the hospital for treatment of an acute poisoning under the guise of an accidental ingestion.

2.  A child presents with signs and symptoms of unknown etiology.

3.  The child presents with recurrent unexplained illnesses (MSBP).

**Table 16-2. Symptoms and Signs Following Intentional Poisoning**

| Symptoms and Signs | Drug | Reference |
|---|---|---|
| *Seizures* | Phenothiazine | Dine, 1965 |
| | Hydrocarbons | Saulsbury et al., 1984 |
| | Salt | Rogers et al., 1976 |
| | Water | Mortimer, 1980 |
| | Cocaine | Rivkin & Gilmore, 1989 |
| *Drowsiness, coma* | Tricyclic antidepressants | Simon, 1980 |
| | Chloral hydrate | Lansing, 1974 |
| | Insulin | Bauman & Yalow, 1981 |
| | Acetaminophen | Hickson et al., 1983 |
| | Salicylates | Pickering, 1976 |
| | Phenothiazines | Schnaps et al., 1981 |
| | Barbiturates | Rogers et al., 1976; Lorber, 1978 |
| | Opiates | Rogers et al., 1976 |
| | Valium | Dine, 1982 |
| | Alcohol | Dine, 1982 |
| | Glutethimide | Dine, 1982 |
| *Apnea* | Tricyclic antidepressants | Watson et al., 1979 |
| | Salt | Rogers et al., 1976 |
| | Pepper | Cohle et al., 1988 |
| *Vomiting* | Ipecac | Sutphen & Saulsbury, 1986 |
| *Diarrhea* | Phenolphthalein | Fleisher & Ament, 1977 |
| | Epsom salts | Fenton et al., 1988 |

4. The child is found dead or near death because of significant time lapse since ingestion.

Given the confusing history, the physician must be alert to the myriad signs and symptoms children can manifest after an ingestion. **Table 16-2** lists common presenting signs and symptoms reported in intentionally poisoned children with their respective etiologies.

## PHYSICAL EXAMINATION

Various drug ingestions in children can rapidly lead to severe depression of the central nervous system and coma. The physical examination can differentiate drug-induced encephalopathy from the other common causes of coma in children, such as mass lesions and seizures. Intact pupillary reflexes to light in the comatose patient indicate a functional midbrain. In most forms of metabolic coma, including drug-induced, pupillary reflexes remain intact.

The physical examination can also enable the physician to identify a specific toxicological syndrome accounting for the patient's unexplained symptoms (**Table 16-3**).

### Table 16-3. Identifying Specific Toxicological Syndrome

| Poison Syndrome | Signs and Symptoms | Drugs |
|---|---|---|
| *Sympathomimetic* | Increased pulse and blood pressure, fever, pupillary dilatation, sweating, agitation, psychosis | Cocaine, barbiturates, phencyclidine |
| *Sympatholytic* | Decreased pulse and blood pressure, hypothermia, small pupils, decreased peristalsis, obtundation, coma | Ethanol, barbiturates, sedative hypnotics, opiates |
| *Cholinergic* | Bradycardia, miosis, sweating, hyperperistalsis, salivation, bronchorrhea, urinary incontinence | Organophosphates, carbamates, nicotine |
| *Anticholinergic* | Tachycardia, hypertension, fever, pupillary dilation, hot dry skin, decreased peristalsis, urinary retention | Tricyclic antidepressants, antihistamines, phenothiazines, atropine, scopolamine |

*(Adapted from Olsen, K, and Banner, W: Emergency Management of Childhood Poisoning. In M Grossman and R Dieckmann, eds: Pediatric Emergency Medicine. Philadelphia, JB Lippincott, 1991, pp. 332-339.)*

## LABORATORY DATA

Laboratory data that can help in arriving at a diagnosis include serum osmolality, electrolytes, glucose, blood urea nitrogen (BUN), and creatinine.

## SERUM OSMOLALITY

*The serum osmolality is normally about 290 mOsm/l. Serum osmolality should be directly measured with a freezing point depression osmometer and can be estimated by calculation using the following equation:*

$$\text{Osmolality} = 2\,(\text{Na})\ [\text{mEq/l}] + \text{Glucose}\ [\text{mg/dl}]\ /\ 18 + \text{BUN}\ [\text{mg/dl}]\ /\ 2.8$$

The difference between the measured and calculated osmolality is known as the osmolar gap. Ethanol ingestion is a common cause of elevated osmolar gap.

## ELECTROLYTES

Serum electrolytes are helpful in determining the presence of a metabolic acidosis associated with an anion gap. **Table 16-4** identifies drugs that can cause an elevated anion gap metabolic acidosis.

### Table 16-4. Drugs Associated with an Elevated Anion Gap Acidosis

Methanol
Ethylene glycol
Phenformin
Isoniazid
Iron
Salicylates
Cyanide
Carbon monoxide

*The anion gap can be calculated as follows:*

$$\text{Anion gap} = \text{Na} - (\text{Cl} + \text{HCO3}) = 8 - 16 \text{ mEq/l in children}$$

## ADDITIONAL LABORATORY TESTS

Serum glucose, BUN, creatinine, and urinalysis should also routinely be measured in the poisoned patient.

## RADIOLOGIC STUDIES

Abdominal radiographs can demonstrate radiopaque tablets in the gastrointestinal tract. Although iron- and enteric-coated tablets can be seen by X-ray, a negative film does not rule out their ingestion. In infants and toddlers, additional radiographs in the form of a skeletal survey (humanogram) should be considered to detect other signs of abuse as indicated. This may be especially helpful in children with certain stigmata of abuse, for example, inflicted burns *(see Chapter 7)*.

## TOXICOLOGY SCREENING

The routine toxicology screening test employed by most hospitals can be valuable in the identification of the poisoning agent if the child has been poisoned with a drug included in the screen. In many recorded cases of intentional poisoning, however, the drug was not part of the standard toxicology screen. It is important for the physician to consider which particular drugs may be responsible and ask the laboratory to perform specific assays for them. If the clinical presentation of the child is particularly confusing, it is wise to preserve samples of blood, urine, and gastric aspirate until a more specific request can be made of the toxicology laboratory. These samples and any samples sent for specific toxicological assays should be prepared in a chain of custody protocol. Urine and blood should be collected in special containers and sealed with tamper-evident seals. Most hospitals and reference laboratories have lists available and policy and procedure manuals for collecting specimens under the chain of custody, which is a system where personnel collecting, transferring, or analyzing biological specimens or controlled substances retrieved from patients (for example, rocks of crack cocaine retrieved in gastric lavage) must sign a legal log for each step in the handling of the specimen. This affords the legal system evidence that is admissible in a court system. The timing of samples is critical and must be noted in the medical record.

Certain substances may require a second analytical method for confirmation. Toxins detected by screening methods such as thin layer chromatography (TLC) or gas chromatography (GC) may need to be confirmed by gas chromatography–mass spectrophotometry (GC-MS). A Regional Poison Center and toxicologist should be consulted for advice in individual cases on the recommended assays for laboratory testing. It is also helpful to discuss the case with the analytical or forensic toxicologist involved with the clinical laboratory that will be analyzing the patient's specimens.

When attempting to identify the potentially offending agent, it could be helpful to contact that parent's physician to determine which drugs have been prescribed for each of the parents. Also, the parent's occupation may give a clue as to which drugs may be present in the home. It should be noted that a negative screen may result from obtaining the sample too late to identify a drug with a short half-life.

## ◆EXAMPLES OF POISONING AGENTS

A few specific poisonings will be discussed to highlight particular aspects of this phenomenon.

## SALT

The literature contains several instances of infants intentionally poisoned with salt (Rogers et al., 1976; Meadow, 1977). These infants presented with multiple episodes of hypernatremia. They exhibited various findings, including seizures, lethargy, ataxia, coma, and dehydration. All had extreme elevations of serum and urine sodium levels. Normal renal function was demonstrated on recovery. Several authors have postulated that these infants would have been able to excrete the excess salt in the urine efficiently, but this mechanism failed probably because they were likely also deprived of water. The clinical and biological findings in these salt-poisoned children are very similar to findings in children with hypernatremic dehydration secondary to intentional withholding of water (Pickel et al., 1970). Mothers were the perpetrators in all cases of salt poisoning, and all had histories of severe psychiatric problems.

## PEPPER ASPIRATION
Eight children dying of pepper aspiration have been reported (Cohle et al., 1988). In each case the child was asphyxiated by forced pepper ingestion as a punishment for some perceived wrongdoing. The children all died due to airway obstruction. Typically, the airways were totally occluded by pepper and mucosal edema. All but one of the victims was under 5 years old, and the perpetrators were all caretakers of various types. Four of the children showed signs of chronic abuse.

## COCAINE
Children clinically intoxicated with cocaine usually have a combination of central nervous system and cardiovascular findings. Seizures are common and frequently difficult to control. Since cocaine can cause fever in children, one might reasonably presume the fever to be the etiology of the seizure. Cardiovascular findings can provide the clue to the true cause of the child's condition. Hypertension, tachycardia, cardiac arrhythmias, and poor peripheral perfusion often are present. As part of the sympathomimetic syndrome induced by cocaine, the pupils may be dilated. It is important to stress that any combination of these findings can be present. The study by Kharasch and associates reminds us that cocaine exposure can be clinically undetectable. In areas where cocaine use is common, its presence in children presenting with unexplained neurological or cardiovascular findings should be explored.

## ALCOHOLS, GLYCOLS, AND HYDROCARBONS
Children intoxicated with ethanol may present to emergency departments with altered mental status, metabolic acidosis, and often hypoglycemia. The source may be half-consumed containers of alcohol (beer or wine coolers) or mixed drinks left after an adult party. Toddlers may access these beverages when there is inadequate supervision or neglect. Furthermore, parents have offered children alcohol to quiet them when the adults are frustrated by the child's "excessive" crying.

Alcohols, glycols, and hydrocarbons are three compounds that should be given special attention when investigating potential child abuse. These three agents are a unique group because they are common to most households and because their dangerous properties are not always realized. In addition, abusive forced ingestion can readily be passed off as accidental injury if the investigator does not probe into this possibility. This is particularly true during "holiday" seasons.

There are cases of intentional ethylene glycol (antifreeze) poisoning in small infants (Saladino & Shannon, 1991; Woolf et al., 1992). Ethylene glycol is sweet tasting and only a small amount is toxic, factors that may contribute to its ease of administration. In fact, cases of animal abuse or accidental poisoning have occurred secondary to these physical characteristics. Infants presenting with anion gap metabolic acidosis of unexplained etiology should be evaluated for infection; toxic overdose from agents such as ethylene glycol, ethanol, methanol, salicylates, and iron; and metabolic conditions such as diabetic ketoacidosis, uremia, and inborn errors of metabolism.

Hydrocarbons in various forms have been associated with intentional poisoning from practices such as lighter fluid administration in an intravenous line (Saulsbury et al., 1984) and recurrent pine oil intoxication in an infant (Hill et al., 1975). An unusual hydrocarbon-type odor and unexplained respiratory failure with pulmonary edema may be clues to this form of abuse.

## ♦ SUMMARY

The intentional poisoning of children is an uncommon but highly dangerous form of child abuse. It can occur in the context of extreme neglect, bizarre means of discipline, or MSBP. The physician must approach the family with as much understanding and compassion as possible. In some instances, what appears to be an attempt to harm a child may instead be the injudicious but well-intentioned use of a folk remedy the family felt too embarrassed to discuss. On the other hand, perpetrators of MSBP may be extremely sophisticated in their ability to conceal their intent.

As always, the duty of the physician is to approach the ill child with a sensitivity to the history and close attention to the physical findings and laboratory studies. When the latter is not explained by the former, child abuse must always be considered. The persistent search for an explanation of those findings, particularly in the intentionally poisoned child, may save that child from future harm and even death.

## ♦ BIBLIOGRAPHY

Bateman, D, and Heagerty, M: Passive freebase cocaine ("crack") inhalation by infants and toddlers, *Am J Dis Child* 143:25, 1989.

Bauman, W, and Yalow, R: Child abuse: Parenteral insulin administration, *J Pediatr* 99:588, 1981.

Bays, J: Substance abuse and child abuse, *Pediatr Clin North Am* 37:881, 1990.

Chaney, NE: Cocaine convulsions in a breast-feeding baby, *J Pediatr* 112:134, 1988.

Chasnoff, IF, Lewis, DE, and Squires, L: Cocaine intoxication in a breast-fed infant, *Pediatrics* 80:836, 1987.

Cohle, S, Trestail, J, and Graham, M: Fatal pepper aspiration, *Am J Dis Child* 142:633, 1988.

Dees, DN, and Dees, DJ: Child abuse by poisoning, *South Dakota J Med* 46(3):91-2, 1993.

Dine, M: Tranquilizer poisoning: An example of child abuse, *Pediatrics* 36:782, 1965.

Dine, M: Intentional poisoning of children: An overlooked category of child abuse: Report of seven cases and review of the literature, *Pediatrics* 70:32, 1982.

Ernst, A, and Sanders, W: Unexpected cocaine intoxication presenting as seizures in children, *Ann Emerg Med* 18:774, 1989.

Fenton, AC, Wailoo, MP, and Tanner, MS: Severe failure to thrive and diarrhea caused by laxative abuse, *Arch Dis Child* 63:978, 1988.

Fischler, R: Poisoning: A syndrome of child abuse, *Am Fam Physician* 28:104, 1983.

Fleisher, D, and Ament, M: Diarrhea, red diapers, and child abuse, *Clin Pediatr* 17:820, 1977.

Friedman, E: Caustic ingestions and foreign body aspirations: An overlooked form of child abuse, *Ann Otol Rhinol Laryngol* 96:709, 1987.

Gotschlich, T, and Beltran, RS: Poisoning of a 21-month-old child by a baby-sitter, *Clin Pediatrics* 34(1):52-3, 1995.

Green, J, Craft, L, and Ghishan, F: Acetaminophen poisoning in infancy, *Am J Dis Child* 137:386, 1983.

Hickson, GB, Greene, J, Ghishan, FK, et al: Apparent intentional poisoning of an infant with acetaminophen, *Am J Dis Child* 137:917, 1983.

Hill, RM, Barer, J, and Leighton, H: An investigation of recurrent pine oil poisoning in an infant by the use of gas chromatographic-mass spectrometric methods, *J Pediatr* 87:115, 1975.

Kempe, CH, Silverman, FN, Steele, BF, et al: The battered child syndrome, *JAMA* 181:17, 1962.

Kharasch, S, Glotzer, D, Vinci, R, et al: Unsuspected cocaine exposure in young children, *Am J Dis Child* 145:204, 1991.

Kharasch, S, Vinci, R, and Reece, R: Esophagitis, epiglottitis, and cocaine alkaloid ("crack"): "Accidental" poisoning or child abuse, *Pediatrics* 86:117, 1990.

Kresel, JJ, and Lovejoy, FH: Poisonings and child abuse. In N Ellerstein, ed: *Child Abuse and Neglect*, Churchill Livingstone, New York, 1981, pp. 307-313.

Lansky, L: An unusual case of childhood chloral hydrate poisoning, *Am J Dis Child* 127:275, 1974.

Levanthal, JM, Garber, RB, and Brady, CA: Identification during the postpartum period of infants who are at high risk of child maltreatment, *J Pediatr* 114:481, 1989.

Lorber, J: Unexplained coma in a two-year-old, *Lancet* 2:680, 1978.

Mahesch, V, Stern, P, and Kearns, G: Application of pharmokinetics in the diagnosis of chemical abuse in Munchausen Syndrome by Proxy, *Clin Pediatr* 27:243, 1988.

McClung, HJ, Murray, R, and Braden, NJ: Intentional ipecac poisoning in children, *Am J Dis Child* 142:637, 1988.

McClure, RJ, Davis, PM, Meadow, SR, and Sibert, JR: Epidemiology of Munchausen syndrome by proxy, non-accidental poisoning, and non-accidental suffocation, *Archives of Disease in Childhood* 75(1):57-61, 1996.

Meadow, R: Munchausen Syndrome by Proxy: The hinterland of child abuse, *Lancet* 2:343, 1977.

Meadow, R: Munchausen Syndrome by Proxy, *Arch Dis Child* 57:92, 1982.

Meadow, R: ABC of child abuse: Poisoning, *Br Med J* 298:1445, 1989.

Mortimer, JG: Acute water intoxication as another manifestation of child abuse, *Arch Dis Child* 55:401, 1980.

Olsen, K, and Banner, W: Emergency management of childhood poisoning. In M Grossman and R Dieckmann, eds: *Pediatric Emergency Medicine*, JB Lippincott, Philadelphia, 1991, pp. 332-339.

Pickel, S, Anderson, C, and Holliday, M: Thirsting and hypernatremic dehydration: A form of child abuse, *Pediatrics* 45:54, 1970.

Pickering, D: Salicylate poisoning as a manifestation of the battered child syndrome, *Am J Dis Child* 130:675, 1976.

Rendle-Short, J: Non-accidental barbiturate poisoning of children, *Lancet* 2:1212, 1978.

Rivkin, M, and Gilmore, H: Generalized seizures in an infant due to environmentally acquired cocaine, *Pediatrics* 84:1100, 1989.

Rogers, D, Tripp, J, and Bentovim, A: Non-accidental poisoning: An extended syndrome of child abuse, *Br Med J* 1:793, 1976.

Rosenberg, D: Web of deceit: A literature review of Munchausen Syndrome by Proxy, *Child Abuse Negl* 11:547, 1987.

Saladino, R, and Shannon, M: Accidental and intentional poisonings with ethylene glycol in infancy: Diagnostic clues and management, *Pediatr Emerg Care* 7:93, 1991.

Saulsbury, FT, Chobanian, MC, and Wilson, WG: Child abuse: Parenteral hydrocarbon administration, *Pediatrics* 73:719, 1984.

Schnaps, Y, Frand, M, Rotem, Y, et al: The chemically abused child, *Pediatrics* 68:119, 1981.

Schwartz, RH, Peary, P, and Mistretta, D: Intoxication of young children with marijuana: A form of amusement for "pot"-smoking teenage girls, *Am J Dis Child* 140:326, 1986.

Schwartz, RH, and Einhorn, A: PCP intoxication in seven young children, *Pediatr Emerg Care* 2:238, 1986.

Simon, F: Uncommon type of child abuse (letter), *J Pediatr* 96:785, 1980.

Sobel, R: The psychiatric implications of accidental poisoning in childhood, *Pediatr Clin North Am* 17:653, 1970.

Sutphen, J, and Saulsbury, FT: Intentional ipecac poisoning: Munchausen Syndrome by Proxy, *Pediatrics* 82:453, 1986.

Tolis, A: Hypoglycemic convulsions in children after alcohol ingestion, *Pediatr Clin North Am* 12:423, 1965.

Watson, JB, Davies, JM, and Hunter, JL: Non-accidental poisoning in childhood, *Arch Dis Child* 54:143, 1979.

Woolf, AD, Wynshaw-Boris, A, Rinaldo, P, et al: Intentional infantile ethylene glycol poisoning presenting as an inherited metabolic disorder, *J Pediatr* 120:421, 1992.

# MUNCHAUSEN SYNDROME BY PROXY

James A. Monteleone, M.D.

*John was followed from birth in the hemophiliac clinic. His mother was a known carrier. She had two brothers with a bleeding disorder. John was found to be a mild bleeder, having only two episodes of bleeds requiring special attention in the emergency room in his first 2 years. The bleeding was controlled easily and required short hospitalization. When he was 2, his mother asked to be taught home care to manage his future bleeds. She was an eager and excellent student. Soon she was calling every day, stating that he had sustained a fall or that she had noted blood in his stool. This was followed by her appearing in the clinic on a daily basis stating that John had fallen or that she had found blood in his stool. No one had ever witnessed the falls. He was hospitalized 37 times and while in the hospital was found to have unexplained drops in his hemoglobin levels. The child was placed in foster care and experienced no bleeds over an extended period of time. The mother was ordered by the court to see a counselor. The child was returned to his mother's care with supervision. He continued to do well.*

## ◆ OVERVIEW

Baron von Munchausen was a teller of outrageous tales who lived in the 18th century. Some of his tales, authored by one of his friends, Rudolph Raspe, were published in a children's book entitled *Baron von Munchausen's Narrative of His Marvelous Travels and Campaigns in Russia* (1936).

In 1951, Asher described an unusual group of patients who went from physician to physician fabricating stories of illness; they were willing to subject themselves to numerous tests and needless surgery. He called this the von Munchausen's (or Munchausen) syndrome. Later, Roy Meadow (1977) described a variant of the Munchausen syndrome in a case report of two hospitalized children. Unlike the original Munchausen syndrome, in this case, the parent fabricated the illness in the child and presented the child to a physician for treatment. Meadow called this phenomenon the *Munchausen Syndrome by Proxy (MSBP)*. Since then, the syndrome has become more widely recognized, although before Meadow coined the name, others (Rogers et al., 1976) had reported incidents in which several mothers had deliberately poisoned their children and then tried to convince their physicians that their children were ill, by either simulating or actually inducing illness in their children.

Naturally, such falsification of medical illness can cause emotional harm by propagating a self-image in the child as chronically ill and causes physical injury with unnecessary medical testing and possible pointless use of medications to treat false symptoms. In some cases, it has led to the child's death.

## ◆ CLINICAL PRESENTATION

### SIGNS AND SYMPTOMS

MSBP affects children of widely varying ages. Children have presented with factitious illness by proxy from as young as neonates (Rogers et al., 1976) to as old as 21 years (Rosenberg, 1987). Perpetrators of MSBP are found in all socioeconomic groups; some deceptions are unsophisticated, while others are complex, requiring complicated investigative techniques to unravel. In general, the child appears to have a persistent or recurrent condition or illness that cannot be explained. There may be abnormal laboratory studies without strong evidence of underlying disease or, conversely, there may be normal laboratory results that do not support the illness reported. Treatments are not well-tolerated or else seem ineffective. For example, a child may develop a rash but is unable to tolerate prescribed drug treatments because of reported vomiting or other untoward reactions. The parent, most often the mother, is willing to have her child undergo diagnostic procedures and medical treatments even when they are invasive. If the child is hospitalized, the situation may go from bad to worse, with the child becoming febrile or lapsing into a coma; on the other hand, with hospitalization the severity of illness simulated or described by the parent may not continue, and the child may appear well. Experienced specialists often remark that they have never seen a case like this before.

Presenting complaints can vary widely, with the parent complaining that the child is tired all the time, that the child stops breathing and becomes cyanotic, or that the child convulses. Deliberate poisoning may be seen, sometimes involving medications prescribed by a physician. Children have also been injected with medications, such as insulin, to produce coma and with foreign substances, such as feces, to produce infection.

### MEDICAL RECORD REVIEW

Typically, when reviewing the history and the medical record, it is noted that there have been numerous visits to the doctor and numerous hospitalizations. The child has undergone many diagnostic procedures, often involving several hospitals and physicians. The perpetrator, again most often the mother, usually denies knowledge of the etiology of the child's illness. The mother may report that she or another child has complained of symptoms similar to the ones she says are being experienced by the child. A rare disease is often diagnosed or strongly considered.

## OCCURRENCE

The frequency of MSBP is difficult to estimate. Most published articles on this syndrome are single case studies that focus on the type of medical deception used by the parent. Meaningful research has been difficult to conduct and is therefore limited in the literature. Still, it may not be as rare as previously thought. For instance, Warner and Hathaway (1984) estimated that 5% of cases evaluated for food allergies were consistent with MSBP.

## ♦ ETIOLOGY

The first significant review of the literature on MSBP was by Roy Meadow. He was the first to recognize and describe MSBP occurring in children. Others had described MSBP symptoms in children, but Meadow made the connection between the symptoms and the syndrome. Meadow reviewed the cases of 19 children from 17 families, 10 boys and 9 girls. The children ranged in age from 4 months to 7 years, with a mean age of 3 years, 2 months. The children had a wide range of signs and symptoms, usually suggesting a multisystem disorder. The false symptoms and signs had occurred for 1 1/2 months to 4 years before diagnosis, the average being 13 months. The most common fabricated sign in Meadow's review was bleeding, which was reported in 12 of the 19 children. Neurological signs were also common (**Table 17-1**). Most of the children had been seen by many different doctors and had many referrals to various specialists. Even though the initial reported symptoms and signs were false, most of the children incurred secondary symptoms and signs as a result of medical investigations, operations, and medications. During their illness, many different diagnoses were considered. Meadow concluded that the doctors who were treating the false illness did the most harm to the child, unknowingly.

| Table 17-1. Summary of Meadow's Results: Fabricated Signs | |
| --- | --- |
| **Number of Cases: 19** | |
| *Bleeding:* | 12 |
| Hematuria | 7 |
| Hematemesis | 5 |
| Hemoptyses | 3 |
| Blood in feces | 3 |
| *Neurological Signs:* | 7 |
| Drowsiness with coma | 5 |
| Seizures | 3 |
| Unsteadiness | 2 |
| *Other Fabricated Signs* | |
| Rashes | 6 |
| Glycosuria | 5 |
| Fevers | 4 |
| Biochemical abnormalities | 4 |
| Feculent vomitus | 2 |

In addition to Meadow's study, Rosenberg's review is significant because all the cases known at the time (1987) were assembled for his study, a total of 117 cases. This review was of greater significance than Meadow's because the number of cases studied was larger.

The patient population was identified as 46% males and 45% females; in 9% of the cases no sex was indicated. The mean age (67 cases) was 39.8 months ± 32.1 months. Mean time of onset of symptoms and signs to the time of diagnosis was 14.9 months ± 14 months. The range of age at diagnosis was 1 month to 21 years. The range from time of onset of symptoms and signs to time of diagnosis was from several days to 20 years.

Presenting symptoms and signs covered a wide range. The most common presentations were bleeding from various sites (44%), seizures (42%), central nervous system depression (19%), apnea (15%), diarrhea (11%), vomiting (10%), fever (10%), and rash (9%). Many children had more than one presenting problem.

## SIMULATED VERSUS PRODUCED ILLNESS

Rosenberg identified two categories of presentation: simulated illness and produced illness. *Simulated illness* is defined as illness that is faked by the mother. An example of a simulated illness would be the mother's contamination of the child's urine specimen with her own blood and her subsequent claim that the child had been urinating blood. *Produced illness* is defined as illness that the mother actually inflicted on the child. An example of a produced illness would be the injection by the mother of a foreign material such as feces or a drug into the child's intravenous line or formula, causing physiological disorders.

In 72 cases in which the presentation was known, 25% involved simulation of illness; in 72% of these cases the simulation took place while the child was in the hospital. Production of illness was found in 50% of the 72 cases; in 95% of this group the production of illness took place while the child was in the hospital. In 25% of the cases, both simulation and production of illness were involved, and in 84% of these cases both the simulation and the production of illness took place while the child was in the hospital.

## PRESENTATION DECEPTIONS

The child's mother was the perpetrator in each of the cases Meadow and Rosenberg reviewed. Meadow found that the mothers in his study were able to accomplish the deception in a number of ways. Bleeding was generally the result of the mother adding her own blood to the child's vomit, urine, or feces. Sometimes blood was smeared on the child's face or perineum. The blood was usually obtained by the mother pricking herself. One mother used blood from an open thigh wound; another stirred a vaginal tampon in the child's urine specimen. A few mothers simulated blood in a specimen from the child by adding paint, cocoa, or phenolphthalein. One mother produced feculent vomitus by adding soft feces, which she stored in a container in her room, to the child's vomit. Fevers were produced by rubbing thermometers or immersing them in hot liquid. Biochemical abnormalities were simulated by adding chemicals, such as salt, to a specimen. To accomplish the deception, various tricks distracted the person who had taken the specimen.

Rashes were fabricated by rubbing the skin repetitively with a fingernail or a sharp object to obtain a bullous lesion, by applying caustic solutions to areas of skin, or by painting with a dye such as phenolphthalein.

The neurological symptoms were the result of the mother giving the child a sedative or tranquilizer that had been prescribed for herself. The mother gave the medications in doses greater than those prescribed for herself. One mother applied pressure to the child's neck to induce seizures.

Seizures are a common presenting complaint in MSBP. Meadow noted that the best way to rule out a convulsive disorder was by taking a careful history. Often the children were said to have had a seizure at school or a similar place, in the presence of a third party or parties; questioning the party or others present at the time of the reported seizure usually revealed that no seizure had happened.

There is a high prevalence of MSBP in the subgroup of apnea patients. These patients have had two or more episodes of apnea that terminated after mouth-to-mouth resuscitation. The episodes have their onset only in the presence of the parent, but are witnessed secondarily by other persons after they have been called for assistance. When these infants die, the presumptive cause of death may be sudden infant death syndrome (SIDS). It may be impossible to distinguish between SIDS and other causes of death even with an autopsy. However, it is essential that all infants with unexplained deaths have an autopsy.

## MULTISPECIALTY INVOLVEMENT

Rosenberg in particular found that many of the children had symptoms involving more than one organ system and saw more than one pediatric subspecialist. The overall problem in such cases is that the subspecialists see only their part of the elephant. Rosenberg felt that the pediatric subspecialists should consider factitious illness in their differential diagnosis and that they could make the correct diagnosis quicker if they reviewed the child's medical record thoroughly and carefully.

# ◆ DEMOGRAPHICS

## PARENTAL CHARACTERISTICS

Certain characteristics seem to be held in common in these families. Most of the mothers, according to Meadow's study, seem loving and caring. They do not appear cruel, negligent, or uncaring. The father is usually distant and minimally involved. If the mother has other children, they are rarely discussed. All her energy is focused on the sick child. The mother spends an excessive amount of time on the hospital ward with the child and refuses to leave the child alone in the hospital even for one hour. She often insists that she is the only one to whom the child can relate and from whom the child will accept food, drink, and medication. The mother, despite her child's problems, does not seem as concerned about her child as are the medical and nursing staff. She may actually be conciliatory about the child's condition with the hospital staff.

The mother is typically familiar with medical terminology and procedures. Many of them have had some nursing education or have worked in a medical setting and may become overly friendly with the hospital staff. The occupations of 40% of the 97 mothers were unknown (**Table 17-2**). There is often conflict among medical professionals in the case, each taking a side as to whether or not the child is ill or, if suspected, a victim of MSBP. The child usually improves when separated from the parent. With parental confrontations the symptoms may stop and the child may improve, or the child may be in greater danger.

Seven of 12 mothers in the Meadow study who were questioned on the subject had a history with some features of Munchausen's Syndrome. Five of 10 mothers had a history within the previous 3 years of symptoms and signs similar to those which she fabricated for the child. Munchausen Syndrome or features of the syndrome were noted in 24% of the mothers in Rosenberg's study.

| Table 17-2. Occupational Distribution Among Mothers in Rosenberg's Study | |
| --- | --- |
| Nurse or training for nursing | 27% |
| Housewife | 20% |
| Unemployed | 4% |
| Medical office worker | 3% |
| Social worker | 2% |
| Schoolteacher | 1% |
| Home helper | 1% |
| Baby food demonstrator | 1% |
| Orderly | 1% |

## FAMILY DYNAMICS

At the time the fabrication was discovered, 15 of the 17 pairs of parents in the Meadow study were living together. Their mean age was 29 years, ranging from 24 to 37 years of age. Most of the mothers lived in the hospital with the child or visited the child for long periods each day. The fathers kept a low profile; 10 of 15 rarely visited the child in the hospital, which was particularly noteworthy in view of the severity of the child's illness. Six of 11 had jobs that required them to be away from home for long periods or in the evenings, and two others were considered extremely unsupportive of their wives. The fathers did not appear to know of the fabrication and had difficulty in believing it when told. In 10 of 15 families, there was a discrepancy between the social and the intellectual level of the parents. In each instance, the wife either came from a higher social background or seemed much more intelligent than her husband. In 15 of 17 families there were other children. In five families a second child incurred the syndrome or died of suspicious circumstances. In 10 families there was nothing to suggest involvement of older or younger siblings.

In describing the 97 perpetrators in her 117 cases, Rosenberg assessed that 98% were biological mothers and 2% were adoptive mothers. Many of the mothers were described as friendly and socially adept. Once the deception by the mother was discovered, evidence of secondary paternal collusion occurred in only 1.5% of all cases. In 15% of the cases the mother admitted completely to the deception; an additional 7% partially admitted; and 18% of the mothers denied the deception. The mother's reaction to confrontation was unknown in 60% of the cases.

***Meadow's Prognoses for Victims of Munchausen Syndrome by Proxy***

*Meadow (1989) listed the following consequences for children who are falsely labeled as ill:*

**1.** *They will receive needless and possibly harmful treatments.*
**2.** *They may develop a genuine disease.*
**3.** *They may die.*
**4.** *They may develop chronic invalidism.*
**5.** *They may develop Munchausen Syndrome as an adult.*

When a psychiatric diagnosis was described, depression was cited most often, and some personality disorders were noted. Many authors made a point of indicating that the perpetrator was not psychotic. Only one mother was described as an hysterical psychopath and one as probably psychotic. Loneliness and isolation were prominent in these women's lives.

## ◆ OUTCOMES

In Meadow's report, 17 of the 19 children survived. One died from presumed poisoning and one from uncertain circumstances. Of the survivors, eight were taken away from the family, and nine remained at home after confrontation with the parents and involvement of social services with arrangements for continued supervision. Seven of these nine children were well and free of all symptoms at follow-up 1 to 4 years later. Two mothers continued to take their children to a variety of doctors with minor complaints, but no harmful fabrication took place.

Ten of the 117 children in Rosenberg's review died, giving a mortality rate of at least 9%. The age at the time of death was known for eight. All were younger than 3 years of age. The causes of death were from suffocation (4), salt poisoning (3), other poisoning (2), and uncertain (1). All the children died in the custody of their mothers. No mother admitted to homicide. In two of the children who died, the parents had been confronted with the diagnosis of MSBP and the children had been sent home with them, subsequently to die. Rosenberg warns that the fact that the parents had been confronted does not preclude the possibility of subsequent murder of the child.

Among the 117 victims reviewed by Rosenberg, 10 siblings had died under unusual circumstances. Those 10 siblings were not included in the original case reports.

### SHORT-TERM MORBIDITY

Rosenberg defined short-term morbidity as pain and/or illness that did not leave permanent disfigurement or permanent impairment of function. One hundred percent of the children studied suffered short-term morbidity. In 75% of the cases the morbidity was caused by both medical staff and the perpetrator. In 25% of the cases the morbidity was caused most directly by the medical staff. The morbidity caused by the medical staff was related to investigations and procedures.

### LONG-TERM MORBIDITY

Rosenberg defined long-term morbidity as pain or illness that caused permanent disfigurement. Of the 107 survivors, 8% had long-term morbidity, including impairment of gastrointestinal function following multiple esophageal surgeries, serious psychiatric problems, destructive joint changes, a limp, and mental retardation with cerebral palsy and cortical blindness. Several had multiple abdominal surgeries for laparotomy, colectomy, or ileostomy. Rosenberg felt the incidence of long-term morbidity was an underestimate, since few of the cases had long-term follow-up.

Twelve of the perpetrators on whom information was available were suicidal. Of these, seven attempted suicide before the disclosure and five after the disclosure; 38 did not attempt suicide. No information was available on 47 of the perpetrators.

## ◆ CATEGORIES OF MSBP

Before examining guidelines for approaching suspected MSBP, it may be helpful to the examiner to be aware of various categories of the syndrome established by researchers. This can sometimes aid in diagnosis of both the syndrome and its degree of severity, which in turn aids in the choice of intervention.

Meadow (1989) and Libow and Schreier (1986) suggest a spectrum of categories for MSBP, including the following. Meadow identifies such categories as Perceived Illness, Doctor Shopping, Enforced Invalidism, and Fabricated Illness. Libow and Schreier classify perpetrators as Help Seeker, Active Inducer, and Doctor Addict. As with all forms of child abuse, it is the degree of abuse that matters. This will influence actions taken by social agencies.

## PERCEIVED ILLNESS

*Perceived illness* describes the anxious mother, inexperienced, under stress and lonely, who needlessly worries that her healthy child is ill. She perceives symptoms in her child that others do not observe. The child is taken to the doctor on many occasions because the mother cannot be reassured, resulting in unpleasant investigations and treatments for the child. This process would not be classified as child abuse unless the mother's persistence and refusal to accept normal results were excessive and the quality of the child's life was seriously impaired.

## DOCTOR SHOPPING

Meadow uses the term *doctor shopping* to describe the parent who seeks help from a succession of different doctors claiming that a healthy child is ill. As each doctor in turn refuses further investigation, she consults yet another doctor. She tells none, in a chain of doctors, that she has seen anyone else for diagnosis or treatment. The result for the child is a series of repetitive investigations. When the parent's convictions about illness reach these proportions, it is child abuse.

## ENFORCED INVALIDISM

*Enforced invalidism* develops when a parent with an ill or disabled child seeks to keep the child ill or increases the degree of disability. If the child has no disability, the parent ensures that the child is regarded as incapacitated and in need of special attention or assistance.

## FABRICATED ILLNESS

*Fabricated illness* results when the parent lies to the doctor about a child's health, giving a convincing history of illness, and fabricates physical signs or alters health records that cause the doctor to perform detailed investigations and prescribe treatment. The parent invents the illness while the child is young and continues and intensifies the story as the years pass. When they are older, some children will participate in the deception. Some have become independent illness addicts and have grown up to have the Munchausen Syndrome.

## HELP SEEKER

The *help seeker*, which would be comparable to Meadow's perceived illness category, fabricates illness in a child on a limited basis, but the desperate request for help with parenting is the clear motivation. These mothers may respond to psychiatric intervention.

## ACTIVE INDUCER

At the other extreme of the Munchausen Syndrome by Proxy is the *active inducer* —the prototype who will make life-threatening assaults on very young children. This type of parent, again usually the mother, is a very dangerous person. This person will go to extreme lengths to actively induce injury or illness.

## DOCTOR ADDICT

The category of *doctor addict*, comparable with Meadow's doctor shopping group, represents the other major class of cases. Neither as dramatic as active inducers in symptomatology and danger, nor as blatant as the help seekers in their request for intervention, the doctor addict mothers are frequently written off as cranks or overanxious and their children as psychosomatic or depressed. They are less likely to be identified than the prototypical cases, since doctor addiction can evade resolution for longer than the prototypical cases in which the victim is hospitalized with an acute condition.

## ◆GUIDELINES WHEN MSBP IS SUSPECTED

If the diagnosis of MSBP is to be made, the physician must remember that sometimes a story is false. A small degree of suspicion should be maintained at all times, especially when the course of a child's condition does not make sense.

*If the attending physician suspects MSBP, he or she should take the following steps:*

1. The child's safety is the primary concern. These children are at risk. Approximately 10% of them will die, and the majority will have long-term morbidity. The physician should continue to behave as if the mother's story of her child's illness is accurate; it may be. Perform whatever diagnostic tests are necessary to confirm the diagnosis, using other professionals, crime labs, veterinarians, or others who might be useful in aiding with the diagnosis. Veterinarians are included in the diagnostic process because they are familiar with animal blood and tissue, which some parents have attempted to pass off as coming from the child. It is often not possible, or necessary, to obtain laboratory evidence to prove MSBP.

2. The child should be separated from the parents for a sufficient length of time to determine if the symptoms and signs occur in their absence. Try to get the parents to leave voluntarily. If not, this action may require legal enforcement and a court order.

3. If the child is verbal, interview him or her alone. An experienced counselor is recommended.

4. Check with other physicians, other hospitals, employers, and schools for details of the history relating to the child and family. Check out the social and work histories as well. It is common for the parent to fabricate details such as schooling, employment, illnesses, and hospitalizations. Check out the parent's history with witnesses to illness in the child and interview them about the facts they have allegedly witnessed. Check past medical records. Do not allow the parent to talk you out of the search. Look for unusual illnesses in siblings of the patient or unusual illnesses in the parents.

5. Pay careful attention to documentation in the medical record. Follow chain of evidence procedures in handling specimens.

6. The possibilities of simulating or producing illness are endless and as diverse as the human imagination. Nothing is farfetched, especially when one suspects poisoning. Decide which poisons are suspected, and obtain specific assays on the appropriate body fluids and exogenously administered fluids. Consider all sources, food, syringes, and intravenous bottles as possible evidence. Save all specimens for toxicological assay. It may be necessary to have more than one reference laboratory assay the specimen. Check the reliability of the signs, that the rash does not wash off with water or alcohol, and that the blood is blood and that it is the child's.

7. An experienced nurse who has been carefully instructed about the problem should be stationed in the room at all times. All specimens must be carefully collected and guarded. No food, drink, or medicines may be brought in by the family. The child should never be left alone with a parent, and the person in attendance should be aware that the parent may try to harm the child; the nurse must watch carefully at all times while the parent is with the child.

8. The child should have a psychiatric and/or psychological evaluation. As with the parents, the purpose of this evaluation is not to confirm the diagnosis (which cannot be done by testing) but to aid with the impact of the situations and to identify other potential problems.

9. Involve local social service and child protective services immediately.

10. The medical team, social service, and protective agencies must work out a plan of action. It is wise for the child protection team to have a protocol outlining the procedures to follow. Remember, the child is not free of risk because he is in the hospital. If the parent is producing illness, there is a 70% chance that he or she will produce it in the hospital. The protective plan may include video monitoring of the child. As in any other child abuse case, the plan should include whether the child should be removed from the home or can remain there under supervision.

11. Be supportive, not accusing when presenting the diagnosis to the family. State the case clearly and simply. Tell the parents that the case has been reported to child protective services. Be prepared to immediately protect the child. Child protective services and the court should be on notice so that a court holding order on the child may be obtained if necessary. The object of presenting the diagnosis to the parents is not to persuade them that it is true or to obtain a confession; it is to inform them that such a diagnosis has been made and that steps will be taken to protect the child and confirm the diagnosis.

12. The parent may be suicidal. Psychiatric care should be made immediately available to the mother and father after disclosure of the diagnosis.

## COMPLICATIONS IN EVALUATION

Sometimes the evaluation is complicated because a genuine organic disease is present in addition to the fabricated illness. The child may actually have a legitimate illness, such as hemophilia, asthma, or convulsive disorder, which the parent uses as a basis for complaints. For example, the parent of a hemophilia patient may precipitate problems by causing a bleed; another might withhold or increase the prescribed medications in the child with an asthmatic or convulsive disorder.

## CHILD SURVEILLANCE

Video surveillance has been effective as a means of confirming the diagnosis of MSBP (Epstein et al., 1987). In answer to the critics of video surveillance who state that it is not ethical, Frost and Glaze (1988) respond that the critics of videotaping forget that it is the patient, the child, who is being watched secretly by the camera, not the mother. Videotaping is performed for the child's protection and is therefore ethical. There is no entrapment, since the presence of the surveillance apparatus does not increase the likelihood that the illegal act will be committed. The method is legal, and the information obtained has been used as evidence in legal proceedings.

## ◆ CONFRONTATION

Meadow suggested that these parents be confronted by the physician immediately after he or she suspects the charade. In his experience the fabrication usually ended following confrontation. He warned that those he did not confront continued the abuse, and in one case he believed it resulted in the death of the child. He further stated that, when confronted, most perpetrators do not acknowledge the abuse but they do stop the actions.

If MSBP is not recognized, the child is at higher risk for morbidity. When the diagnosis is being considered, the hospital is the best place to confirm the diagnosis, if necessary. The child's involvement in the pretense can result in his or her death.

◆ BIBLIOGRAPHY

Amegavie, L, Marzouk, O, Mullen, J, Sills, J, and Gauthier Le Tendre, JBM: Munchausen's Syndrome by Proxy: A warning for health professionals, *Br Med J* 293:855-856, 1986.

Asher, R: Munchausen Syndrome, *Lancet* 1:339-341, 1951.

Blix, S, and Brack, G: The effects of a suspected case of Munchausen's Syndrome by Proxy on a pediatric nursing staff, *Gen Hosp Psychiatry* 10:402-409, 1988.

Clark, GD, Key, JD, Rutherford, P, and Bithoney, WG: Munchausen's Syndrome by Proxy (child abuse) presenting as apparent autoerythrocyte sensitization syndrome: An unusual presentation of Polle syndrome, *Pediatrics* 74:1100-1102, 1984.

Drell, MJ: More on Munchausen by Proxy, *J Am Acad Child Adolescent Psychiatry* 27:140, 1988.

Epstein, MA, Markowitz, RL, Gallo, DM, Holmes, JW, and Gryboski, JD: Munchausen Syndrome by Proxy: Considerations in diagnosis and confirmation by video surveillance, *Pediatrics* 80:220-224, 1987.

Frederick, V, Luedtke, GS, Barrett, FF, Hixson, D, and Burch, K: Munchausen Syndrome by Proxy: Recurrent central catheter sepsis, *Pediatr Infect Dis J* 9:440-442, 1990.

Frost, JD, and Glaze, DG: Munchausen's Syndrome by Proxy and video surveillance, *Am J Dis Child* 142:917-918, 1988.

Griffith, JL, and Slovik, LS: Munchausen Syndrome by Proxy and sleep disorders medicine, *Sleep* 12:178-183, 1989.

Guandolo, VL: Munchausen Syndrome by Proxy: An outpatient challenge, *Pediatrics* 75:526-530, 1985.

Herzberg, JH, and Wolff, SM: Chronic factitious fever in puberty and adolescence: A diagnostic challenge to the family physician, *Psychiatr Med* 3:205-212, 1972.

Holborow, PL: A variant of Munchausen's Syndrome by Proxy, *J Am Acad Child Psychiatry* 24:238, 1985.

Hosch, IA: Munchausen Syndrome by Proxy, *Am J Maternal Child Nurs* 12:48-52, 1987.

Jones, JG, Butler, HL, Hamilton, B, Perdue, JD, Stern, P, and Woody, RC: Munchausen Syndrome by Proxy, *Child Abuse Negl* 10:33-40, 1986.

Kahan, BB, and Yorker, BC: Munchausen Syndrome by Proxy, *J Sch Health* 60:108-110, 1990.

Kurlandsky, L, Lukoff, JY, Zinkham, WH, Brody, JP, and Kessler, RW: Munchausen Syndrome by Proxy: Definition of factitious bleeding in an infant by 51Cr labeling of erythrocytes, *Pediatrics* 63:228-231, 1979.

Lazoritz, S: Munchausen Syndrome by Proxy or Meadow's syndrome, *Lancet* 2(8559):631, 1987.

Libow, JA, and Schreier, HA: Three forms of factitious illness in children: When is it Munchausen Syndrome by Proxy? *Am J Orthopsychiatry* 56:602-611, 1986.

Light, MJ, and Sheridan, MS: Munchausen Syndrome by Proxy and apnea (MBPA), *Clin Pediatr* 29:162-168, 1990.

Liston, TE, Levine, PL, and Anderson, C: Polymicrobial bacteremia due to Polle syndrome: The child abuse variant of Munchausen by Proxy, *Pediatrics* 72:211-213, 1983.

MacDonald, TM: Myalgic encephalomyelitis by proxy, *Br Med J* 299:1030-1031, 1989.

Makar, AF, and Squier, PJ: Munchausen Syndrome by Proxy: Father as a perpetrator, *Pediatrics* 85:370-373, 1990.

Malatack, JJ, Wiener, ES, Gartner, JC, Zitelli, BJ, and Brunetti, E: Munchausen Syndrome by Proxy: A new complication of central venous catheterization, *Pediatrics* 75:523-525, 1985.

Masterson, J, Dunworth, R, and Williams, N: Extreme illness exaggeration in pediatric patients: A variant of Munchausen's by Proxy? *Am J Orthopsychiatry* 58:188-195, 1988.

McGuire, TL, and Feldman, KW: Psychologic morbidity of children subjected to Munchausen Syndrome by Proxy, *Pediatrics* 83:289-292, 1989.

McKinlay, I: Munchausen's Syndrome by Proxy, *Br Med J* 293:1308, 1986.

Meadow, R: Munchausen Syndrome by Proxy: The hinterland of child abuse, *Lancet* 2:343-345, 1977.

Meadow, R: Munchausen Syndrome by Proxy, *Arch Dis Child* 57:92-98, 1982.

Meadow, R: Munchausen Syndrome by Proxy and pseudo-epilepsy, *Arch Dis Child* 57:811-812, 1982.

Meadow, R: Munchausen by Proxy and brain damage, *Dev Med Child Neurol* 26:672-674, 1984.

Meadow, R: Management of Munchausen Syndrome by Proxy, *Arch Dis Child* 60:385-393, 1985.

Meadow, R: Munchausen Syndrome by Proxy, *Br Med J* 299:248-250, 1989.

Meadow, R, and Lennert, T: Munchausen by Proxy or Polle syndrome: Which term is correct? *Pediatrics* 74:554-556, 1984.

Money, J: Paleodigms and paleodigmatics: A new theoretical construct applicable to Munchausen's Syndrome by Proxy, child-abuse dwarfism, paraphilias, anorexia nervosa and other syndromes, *Am J Psychother* 43:15-24, 1989.

Nicol, AR, and Eccles, M: Psychotherapy for Munchausen Syndrome by Proxy, *Arch Dis Child* 60:344-348, 1985.

Orenstein, DM, and Wasserman, AL: Munchausen Syndrome by Proxy simulating cystic fibrosis, *Pediatrics* 78:621-624, 1986.

Palmer, AJ, and Yoshimura, GJ: Munchausen Syndrome by Proxy, *J Am Acad Child Psychiatry* 23:503-508, 1984.

Pickford, E, Buchanan, N, and McLaughlan, S: Munchausen Syndrome by Proxy: A family anthology, *Med J Aust* 148:646-650, 1988.

Raspe, RE: *The Adventures of Baron Munchausen*, Grosset & Dunlap, New York, 1936.

Richardon, GF: Munchausen Syndrome by Proxy, *Am Fam Physician* 36:119-123, 1987.

Rogers, D, Tripp, J, Bentovim, A, Robinson, A, Berry, D, and Goulding, R: Non-accidental poisoning: An extended syndrome of child abuse, *Br Med J* 1:793-796, 1976.

Rosen, CL, Frost, JD, Bricker, T, Tarnow, JD, Gillette, PC, and Dunlavy, S: Two siblings with recurrent cardiorespiratory arrest: Munchausen Syndrome by Proxy or child abuse? *Pediatrics* 71:715-720, 1983.

Rosenberg, DA: Web of deceit: A literature review of Munchausen Syndrome by Proxy, *Child Abuse Negl* 11:547-563, 1987.

Senner, A, and Ott, MJ: Munchausen Syndrome by Proxy, *Issues Compr Pediatr Nurs* 12:345-357, 1989.

Sheldon, SH: Munchausen Syndrome by Proxy, *Pediatrics* 76:855-856, 1985.

Sheridan, MS: Munchausen Syndrome by Proxy, *Health Soc Work* 14:53-58, 1989.

Sigal, M, Gelkopf, M, and Meadow, RS: Munchausen by Proxy Syndrome: The triad of abuse, self-abuse, and deception, *Comp Psychiatry* 30:527-533, 1989.

Sigal, MD, Altmark, D, and Carmel, I: Munchausen Syndrome by adult proxy: A perpetrator abusing two adults, *J Nerv Ment Dis* 174:696-698, 1986.

Sutphen, JL, and Saulsbury, FT: Intentional ipecac poisoning: Munchausen Syndrome by Proxy, *Pediatrics* 82:453-456, 1988.

Waller, DA: Obstacles to the treatment of Munchausen by Proxy Syndrome, *J Am Acad Child Psychiatry* 22:80-85, 1983.

Warner, JO, and Hathaway, MJ: Allergic form of Meadow's syndrome (Munchausen by Proxy), *Arch Dis Child* 59:151-156, 1984.

Wood, PR, Fowlkes, J, Holden, P, and Casto, D: Fever of unknown origin for six years: Munchausen Syndrome by Proxy, *J Fam Pract* 28:391-395, 1989.

Woody, RC, and Jones, JG: Neurologic Munchausen-by-Proxy Syndrome, *South Med J* 80:247-248, 1987.

Zitelli, BJ, Seltman, MF, and Shannon, RM: Munchausen's Syndrome by Proxy and its professional participants, *Am J Dis Child* 141:1099-1103, 1987.

# Neglect and Abandonment

Wayne I. Munkel, M.S.W., L.C.S.W.

*This chapter cannot begin to explain the complex issue of neglect but can only look at the outcomes. Usually, if there is no unfortunate outcome, neglect goes undetected and unreported. It takes a death or shocking evidence before many cases of neglect are brought to light.*

*A severely malnourished 7-year-old boy was taken to the emergency room by ambulance. The child's mother found him unresponsive in bed and not breathing. The mother stated that the child had had a cold for the past few days and appeared to be recovering.*

*He was emaciated and dirty, he had bed sores on his buttocks and hips, and the soles of his feet were crusted with dirt that had to be scraped off. Under the dirt were several infected wounds, one looking like a cigarette burn. Attempts at resuscitation were successful, and he was intubated and given fluids and antibiotics. He had severe bilateral pneumonia. After several hours in the hospital, he suffered cardiac arrest. Attempts at resuscitation were futile.*

*There were three other children in the family. All, although poorly clothed, were well nourished and healthy. The mother was single, and none of the children had the same father. The mother was receiving public aid and had been reported for abuse and neglect several times in the past. She was regularly visited by state*

*child protection services, the last visit the week before the child's admission. The worker did not see the child during the visit, although he was supposedly sick and in bed at that time.*

*The school was contacted. The three siblings had been to school regularly. The dead child had missed a number of days in the past and had been absent for the previous 2 weeks. One of the teachers stated that on several occasions the child had come to school in obvious distress. He was dirty, malnourished, and unable to work on his school assignments. On one occasion the child was so weak he had to crawl up the stairs. His teacher had suggested they report the child to the Division of Family Services. The school principal decided that since the other children seemed to be doing well, he would just send the child home.*

*The media caught wind of the story and took pictures of the home, which should have been condemned. But as we review the case it is clear that the media had chosen this family as a scapegoat for the child protection system itself. In truest perspective, the system was the cause of the child's death. Had the mother received better services, the child would have survived and thrived. The school's role in the tragedy, although understandable, compounded the situation.*

Given this history, typical of so many cases, it is easy to see that neglect resulted in death. But too often the causative responsibility is shared among several factors that can be difficult to define. Furthermore, neglect is often difficult to prevent. This chapter will attempt to identify the various forms of neglect and abandonment as they are seen in the medical setting, just touching on the *"who"* and the *"why,"* which constitute a social problem beyond the scope of this chapter.

As is true with most problems, there is a spectrum of neglect that ranges from mild to severe. It is easy to agree on what constitutes severe neglect and what should be done about it. Beyond that, unless an obviously bad outcome is brought to light, nothing is done or, in most cases, can be done.

*The following case illustrates this point:*

*A 2-month-old child was found dead in his crib by his mother. The cause of death was suffocation. The child shared the crib with two siblings who were 2 and 4 years old. The medical examiner decided the cause of death was accidental. One of the siblings, while sleeping, probably laid on the child to cause the suffocation.*

Was neglect involved here? Who was neglectful? The mother? No one told her the child would be in danger if he slept with others. If the mother had had more money, she could have afforded beds for each child. If she had been better educated, she might have known better.

*A mother leaves seven children in the home while she goes on a date. The eldest is 8 years old. He has been told not to play with matches and had been reprimanded for this very thing. While the mother is gone, there is a fire and all of the children are killed. It is declared an accident caused by a child playing with matches. The neighbors and firemen had trouble reaching the children because the windows were barred and the door had a "deadman" board against it. The family was known to the state protective services.*

This case certainly illustrates neglect and shows that the neglect must be shared among the mother, the landlord, the neighbors who were aware that the mother would often leave the children alone, the fire inspector, and the state protective system.

Some feel that the consideration of neglect should be simplified. Missouri law defines neglect as "**reckless** failure to provide, by those responsible for the care, custody, and control of the child, the proper or necessary support, education as required by law, nutrition or medical, surgical, or any other care necessary for his well-being; and **food, clothing or shelter sufficient for life or essential medical and surgical care.**" This definition in the law clearly allows for broad interpretation by the courts.

## ◆ INCIDENCE AND DEFINITIONS

In 1980, neglect reports accounted for 48% of all child maltreatment reports (NIS-1, 1981). A change in definition expanded the percentage to 63% in 1986 (NIS-2, 1988). With an increased percentage of reports defined as neglect, one could assume that an increased focus on this problem would appear in the professional literature. However, there is a conspicuous lack of research on neglect as compared to other forms of abuse. Neglect is often noted as a component in some studies of other forms of abuse, but the concept of neglect as a separate entity for study is poorly defined. This is still true as we see the challenge of preventing neglect growing even greater in a climate of uncertain economic conditions and changing political realities.

Simply stated, neglect is the failure of caretakers to provide for the basic needs of their children. Failure to meet these needs may vary in degree from mild to severe and can be acute or chronic. No workable definition that quantifies the degree of neglect has yet been found. While there is general agreement on what constitutes extreme neglect, little agreement has been reached concerning what constitutes milder forms of neglect and the harm caused by neglect.

## DEVELOPING CRITERIA TO DEFINE NEGLECT OBJECTIVELY

The degree of harm suffered by the child was the impetus for the first national study on the incidence of child neglect. The National Study of the Incidence and Severity of Child Abuse and Neglect (NIS-1, 1981) defined neglect as a situation in which it could be shown that, as a result of caretaker inattention to the child's basic needs for care, protection, or control, the child experienced predictable injury or impairment of serious or greater severity.

*In addition, an affirmative answer had to be obtained for the following questions:*

1.  Had the caretaker been informed of the child's need or problem by a competent professional, or under the circumstances of the situation, would the child's need have been apparent to most reasonably caring and attentive adults?

2.  Was the caretaker physically and financially able to obtain or provide the needed care, protection, or supervision? (Mayhall & Norgard, 1983)

Using an expanded definition the Department of Health and Human Services (NIS-2, 1988) added a category titled "endangered." This new category allowed for reporting children who had no present evidence of abuse through neglect but for whom it was reasonable to suspect there was the risk of injury as a result of neglect. This change added a substantial number of children who were considered to be neglected. While the risk of harm or endangerment is a category of neglected children that may need intervention to prevent future neglect, the lack of sufficient resources available to child protective services (CPS) and other human services leaves this category of neglect unserved in many states. The dramatic 55% increase in child abuse and neglect reports between 1980 and 1986 was accompanied by a meager 4% increase in funding (Krugman, 1990). During the same period the substantiation rates for child protective services declined (Besharov, 1985; Eckenrode et al., 1988; Kessler & New, 1989). The NIS-2 (1988) concluded that CPS were more selective in the reports investigated.

Overreporting, which is defined as reported cases that are investigated and closed without services being provided (Berger et al., 1989), has led some parent groups to advocate for changes in laws to redefine abuse and neglect and to protect parental rights. Others feel that rather than redefine abuse and neglect, children and parents would be better served by expanding the support and resources of the child protection system and the training of child protection workers.

The following discussion uses the NIS-1 definition of "demonstrable harm," which provides the physician with a workable definition. This facilitates reporting of children who are endangered by neglect, in the judgment of the reporter, in accordance with reporting statutes.

## ◆ TYPES OF NEGLECT

When a child presents with an injury or other signs that potentially result from neglect, it is the responsibility of the physician to find a mechanism to explain the physical signs. For example, a child who falls and is seriously injured may reasonably appear to have suffered an accident. When the physician has suspicions about the cause, a good social history is necessary to determine if it was, in fact, an accident or if neglect or intent played a role in the event.

It is not uncommon to hear or read accounts of children found living in squalid conditions. These reports have common themes: children who are not fed or bathed, extremes of temperatures, and a building filled with debris and contaminated with urine, feces, and vermin. The conditions are described by investigators as the worst they have encountered. In the following sections, conditions that constitute or contribute to the neglect of children are discussed. These conditions may be seen first-hand by workers going into the home or may be inferred when children are examined outside their home environment. The neglect these children suffer may be revealed through their physical appearance, health status, or injuries, or, in some cases, by their deaths.

## PHYSICAL ENVIRONMENT

### INADEQUATE SHELTER

Frequently a house where neglect exists is overcrowded with people, furnishings, trash, or garbage; for example, 25 persons may live in a four-bedroom house. The children simply get lost in the house because of the adults' inattention. They are not supervised because each adult assumes someone else is managing the child's care.

### INADEQUATE SLEEPING ARRANGEMENTS

When a child does not get adequate sleep, he or she may appear as chronically fatigued or listless, particularly as noted by schoolteachers or neighbors. The child's need for sleep may not be met because there are too many people living in the house, too much noise, too many people sleeping in one bed, or no beds available. The practice of allowing or forcing children to sleep with adults can contribute to sexual abuse of the child. This is frequently exacerbated by the lack of consideration for personal boundaries and/or poor self-control (often as a result of drug or alcohol use). Another problem involves bedding that is inadequate for cold weather or soiled with feces or urine. Furthermore, the child may be denied privacy from opposite-sex children or adults, contributing to a sense of shame that can lead to a lack of sleep. Another source of anxiety results from fear when different people are free to roam the premises, posing a threat to the child's security.

### UNSANITARY CONDITIONS

As noted, often in neglect cases the house is filled with an accumulation of garbage and trash. Toilets are unusable, and there may be animal and/or human feces on the floors. Often uncontrolled vermin—rats, spiders, cockroaches—are present. Food preparation under these circumstances is unhealthy and can cause ongoing illness in the child as well as others in the house.

### STRUCTURAL HAZARDS

Not uncommonly, the house or dwelling has partially collapsed. Stairs may have broken steps and railings may be missing, as well as protective barriers on porches or balconies. Windows and doors are in poor repair, with broken or jagged glass. The doors and windows are without screens, and floors and ceilings have holes. Badly worn floors may be covered with large splinters.

### HOUSEKEEPING PROBLEMS

The condition of the house and furniture indicates the lack of even minimal care. Dirt and filth cover the surfaces, especially in the kitchen and bathroom. Clutter and trash are everywhere, obviously having accumulated over a long period of time.

## ENVIRONMENTAL HAZARDS

### FIRE HAZARDS

Exposed or frayed wiring is frequently found in the home. Fuel containers are stored in living areas, and combustible materials are placed near heat sources. Beds are too close to heat sources, which could result in burns of unaware children, as well as fires. Metal bars on windows and "deadman" props against doors impede evacuation should a fire occur in the house.

## Substance Accessibility and Use

Chemicals or drugs may be within reach or easy accessibility of children who can climb up to storage areas. Illicit drugs in the house or the use of the house in drug traffic are particularly hazardous to children and often accompany neglect.

## Excessive Hot Water Temperature

In houses where neglect is practiced, the hot water available at the tap may be greater than 130° Fahrenheit. The time required to burn skin with water at this temperature is less than 30 seconds; if the water is at 140° F a burn can occur in 3 seconds; at 147° F it only takes 1 second for a burn to be inflicted (Johnson, 1990). Thus if an unsupervised child accidentally turns on the hot water tap, a serious burn can result in 1 second.

## Inadequate Care Standards

### Nutrition

The food may be of poor quality and lacking in nutritional value. The diet is inadequate with regard to the basic food groups and does not offer any variety, indicating a lack of meal planning or haphazard planning. Often no adult caretaker prepares meals on a consistent basis. The food provided may also be inappropriate for the child's age and developmental abilities. Food found stored in either a cupboard or a refrigerator may be spoiled. Unfortunately, in many cases no food is available. The mealtime itself may be marked by chaos or unpleasant routines for the child, further adversely affecting his or her nutritional status.

### Clothing

Clothing for neglected children is inadequate and inappropriate for the weather and season. It may also be dirty, ill-fitting, or in a poor state of repair. The child's footwear can be inadequate for the season, too small, too large, or in poor repair.

### Personal Hygiene

Neglected children often show evidence of not having bathed for a lengthy period of time, smelling of urine, feces, or sweat, covered with crusted dirt, and hair unkempt. The child often states that he or she has not bathed. Poor dental hygiene is evident by severe dental caries and mouth odor. When asked, the child may state that he or she does not brush his or her teeth. Furthermore, neglect is evident when there is the persistent presence of lice.

### Health Care

Neglect implies that even minimal health care is not obtained and the child lacks immunizations. The adult either overuses emergency services, going to the hospital for even slight problems, or does not use them at all, even with severe injury and illness. When medicine or rehabilitative equipment is prescribed, the prescription goes unfilled. Dental caries and other dental needs remain untreated. Regimens recommended for the treatment of chronic illness are not followed or compliance is poor. Prescribed psychological help is not obtained.

### Supervision

The lack of supervision by the parent and/or caretaker can lead to injuries that could have been avoided and to repeated injuries. The key question to be answered is whether the behavior of the parent and/or caretaker contributed significantly to the child's injury.

## Developmental Neglect

### Education

Neglected children are often not enrolled in school after the state-required age. The adult caretaker permits chronic truancy and fails to provide encouragement for the educational process. The adult caretaker also fails to provide the necessary control, discipline, or role model for learning, socialization, and responsible behavior.

### EMOTIONAL GROWTH

When there is emotional neglect, the child's needs for emotional support and encouragement are not provided by the adult caretaker. The adult caretaker is unavailable emotionally, is indifferent, or rejects the child. Because there is inadequate supervision, the child engages in dangerous behaviors for long periods of time. The child's need for emotional security is not met.

## ♦ ATTACHMENT DISORDERS

Attachment disorders are defined as the caregiver's rejection of the child and the parental role. Abandonment can occur because attachment to the child, or bonding, which normally develops during the prenatal or immediate antenatal period, fails to occur. The parent has no feelings of attachment to the child and no sense of responsibility for providing for the child's basic needs.

### ABANDONMENT

In general, abandonment is a legal term with legal implications that refers to the physical aspects of neglect and fulfills certain rigid criteria. However, in addition to physical abandonment, which frequently results from attachment disorders, there is emotional abandonment, which, in the long run, is potentially more devastating. In emotional abandonment the parent, usually the mother, in one way or another completely withdraws from nurturing and meeting the child's needs for security. This parallels the general aspects of abandonment, where the caregiver does not meet the child's needs for physical security. The child's needs are either not met or are provided for by others.

Parental characteristics, rather than those associated with the child, and environmental factors are the best predictors of the potential for abandonment. Among the predisposing characteristics are sexual promiscuity with or without alcoholism, financial problems, and relatively poor state of health. Depression, especially when severe, can be a factor in causing abandonment (Martin & Walters, 1982).

*The circumstances and conditions associated with abandonment can be categorized by the following six types:*

1. Fatal or near-fatal abandonment
2. Abandonment with physical needs provided by others
3. Throwaways
4. Parental custody refusal
5. Lack of supervision
6. Emotional abandonment

### FATAL OR NEAR-FATAL ABANDONMENT

Children abandoned with the intent to kill either die or are saved by fortuitous circumstances. Abandonment at its worst is abandonment infanticide. In these instances the child is left to die or is left in conditions likely to result in his or her death. Children can also be abandoned in places where they are likely to be found and subsequently cared for. Sometimes, however, they are not found in time to prevent serious health problems or death.

*A set of twins was put in trash bags and placed in a dumpster by the mother, who then called the father and told him where they were.*

*A young mother placed her child in a gangway in subzero weather where the baby would be found by a passerby.*

*A 2-year-old was found, bound hand and foot, in a suitcase under a hospital dumpster by a security guard. The child's gag had been slipped off her mouth and the zipper of the suitcase was left open so the child's cries could be heard.*

*A newborn infant was found by an alert security guard in a gym bag on an icy street in a public park.*

These children and their parent(s) obviously had great need of protective services. Fortunately, most children are found in time to prevent serious health problems or death.

### ABANDONMENT WITH PHYSICAL NEEDS PROVIDED BY OTHERS

Children can be abandoned under conditions that result in the child's physical needs being met by others (Heger & Yungman, 1989). These children are left at hospitals, sitters, relatives, friends, neighbors, licensed providers, or extended care facilities. Children who are not picked up 2 days after the agreed upon or arranged pickup are considered abandoned. *(NOTE: This time may vary from state to state.)* In other cases, hospitals and extended care facilities care for children for various periods of time and the caregiver has little responsibility, if any, for providing basic needs. These interludes of absence initiate separations between parent and child and provide an opportunity for parents to abandon the child. Handicapped children are especially susceptible. Prematurely born children often have serious health problems that require lengthy hospitalizations in high technology environments. In some cases, no attachment is formed between the parent and child. Temporary abandonments by parents because of incarceration or emergency hospitalization without care plans are not considered legal abandonment unless there is a previous history of physical abandonment.

### THROWAWAYS

Some children, particularly adolescents, are thrown out of their homes by their parents or caregivers. They may be physically thrown out, locked out, or refused admittance to the home upon their return after having run away or after delinquent behavior or becoming pregnant. Some children choose to leave the home and parental care. In some cases the parents or caregivers relinquish parenting and turn legal custody of the child over to juvenile authorities. The child's delinquent or incorrigible behavior is often cited as the reason for this action rather than the parents' inability to parent. These children are emancipated prematurely and abandoned to others for care. They are vulnerable to exploitation, often wander the streets, and are totally left to their own resources to provide for their care and survival.

### PARENTAL CUSTODY REFUSAL

Some parents are unable or unwilling to accept custody responsibilities for their children. The children in these circumstances live an uncertain existence. They spend days or weeks with different relatives, parents' friends, or even total strangers. The shuffling of children from one caregiver to another is a chronic situation and is usually based on the parents' unwillingness to parent rather than an acute financial or housing problem. The child's need for a stable environment is not met. Financial and housing difficulties, however, do occur among these families and can play a significant role. Each case must be investigated individually.

### LACK OF SUPERVISION

Children who are unsupervised for long periods of time, who engage in dangerous activities, or who stay away from home overnight—and the caregiver does not know where they are and makes no attempt to locate them—are in a sense abandoned. They may become throwaways later in life, or their parents or caregivers may refuse custody when these children get into predelinquent or delinquent activities.

### EMOTIONAL ABANDONMENT

Emotional abandonment has been described in the backgrounds of many adults. As children, they did not form secure attachments (Armsworth, 1990). The parent may have been physically present but emotionally absent or unavailable to the child. Often these were severely dysfunctional families in which these individuals describe periods of emotional abandonment and then overcontrol. Some experienced physical abandonment in conjunction with the emotional absence. Often these adults were sexually victimized as children and later by others. The dynamics present in these emotionally scarred adults can be found in members of other severely dysfunctional families where physical abuse and neglect occur.

The effects of the parents' behavior, through abandonment, leave the child in a confused, emotionally stressed state. The child's sense of trust in an adult's availability to meet his or her needs is severely shaken. This lack of trust may have lifelong consequences in relationships with others. As adults, these victims may exhibit no understanding of what is right and what is wrong. They often experience difficulty bonding to their own offspring and may have marital problems. If their youth included juvenile delinquency, this can be carried into adulthood as antisocial behavior. Unless they receive treatment, a cycle of emotional and/or physical abandonment can continue.

## ♦ FAILURE TO THRIVE

Nonorganic failure to thrive is an interactional disorder in which parental expectations, parental skills, and the resulting home environment are intertwined with the child's developmental capabilities. Spinner and Siegel (1987) have found that an effective approach to this syndrome must consider the multiple etiologic factors involved.

Nonorganic failure to thrive in some instances relates to child abuse or neglect. This syndrome can be associated with maternal deprivation or emotional abuse and for that reason has also been referred to as psychosocial dwarfism. Nonorganic failure to thrive is characterized by physical and developmental retardation associated with a disturbed mother-infant relationship.

Berkowitz and Senter (1987) published a study that quantified the differences noted in interactions between a mother and her failure-to-thrive infant whose condition was not induced by organic causes. These mother-infant pairs were videotaped and evaluated in comparison to a control group of mother-thriving infant pairs. Twenty-one different behavioral categories were assessed, and statistically significant differences were noted in five.

A high percentage of failure-to-thrive cases, where children are slow to develop or learn, involve victims of deprivation and neglect. Cooper (1978) highlighted the importance of underdiagnosing the incidence of failure to thrive without organic cause. She emphasized that growth retardation is more readily demonstrated in the first 3 years of life when growth is most rapid (Lacey & Parkin, 1974). Pediatricians must evaluate the psychosocial environment of children who are not growing properly. Often the reason given is that the parents were also small, but in many instances the parents were small for the same psychosocial reasons. In evaluating children with failure to thrive without organic cause, Lacey and Parkin mentioned that the typical child's height is below the third percentile for his age and birth weight. He is thin and even emaciated. Pot belly, hypotonia, episodes of diarrhea, tension, misery, and cold, dull, pale, and mottled skin are characteristic. These children are apathetic and withdrawn, avoid personal contact, and are emotionally and verbally unresponsive, often avoiding eye contact. They may have short temper tantrums. Many appear to be insensitive to pain and have self-inflicted injuries. Some are encopretic and enuretic. Insomnia and disrupted sleep are common, with the result that they often roam the house at night, probably searching for food. Some eat and drink inappropriate substances from the garbage can, toilet bowl, or a dog's or cat's dish. Questions regarding their behavior in the home must be evaluated cautiously because families usually hide any psychological harassment and physical abuse of children. Lacey and Parkin summarize the definition of "deprivation dwarfism" in **Table 18-1**.

| Table18-1. Findings in Deprivation Dwarfism |
| --- |
| *The Child's Appearance* <br>     Short stature <br>     Usually thin <br>     Infantile proportions <br>     Pot belly (with episodes of diarrhea) <br>     Skin dull, pale, and cold <br>     Limbs pink or purple, cold, and mottled <br>     Edema of the feet, legs, hands, and forearms <br>     Poor skin care, excoriations, abrasions, and ulcers <br>     Sparse, dry hair with patches of alopecia <br>     Dejection and apathy <br>     May have bruises, small cuts, burns, or scars <br><br> *The Child's Behavior* <br>     Passive with or without catatonia <br>     Rocking or head banging <br>     Retarded speech and language <br>     Delayed development <br>     Solitary and unable to play <br>     Easily bullied <br>     Gorging food and scavenging from wastebaskets, etc. <br>     Particularly notable—during their convalescent stay in a hospital they have marked growth spurts that relapse as soon as they return to their home environment. <br><br> *The Child's Progress in the Hospital* <br>     Rapid recovery of growth and liveliness <br>     Slower progress with speech and language <br>     Affection seeking, but may be shallow or even promiscuous <br>     Attention seeking <br>     Severe tantrums at the slightest frustration <br>     Rocking and head banging when upset <br>     Remain greedy and scavenge food <br><br> *The Child's Later Behavior* <br>     Speech and language immaturity <br>     Gorging of food that may last 6 months or more <br>     Restlessness with short attention span <br>     Rocking and head banging if stressed <br>     Difficulties with peer group and learning in school <br>     Soiling and wetting <br>     Stealing and lying <br>     Tantrums and aggression |

The characteristic endocrine abnormality of these children is a deficient growth hormone response to insulin-induced hypoglycemia. Most have a deficient growth hormone response to arginine infusion and to exercise. Apparently a deficit also exists in slow-wave sleep associated with the deficiency in growth hormone secretion (Guilhaume et al., 1982). Although failure to thrive can be caused by a number of organic conditions, failure to thrive caused by parental behavior is clearly defined. With nutritional neglect or deprivation the child does not consume enough calories and other nutrients to grow and develop at the expected rates (Helfer, 1984). In failure to thrive the child is found to be below the third percentile on standardized growth grids and is not growing at the expected rate; he may, in fact, lose weight and show no change in length or height. In some cases the child may receive sufficient calories, but because of emotional deprivation he still does not thrive. This phenomenon has been called maternal deprivation or psychosocial dwarfism.

## FAMILY DYNAMICS

Family dynamics have been researched in an attempt to understand failure to thrive. Although stress, parental skill and education, and personality each play a role in failure to thrive, parental interaction with the child, the family support system, and parental relationships are more basic to the problem (Heger & Yungman, 1989).

Since the mother is the primary caretaker in most families, many studies have focused on the maternal role. The concept of parental deprivation was used by Gagan to explain the dynamics in his study (Gagan et al., 1984). He concluded, "It is parental deprivation and deficient social support networks for the mother, rather than maternal deprivations, which are central to the etiology of non-organic FTT."

Alderette and deGraffenried (1986) found nonorganic failure to thrive in families whose interactional style was described as disengagement. These families had poor communication between all members, and there was minimal interaction among family members. The preexisting disengaged style is responsible for the lack of parental bonding. The pervasive lack of nurturing and attachment by the parents causes the child to respond similarly. The child responds with a feeding and behavioral problem. Infants in these families adopt the disengaged style by becoming withdrawn, undemanding, and unresponsive. Thus the failure-to-thrive infant is viewed as the symptom of a breakdown in the family system.

Parental denial of the physical and behavior problems in failure-to-thrive children was found to be significant (Ayoub & Milner, 1985); "the absence of attachment pervaded the parent-child encounters." The more severe the family dynamics problem, the more likely it is that the child will have a reactive attachment disorder.

## CHILDREN AT RISK

Children begin an interactive role at age 4 months. The mother-child interactional roles are defined when the child is between 5 and 12 months of age. During this first year of life, most children are initially admitted to hospitals for nonorganic failure to thrive, with 25% admitted during the first month of life (Gagan et al., 1984). These children are most vulnerable at this time and at the highest risk for morbidity and mortality.

Failure-to-thrive children can also be targeted for abuse if the family situation is left untreated. Koel (1969) reported several failure-to-thrive children who were victims of violent deaths when they were sent back to parents who had not been treated or counseled.

## ♦ FETAL NEGLECT

Included in good prenatal care are instruction in nutrition management, medical checkups to monitor fetal development and the mother's health, and education regarding the avoidance of toxins harmful to the developing fetus. Poor nutrition and cigarette smoking are well known to cause lower birth weights. In addition, fetal alcohol syndrome is a recognized result of alcohol abuse by the mother during her pregnancy. Heavy metal intoxication causes brain damage and adversely involves other systems of the developing fetus. Rubella is known to cause birth defects. The effects of illicit drugs (e.g., heroin, marijuana, amphetamines, cocaine) and crack cocaine have been documented for harm caused to the developing fetus as well as for contributing to inadequate parenting skills and interest on the part of the mother. Cocaine use during pregnancy specifically results in newborn infants with growth retardation and microcephaly (Doberczak et al., 1987; Hadeed & Siegel, 1989); increased rates of anomalies of the genitourinary, cardiac, and central nervous system (Bays, 1990); renal malformation; and cerebral cortical atrophy (Cregler & Mark, 1986), among numerous other harmful effects.

Two issues emerge regarding neglect in the prenatal period of development. First, what level of responsibility does a mother have toward her developing fetus? Second, what should society do about mothers who ingest harmful toxins and injure their developing child? These questions are especially pertinent when the majority of infants exposed to drug or alcohol are discharged to addicted families where they are at risk for further abuse and/or neglect (Bays, 1992). Opinions differ as to the rights of the fetus (Risenberg, 1989) and the rights of the pregnant woman (Fleisher, 1987, 1988). The debate over this topic is unlikely to conclude soon.

The significance of fetal neglect becomes clear after examining the growing body of knowledge about preventive and prenatal predictors of child maltreatment. Lally (1984) pointed out that the emotional relationship between parent and child begins before the child is born and is particularly malleable throughout pregnancy and during the first year of life. Research has shown that prevention efforts are effective at these early stages. Murphy et al. (1985) found that prenatal testing of pregnant women could predict which women were at risk for neglecting their yet unborn child. Main and Goldwyn (1984) observed child-mother relationships. They found that mothers whose children avoided them gave descriptions of their own childhood experiences that had cognitive distortions of their relationships with their mothers. These researchers inferred that mothers who have been rejected by their mothers, in turn, reject their own children.

# ◆Drugs and Alcohol

In addition to the physical effects in the developing fetus, drug and alcohol use is a significant contributing factor in the maltreatment of children. Parents and/or caretakers under the influence of these toxins commit thousands of neglectful and abusive acts each year. Drugs and alcohol facilitate the sexual abuse of children by lowering inhibitions in both the adult and the child. Their contribution to the problem of neglect is considerable. The purchase of drugs and alcohol by a parent or caretaker diverts financial resources, often a scarce commodity, from providing for the basic needs of the family—food, shelter, and warmth. Under the influence of these substances, the parent or caretaker cannot provide optimum care for the children. The level of care declines; for infants the lack of care can be catastrophic.

The presence of illicit drugs in a child's environment produces the risk of serious harm. Children and infants may become intoxicated themselves through deliberate poisoning, passive inhalation, accidental ingestion of drugs or alcohol, or accepting drugs proffered by an adult or older child (Schwartz & Einhorn, 1986). Cases involving children who have been healthy but who come seeking medical attention with unexplained neurologic symptoms or seizures, children who apparently fall victim to sudden infant death syndrome (SIDS), or those who die unexpectedly in other situations should be screened for the presence of alcohol or drug intoxication (Bays, 1990).

## ◆THE EFFECTS AND OUTCOMES OF CHILD NEGLECT

Neglected children suffer hurts in their bodies, their minds, their emotions, and their spirits. The hurts in their bodies mend and heal, but the hurts in their minds, emotions, and spirits have far-reaching ramifications. Neglect of their minds can be recognized through delayed intellectual development that affects performance in preschool and school. Emotional hurts can be exhibited by aggression and depression. When the spirit is hurt, the child no longer tries to succeed, instead withdrawing from life. The joy of childhood is lost.

### DEVELOPMENTAL EFFECTS

The early years of life are critical periods of development for the child. Neglect during this time can cause development to stop, freeze permanently, or even fail to occur (Helfer et al., 1976). The body, mind, and emotions of children operate on a developmental timetable that is individually determined. These developments cannot be put in an emotional deep freeze or placed on hold while parents work through problems sufficiently to make it safe for the child to live in the home (Kempe, 1976). Some families are untreatable or cannot be treated in time to meet the developmental needs of the child (Jones, 1987).

Each neglected or maltreated child needs an individual treatment plan to meet his or her needs. Often the treatment services provided by CPS are parent oriented rather than child oriented. Services are dropped when the crisis appears to have resolved (Alfaro, 1984). But some children need help from the day they are born (Brazelton, 1990), and still others may need a lifetime of treatment services.

### LONG-TERM EFFECTS OF NEGLECT

The long-term effects of neglect reveal extreme variations in the child's behavior or illness. Extreme neglect can result in child fatalities. One-fifth of unexpected child deaths (defined as those occurring before arrival at the hospital or within 10 days of being hospitalized) were suspicious for abuse or neglect (Christoffel et al., 1985). Children who do not die from abuse or neglect may suffer long-term sequelae. The effects of malnutrition, for example, include lower intelligence, slowed growth, poor teeth, deformities, and life-long poor health.

Children who have been neglected have an increased incidence of psychopathology. They tend to be slow and cognitively impaired (Vondra, 1990), have difficulty relating to others, and have an increased frequency of unsocialized conduct disorders (Rogeness et al., 1986). Adults who were neglected as children may be unable to trust others, develop problems with anger, suffer feelings of low self-esteem, have a decreased ability to form enduring, satisfying relationships, and exhibit impaired social skills (Tower, 1989). Mothers who neglect their children seem unable or unwilling to provide for the health, safety, or well-being of their children. In turn, their children have difficulty mustering the energy or resources to deal with various tasks. As preschoolers they are dependent, have poor ego controls, are negativistic, and frequently are noncompliant (Egeland et al., 1983).

Another widely studied effect of physical abuse and neglect is the link to delinquency and adult criminality. Most studies link abuse and neglect in some combination. One study, however, separates neglect and its outcomes (McCord, 1983). In McCord's findings, 45% of abused and neglected boys had been convicted of serious crimes, become alcoholics or mentally ill, or died before age 35. If there was a history of abuse or neglect, juvenile delinquency tended to result. This finding is similar to the bidirectional relationship between child abuse and delinquency (Howing et al., 1990).

Victimization in childhood has demonstrable consequences in adult criminal behavior. In one study, individuals who were abused or neglected as children had higher arrest rates as adults than did control subjects (Widom, 1989). While there is a clear relationship between childhood victimization and later adult criminal behavior, the majority of subjects in both the McCord (53%) and Widom (71%) studies did not demonstrate extreme behavioral problems or damage. Widom points out the need to look for more subtle forms of damage in evaluating these cases.

Among the outcomes in those with subtle forms of damage, we see the developmentally frozen child or the untreated, neglected child becoming the neglecting parent in the next generation of the cycle of neglect. Whether extreme or subtle, the effects of neglect create unhappy, unproductive, and sometimes violent adults. The cycle can be broken through the treatment of neglected children and neglecting families as well as the prevention of neglect.

## ♦ PREVENTION

Although it may not always be possible to break the intergeneration cycle of neglect, an effort should be made. Primary prevention of neglect involves finding those at risk and connecting them with resources that provide supportive programs aimed at preventive measures. However, most current efforts in preventing neglect involve secondary prevention. Thus the system waits until a neglected child is recognized before efforts are made to prevent further neglect and to treat the harm already done to the child. Prenatal and perinatal predictors of neglect that have been identified could form the basis of primary prevention programs. Early diagnosis of attachment disorders (Caffo et al., 1982; Call, 1984; Harris et al., 1989), problem parenting, family stress, failure to thrive, and parental rejection of the current parent point to areas where preventive efforts may be directed to help both the infant and the family (Gagan et al., 1984; Main & Goldwyn, 1984; Ayoub & Milner, 1985; Murphy et al., 1985; Avison et al., 1986; Edwards et al., 1990).

Truly effective programs addressing primary prevention of neglect are generations away even if we start now. However, if we treat the victims of neglect today, we can be accomplishing primary prevention for a future generation. Treatment of the neglecting parent or caretaker can also decrease the damage at the present time.

Families are only one context in which neglect occurs. These families live in a society that neglects children. The social welfare infrastructure developed to offer support for families has been reduced or dismantled by budget cuts over the last decade. Many of these services reduced stress factors known to be associated with neglect, such as insufficient income, inadequate housing, social isolation, family discord, and the use of drugs and alcohol. The loss of these supportive services has stressed families even more. Cuts in funding for education, mental health, public medical care, and limited access to this medical care have exacerbated the neglect of children. As stated earlier, the drug problem and associated crime have led to the deaths of children and extreme physical neglect. In addition, the economic changes noted have led to neglect in families involved with traditionally secure professions, such as farming and manufacturing.

The child protection system was designed to evaluate families and to provide services to aid in correcting conditions known to produce neglect and abuse (Krugman, 1990). Yet it has not met the increasing demands for investigation, treatment, and prevention services that we have seen over the past decade. The result has been the loss of trained, clinically oriented workers; decreased treatment capabilities; and poor general ability to perform the functions mandated by statutes. The impact of the cocaine and crack epidemic has overwhelmed child protection services as well as the foster care system. There is a crisis in the child protection system that now represents a national emergency (U.S. Advisory Board on Child Abuse and Neglect, 1990).

During the last decade the issue of prevention gained legislative attention. Forty-nine states now have trust funds for prevention programs. In 1988 the funds for prevention programs totaled $32 million (Krugman, 1990). These monies are earmarked for programs aimed at prevention of abuse.

Treating and preventing chronic neglect consumes both time and resources. It is frustrating to work with neglectful families, and success comes slowly, if at all. As stated earlier, some families are untreatable (Jones, 1987). Focusing prevention or treatment on the individual neglected child or neglecting parent will not guarantee that neglect will not occur.

## PHYSICIAN ROLES

The prevention of child neglect must be addressed at the level of the individual, family, society, and culture. The prevention of neglect requires a concentrated effort at each of these levels and a long-term commitment to accomplish its goals. Leadership is needed in this effort, and the physician can play a key role in preventing and treating neglect.

The physician recognizing neglect is legally responsible for reporting it to CPS. The physician's evaluation of the child provides direct evidence of neglect as well as signs that point to neglectful conditions in the child's environment. The American Medical Association issued guidelines to assist physicians in evaluating and reporting child abuse and neglect (Council on Scientific Affairs, 1985). Immunity has been granted to physician reporters and penalties provided for failure to report.

Physicians still fail to recognize and report child maltreatment. Some physicians do not report it because experience has caused them to question the ability of CPS to protect children or to follow through with appropriate intervention for neglected children (Helfer, 1990; Krugman, 1990). Their reluctance to report abuse and neglect may also result from lack of training and fear of potential loss of patients. Pollack and Levy (1989) state that countertransference (also referred to as vicarious traumatization [McCann & Pearlman, 1990], where the therapist takes on the symptoms of trauma of the child and reacts to them adversely), is an inevitable part of work with child abuse and neglect cases and recommend education and training so that all persons employed in this field better understand these reactions.

## CHILD ADVOCATE

By virtue of their knowledge and expertise, physicians are in a unique position to impact outcomes for abused and neglected children. The role of child advocate accompanies the recognition and reporting roles. Most physicians are reluctant to be involved in the court system, viewing it as a possibly unpleasant experience. Yet the physician's testimony in court can be the determining factor in helping the court decide whether abuse or neglect occurred, what degree of harm the child has suffered, and future problems the child could face related to this harm. The physician can and should make recommendations regarding the child's safety and protection.

Physicians can also impact the legislative process on behalf of children. They can speak to the needs of children, the effects of abuse and neglect, and the effects of specific public policies on children. In this period of declining resources, children need articulate spokespersons who are willing to represent them at all levels of government.

## ◆ REGIONAL CENTERS

Programs or regional centers have been developed to address the unique needs posed by premature infants, genetic disorders, hemophilia, and learning disabilities. Many child protection workers feel that regional child abuse centers could concentrate resources and expertise to manage and treat child abuse and neglect more effectively. These centers can gather research data and information for prevention and treatment programs (Heger & Stewart, 1988; Kessler & New, 1989). Regional centers could be located in medical facilities or be freestanding. A multidisciplinary center can bring together all the agencies involved in the investigation, coordination, treatment, and prevention of child abuse and neglect. In view of the current lack of funding in numerous fields, the regional center concept may be the most cost-effective means to manage the existing problem of child abuse and neglect and to further advance the knowledge base related to the problem.

## ◆COMMUNITY FAMILY SUPPORT CENTERS

Another approach that shows promise in providing the necessary integration and coordination of services is the development of community family support centers. Several authors have urged the development of a single site for services delivery (Greenspan, 1987; Cicchetti and Roth, 1995). Family support centers can be found in a number of states. Legislation in Missouri has enabled the Division of Family Services to pilot a number of such projects throughout the state and will select models for state-wide implementation at a later date.

## ◆BIBLIOGRAPHY

Alderette, P, and deGraffenried, DF: Non-organic failure-to-thrive syndrome and the family system, *Soc Work* May-June:207, 1986.

Alfaro, J: Helping children overcome the effects of abuse and neglect, *Pediatr Ann* 13:778, 1984.

Armsworth, M: A qualitative analysis of adult incest survivors' response to sexual involvement with therapists, *Child Abuse Negl* 14:541, 1990.

Avison, W, Turner, RJ, and Nolt, S: Screening for problem parenting: Preliminary evidence on a promising instrument, *Child Abuse Negl* 10:157, 1986.

Ayoub, C, and Milner, JS: Failure to thrive: Parental indicators, types and outcomes, *Child Abuse Negl* 9:491, 1985.

Bays, J: Substance abuse and child abuse: Impact of addiction on the child, *Pediatr Clin North Am* 37:881, 1990.

Bays, J: The Care of Alcohol and Drug-Affected Infants, *Pediatr Ann* 218:485-495, August, 1992.

Berger, D, et al: Child abuse and neglect: An instrument to assist case referral decision making, *Health Soc Work* 14:60, 1989.

Berkowitz, CD, and Senter, SA: Characteristics of mother-infant interactions in nonorganic failure to thrive, *J Fam Practice* 25(4): 377-381, 1987.

Besharov, DJ: Doing something about child abuse: The need to narrow the grounds for state intervention, *Harvard J Law Pub Pol* 8:539, 1985.

Brazelton, T: Why is America failing its children? *NY Times Magazine* Sept 9, 1990.

Caffo, E, et al: Prevention of child abuse and neglect through early diagnosis of serious disturbances in the mother-child relationship in Italy, *Child Abuse Negl* 6:453, 1982.

Call, JD: Child abuse and neglect in infancy: Sources of hostility within the parent/infant dyad and disorders of attachment in infancy, *Child Abuse Negl* 8:185, 1984.

Christoffel, KK, Zieserl, EJ, and Chiaramonte, J: Should child abuse and neglect be considered when a child dies unexpectedly? *Am J Dis Child* 139:876, 1985.

Cicchetti, D, and Toth, SL: A developmental psychopathological perspective on child abuse and neglect, *J Am AcAD Child Adolesc Psychiatry* 34:51, May, 1995.

Cooper, CE: Child abuse and neglect: Medical aspects. In SM Smith: *The Maltreatment of Children*, University Park Press, Baltimore, 1978.

Council on Scientific Affairs: AMA diagnostic and treatment guidelines concerning child abuse and neglect, *JAMA* 254:796, 1985.

Cregler, LL, and Mark, H: Medical complications of cocaine abuse, *N Engl J Med* 315:1495, 1986.

Doberczak, DM, Thornton, JC, Bernstein, J, et al: Maternal drug dependency and growth impact, *Am J Dis Child* 141:1163, 1987.

Eckenrode, J, et al: Substantiation of child abuse and neglect reports, *J Consult Clin Psychol* 56:9, 1988.

Edwards, A, et al: Recognizing failure to thrive in early childhood, *Arch Dis Child* 65:1263, 1990.

Egeland, B, Stroufe, LA, and Erickson, MA: The developmental consequences of different patterns of maltreatment, *Child Abuse Negl* 7:459, 1983.

Fleisher, LD: Wrongful birth: When is there liability for prenatal injury? *Am J Dis Child* 141:1260, 1987.

Fleisher, LD: Fatal neglect as child abuse, *Am J Dis Child* 142:914, 1988.

Gagan, R, Cupoli, JM, and Watkins, AH: The families of children who fail to thrive: Preliminary investigation of parental deprivation among organic and non-organic cases, *Child Abuse Negl* 8:93, 1984.

Greenspan, S: A model for comprehension preventive intervention services for infants, young children and their families. In SI Greenspan, S Weider, A Lieberman, R Nover, R Louri, and M Robinson, eds: *Infants in Multi-risk Families*, International Universities Press, New York, 1987, pp. 377-390.

Guilhaume, A, Benoit, O, and Gourmelen, M: Relationship between sleep IV deficit and reversible HGH deficiency in psychosocial dwarfism, *Pediatr Res* 16:299-303, 1982.

Hadeed, AJ, and Siegel, SR: Maternal cocaine use during pregnancy: Effect on the newborn infant, *Pediatrics* 84:205, 1989.

Harris, ES, Weston, DR, and Lieberman, A: Quality of mother-infant attachment and pediatric health care use, *Pediatrics* 84:248, 1989.

Hathaway, P: Failure to thrive: Knowledge for social workers, *Health Soc Work* May:122, 1989.

Heger, A, and Stewart, D: *Sexual abuse: The pediatrician's role*. Paper presented at the American Academy of Pediatrics, Spring Session, 1988, New York.

Heger, RL, and Yungman, JJ: Toward a causal typology of child neglect, *Child Youth Services Rev* 11:203, 1989.

Helfer, RE: The epidemiology of child abuse and neglect, *Pediatr Ann* 13:745, 1984.

Helfer, RE: Where to now, Henry? A commentary on the battered child syndrome, *Pediatrics* 76:993, 1985.

Helfer, RE: The neglect of our children, *Pediatr Clin North Am* 37:923, 1990.

Helfer, RE, McKinney, JP, and Kemper, R: Arresting or freezing the developmental process. In Child Abuse and Neglect: *The Family and the Community,* Ballinger Publishing Co, Cambridge, MA, 1976.

Howing, P, et al: Child abuse and delinquency: The empirical and theoretical links, *Soc Work* May:244, 1990.

Howze, DC, and Kotch, JB: Disentangling life events, stress and social support: Implications for the primary prevention of child abuse and neglect, *Child Abuse Negl* 8:401, 1984.

Johnson, CF: Inflicted injury versus accidental injury, *Pediatr Clin North Am* 37:791, 1990.

Jones, DPH: The untreatable family, *Child Abuse Negl* 11:409, 1987.

Justice, B, Calvert, A, and Justice, R: Factors mediating child abuse as a response to stress, *Child Abuse Negl* 9:359, 1985.

Kempe, CH. In H Martin and CH Kempe, eds: *The Abused Child: Multidisciplinary Approach to Developmental Issues and Treatment,* Ballinger Publishing Co, Cambridge, MA, 1976, pp. xi-xiii.

Kessler, DB, and New, M: Emerging trends in child abuse and neglect, *Pediatr Ann* 18:471, 1989.

Koel, BS: Failure to thrive and fatal injury as a continuum, *Am J Dis Child* 118:565, 1969.

Krugman, RD: Future role of the pediatrician in child abuse and neglect, *Pediatr Clin North Am* 37:1003, 1990.

Lacey, KA, and Parkin, JM: The normal short child, *Arch Dis Child* 49:417, 1974.

Lally, JR: Three views of child neglect: Expanding visions of preventive intervention, *Child Abuse Negl* 8:243, 1984.

Main, M, and Goldwyn, R: Predicting rejecting of her infant from representations of her own experience: Implications for the abused-abusing intergenerational cycle, *Child Abuse Negl* 8:203, 1984.

Martin, MJ, and Walters, J: Familial correlates of selected types of child abuse and neglect, *J Marriage Fam* 44:267-276, 1982.

Mayhall, PD, and Norgard, KE: *Child Abuse and Neglect: Sharing Responsibility,* John Wiley & Sons, New York, 1983.

McCann and Pearlman, LA: Vicarious traumatization: A framework for understanding the psychological effects of working with victims, *J Trauma Stress* 3:133, 1990.

McCord, J: A forty-year perspective on effects of child abuse and neglect, *Child Abuse Negl* 7:265, 1983.

Murphy, S, Orkow, B, and Nicola, RM: Prenatal prediction of child abuse and neglect: A prospective study, *Child Abuse Negl* 9:225, 1985.

Pollack, J, and Levy, S: Countertransference and failure to report child abuse and neglect, *Child Abuse Negl* 13:515, 1989.

Rekowitz, CD, and Senter, SA: Characteristics of mother infant interactions in nonorganic failure to thrive, *J Fam Pract* 25(4):377-381, 1987.

Risenberg, HM:  Fetal neglect and abuse, *NY State J Med* March:148, 1989.

Rogeness, GA, et al:  Psychopathology in abused and neglected children, *J Am Acad Child Psychiatry* 25:659, 1986.

Schwartz, RH, and Einhorn, A:  PCP intoxication in seven young children, *Pediatr Emerg Care* 2:238, 1986.

Spinner, MR, and Siegel, L:  Nonorganic failure to thrive, *J Prevent Psychiatry* 3:279-287, 1987.

Study Findings (NIS-1):  National study of the incidence and severity of child abuse and neglect, US Department of Health and Human Services, 1981.

Study Findings (NIS-2):  Study of the national incidence and prevalence of child abuse and neglect, US Department of Health and Human Services, 1988.

Tower, CC:  The neglect of children. In *Understanding Child Abuse and Neglect*, Allyn and Bacon, 1989.

US Advisory Board on Child Abuse and Neglect:  Child abuse and neglect: Critical first steps in response to a national emergency, US Department of Health and Human Services, 1990.

Vondra, JI:  Self-concept, motivation, and competence among preschoolers from maltreating and comparison families, *Child Abuse Negl* 14:525, 1990.

Widom, CS:  Child abuse, neglect, and adult behavior:  Research design findings on criminality, violence, and child abuse, *Am J Orthopsychiatry* 59:355, 1989.

# FAILURE TO THRIVE: A RECONCEPTUALIZATION

PASQUALE J. ACCARDO, M.D.

*"Myth No. 1: Failure to thrive is not an emotional disorder." (Frank, Silva, & Needlman, 1993)*

*The Division of Developmental Pediatrics was asked to evaluate a 6-month-old white male who had been admitted for an assessment of his failure to thrive. Since this was the third documented episode of growth failure within the first year of life for this child, the state Department of Protective Services had begun legal proceedings to terminate parental rights.*

*When the consultants arrived at the numbered hospital room where the infant was located, one crib was empty. The other bed was occupied by a plump, happy baby who physically and developmentally appeared to be at a 6- to 8-month-old level. The infant was interested and alert and playfully interacting with a woman who was behaving very appropriately with him. If it would be sexist to describe the young woman as beautiful, it would be accurate to describe this mother-infant dyad as beautiful. A videotape of their interactions could be used educationally as a textbook case of the ideal mutual response pattern for mothers and infants. Certainly the failure-to-thrive patient must be the occupant of the other crib. This was, in fact, not the case.*

*The history obtained from the mother was documented by a copy of the primary care physician's office notes in the baby's chart. The mother was 17 years old, married,*

*and living with her husband in a trailer park. The father was employed. The mother was a primigravida who had received prenatal care. The pregnancy, labor, and delivery were unremarkable; the baby's birth weight was 7 pounds. At 5 weeks of age, the baby developed an ear infection with fever and vomiting. At the acute care office visit, it was noted that his weight was slightly down from what it had been at his well-child checkup a week earlier. The otitis cleared quickly in response to medication. He was growing and developing normally at his 2- and 4-month visits, and his immunizations were up to date. At 4-1/2 months, he developed an acute viral gastroenteritis and showed up in the physician's office mildly dehydrated with some weight loss. He was placed on clear liquids, and the gastroenteritis resolved within a few days. Whether the doctor had not specifically prescribed a time limit on the dietary change or the mother did not fully understand his instructions, she kept the baby on clear fluids for the next 2 weeks, after which the infant appeared in the office with weight loss. This was diagnosed as failure to thrive and, since this was noted to be the third episode of such poor weight gain, it was reported to the Division of Protective Services. With such strong medical documentation of maternal incompetence, the decision was made to apply for termination of parental rights.*

What went wrong here? The state's handbook with guidelines for caseworkers included as a criterion for grossly inadequate parenting three episodes of failure to thrive occurring in the first year of life. The establishment of such a rule reflected (1) the social agency's ignorance of the complexities involved in making such a diagnosis and (2) an erroneous assumption that something called "failure to thrive" is pathognomonic of child neglect, if not child abuse.

This chapter will attempt to address the complexities surrounding the poorly defined clinical entity of failure to thrive within the context of a brief history of how all failure-to-thrive cases became confused with child abuse. Throughout this revisionist interpretation, it must be remembered that many infant victims of abuse will exhibit all the signs and symptoms of failure to thrive, and therefore failure to thrive may, in selected cases, occupy a position on the spectrum of child abuse. Similarly, many severely abused infants will exhibit none of the signs or symptoms of failure to thrive. One of the main goals of this chapter will be to caution against an overreliance on this association. To highlight the difficulties of the concepts involved, the acronym FTT will not be used; its use too readily facilitates the reification of an entity that may not exist.

## ◆ Definition

Severe malnutrition in children goes by several names: *marasmus* ("withering"), *kwashiorkor* ("red hair"), *athrepsia* (alpha privative + threpsis = nourishment), *shibi gachaki* (Japan), *Mehlnarschaden* (Germany), and *obwosi* (illness relating to breast feeding during pregnancy [Ainsworth, 1962]). Many of the clinical signs of malnutrition are nonspecific. However, the malnourished child is not simply a smaller version of the well-nourished child; a relative sparing of brain growth produces the appearance of hydrocephalus that, in combination with the distribution of fat loss, leads to a more infantile, premature, or even fetal habitus.

Failure to thrive is not a diagnosis but a presenting symptom, a chief complaint of initial impression. Although some degree of growth failure is an obligatory part of the syndrome, both the perception of illness and the absence of an obvious etiology, either treatable or nontreatable, are also required (Accardo, 1982; Accardo, Morrow, & Whitman, 1991).

### Growth Failure

A weight (in younger infants) or a height (in older children) persistently below the third percentile (2 standard deviations below the mean) for age, a weight less than 80% of the ideal weight for age or height, and failure to maintain a previously established growth pattern are several suggested criteria for growth failure. The crossing of percentile curves by 2 standard deviations is probably the only absolute indicator of growth failure. The child who is small but gaining steadily, following his own growth curve, and whose development is within normal limits, should not be considered as failing to thrive. If an appropriate history is obtained and growth parameters are plotted, constitutional short stature and intrauterine growth retardation should not be confused with failure to thrive. The onset of weight gain in the hospital is an unreliable point to exclude an underlying organic etiology to the growth failure.

Routine growth measures performed at well-child visits must not be performed with a "routine" attitude. Such measurements are critical indicators of an infant's health status. If, as part of a well-child checkup, one of the physical growth parameters (weight, height, or head circumference) demonstrates a marked deviation from normal, the accuracy of that same measurement obtained several months previously at the child's last examination becomes imperative. One cannot go back in time to remeasure. The frequency of errors in such routine measurements of squirming, uncooperative, crying babies is understandable but unacceptable. The importance of accurate body measures is so vital that perhaps every child should be weighed and measured twice at each visit, with a third set of measurements to correct any discrepancies between the first two sets of numbers.

Merely reporting a weight of "below the third percentile" does not provide sufficient detail for comparison or clinical decision making. The growth measures of height, weight, and head circumference should all be plotted on a growth grid so that they may be compared with respect to percentiles, growth ages, and standard deviations from the mean.

Finally, for the growth failure to be compatible with failure to thrive, it must be persistent rather than acute; in infants up to 5 months of age a duration of 56 days and in infants over 5 months a duration of 90 days have been suggested. Most acute illnesses will present with weight loss of shorter duration and should not be considered as failure to thrive. Clusters of recurrent acute episodes of disease may present the clinician with greater diagnostic difficulty.

## PERCEPTION OF ILLNESS

Failure to thrive is growth failure about which the physician is concerned. The suspicion of illness that a particular case of growth failure raises for the experienced clinician is not necessarily one relating exclusively to organic disorders. The concern is that, if this growth failure continues untreated, the child's general health and well-being will be compromised. Mild developmental delay along with apathy and absent to decreased responsiveness to either nurturant or intrusive stimuli are several components of this clinical perception. Such an impression is frequently but not always absent in a child whose primordial or postnatal growth deficiency is secondary to a genetic etiology.

Mitchell, Gorell, & Greenberg (1980) reported an incidence of 9.6% growth failure in a primary care setting and argued a generally benign course for such growth delay. Using weight as the sole criterion for failure to thrive seems more objective, but in fact it produces a completely different population of infants. It is probable that none of these cases would have satisfied the criterion of "perception of illness." The 1% incidence of failure to thrive in hospitalized children (English, 1978) was associated with a much higher morbidity. If failure to thrive is considered a developmental symptom, a comparison with mental retardation might be instructive. Although intelligence quotients (IQs) are still an essential component of the diagnosis, mental retardation cannot be diagnosed by an IQ number alone. Multiple other medical and support factors must be taken into account.

## ABSENCE OF OBVIOUS ETIOLOGY

That the reason for the growth failure should not be immediately apparent to the responsible clinician after a careful history and physical examination is the single criteria contributing most to the vagueness of the syndrome. Some of the rarest causes of growth failure will be immediately recognized by one physician, whereas a less esoteric etiology will lead another practitioner to seek hospitalization and consultation for the child. Most of the large tertiary pediatric hospital studies of failure to thrive were based on populations evaluated before the early 1970s and would therefore not include fetal alcohol syndrome (FAS) in their differential diagnosis. They would have then noted significant family problems in these cases whether or not the maternal alcoholism was diagnosed.

The term *failure to thrive* was originally derived to specifically avoid the implication of any specific etiology and to not prejudice the clinician in a given direction. Traditional approaches discriminated organic failure to thrive from nonorganic failure to thrive. In its evolution, what was intended as a nonjudgmental descriptor evolved into being synonymous first with nonorganic failure to thrive and then with maternal psychopathology. This is perhaps best reflected in the change in descriptive terms used in the American Psychiatric Association's *Diagnostic and Statistical Manual of Mental Disorders,* editions 3 (1980) and 4 (1994), which went from "Lack of the type of care..." in DSM-III to "Pathogenic care....Persistent disregard..." in DSM-IV. Such an historic development has inappropriately dislocated the focus away from the sick child who is failing to thrive.

## ♦ EVALUATION

In no diagnostic problem in pediatrics is the following classic medical maxim more appropriate: 75% of diagnoses are ascertained from the history and 25% from the history combined with the physical examination, with the laboratory being used as needed to confirm these diagnostic impressions or to monitor treatment.

The detailed medical history should focus on feeding, development, previous and familial growth patterns, and feeding problems, as well as a careful review of systems for signs of rare syndromes or unusual presentations of more common conditions. Low birth weight (with the baby being small for gestational age) should make the physician suspect an intrauterine cause for the growth failure, such as congenital infection or generic defect.

Although the importance of a detailed history cannot be overemphasized, some parents will be poor historians. A lack of health care continuity frequently makes obtaining old medical records difficult and unrewarding. An adequate history should prevent patients with simple feeding problems and constitutional short stature from receiving complex medical evaluations or being referred to social agencies for child neglect.

A small percentage of infants do not cry when they are hungry and thus give no indication that they are being underfed. With bottle-fed babies, the deficit in their intake can be readily calculated, but this is more difficult with breast-fed babies.

Height, weight, head circumference, and ponderal index must be plotted on a growth grid appropriate for sex and race and compared with one another. The pattern generated by these plots when they correlate past, present, and follow-up growth data with life history events, onset of clinical signs, and responses to different therapeutic interventions is the single most important contribution to confirming a diagnosis. Special growth grids are available for several different situations (e.g., Guo et al., 1996), including specific genetic syndromes (Cronk et al., 1988). In infancy, if malnutrition persists over time, weight is affected first, length next, and head circumference last. Height will be affected more than weight in endocrine disorders and constitutional short stature, but there is a proportional reduction of both height and weight in growth disturbances secondary to primordial dwarfism or severe central nervous system lesions. Severe, especially disproportionate, microcephaly should always focus attention on the central nervous system. The possibility of recovery of weight, height, and head circumference depends on the underlying cause as well as the duration of the untreated state. Major organ system involvement and minor malformations consistent with suspected syndromes should be sought diligently. When a child presents with height, weight, and head circumference all below the third percentile, there is an increased probability for an organic etiology. Many of the physical and behavioral signs seen in failure to thrive are nonspecific and merely reflect the child's malnourished state (**Table 19-1**).

There is no routine laboratory test battery for failure to thrive. Sample suggested tests to be considered are presented in **Table 19-2**, but which if any of these items are appropriate depends on specific indicators derived from the history and physical examination. Again, it must be remembered that many abnormal laboratory findings reflect the infant's nutritional state rather than any underlying disease process. The large variety of interview instruments and surveys to assess family (almost always identified with the mother) functioning and maternal psychopathology must be considered supportive evidence, but not diagnostic. What most of these tools measure is *risk*. A mother who has suffered a great deal of stress and loss during her pregnancy may be at risk for poor nurturance, but the babies of most such mothers thrive.

## Table 19-1. Signs of Malnutrition

Decreased weight, decreased skinfold thickness, prominent ribs, "skin and bones" appearance

Hair sparse, thin, dry, lifeless, easily pulled out, dull brown/reddish yellow

Pallor (and possibly heart murmur) secondary to anemia ("pastel children")

Excessive perspiration, especially about the head

Facies: lined, aged, pinched appearance with sharp features and sunken cheeks from loss of the suctorial fat pads of Bichat ("fish mouth of misery")

Skin: an "old look," wrinkled, poor turgor, folds hanging on inner thighs and buttocks

Protuberant abdomen, edema ("sugar baby")

Disturbed sleep cycle

Constipation or diarrhea

Hypothermia

Apathy, lethargy, withdrawal

Hypotonia ("floppy baby"), tonic immobility, plastic rigidity

Developmental delay

Affect: quiet, wide-eyed gaze, sad, wary, decreased stranger anxiety, indiscriminate affect, self-stimulatory behavior

## Table 19-2. Medical Evaluation of Failure to Thrive

History

Physical examination

Neurologic assessment

Developmental evaluation

Calorie count (plus intake and output, frequent weight measurements)

Complete blood count (hemoglobin, hematocrit, differential count, and indices)

Blood chemistries (Na, K, C1, $CO_2$ content, urea nitrogen, creatine, Ca, P, alkaline phosphatase, bilirubin, blood sugar, glucose tolerance test)

Urinalysis (pH, specific gravity, reducing substances, ketones, protein, blood, microscopic examination, culture, creatinine, amino acids)

Stool examination (pH, reducing substances, fat balance)

Radiologic examination (chest, intravenous pyelography, upper and lower gastrointestinal series, trauma survey, bone age)

Endocrine tests (thyroid, growth hormone)

Sweat chloride

Serology (VDRL, immunoglobin levels, HIV)

Electrocardiography

Chromosomes studies/genetics consultation

Failure to thrive in infancy and early childhood can be caused by various developmental anomalies, organic diseases, and environmental disorders. An exhaustive listing of potential etiologies is impossible, since growth represents a final common pathway for the impact of multisystem and environmental factors on the child. *Retrospective studies have highlighted certain general conclusions:*

1. A shotgun approach to medical diagnosis is almost always unrewarding.

2. Among organic etiologies, neurologic and neurodevelopmental diagnosis (including mental retardation syndromes) always rank the highest.

The older distinction between organic and nonorganic failure to thrive demonstrated an incidence of organic etiologies ranging from 20% to 50%, depending on study entrance criteria. Sills (1978) found a 10:1 incidence of environmental deprivation compared to simple feeding problems, while Hannaway (1970) reported that feeding problems outnumbered deprivation by a factor of 2:1. Thus even the breakdown among nonorganic failure to thrive has been inconsistent.

Truly pathologic mothering must be considered as very rare and the exception rather than the rule. When it does occur, many of the behavioral features of psychosocial dwarfism (PSD) are evident: polydipsia, polyphagia, food refusal, food hoarding, drinking from the toilet bowl, eating from garbage cans, a disturbed sleep pattern, encopresis, pain agnosia, self-injurious behavior, and reversibly lowered growth hormone levels (hyposomatotropinism).

Although certain cases of failure to thrive will fall along the continuum of child abuse (Koel, 1969), many disorders of parenting and feeding are very inappropriately described by referring to "maternal deprivation." Rutter (1972) commented that maternal deprivation is neither maternal nor deprivation. The presumption that all lower social class environments are inferior and either abusive or neglectful, if not both, is inappropriate. The vague conceptualization of maternal deprivation has nevertheless persisted and resurfaced in altered dress in the form of an extensive literature on maternal bonding.

## ♦ INTERACTIONAL AND NEURODEVELOPMENTAL ASPECTS

Cases of failure to thrive may have multiple etiologies. For example, infants with low body weights before the development of gastroenteritis are more susceptible to a secondary disaccharide intolerance. Since malnutrition impairs the body's ability to respond to infection, marginal undernutrition with a supervening infection may more rapidly progress to overt malnutrition. This interaction between etiologies need not be restricted to organic factors.

A high prevalence of either mental retardation or other significant neurodevelopmental disabilities (with up to two thirds of such children exhibiting significant developmental delay) is reported either during the initial assessment or as part of the long-term follow-up of children with failure to thrive (Ambuel & Harris, 1963; Elmer, Gregg, & Ellison, 1969; Glaser et al., 1968; Ripley et al., 1968; Hufton & Oates, 1977). A large percentage of cases classified as nonorganic failure to thrive may mask a hidden neurodevelopmental component.

This raises the question of whether it is possible to distinguish between brain damage existing before (and contributing to the development of) malnutrition and brain damage secondary to severe malnutrition. Although there are no true "critical periods" in human development, the impact of severe, prolonged malnutrition on the developing infant brain may reflect a "sensitive period" of increased vulnerability. The possibility that such malnutrition will affect brain development does not receive strong support from studies of recovery from severe nutritional deficiency in Third World countries (Southeast Asia, Guatemala, etc.), which describe a relatively rapid developmental catch-up after realimentation, followed by minimal long-term developmental impact. The limitation of this body of research lies in the relatively crude indices of outcome used as well as the lowered expectations for "good" outcomes.

On the other hand, transient neurologic findings such as hypotonia ("floppy baby") or hypertonia (in a pattern suggestive of spastic diplegia) are common in infants who are severely malnourished on whatever basis. Cerebral palsy with or without oral motor involvement is both difficult to diagnose in children under 18 months of age and quite commonly associated with poor physical growth.

Similarly for cognition, the child with failure to thrive tends to exhibit psychomotor retardation that responds to refeeding; the undiagnosed child with mental retardation may feed poorly, interact poorly with the caretaker, and significantly contribute to his or her own poor growth. Some babies simply seem not to respond to what otherwise would be considered adequate mothering. These children might be considered to have difficult temperaments or to be exhibiting subtle but not insignificant neurologic abnormalities.

The neurodevelopmental component of most of these cases of failure to thrive is often minimized if not neglected (Goldson, 1989). Such a focus on the neurodevelopmental components of failure to thrive does not place the physician under any obligation to use an expensive battery of invasive tests and may indeed help relieve the pressure to do so. Neither does a focus on the neurodevelopmental aspects excuse the physician from addressing relevant psychosocial factors. The combined emphasis on neurodevelopmental and emotional/interactive aspects represents instead the optimal application of clinical skills. Close observation of feeding sometimes supplemented by radiographic studies of swallowing are often available through feeding teams and skilled occupational therapists located at tertiary children's hospitals (Arvedson, 1993).

Casey et al. (1994) randomized 914 preterm infants into multifaceted intervention and control groups; 64 (20%) in the treatment and 102 (22%) in the control groups developed failure to thrive. Intensity of and cooperation with the center-based component of the intervention correlated with developmental outcome. Significantly, prospectively addressing precisely those maternal factors presumed to influence the development of nonorganic failure to thrive had had no impact on the incidence of growth failure, which was identical in both the treated and the untreated groups.

Recognizing the importance of a multidisciplinary approach, Skuse (1985) found a 50% rate of oral motor dysfunction in growth-retarded 4-year-old children from inner city disadvantaged environments (Heptinstall et al., 1987) and upward of 66% of immature and abnormal oral findings in a *controlled* detailed study of nine inner city infants with failure to thrive (Mathisen et al., 1989). Oral hypotonia was present in six of nine cases, oral tactile aversion in eight of nine, and facial tactile aversion in all nine cases. It would be difficult to underestimate the significance of this research to the understanding of the pathogenesis of growth failure in infancy. The accepted wisdom of the past several decades has here been inverted.

In addition, this last study reported less successful nonverbal communication skills surrounding feeding in their failure-to-thrive infants. It is precisely such behaviors that in the past were used to support psychiatric diagnoses applied to the mothers of infants with failure to thrive. A careful study of verbal and nonverbal communication skills in both mothers and children with failure to thrive must be carried out. It might be reasonably hypothesized that a significant subset of children with failure to thrive will ultimately be reclassified as having neurologically based communication disorders impacting on feeding. It should be noted that language delays have always been more prevalent and more persistent in abused children (Lynch & Roberts, 1982).

While only a quarter of cases of failure to thrive may be "organic" in nature, more than half of the remaining "nonorganic failure to thrive" cases can now be recognized as examples of subtle oral motor (and possibly communication) deficits even in inner city infants from "deprived" homes and underprivileged family environments.

The present age has increasingly generated both the breakup of the extended family and the dissolution of the nuclear family; these developments have produced a growing number of single-parent families headed by mothers with little or no support networks. When one allows that many of the cases once classified as nonorganic failure to thrive are in fact feeding and nutrition education problems rather than parent-child interaction disorders, then one is left with a low incidence of pure nonorganic (i.e., emotional interaction) failure to thrive. **Table 19-3** presents this more complex categorization of failure to thrive.

| **Table 19-3. Etiologic Matrix for Failure to Thrive** | | |
|---|---|---|
| **Organic** <br> (focus on baby) | | **Nonorganic** <br> (focus on mother) |
| Organ system disease [22] | *Independent* <br> *Rare* <br> *Severe* | Parenting disorder [20] |
| Spectrum of neuro-developmental disability, including feeding/language disorders [20] | *Interactive* <br> *Common* <br> *Mild* | Nutritional education deficit, including parental cognitive or language deficit [26] |

*The numbers in brackets are derived from Hull (1976), with the added interpretation that the 20 cases under common organic conditions were classified by him as of undetermined etiology. It might be best for clinicians to approach the clinical problem of growth failure in young children with no preconceived notions that one subtype, category, or etiology is predominant.*

The possibility of neurodevelopmental disorders in the parents of children with failure to thrive has not received sufficient investigation. Maternal intelligence (Sheridan, 1956), social stresses, prematurity, and physical deformity can contribute to a mother's reaction to a baby who may also have an organic condition contributing to growth failure. Such an association can, however, be problematic. Accardo and Whitman (1990) did not observe an unusually high incidence of growth failure in children of mothers with mental retardation, and in the classic study by Skeels and Dye (1930), infants who typically failed to thrive in institutions blossomed and did quite well when nurtured by female inmates who were mentally retarded.

## ♦ CONCLUSION

At the beginning of the twentieth century, pediatric medicine developed expertise in the complexities of infant feeding. By mid-century, the science of pediatrics was able to mount an impressive array of laboratory investigations in the event that a baby did not grow appropriately. During the next quarter of a century, within the medical profession, criticisms were leveled for an overuse of such laboratory measures without clinical indications and for a neglect of some of the most obvious and bizarre examples of child abuse masquerading as growth failure. This resulted in the pendulum swinging to the opposite extreme, with most failure to thrive being considered a sign of maternal pathology.

Pediatricians were too ready to interpret failure to thrive as a mild variation on Chapin's (1915) "cachexia of hospitalism," Goldfarb's (1945) "affect hunger," and their numerous progeny. The clinical picture of a malnourished child who is too quiet, passive, anxious, listless, apathetic, without enthusiasm, rarely smiling, and exhibiting waxy immobility and a flexion posture of tonic immobility (Krieger and Sargent, 1967) was reported over and over again under different names and with slight variations that tended to focus increasingly on and offer varying interpretations regarding an assumed underlying maternal psychopathology (**Table 19-4**).

Historically this evolution coincided with (and sometimes became inextricably mixed up with) a long overdue prominence given to the broad spectrum of manifestations of child abuse. Certainly, many children who are abused exhibit signs of failure to thrive, but the two conditions are both too complex to allow a simplistic identification. It is only in the past decade that research data have finally allowed a more reasoned approach to this most complex of pediatric health problems. The point of balance is not simple.

---

**Table 19-4. The Conceptual Matrix for Nonorganic Failure to Thrive**

Hospitalism (Chapin, 1915; Bakwin, 1942; Spitz, 1945)

Anaclitic depression (Spitz, 1946)

Psychological deprivation in infancy (Goldfarb, 1945)

Infants in institutions/institutional syndromes (Gesell & Amatruda, 1941;
  Provence & Lipton, 1969; the Creche in Beirut, Lebanon, [Dennis, 1973])

Environmental retardation (Coleman & Provence, 1957)

Social deprivation in monkeys (Harlow, 1973)

Maternal deprivation (Levy, 1931; Lowrey, 1940; Ribble, 1943; Ainsworth,
  1962; Patton & Gardner, 1963)

Attachment and loss (Bowlby, 1951, 1969, 1973, 1980)

Psychosocial deprivation

Marasmus

Kwashiorker

Battered child syndrome (Kempe et al., 1962)

Maltreatment syndrome (Fontana, 1964)

Deprivation dwarfism, psychosocial dwarfism (Powell, Brasel, & Blizzard,
  1967; Silver & Finkelstein, 1967)

Shaken baby syndrome (Caffey, 1957)

Nonorganic failure to thrive (Hufton & Oates, 1977)

Psychological short stature (Tanner, 1967)

Buchenwald baby syndrome (Jacobs, 1979)

Maternal-infant bonding (Klaus et al., 1972)

Munchausen's syndrome by proxy (Money & Werlwas, 1976)

Reversible hyposomatotropinism (Money, 1977)

Abuse dwarfism (Money, 1977)

Infants and mothers at risk

Kaspar Hauser syndrome (Money, 1992)

---

Since growth is a linear variable, the measurement of failure to grow is also linear. Failure to thrive, however, is not linear but discontinuous. If one were to take 80% of ideal weight (or any similar number) as the cutoff point for diagnosing growth failure, there would be infants who at 81% of their ideal weight would appear sickly and qualify as failure to thrive. There would also be other infants at 79% of their ideal weight who appear so healthy and energetic that only routine health supervision would be indicated.

The linear nature of growth measurements contributes to a misleading impression of a continuum. Failure to thrive in infants has been considered to occupy one end of the spectrum of child abuse. This conceptualizes physical abuse to be at the severe end, while neglect leading to malnutrition and severe emotional pathology leading to poor feeding are considered to be problems at the mild end of this single spectrum. Children with severe growth failure who starve to death cannot occupy the mild end of any hypothetical spectrum. There is severe and mild physical abuse; there is severe and mild nutritional neglect.

More insidiously, the spectrum analogy has been applied to mothering itself. It cannot be stated too strongly that good mothering and bad mothering do not occupy the extreme ends of the same continuum of mothering. Good mothering is not bad mothering with a little extra tender loving care added to produce a qualitative or quantitative difference. Good mothering and pathologic disorders of mothering represent two completely different continua. The analogy of a single continuum of mothering is as fallacious as the analogy of bonding (Eyer, 1992).

Many of the variations in the etiologic distribution of failure to thrive derive from the definitions employed and the resulting differences in the patients identified. The neurologically impaired infant is at high risk for failure to thrive. Although a specific subset of failure-to-thrive cases are associated with maternal psychopathology and can be located on the continuum of child neglect and abuse, it is imperative that such a diagnosis not be entertained in the absence of positive evidence. Feeding problems resulting from lack of maternal education, oral motor disorders in the infant, or some combination of the two account for a significant proportion of what in the past was called nonorganic failure to thrive.

This reconsideration of failure to thrive fits in with a more positive trend to avoid "blaming the mother" as a first principle of failure-to-thrive management. Growth failure does not automatically and indeed does not usually occupy a place on the spectrum of child neglect and abuse.

## ◆ BIBLIOGRAPHY

Accardo, P, ed: *Failure to Thrive in Infancy and Early Childhood: A Multidisciplinary Team Approach*, University Park Press, Baltimore, 1982.

Accardo, P, and Whitman, BY: Children of parents with mental retardation, *Am J Dis Child* 144:69-70, 1990.

Accardo, P, Morrow, J, and Whitman, BY: Failure to thrive. In RB Conn, ed: *Current Diagnosis* 8, WB Saunders, Philadelphia, 1991, pp. 1280-1284.

Ainsworth, MD: The effects of maternal deprivation: A review of findings and controversy in the context of research strategy. In *Deprivation of Maternal Care: A Reassessment of its Effects*, Public Health Papers, No. 14, World Health Organization, Geneva, 1962, pp. 97-165.

Ambuel, JP, and Harris, B: Failure to thrive: A study of failure to grow in height or weight, *Ohio Med J* 59:907-1001, 1963.

American Psychiatric Association: *Diagnostic and Statistical Manual of Mental Disorders, Third Edition (DSM-III)*, American Psychiatric Association, Washington, DC, 1980.

American Psychiatric Association: *Diagnostic and Statistical Manual of Mental Disorders, Fourth Edition (DSM-IV)*, American Psychiatric Association, Washington, DC, 1994.

Arvedson, JC: Management of swallowing problems. In JC Arvedson and L Brodsky, eds: *Pediatric Swallowing and Feeding: Assessment and Management*, Singular Publishing Group, San Diego, CA, 1993, pp. 327-387.

Bakwin, H: Loneliness in infants, *Am J Dis* 63:30-40, 1942.

Bowlby, J: Maternal care and mental health, *Bull WHO* 3:355-534, 1951.

Bowlby, J: *Attachment and Loss, I: Attachment*, Basic Books, New York, 1969.

Bowlby, J: *Attachment and Loss, II: Separation and Anxiety*, Basic Books, New York, 1973.

Bowlby, J: *Attachment and Loss, III: Loss: Sadness and Depression*, Basic Books, New York, 1980.

Caffey, J: Traumatic lesions in the growing bones other than fractures and dislocations—clinical and radiological features. MacKenzie Davidson Memorial lecture, *Br J Radiol* 30:225-238, 1957.

Casey, PH, Kelleher, KJ, Bradley, RH, Kellogg, KW, Kirby, RS, and Whiteside, L: A multifaceted intervention for infants with failure to thrive: A prospective study, *Arch Pediatr Adolesc Med* 148:1071-1077, 1994.

Chapin, HD: Are institutions for infants necessary? *JAMA* 64:175-177, 1915.

Coleman, RW, and Provence, S: Environmental retardation (hospitalism) in infants living in families, *Pediatrics* 19:285-292, 1957.

Cronk, C, Crocker, AC, Pueschel, SM, Shea, AM, Zackai, E, Pickens, G, and Reed, R: Growth charts for children with Down syndrome: 1 month to 18 years of age, *Pediatrics* 81:102-110, 1988.

Dennis, W: *Children of the Creche*, Appleton Century Crofts, New York, 1973.

Elmer, E, Gregg, GS, and Ellison, P: Late results of the "failure-to-thrive" syndrome, *Clin Pediatr* 8:584-589, 1969.

English, PC: Failure to thrive without organic reason, *Pediatr Ann* 7:774-781, 1978.

Eyer, DE: *Mother-Infant Bonding: A Scientific Fiction*, Yale University Press, New Haven, CT, 1992.

Fontana, VJ: *The Maltreated Child: The Maltreatment Syndrome in Children*, Charles C Thomas, Springfield, IL, 1964.

Frank, DA, Silva, M, and Needham, R: Failure to thrive: Mystery, myth, and method, *Contemp Pediatr* February 1993, pp. 114-133.

Gesell, A, Amatruda, CS: *Developmental Diagnosis: Normal and Abnormal Child Development. Clinical Methods and Pediatric Applications*, Paul B Hoeber, New York, 1941.

Glaser, HH, Heagarty, MC, Bullard, Jr, DM, and Pivchik, EC: Physical and psychological development of children with early failure to thrive, *J Pediatr* 73:690-698, 1968.

Goldfarb, W: Effects of psychological deprivation in infancy and subsequent stimulation, *Am J Psychiatry* 102:18-33, 1945.

Goldson, E: Neurological aspects of failure to thrive, *Dev Med Child Neurol* 31:816-826, 1989.

Guo, SS, Wholihan, K, Roche, AF, Chumlea, WC, and Casey, PH: Weight-for-length reference data for preterm, low-birth-weight infants, *Arch Pediatr Adolesc Med* 150:964-970, 1996.

Hannaway, PJ: Failure to thrive: A study of 100 infants and children, *Clin Pediatr* 9:96-99, 1970.

Harlow, HF: *Learning to Love*, Ballantine Books, New York, 1973.

Heptinstall, E, Puckering, C, Skuse, D, Dowdney, L, and Zur-Szpiro, S: Nutrition and mealtime behavior in families of growth-retarded children, *Hum Nutr Appl Nutr* 41a:390-402, 1987.

Hufton, IA, and Oates, RK: Nonorganic failure to thrive: A long-term follow-up, *Pediatrics* 59:73-77, 1977.

Hull, D: Some nutritional problems in infants. In AW Wilkinson, ed: *Nutrition and Later Development*, Year Book Medical Publishing Co, Chicago, 1976, pp. 134-139.

Jacobs, JC: Breast-feeding and malnutrition, *Am J Child* 133:756, 1979.

Kempe, CH, Silverman, FN, Steele, BF, Droegemueller, W, and Silver, HK: The battered-child syndrome, *JAMA* 181:17-24, 1962.

Klaus, M, Jerauld, P, Kreger, N, McAlpine, W, Steffa, M, and Kennell, J: Maternal attachment: Importance of the first postpartum days, *N Engl J Med* 286:460-463, 1972.

Koel, BS: Failure to thrive and fatal injury as a continuum, *Am J Dis Child* 118:565-567, 1969.

Krieger, I, and Sargent, SA: A postural sign in the sensory deprivation syndrome in infants, *J Pediatr* 70:332-339, 1967.

Levy, DM: Maternal overprotection and rejection, *Arch Neurol Psychiatry* 25:886-889, 1931.

Lowrey, LG: Personality distortion and early institutional care, *Am J Orthopsychiatry* 10:576-585, 1940.

Lynch, MA, and Roberts, J: *Consequences of child abuse*, Academic Press, London, 1982.

Mathisen, B, Skuse, D, Wolke, D, and Reilly, S: Oral-motor dysfunction and failure to thrive among inner-city infants, *Dev Med Child Neurol* 31:293-302, 1989.

Mitchell, WG, Gorrell, RW, and Greenberg, RA: Failure-to-thrive: A study in a primary care setting: Epidemiology and follow-up, *Pediatrics* 65:971-977, 1980.

Money, J: The syndrome of abuse dwarfism (psychosocial dwarfism or reversible hyposomatotropinism), *Am J Dis Child* 131:508-513, 1977.

Money, J: *The Kaspar Hauser Syndrome of "Psychosocial Dwarfism": Deficient Statural, Intellectual, and Social Growth Induced by Child Abuse*, Prometheus Books, Buffalo, NY, 1992.

Money, J, and Werlwas, J: Folie a deux in the parents of psychosocial dwarfs: Two cases, *Bull Am Acad Psychiatry Law* 4:351-362, 1976.

Patton, RG, and Gardner, LI: *Growth Failure in Maternal Deprivation*, Charles C Thomas, Springfield, IL, 1963.

Powell, GF, Brasel, JA, and Blizzard, RM: Emotional deprivation and growth retardation simulating idiopathic hypopituitarism. I. Clinical evaluation of the syndrome, *N Engl J Med* 276:1271-1278, 1967.

Powell, GF, Brasel, S, Raitti, JA, and Blizzard, RM: Emotional deprivation and growth retardation simulating idiopathic hypopituitarism. II. Endocrinological evaluation of the syndrome, *N Engl J Med* 276:1279-1283, 1967.

Provence, S, and Lipton, RC: *Infants in institutions,* International Universities Press, New York, 1969.

Ribble, MA: *The Rights of Infants: Early Psychological Needs and Their Satisfaction,* Columbia University Press, New York, 1943.

Riley, RL, Landwirth, J, Kaplan, SA, and Collip, PJ: Failure to thrive: An analysis of 83 cases, *Calif Med* 108:32-38, 1968.

Rutter, M: *Maternal Deprivation Reassessed*, Penguin Books, Baltimore, 1972.

Sheridan, MD: The intelligence of 100 neglectful mothers, *Br Med J* 1:91-93, 1956.

Sills, RH: Failure to thrive: The role of clinical and laboratory evaluation, *Am J Dis Child* 132:967-969, 1978.

Silver, HK, and Finkelstein, M: Deprivation dwarfism, *J Pediatr* 70:317-324, 1967.

Skeels, HM, and Dye, H: A study of the effects of differential stimulation on mentally retarded children, *Proc Am Assoc Ment Defic* 44:114-136, 1939.

Skuse, D: Non-organic failure to thrive: A reappraisal, *Arch Dis Child* 60:173-178, 1985.

Spitz, RA: Hospitalism: An inquiry into the genesis of psychiatric conditions in early childhood, I. In *Psychoanalytic Study of the Child*, vol 1, International Universities Press, New York, 1945, pp. 53-64.

Spitz, RA: Anaclitic depression: An inquiry into the genesis of psychiatric conditions in early childhood, II. In *Psychoanalytic Study of the Child*, vol 2, International Universities Press, New York, 1946, pp. 313-342.

Tanner, JM: Resistance to exogenous human growth hormone in psychosocial short stature (emotional deprivation), *J Pediatr* 71:317-324, 1967.

# PSYCHOLOGICAL ABUSE

PEGGY S. PEARL, ED.D.

*As far back as anyone can remember, Carol has regularly told Mary how lazy and stupid she is. Everywhere they go, Carol is heard telling Mary what she is doing wrong. Carol routinely tells Mary, as well as anyone else who will listen, that all of Carol's problems began when Mary was born. Carol has long complained that she couldn't keep a job because Mary was so demanding. When Mary entered school, she was behind her age-mates, wouldn't attempt new assignments, and did not appear to enjoy any activity. At the first parent conference, Carol told the teacher that she had always recognized that Mary was lazy, stupid, and a troublemaker. Mary had a very short attention span. In third grade, Mary was referred to the school psychologist for depression. Later that year she was found sitting on the playground in below-zero-degree temperatures without a coat, gloves, or hat. When asked what was wrong she said, "Nothing...," without looking at the teacher. Although Mary never complained to anyone, another student called the teacher's attention to the fact that Mary's hands "looked weird." The school nurse referred Mary to a pediatrician. Mary had frostbite.*

Psychological abuse is the core issue and major destructive factor in the broader topic of child maltreatment, and, therefore, it exists in all types of neglect, physical abuse, and sexual abuse (Dean, 1979; Garbarino, 1987; Straus & Kantor, 1987; Szur, 1989; Edmundson & Collier, 1993). Psychological maltreatment of children and youth consists of acts of omission and commission that are psychologically damaging. Psychological abuse is the presence of hostile behaviors as well as the absence of positive parenting. Such acts damage immediately or ultimately the behavioral, cognitive, affective, or physical functioning of the child. Emotional abuse is a concerted attack on a child's development of self and social competence. It may or may not be a conscious act by the parents or other caregivers. Emotional abuse damages the child's psychological development and emerging personal identity (Brassard, Hart, & Hardy, 1993; O'Hagan, 1995). Emotions are primary to cognition and precede cognitive processing (Zanjonc, 1980). Hence the assessment of cognitive skills serves as evidence of psychological abuse. Emotional neglect can take place anywhere and may be relatively more prevalent in wealthier countries (Ney, Fung, & Wickett, 1993).

Regardless of the intent, the consequences to the child are the same. A pattern of psychologically destructive behavior by an adult can involve ignoring the child, or repeatedly telling the child that he or she is stupid. It is the most elusive and damaging of the types of maltreatment (Green, 1978; Dean, 1979; Yates, 1982; Fortin & Reed, 1984; Garbarino et al., 1986; Hickox & Furnell, 1989; Burgess et al., 1990). Emotional abuse interrupts the process of attachment, affective development, and the evolution of empathetic capacities. As a result of the child's failure to develop empathy, the child is impaired in his or her ability to appropriately receive and transmit emotional information. Some researchers think that lack of attachment, continual attack on the child's sense of worth, and failing to provide emotional nurturance, coupled with neglect and perhaps early physical abuse, impair the child's total capacity to respond emotionally (Brothers, 1989). An inability to consciously experience and communicate feelings has been linked to primate studies in deprivation (Sackette, 1966) and appears to be linked to human maternal deprivation. Mullen et al. (1996) concluded that "the impact of emotional abuse varied with the gender of the abuser. Those emotionally abused by their female caregivers were more prone to psychiatric difficulties in adult life whereas such abuse from male parent figures was particularly deleterious to adult sexuality." Since affective development must precede cognitive and physical development, early diagnosis and treatment of emotional abuse are important to minimize an individual's developmental damage and maturational impairment. Early diagnosis and treatment are the most effective means of reducing societal costs of emotional abuse and increasing the likelihood that the victim will live a fuller and more productive life.

### ◆ FORMS OF PSYCHOLOGICAL ABUSE

Psychological abuse can take many forms. It is always involved in the adult's struggle for absolute control over the child. The younger the child

---

**Table 20-1. Categories of Psychological Abuse**

1. *Ignoring* the child and failing to provide necessary stimulation, responsiveness, and validation of the child's worth in normal family routine.

2. *Rejecting* the child's value, needs, and requests for adult validation and nurturance.

3. *Isolating* the child from the family and community; denying the child normal human contact.

4. *Terrorizing* the child with continual verbal assaults, creating a climate of fear, hostility, and anxiety, thus preventing the child from gaining feelings of safety and security.

5. *Corrupting* the child by encouraging and reinforcing destructive, antisocial behavior until the child is so impaired in socioemotional development that interaction in normal social environments is not possible.

6. *Verbally assaulting* the child with constant name-calling, harsh threats, and sarcastic put-downs that continually "beat down" the child's self-esteem with humiliation.

7. *Overpressuring* the child with subtle but consistent pressure to grow up fast and to achieve too early in the areas of academics, physical/motor skills, and social interaction, which leaves the child feeling that he or she is never quite good enough.

and the less developed the child's sense of self and identity, the more serious are the physical, social, and emotional consequences. When a child experiences the emotion of fear or distress, a parent normally responds with compassion, love, and physical comforting. Such emotionally interactive appropriateness is a core component of "attachment" (Ainsworth, 1980; Crittenden & Ainsworth, 1989; Crittenden, 1990; Wright, 1993). But when the parents repeatedly respond to the child's fear and distress with anger and rejection, attachment does not occur and the child experiences psychological maltreatment. Psychological abuse of older children with a well-established sense of self may have less impact than the same action on a younger child or a previously maltreated child.

Psychological abuse varies in intensity from occasional to mild to extreme over a sustained period of time. Categories of psychological abuse include ignoring, rejecting, isolating, terrorizing, corrupting, verbally assaulting, and overpressuring (**Table 20-1**).

In most dysfunctional families, children experience many types of maltreatment. In some families, all children are treated or mistreated similarly, while in others, each child is treated uniquely and is individually affected. The child's developmental stage influences both the parent-child interaction and the impact of the interaction on the child. The more nurturing the child has had before the maltreatment and the more secure the child's attachment is to his or her caregiver(s) early in life, the less impact the maltreatment will have on the child.

| Table 20-2. Parental Ignoring Behaviors |
|---|
| Does not respond to child's needs |
| Fails to stimulate child in appropriate manner |
| Does not look at child |
| Does not call child by name |
| Does not attach or bond to child |
| Fails to recognize child's presence |
| Shows no affection for child |
| Is psychologically unavailable for child on consistent basis |
| Fails to allow child normal and appropriate privacy |

## ◆ IGNORING

Ignoring parents or other caregivers fail to acknowledge the child's presence or needs (**Table 20-2**). The ignoring parent is neither physically nor psychologically available for the child, either consistently or on an unpredictable basis. Ignoring is often part of serious physical neglect where the child is not fed, clothed, sheltered, bathed, supervised, or acknowledged as needing these basics.

### CASE EXAMPLE

*Martha seldom if ever calls any of her children by name. She neither talks to them nor looks at them. Martha's house is spotlessly clean, but meals are rarely prepared and seldom is there food that the children can readily prepare for themselves. Following a visit with her daughter, Martha's mother brought the youngest child to the emergency room, concerned about the child's lack of appetite. He was diagnosed as having nonorganic failure to thrive. On examination of the other children, each child was found to be in the lowest percentile on growth charts, with abnormally short limbs, poor skin coloring, and extreme delays in muscle development. A visit to the school found the oldest child was barely passing, had poor social skills, and was withdrawn and passive. Discussion with Martha revealed that her husband, Tom, is a workaholic, a very successful lawyer who spends long hours at the office. His income is one of the highest in the community, from which he generously provides for his family. However, he spends little time at home and little of that time with his children. Even from cursory observation of Martha, she appears depressed and merely says that she misses her husband's company.*

Studies of ignored children in institutions describe socioemotional deprivation severe enough to cause infant mortality of more than 33% (Spitz, 1945, 1946). Because of medical intervention, however, each year the number of failure-to-thrive cases is growing.

### CASE EXAMPLE

*Jane is a 21-year-old single mother of three children. She has had normal pregnancies, and each child was observed as normal at birth. However, each child now appears developmentally delayed and malnourished. Their skin is dry with little resiliency and a pale color. Their hair is dull, dry, and brittle. Their scalps are very dry. The children*

---

**Table 20-3. Signs of Munchausen Syndrome by Proxy**

1. Persistent symptoms and/or illnesses for which a cause cannot be found.

2. Unusual symptoms, signs, and/or laboratory findings that do not make sense.

3. A diagnosis of disorders that are less common than MSBP.

4. Symptoms and signs that go away when the child is not with the mother or appear when only the mother is present.

5. Overly attentive parent. Parent becomes attached to medical staff, seems less concerned about child's condition than medical staff, and is highly involved in the care of other patients.

6. Affect of parent inconsistent with the apparent seriousness of the child's condition.

7. In a two-parent functional home, father absent or uninvolved in making medical decisions for what appears to be a seriously ill child.

8. Parental suggestions for or welcoming of medical tests even when painful for the child, including excessive pelvic examinations.

---

**Table 20-4. Substances and Maneuvers Creating or Simulating Illness in Victims of Munchausen Syndrome by Proxy**

**Psychoactive Drugs**

| | |
|---|---|
| Phenothiazines | Chloral hydrate |
| Imipramine | Methaqualone |
| Amitriptyline | Amphetamines |
| Codeine | Barbiturates |

**Drugs/Substances Altering Fluid and Electrolyte Balance**

| | |
|---|---|
| Excessive table salt | Phenformin |
| Excessive water | Salicylates |
| Insulin | Theophylline |
| Furosemide | Chlorthalidone |

**Miscellaneous Toxins**

| | |
|---|---|
| Pepper | Laxatives |
| Naphtha | Lye |
| Warfarin | |

**Other Mechanisms**

Starvation

Suffocation

Fabricated history of previous diagnosis of serious illness, e.g., operable cardiac disease or epilepsy

Inflicted vaginal/rectal injury to produce bleeding

Altered laboratory studies, e.g., simulation of cystic fibrosis by altering sputum samples, putting salt in collection for sweat test, adding fat to stool collection

Injection of contaminated material into intravenous lines

Putting parent's blood into urine

Removal of blood from child's central venous line

*(From Wissow, 1991.)*

---

*appear lethargic, as if drugged. The oldest child, 3 years 6 months old, lacks language. In the doctor's waiting room, nurses observed the eldest child feeding the 6-month-old infant. The mother sat nearby, ignoring the children and their activities.*

## RESULTING CHARACTERISTICS

Once treated, failure-to-thrive infants remain apathetic and lethargic. They are developmentally delayed, both physically and behaviorally. After they begin to look normal physically, behavioral problems remain for children who were failure-to-thrive infants. They experience a higher frequency of temper tantrums at all ages, isolation, and socioemotional delay, and they commit more petty theft (Bullard et al., 1967; Gardner, 1972). MacCarthy (1979) described these children as engaging in attention-seeking behavior, superficial displays of affection, selfishness, and spiteful actions.

Other physical conditions are linked to severe emotional neglect during childhood. These conditions include psychosocial and deprivation dwarfism, sleep and eating disorders, and motor abnormalities (Powell et al., 1967; Gardner, 1972). Egeland et al.'s study (1983) of psychologically unavailable parents found that the children failed to thrive and develop normally. These children were both emotionally and cognitively delayed. One extreme form of parental ignoring is Munchausen Syndrome by Proxy (**Table 20-3 and Chapter 17**). The child's needs are ignored as the parent attempts to meet her own needs. In this syndrome a parent, usually the mother, fabricates symptoms for the child, or actually causes illnesses, that result in unnecessary medical procedures (**Table 20-4**). Extreme lack of concern for the needs of the child is also seen in the behaviors of caregivers obsessed with the sexual maltreatment of their child, which are now termed, "Contemporary-type Munchausen Syndrome by Proxy." The caregiver, usually the mother, allows or requires that the child go through multiple, unnecessary sexual abuse evaluations and pelvic examinations (Rand, 1993).

| Table 20-5. Parental Rejecting Behaviors |
| --- |
| Refusing to allow child to get needed psychological or medical treatment or educational services |
| Belittling and ridiculing child |
| Purposefully and continually embarrassing child |
| Singling child out for criticism and punishment |
| Failing to allow child to develop autonomy or independence |
| Confusing child's sexual identity |
| Undermining attachment of child with others |
| Routinely rejecting child's ideas |
| Ridiculing or punishing age-appropriate behaviors as too immature |
| Routinely calling child dumb, stupid, freak, nerd |
| Privately and publicly routinely putting child down |
| Inappropriately attributing undesirable characteristic(s) to child |
| Continuing to treat adolescent as young child |
| Denying child's needs and making child meet adult needs |
| Making child perform household tasks because the parent finds the task undesirable |

In addition to the physical harm, the child learns to live under absolute control with adults who cannot be trusted (McGuire & Feldman, 1989). Children of depressed mothers who were emotionally unavailable to their children on a consistent basis showed both emotional and cognitive developmental delay (Polanky et al., 1981). The schizophrenic parent or character disorder parent also is in such need emotionally that she or he is consistently unavailable to the child. Ignoring is an act of omission, passive and neglectful, as compared to rejecting, which is an act of commission, active and abusing.

## ♦ REJECTING

Rejecting parents refuse to touch or show affection to their child and/or do not acknowledge this child's presence or accomplishments as well as constantly "rejecting and demeaning" age-appropriate behaviors. **Table 20-5** lists parental rejecting behaviors.

With an infant the parent refuses to form an attachment. The parent does not respond to the child's behaviors to have basic needs met, such as when the child cries for food or with a wet diaper. Nor does the parent respond to the child's smiles and vocalizations of pleasure. As the child grows the parent does not talk with the child or get involved in the preschooler's activities. The child is not included in family activities. The child may spend long periods of time in solitary play, often in another room with the door closed. As the child develops, the parent consistently communicates a negative definition of self to the child. The parent belittles the child and his or her accomplishments, both privately and publicly calling the child "dummy, clumsy, dunce, nerd," and/or "freak." The parent has very low expectations of the child in school, telling the child that he or she can't expect to pass or do well in school because he or she is too dumb. The school-aged child or adolescent is treated like a small child and not allowed to act in age-appropriate ways. The parent does not acknowledge, or openly rejects, the changes associated with adolescence, including social roles, physical size, sexual development, or increased cognitive ability. The child is told of his failures and seldom if ever included as a valued individual within the family. The parent commonly fails to have empathy for the child's needs (Rohner & Rohner, 1980; Trowell, 1983).

**Table 20-6. Family Circumstances Associated with Increased Risk for Rejection**

Unwanted pregnancies

No opportunity for caregiver to spend time alone

Lack of involvement by father in child rearing

Marital discord

Social and instrumental isolation of family from the community

Rejecting parents generally appear overwhelmed by the convergence of social and economic hardships. Commonly, rejecting parents are reacting to large families, limited material resources, limited education and job skills, and few emotional and social supports, all of which stress the parents and limit their ability to nurture their children (**Table 20-6**). These parents feel materially and psychologically unable to move beyond concern for themselves to concern about their role as caregivers, teachers, and providers of emotional support for their children (Pemberton & Benady, 1973; Trowell, 1983; Garbarino et al., 1986).

## CASE EXAMPLE

*Jane feeds her son regularly on schedule but seldom if ever holds him while she feeds the child his bottle. She lays him on the sofa and props the bottle, telling him and others how much of her time he takes and what better things she could be doing than taking care of him. When she feeds him baby food, she fails to make eye contact or talk to him. When she changes his diaper, the only comments she makes are in disgust at how terrible it smells and what a mess he has made that she must clean up. She is seldom in the same room as the child and does not talk to him or play with him when they are physically near each other. She describes him as a "troublesome baby." However, other family members comment that he is a good baby, since they never hear him cry.*

## RESULTING CHARACTERISTICS

Children who have been psychologically and/or physically rejected by parents or other primary caregivers are hostile and aggressive, have impaired self-esteem, and show either excessive dependency on parents and/or other adults or "defensive independence" (Rohner & Rohner, 1980; O'Hagan, 1995). These children and teens appear emotionally unstable and unresponsive, eventually perceiving the world in negativistic terms (Pemberton & Benady, 1973). They see themselves as having few strengths and skills. They view the world as being hostile and unwilling to assist them. They feel isolated and in turn reject others, including their own children.

**Table 20-7. Parental Isolating Behaviors**

Not allowing child to participate in normal family routine

Not allowing child normal contact with peers

Physically separating child from family unit

Failing to allow child to participate in the social aspects of school

Avoiding physical contact with child, e.g. hugging, touching, holding

Routinely teaching child to avoid and distrust peers

Locking child in room, basement, attic

Punishing requests for interaction with family or others

Binding or gagging child to prevent interaction

Refusing, without justifiable reason, to allow child contact with noncustodial parent, grandparent, or siblings

Hiding child from outside world

## ♦ISOLATING

Isolation of children can come from a variety of parental motivations, but the resulting behavior prevents children from having normal opportunities for social relations with both adults and peers. **Table 20-7** lists parental isolating behaviors. Some isolating parents are themselves fearful of the outside world and want to protect their children from the dangers they believe exist from contact with others. These families usually have a very limited amount of social contact, which deprives the children of learning social skills with a variety of individuals. Isolation is also present in sexually abusive families and in families where ritualistic abuse occurs. The isolation is to keep what happens in the family a secret and to keep the children from learning that there is any other way of life. Other isolating parents are themselves without social skills and merely lack social contacts and/or supports and do not provide the opportunity for their children.

## CASE EXAMPLE

*Neither Maria, 14, nor Christine, 10, are allowed to have friends over to play or go to other homes to play. Their mother believes that other children will introduce her girls to drugs and other "evils of the world." The girls were home-schooled until recently when their mother had to go to work to help pay off some medical and home repair bills. Since entering the public schools the girls have not made friends. Christine has had problems doing group social studies and language arts. Both girls are excessively anxious about trying new experiences at school. They worry about someone taking advantage of them, and as a result peers tease them.*

## RESULTING CHARACTERISTICS

Isolating families often directly teach their children that contact outside the family is undesirable. School-aged children are not allowed to participate in co-curricular school activities, youth activities, or neighborhood play groups. Adolescent children are given home responsibilities and are prohibited from participation in school activities. Some families even remove children from school or do not encourage school attendance. Frequently, children who have been isolated for long periods of time lack the social competence to experience success or enjoyment at school and therefore do not like to attend (Rohner & Rohner, 1980; Garbarino et al., 1986).

## ♦ TERRORIZING

Terrorizing involves threatening the child with extreme or frightening punishment. **Table 20-8** lists parental terrorizing behaviors. The parent intentionally stimulates intense fear, creates a climate of unpredictable threat, or sets unattainable expectations and punishes the child for not attaining them. The discipline techniques are often arbitrary or beyond the child's ability to understand. The parent may tease or scare a young child in the name of humor, but the results terrorize and confuse the child. The parent disciplines the child by playing on fears that are normal for that age, such as loud noises or the dark. The terrorizing parent uses the feared situation "to scare the child into behaving." Parents may tell preschool-aged children that if they don't behave the "monsters will drag them away in the night," or the night-light is "watching and if you're not good, the night-light will zap you." One of the normal fears of adolescents is that their peers will see them as different or that they will not fit into social settings. The terrorizing parent threatens the adolescent with "public humiliation" (Garbarino et al., 1986).

### Table 20-8. Parental Terrorizing Behaviors

Excessive threats and psychological punishment

Threatening and frightening child with guns, knives, whips, etc.

Bizarre means of discipline

Excessive use of guilt-producing activity

Chaotic behavior to frighten child

Laughing at or ridiculing child when frightened, or putting child down for expressing normal fears

Punishing child by playing on normal childhood fears

Refusing to comfort infant in distress

Inconsistent and capricious disciplining of child

Continually threatening suicide or to leave child

Threatening to harm others in child's presence

Knowingly permitting child to view or be involved in violent behavior

Routinely engaging in fights and frightening behavior in front of child

Binding and/or gagging child

Permitting others to terrorize child

Failing to provide shelter, consistency, and safety for child

## CASE EXAMPLE

*Sam repeatedly has had his dad threaten him and other family members with a gun, a bullwhip, and a switchblade. He has never seen them used on a family member but regularly hides so he cannot be found in case his dad comes home mad.*

## RESULTING CHARACTERISTICS

Terrorizing parents play mind games with older children. These games are designed to be no-win situations where the child becomes very anxious, fearing the consequences. When parents place the child in the middle of arguments, as often happens in divorces, the child also becomes terrorized by the no-win situations. A child may be blamed for everything that goes wrong in the family, regardless of whose behavior is inappropriate. Constant criticism often leaves children so traumatized that they will not act because they fear they will be criticized.

## ◆ RITUALISTIC ABUSE

Ritualistic or multiple-victim, multiple-perpetrator abuse is one of the most damaging forms of abuse (Burgess et al., 1990; Snow & Sorensen, 1990). It is the systematic, bizarre misuse of the child physically, socially, sexually, and emotionally that includes some supernatural and/or religious activities by a group of adults. Ritualistic abuse is "carefully integrated and linked with a symbol of overriding power, authority, and purpose," such as a religion or pseudo-religion (Burgess et al., 1990). In this type of abuse, children are routinely involved in ceremonial sexual activity with adults, other children, and to a lesser extent with animals. Use of bondage, excessive threats, and force can be present. This activity is usually performed in front of other adults and children. Children are physically tortured, drugged, and forced to ingest drugs, human and/or animal feces, urine, blood, and flesh. They are buried alive in boxes and bound to crosses, and some stories are told of sacrificing children to the devil (**Table 20-9**).

The children, as well as the adults involved in this activity, are removed from normal social interaction and activity and are taught a very antisocial value system. The "family" environment is one of absolute control by one individual. The children are told that what is happening to them is because of their bad behavior or sin and that they must be punished or they must cleanse themselves during the ceremonies. Children are systematically told they are of no value except for how they can be used by the "all-powerful one," the group leader (Kelley, 1988; Burgess et al., 1990; Snow & Sorensen, 1990; Young et al., 1991).

---

**Table 20-9. Common Behaviors and Interests of Ritualistically Abused Children**

Excessive masturbation

Preoccupation with feces and urine

Detailed, age-inappropriate sexual knowledge

Spontaneous sexual offers to adults

Somatic complaints

Night terrors

Frequent sexual interplay between children

Preoccupation with death and burial

Extreme fears of death, confinement, and abduction

Stories of being buried

References to the devil and magic

Bizarre treatment of animals or talking of the bizarre treatment

Fear of rituals, candles, chants

Multiple personalities

Lack of traditional belief system

Delinquent, often bizarre, behavior

---

In ritualistic abuse cases, children are systematically terrorized into participation and silence. Initially the victim appears normal and denies any ritualistic involvement or multiple-perpetrator activity. Over time when the child feels safe, the child is able to recall memories and begins to describe experiences to a therapist or other trusted individual. The following are commonly used methods of terrorizing children to silence in ritualistic abuse:

Preschool-aged children are given a "mock operation." The child is laid blind-folded and nude on a table. The stomach is brushed with either a local antiseptic or a very cold liquid. Then a sharp pointed object is used to draw an outline on the child's stomach. The child is told that an animal is being placed in his stomach, and if he tells anything that has happened to him the animal or demon will eat the child up to protect the secret. The child may be drugged to drowsiness before the "operation" and then given additional drugs to induce sleep. On waking, the child is asked what has just happened to check for effectiveness and to begin the terrorizing.

Children of any age can be systematically programmed so that when they see a specific thing or hear a specific word they will "forget everything" they know or they will remember specific bizarre threats of what can happen to them if they tell. The word or object is usually something that the child frequently hears, or sees, such as a postal truck or the word "light."

Children are taught to believe that others can "read" their minds to always know what they are thinking. They are also taught to believe that "good is bad and bad is good, hate is smart and love is dumb."

## ♦ SEXUAL ABUSE

Sexual abuse of children involves different types of psychological abuse. Commonly, children are terrorized with extreme threats and the excessive use of power and control. The adult uses extreme methods to both gain and maintain control over the child's mind. The child is told that if he or she tells anyone about the abusive events, the parent or perpetrator will go to jail, the child will be taken away and never be allowed to see family members again, the child will become very ill and die, or some family member or beloved pet will die. Victims experience psychological trauma from shame, guilt, uncertainty, and fear of breaking up the family. The role changes in the incestuous family do not conform with societal norms. The common use of sexual exploitation within the family teaches the child socially inappropriate interpersonal communication skills. Corrupting also occurs in incestuous families as the child is taught inappropriate adult and child behaviors that do not conform with the community standards (Kelley, 1988; Burgess et al., 1990; Snow & Sorensen, 1990).

## ♦ CORRUPTING

Corrupting parental behaviors (**Table 20-10**) teach and reinforce antisocial or deviant patterns that tend to make the child unable to function in a normal social setting. In milder forms the parents convey approval of or encourage the child's precocious interest and/or behavior in the area of sexuality, aggression, violence, or substance abuse. In the more serious forms the parents continue to encourage and reinforce as the child's antisocial behavior grows more intense and destructive to self, others, or property. Reinforcing or ignoring delinquent behavior is parental corrupting behavior.

| Table 20-10. Parental Corrupting Behaviors |
|---|
| Allowing and/or forcing child to watch pornographic materials |
| Teaching child sexually exploitative behaviors |
| Teaching child illegal activity |
| Knowingly allowing others to teach illegal activity to child |
| Praising child for antisocial/delinquent behavior |
| Positively responding to child's antisocial behavior |
| Instructing child in antisocial/illegal activity |
| Assisting child in delinquent behavior |
| Failing to discipline child for delinquent behavior |
| Teaching child that "bad is good and good is bad" |
| Giving drugs or other contraband to child |
| Exposing child to harmful influences or situations |
| Using child as a spy, ally, or confidante in parent's romantic relationships or marital or divorce problems |

Corrupting can begin with rewarding the infant for oral sexual contact, creating drug dependence, encouraging violence toward peers, laughing at antisocial behaviors, and continuing to encourage these behaviors as they grow more habitual and serious. Common parental corrupting behaviors include allowing adults to use their children for sexual activity including prostitution and child pornography, allowing children to sell and deliver drugs, and encouraging drug use. In ritualistic abuse cases, often children reveal, after they feel very safe, that they were encouraged to have sex with younger children.

Parents who knowingly allow children to engage in any illegal activity are corrupting those children. Corruption is also occurring, however, when parents merely fail to teach their children the social skills necessary for successful interaction in the world around them and leave them vulnerable to learn inappropriate behaviors from those who would take advantage of them (Garbarino et al., 1986; Burgess et al., 1990).

In families where parents are corrupting their children, the parents could be repeating the parenting cycle. They pass on the type of parenting they received. Parents who themselves have antisocial behaviors commonly transmit those values, actions, and attitudes to their children. These parental behaviors result from some events or series of events in their own lives. Research suggests that most antisocial and criminal behavior is a consequence of child maltreatment (Cerce et al., 1988).

## CASE EXAMPLE
*Katrina's mother has had a series of boyfriends living in the home for many years, most of whom have had substance abuse problems. Both alcohol and drugs are common in the home. Katrina, 16, tells her friends that she can supply them with almost any drug they want anytime they want it. Katrina has her own car and no curfew. This year her school attendance record has been poor, but she has notes from her pediatrician, who is her grandfather, to "excuse" each absence.*

## RESULTING CHARACTERISTICS
Children who are mistreated during the first year of life fail to develop a basic sense of trust and, therefore, see the world around them as negative. They believe that people are not to be trusted or valued. These children frequently are taught that you have to take care of yourself—"take or get taken." This lack of respect for others leads them to have no respect for themselves. The consequence of corrupting children is that from an early age the children demonstrate antisocial behavior. These children have a pseudo-mature behavior unlike normal behavior of age-mates. They are "street-smart kids." From a very young age, they demonstrate few positive emotions and an inability to play in an age-appropriate manner. They are often rewarded for stealing and assaulting peers. As a result, they are unaware that their behavior is inappropriate. Commonly these families devalue formal public education and fail to send their children to school on a regular basis or fail to discourage school absences, further isolating the children from learning appropriate social skills, values, and attitudes.

| Table 20-11. Parental Verbally Assaulting Behaviors |
| --- |
| Continuous verbal attacks, especially in loud voice |
| Failing to protect child from verbal attacks of others |
| Constant belittling |
| Excessive criticism |
| Routinely humiliating the child |
| Openly telling the child he or she is worthless and no good |
| Excessive name-calling |
| Scapegoating the child |
| Calling child derogatory or demeaning names |
| Cursing child |
| Continually yelling at child |
| Attributing to child behaviors or characteristics that are totally unacceptable to child |

## ◆ VERBAL ASSAULTING
Verbally assaulting the child with constant name-calling, harsh threats, and sarcastic put-downs that continually "beat down" the child's sense of worth with humiliation is a type of emotional abuse. **Table 20-11** lists parental verbally assaulting behaviors. In the verbally assaultive family, words are used to humiliate and control. Repeatedly, the child is told of the things that he is doing wrong without regard for what he does well. The child is often unfavorably compared with other family members or with downcast individuals. The child is regularly called derogatory names. The verbal put-downs and attacks can occur in the privacy of the home. Frequently, however, the child is publicly told what she has failed to do and how worthless she is. The verbally assaultive behavior is so pervasive in the family's functioning that child care professionals routinely hear the verbal assaults. These verbal assaults are usually delivered in a loud voice that further accents their negativeness (Rohner & Rohner, 1980; Trowell, 1983; Vissing et al., 1991).

## CASE EXAMPLE
*Phil is 3 years old. He had been developing normal language, but a radical change has occurred. The neighbor is worried; she hears Phil's dad continually telling Phil to shut up all of that chattering and not to talk when the television is on. "No one wants to hear you talk; we want to listen to the television." Phil's mom is telling all her friends, in front of Phil and whomever else is around, that he's "just retarded, can't talk, and the most awkward child she has ever seen."*

## RESULTING CHARACTERISTICS

As a consequence of verbal battering, children have a flat or negative affect, low self-esteem, and often self-mutilating behavior. These children are withdrawn and shy and have no sense of initiative. The children feel they are incapable of any achievements. They are unable to recognize positive social feedback when it is given to them. In some families, one child is scapegoated and routinely verbally assaulted or the brunt of routine family sarcasm while other children receive no emotional abuse. The scapegoated children are a high risk for failure to thrive, psychological dwarfism, childhood depression, and suicide. Usually the child's physical appearance is one of poor posture and flat affect or excessive acting-out behavior (Pemberton & Benady, 1973; Baily & Baily, 1983; Egeland et al., 1983; Burgess et al., 1990).

## ♦ OVERPRESSURING

Primarily a middle-class phenomenon, overpressuring parents consistently have inappropriately high expectations for their children. As David Elkind described in *The Hurried Child: Growing Up Too Fast Too Soon* (1982), many parents today tend to be more concerned about a child's intellectual achievements than his or her psychological well-being. Children are expected to perform intellectual tasks early to prevent being "normal or average" as compared to peers. Instead of facilitating cognitive development as intended by the parent(s), these parental behaviors actually impair both cognitive and emotional development. **Table 20-12** lists parental overpressuring behaviors. Overpressuring begins when parents toilet train too early or attempt to teach 3- and 4-year-old children to read, count, and work on computers and continues with inappropriate "pressuring and hurrying" throughout the child's life.

Graduating tenth rather than first in the high school class or obtaining an ACT score of 25 is seen as failure by the parent. The parent views the child's consistently coming in second in a swimming meet or a golf tournament as not really trying rather than having done a "good job." The overpressured child is praised and valued for what is accomplished but not for just being.

### CASE EXAMPLE

*Sara's parents expected her to be "Harvard material." She was expected to do well in everything: playing the piano, sports, and academics. But she was average. Her parents regularly expressed their expectations and disappointment with her level of achievement, her appearance, and choice of friends. At 15, she was convinced that she was a failure and attempted suicide "to save her parents the embarrassment," the note said.*

### RESULTING CHARACTERISTICS

Parents can set high standards for their children and still demonstrate acceptance and love. Nurturing parents demonstrate positive feelings to their children, recognize their achievements, and convey pride. Overpressuring parents, however, fail to demonstrate that they feel acceptance, love, and pride toward their children. As a result the overpressured child feels worthless, discouraged, lazy, unreliable, unacceptable, and inferior. The child feels inadequate or unacceptable as she is, since parents are always trying to change her. The child's identity is in terms of accomplishments rather than herself.

Stress-related illnesses are common in these children. Because they lack parental support and good self-esteem, they are more vulnerable to negative experiences.

| Table 20-12. Parental Overpressuring Behaviors |
| --- |
| Excessively advanced expectations of child |
| Excessively critical of age-appropriate behaviors as inadequate |
| Punishes child for acting in age-appropriate manner, calls child "immature" |
| Ostracizes child for not achieving far above normal abilities |
| Does not provide assistance with remedial work, refusing to acknowledge that child would need assistance with such "simple" materials |
| Refuses to provide age-appropriate experiences, insisting on providing experiences that are advanced |
| Begins toilet training very early and insists that child control body functions |
| Makes comparisons of child to those who are very advanced, consistently leaving child "poor by comparison" |
| Routinely buys toys that are far too advanced for child with clear expectations that the toy will be used appropriately, setting the child up for almost certain failure |

These children commonly suffer from depression and are at high risk for eating disorders, suicide, and poor peer relationships throughout their lives.

## ◆TOILET TRAINING

Beginning to toilet train too early (clearly before 18 months of age, but may be later in some children) says to the child "you are not acceptable as you are and need to change." Often parents combine the age-inappropriate toilet training with terrorizing and threats of what will happen to the child if she or he does not gain control of bowels and bladder. These children may later be seen in the physician's office with extreme constipation and/or urinary tract infections as the child continues to try to gain control of the "environment" by control of body functions. When children repeatedly hear parents or grandparents say, "Your dad or mother was potty trained at 9 months," they feel the pressure to be toilet trained but lack the muscle control The children feel inferior because they are unable to perform as wanted by these significant adults. To the child this is a subtle but consistent put-down for not performing at the same level as the parent. When this put-down is combined with other forms of overpressuring, the results are frequently stress-related illnesses and excessive anxiety.

## ◆CAUSES OF EMOTIONAL ABUSE

Many theories exist regarding the causes and correlates of child abuse. The four theories discussed here are (1) the psychiatric approach, (2) the social approach, (3) the developmental approach, and (4) the ecological approach.

### PSYCHIATRIC APPROACH

The psychiatric approach to emotional abuse of children assumes that the perpetrating parent suffers from some mental illness. Kempe and Kempe (1978) estimated that 10% of all maltreating parents are psychopathic or sociopathic. Studies of mentally ill patients show they are at high risk for failing to meet a child's psychological needs because of the amount of effort they must expend to meet their own emotional needs. As compared to a control group, emotionally abusive parents showed significantly more psychosocial problems, more difficulty coping with stress, more difficulty building relationships, and more social isolation (Pemberton & Benady, 1973). According to one study, emotionally abusive parents described themselves as having poor child management techniques and being victims of maltreatment in their childhoods (Hickox & Furnell, 1989). The mother who is overwhelmed with her own depression and psychologically stressed after childbirth lacks the physical or emotional energies to give the child what is needed. The parent preoccupied with the death of a parent, sibling, or spouse may also be unable to meet a child's needs. Although postpartum depression and grief tend to be short-term and reversible, they negatively impact the parent-child relationship and can adversely affect the developing child. Mothers who are psychologically unavailable to their children appear to impair both socioemotional and cognitive development of the children (Polanky et al., 1981; Erickson et al., 1986). Emotional abuse stemming from the mental illness of parents is one possible explanation but explains only a small number of emotional abuse cases.

### SOCIAL APPROACH

Social approach theory places emphasis on the role of stress as a force impacting the family dynamics and causing emotional abuse. Fifty-nine percent of all abuse cases were associated with stress (Gil, 1970). Social stress interacting with other variables leads to aggression in the form of emotional abuse. The stressors for all families include limited resources, problems at work, death of the significant other, unemployment, health problems, overcrowding, isolation, substance abuse, high levels of mobility, poverty, and marital problems (Newberger & Newberger, 1982).

Individuals respond differently to stress. Women as a group demonstrate a tendency toward depression rather than violence as a response. Men as a group respond to stress with violence. Stressed women usually are psychologically unavailable to their children, thus ignoring, rejecting, or isolating them. Men, on the other hand, have a tendency to physically or verbally assault their children. The family's socialization to violence determines if the father is physically or verbally assaultive (Straus & Kantor, 1987). *Since all parents experience stress, the following mediating variables can assist in identifying which parents will abuse their children and which will not:*

1. Presence or lack of appropriate coping mechanisms

2. Degree of family integration or isolation

3. Presence or absence of positive social networks

These mediating variables and the underlying causes of the stress determine the length and degree of the psychological abuse and, consequently, the amount of damage to the child's development (Newberger & Newberger, 1982; Straus & Kantor, 1987; Hickox & Furnell, 1989; Casanova et al., 1992).

## DEVELOPMENTAL APPROACH

The developmental approach to psychological abuse is based on a theory that parenting attitudes and behaviors parallel Piaget's stages of cognitive development and Kolberg's stages of moral development. The stages require increasing cognitive sophistication and moral reasoning. At the lower developmental level, behavior is marked by immediate, direct, and unmodulated responses to external stimuli and internal need states. At higher levels of maturation, behavior is characterized by the appearance of indirect, ideational, conceptual, and symbolic or verbal behavior.

---

**Table 20-13. Cognitive-Developmental Stages of Parental Reasoning**

**Egoistic (Self) Orientation**
The basis for parental activity and for understanding of the child is the child's actions in relation to the parent's needs. Child care tasks and parenting are seen as being carried out in response to external cues that affect the parent's emotional and physical comfort, or which offer approval to the parent. Intentions of the child are recognized, but as a projection of parental feelings, and are not separate from actions. The organizing principle is achieving what the parent wants, and the object of socialization of the child is to maximize parental comfort.

*Examples:*

> *What do you feel children need most from their parents?*
> Love and attention
>
> *When you say love, what do you mean?*
> Holding them, telling them you love them, making them behave so they won't get on that dope and stuff when they get older. I want my kids to feel proud of me. I know eventually when they get older maybe I'll fail, but I'm gonna try my darndest when they're younger and just hope they don't turn out that way.

**Conventional (Norms) Orientation**
The basis for parental activity and for understanding of the child is the child's actions and inferred intentions in relation to preconceived, externally derived expectations. The child is conceived as having internal states and needs that must be acknowledged, but the parent conceives of the child's subjective reality in a stereotypical way. The child is not seen as unique, but as a member of the class of "children" and the parent draws upon tradition, "authority," or conventional wisdom, rather than solely upon the self, to inform expectations and practices. The parent and child are understood to have well-defined roles that are their responsibility to fulfill. The parent-child relationship is conceived as mutual fulfillment of role obligations.

*Examples:*

> *What do you feel children need most from their parents?*
> Love

**Table 20-13. Cognitive-Developmental Stages of Parental Reasoning—*Continued***

*Explain.*
Just letting them know you love them. Letting them know you care, that you are concerned about what they do, and just trying to be the best parent you can.

*Why do you think that is most important, conveying that love?*
Because if children know they have love, then they are secure.

### Individualistic (Child) Orientation

Each child is recognized to have unique as well as universally shared qualities and is understood in terms of his or her own subjective reality. The parent tries to understand the child's world from the child's particular point of view, and conceptualizes the parent-child relationship as an exchange of feelings and sharing of perspectives, rather than only fulfillment of role obligations.

*Examples:*

*What do you think children need most from their parents?*
Love and time, they need to have their needs considered, that they aren't always happy with things that we do and with the things that we want to make them do and with the things we want to make them happy. You have to look at them and if they don't tell, you have to ask them. You have to really try to find out what each child wants and what is going on in their heads.

### Analytic (Systems) Orientation

The parent can view the relationship between parent and child as a mutual and reciprocal system and understand that the child has a complex psychological self-system. The parent can understand that the motives underlying a child's actions may reflect simultaneous and conflicted feelings. The parent can also recognize that there may be ambivalence in his or her own feelings and actions as a parent and still love and care for the child. Individuals and relationships are understood not only in terms of their stable elements, but also as a continual process of growth and change. The parent-child relationship is built not only on shared feelings, but also on shared acceptance of each other's faults and frailties as well as virtues and each other's separateness as well as closeness.

*Examples:*

What do you feel children need most from their parents? I will say love and you will say to me, "What do you mean by love?" and I will say, "I think it is an acceptance, unqualified, for what that person is in time...." It has nothing to do with grades or cleanliness. I would like her to be clean and tidy, but it has nothing to do with love and feeling that someplace in this world you are loved for what you are by the people who know you best and nevertheless love you. I think that it is something that will help the children begin to love themselves.

What do you mean to begin to love itself? Well, I think that people can be so cruel to themselves, "Oh, I'm dumb, I'm stupid." Words that tear down instead of build up. And I think one way to serenity about the way you are and the way you see the world, even if life is difficult, is if you can be gentle with your errors and failures and see them as part of a process. Then I think you will have a kind of stability and mental health that is a legacy from parents who love you unqualified.

*(Newberger & Cook, 1983)*

Parents at the higher levels are more apt to use words and reasoning as part of parenting. Parents at the higher levels look at each child as an individual and at what is best for that individual. Parents at the lower levels are more impulsive, directive, and physical in their parenting. Parents at the lower levels parent from their own point of view and to make themselves feel good (Newberger & Cook, 1983). Abusive parents, therefore, are parenting at their developmental level (Zigler & Hall, 1989).

The orientations toward the parent-child relationship as identified by Newberger and Cook (1983) are egoistic, conventional, individualistic, and analytic orientations. **Table 20-13** describes the characteristics of parental reasoning at each of these cognitive-developmental stages.

## ECOLOGICAL APPROACH

The ecological approach to the psychological abuse of children includes all of the various aspects of the family's life, including what the parents bring to the relationship, the child, the social context of the family and its support system, and the total societal influences and values. The parents bring to the parent-child relationship various influences, including how they were parented, their parental developmental level, their feelings toward the child, their knowledge of child development, their marital relationship, and their individual mental health. The child influences how he or she will be parented. The child's health, temperament, ordinal position in the family, and other family relationships all influence how a child will be parented. Additionally, the support systems of the family and the total societal expectations are influencing factors. The interaction of all the influencing factors determine the type of parenting (Polanky et al., 1981; Hickox & Furnell, 1989; Zigler & Hall, 1989).

---

**Table 20-14. Indicators of Psychological Abuse**

**Socioemotional Indicators**
Impaired capacity to enjoy life
Refuses to defend self
Pseudo-mature behavior
Sexually precocious behavior
Lies notably when it is not to protect self but often in circumstances when there is nothing to lose by telling the truth
Cheats, steals
Refuses to accept responsibility for actions; blames others
Psychiatric symptoms
Tantrums
Bizarre behavior
Low self-esteem
Withdrawal
Opposition
Compulsivity
Aggressive, defiant, domineering
Controlling but lacks self-control
Extreme behaviors

Seeking love, acceptance, and affection outside of home
Pregnant adolescent wanting her baby to love her
Apathy

**Cognitive Indicators**
School learning problems
Short attention span
Hypervigilance
Hyperactivity, attention deficit
Language delayed
Motor delayed
Lack of exploration and curiosity

**Physical Indicators**
Nonorganic failure to thrive
Slowed growth in trunk and distinctly short limbs, dwarfism
Circulatory problems
Accident prone
Awkwardness
Small abrasions that heal slowly on limbs

Coarse, dry, brittle hair and dry scalp
Self-destructive both physically and socially
Eating disorders, anorexia nervosa, bulimia, obesity
Gastrointestinal and bowel problems including chronically loose stools, refusal to void
Poor posture
Reduced energy level, lethargy
Catatonia
Sleep disorders

---

## ◆IDENTIFYING PSYCHOLOGICAL ABUSE

Psychological abuse, although the core of all types of maltreatment, is very difficult to specifically identify and diagnose. With careful multidisciplinary documentation, each professional can provide a valuable part of the total picture (Fortin & Reed, 1984). Many young emotional abuse victims, especially ritualistically abused victims, may initially have few overt indicators. The complete picture becomes evident as the child feels safe with more professionals. The assessment of the child's situation begins with a professional seeing some minor abnormalities and then becoming more concerned as he or she obtains additional information. **Table 20-14** summarizes indicators of emotional abuse in children. Psychological abuse results in reduced cognitive and emotional functioning. The reduced cognitive functioning is more easily identified than the reduced emotional development and functioning. Usually both are present. However, it should not be assumed that cognitive ability will always be impaired.

## ♦ BEHAVIORAL INDICATORS

The emotionally abused child's behavior is characterized by a wide range of behaviors, including apathy, crying and irritability, refusal to be calmed, and avoidance of eye contact with adults, especially parents.

### NEGATIVE AFFECT

Emotionally maltreated infants commonly show a negative affect to anyone in the environment. They also fail to grimace or show pain when appropriate, such as not crying after a fall or a shot. They do not respond as other children would when things such as toys or food are taken away from them. In situations in which a normal child would cry or seek comfort, these children have no emotional response, appearing indifferent.

### FAILURE TO THRIVE

In extreme cases of psychological abuse the infant can undergo the process of nonorganic failure to thrive characterized by insufficient weight gain, impaired health, slow physical growth, retarded language development, distorted social responses, irritability, an anxious attachment, apathetic solitariness, and catatonia.

### PASSIVITY

Abused children appear numb to either negative or positive environmental stimuli. If left alone with familiar objects, they do not have normal age-appropriate play skills and do not demonstrate normal pleasure and satisfaction from either solitary play or play with adults. They are excessively passive and obedient (MacCarthy, 1979; Trowell, 1983).

### NEGATIVE SELF-IMAGE

Young children who have experienced emotional abuse demonstrate a negative view of their world and themselves. They see themselves as unworthy and view the world as a hostile place. They are fearful, angry, anxious, aggressive, and sometimes violent. They may engage in both physically and socially self-destructive behavior. They are often depressed, withdrawn, passive, and shy, exhibiting poor interpersonal communication skills. These children are often suicidal. They may frequently complain of headaches and sleep disturbances.

Children who externalize their feelings tend to be disobedient, impulsive, and overactive. They lack self-control and often are violent toward other people and their environment. Maltreated children who are aggressive exhibit a continuous and generalized aggression. The aggression is a state of being rather than a response to a specific action or individual. They behave according to impulses rather than social norms (Fontana, 1973; Rohner & Rohner, 1980). Children who internalize their feelings are withdrawn, indifferent, submissive, and hostile (Egeland et al., 1983).

### ABNORMAL RESPONSES

Some emotionally maltreated children have low levels of social responsiveness or hesitant response patterns. They approach unfamiliar adults indiscriminately, seeking attention while avoiding physical contact with them (Harter & Zigler, 1974; Balla & Zigler, 1975). Other emotionally maltreated children cling to adults other than their parents and remain distant from peers (MacCarthy, 1979). In both instances the child's social behavior can be situationally inappropriate. In most instances the child cannot respond to environmental rewards, such as children asking them to join in group activities, smiles, and verbal praise (Watkins & Bradbard, 1982). The child is often indifferent to positive feedback about his or her own success and responds negatively with social challenges or peer rejection.

### Table 20-15. Extreme Behaviors of Victims of Child Abuse

Compulsively neat and meticulously clean, or destructive and extremely messy

Very polite, compliant, or very noncompliant and belligerent

Overly obedient, willing to do anything to please, or overly controlling, resistant

Socially very polite, kind, overly generous, or egocentric, revengeful, self-centered, antisocial

Passive, or openly hostile and angry

Indiscriminately friendly, "shows affection" to or hugs anyone, or cold, indifferent, avoids peers, family, strangers

Overly obedient, helpful, "loving," or extremely disagreeable, angry, "purposefully hurts others"

Maltreated children respond negatively to parents and/or merely attempt to avoid the parent and thereby avoid more maltreatment. The child may also try to take care of the parent's needs to reduce the instance and degree of maltreatment in the future. In the home, as in other social environments, the child may rebel and aggressively act out or may withdraw and attempt to escape physically or emotionally.

### BEHAVIOR EXTREMES

Child abuse victims characteristically exhibit behavior at the extremes of the normal spectrum (**Table 20-15**). These children have no moderation in their behavior. One child can be at both extremes on the spectrum in different areas of behavior, but is more likely to be consistently on one end of the spectrum in all areas of development.

## ♦ CHILD AND FAMILY ASSESSMENT

The early indicators of emotional maltreatment should alert child care professionals to possible problems, prompting early intervention and treatment. Assessment tools combined with observational data from all professionals who work with a child and his or her family can give an accurate evaluation of family functioning. Most cases of psychological abuse are mild and will not enter the protective services system; instead, the family in trouble will seek assistance with its own problems. If protective services and the courts become involved, the case should include professional summaries from various professionals and an assessment by a psychologist with at least three of the assessment tools listed in **Table 20-16**.

Although many different professionals can observe behavioral indicators of emotional abuse, assessment for state involvement either by the protective services agency or the courts commonly requires that the case records include assessment by a licensed psychologist (Garbarino, 1978; Yates, 1982; Furnell, 1986). The multidisciplinary assessment of child maltreatment involves a psychologist who has specialized training in administering developmental tests to evaluate (1) the child's cognitive developmental level, (2) the child's personality characteristics, and (3) the quality of the parent-child interaction. The most commonly used instruments for personality assessment are the Minnesota Multiphasic Personality Inventory (MMPI), Rorschach Test, Thematic Apperception Test, and Draw-a-Person Test. A variety of instruments can be used for assessing infant, child, and adolescent psychological maltreatment and parent-child interaction.

## ♦ PARENTAL AND ENVIRONMENTAL INDICATORS

Most researchers and practitioners caution against overemphasis on identifying potential child abusers. Professionals, however, should be aware of parental behaviors and family dynamics that foster the child's behaviors indicating that psychological abuse could be occurring. Emotionally abusive parents as a group share some common characteristics (**Table 20-17**), although nonabusing parents can also have some of these same characteristics. Because parents have some of the identified characteristics does not mean that they are or will become abusing parents, but it denotes the potential for abuse.

### PARENTS MALTREATED AS CHILDREN

Not all maltreated children grow up to maltreat their children. Parents who were maltreated as children, however, lack the role model of appropriate parenting and

---

**Table 20-16. Instruments Used to Assess Psychological Maltreatment and Child-Parent Interaction**

Bayley Scales of Infant Development (Bayley, 1969)

Tennessee Self-Concept Scale (Fitts, 1965)

State-Trait Anxiety Inventory (Spielberger, 1971; Spielberger et al., 1970; Rohner et al., 1978)

Child Behavior Checklist (Achenbach, 1978; Achenbach & Edelbrock, 1979)

Child Assessment Schedule (Hodges, 1982)

---

**Table 20-17. Characteristics Common to Psychologically Abusive Parents**

Emotionally abused as children

Stressed

Lack of appropriate coping skills

Mental illness, e.g., schizophrenia, character disorder, depression

Angry

Hostile

Ambivalence toward parenthood

Few resources, financial, social, etc.

Inappropriate expectations of children

Lack of knowledge of normal child development

Marital problems

Lack of impulse control

---

can suffer from lowered self-esteem, higher anxiety levels, and a more negative view of the world, all conditions that may have a negative impact on their child-rearing practices (Pemberton & Benady, 1973; Burgress & Conger, 1978; Caffo et al., 1982; Baily & Baily, 1983; Straus & Kantor, 1987; Claussen & Crittenden, 1991).

## MENTAL ILLNESS AND CRIMINAL BEHAVIOR

Parents with a history of mental illness or criminal behavior, especially violent criminal behavior, should alert protective service workers and other professionals to the possibility of child maltreatment. Many individuals involved in criminal activity corrupt and/or terrorize their own children (Garbarino, 1977; Burgress & Conger, 1978; Caffo et al., 1982).

## PARENT-CHILD INTERACTION PATTERNS

*A recent study identified the following pattern of parent-child interaction that consistently appeared in emotional abuse cases:*

1. Verbal communication between mother and child was virtually one-way, with the mother using words as commands rather than initiating or allowing dialogue.

2. The mother repeatedly gave confused messages to the child about what was wanted; contradictions sometimes occurred within seconds.

3. The mother carried out activities for the child (for example, putting clothes on a doll) at the child's instigation. This was done without involving the child in the task and consequently did not lead to play or the teaching of skills.

4. The child was not involved in "doing things together with baby." The situation provided numerous (missed) opportunities for activities likely to provide environmental benefit for the child and also to facilitate interaction between the child and her younger brother (Furnell, 1986, p. 182).

---

**Table 20-18. Characteristic Responses of Abusive Parent to Infant**

Considered abortion or giving child up for adoption

Excessively irritated by baby's crying

Repulsed and irritated at having to change diapers

Describes the child in negative terms—ugly, deformed, makes repulsive sounds

Passive, unconcerned about child's needs

Disciplines—spanks, slaps, yells at—infant under 6 months for "bad" behaviors

Does not talk to the child

Tells others of disappointments with appearance, sex of infant

States that the infant does "things on purpose to irritate or to get even with parent(s)"

Not involved with child

Plays very little with child

Very concerned about how soon infant will have control of bowels and bladder

Calls the child derogatory names, e.g., little bastard, fart-head, freak

---

Psychologically abusive parents, as all maltreating parents, have a negative view of their children and their children's behavior. This negative view of their children will be obvious to professionals working with the family. Some of the characteristic responses of abusive parents to their infants are listed in **Table 20-18**. The negative

**Table 20-19. Summary of Parental Behaviors that Indicate Potential for Psychological Abuse**

Seldom shows emotions; when present, emotions tend to be negative

Routinely ignores or denies child's basic needs

Belittles child or calls child derogatory names in public

Consistently yells at child rather than talking in normal tone

Isolates child from normal contact with peers and community

Routinely ignores child behaving inappropriately

Fails to define appropriate behavior for child; instead punishes

Routinely verbally assaultive in public

Consistently demonstrates inappropriate expectations from child

Demonstrates a lack of basic knowledge of normal child development

Demonstrates sadistic behavior toward child

Threatens child with guns, knives, bondage, abandonment

Routinely humiliates child in public or in front of peers

Scapegoats the child

Consistently demonstrates impulsive behavior

Routinely places own needs before child's to child's detriment

Consistently uses bizarre or frightening form of punishment

Teaches child antisocial or criminal activity

Knowingly allows child to engage in antisocial or criminal activity

Sexualizes activities with child

Consistently criticizes or calls child a "baby" when child behaves in age-appropriate manner

Begins toilet training very early and harshly disciplines child for "accidents"

Demonstrates jealous behavior toward child

Has diminished capacity due to mental retardation, psychopathology, substance abuse

Feels his or her life is out of control

Has history of violent behavior

Lives in poverty

Describes self as "no good"

Lacks parental warmth toward child

attitudes toward infants will persist as the child grows and develops if conditions remain the same. Professionals can observe similar parent-child interaction with children of any age. As compared to control groups of parents, the abusive parent sees the infant as purposefully acting in ways to "get even with" or "annoy" the parent (Hickox & Furnell, 1989). This may result from the parent's lack of knowledge about child growth and development, as well as the parent's alexithymia and lack of trust of others.

**Table 20-19** summarizes the parental behaviors that may indicate emotional abuse (Giovannoni & Becerra, 1979; Rohner & Rohner, 1980; Baily & Baily, 1983; Burgess et al., 1990).

## ♦ CONSEQUENCES OF PSYCHOLOGICAL ABUSE

The consequences of psychological abuse vary with the child's age, relationship to

## Table 20-20. Consequences of Emotional Abuse

Psychiatric disorders—depression, character disorder, borderline personality disorder, multiple personality disorder, attention deficit

Self-destructive behaviors

Antisocial and delinquent behaviors, often violent

Increased vulnerability

Language delayed

Cognitive delayed

Fine and gross motor delayed

Decreased exploratory activity

Relationship problems

Low self-esteem

Negative view of self and others

Sleep disorders

Eating disorders

Maternal deprivation syndrome

Deprivation dwarfism

Nonorganic failure to thrive

Circulatory problems

Munchausen Syndrome by Proxy

Learned helplessness

---

the abuser, and level of development of the self at the time the abuse occurs. **Table 20-20** lists some of the common consequences of psychological abuse. The consequences of the maltreatment become evident by differing behaviors as the child progresses through different developmental stages. When psychological abuse is combined with sexual maltreatment, the psychopathology appears to be most evident before puberty. Disturbances in body functions as a result of maltreatment are most evident in children under the age of 4 years, whereas psychoneurotic conflicts mostly manifest during preadolescence. Behavior disorders and psychomotor delays appear at all ages (Martinez-Roig et al., 1983; Cerce et al., 1988; Hartman & Burgess, 1989; O'Hagan, 1995). Longitudinal research has prospectively related psychologically unavailable caregiving and verbal hostile caregiving to the development of child deviance and delay (Egeland & Erickson, 1987).

Ignoring and rejecting a child's basic needs appears to result in children who are destructive, impulsive, low in ego control, passive, low in impulse control, less flexible, less creative, less persistent, and those who avoid mothers. These young children lack the self-esteem and trust necessary to explore the environment or attend to cognitively oriented tasks (Egeland et al., 1983). Since individuals view themselves as they believe "significant others" view them, and parents are the most "significant others" of young children, rejected children view themselves as unworthy of love and inadequate as individuals. Negative self-esteem and negative self-adequacy lead children to be less tolerant of stress, less emotionally stable, emotionally insulated, more dependent (clingy, intensely possessive), more defensive, more emotionally detached, and angrier. Rejected children in all cultures view God, the gods, or whatever form the supernatural takes, as being malevolent. They believe that God is hostile and punitive and inflicts death, sickness, and misfortune (Rohner & Rohner, 1980).

### INCREASED VULNERABILITY

Threats, trauma, or deprivation in a child's life increase vulnerability to other maltreatment. For instance, the emotionally deprived child is more vulnerable to negative experiences in day care than are children from enriched home environments (Gamble & Zigler, 1985). Children can overcome the experiences of physical assault or sexual abuse provided they have been nurtured and valued by psychologically supportive parents (Finkelhor, 1984).

### EATING DISORDERS

Anorexia nervosa, bulimia, obesity, and other eating disorders in individuals at all ages are common consequences of emotional abuse. The food behaviors of an abuse victim can range from refusing to eat or holding food in the mouth but refusing to swallow, to gulping food down, scavenging, stealing, and hoarding. These children are enuretic and encopretic; loose stools are common. Victims of emotional abuse commonly attach more emotional than physical significance to food.

### MUNCHAUSEN SYNDROME BY PROXY

Munchausen Syndrome by Proxy victims manifest psychologically impaired development. These infants fail to develop a basic sense of trust in infancy and therefore are developmentally impaired throughout life. The children develop eating disorders, become withdrawn or hyperactive, and develop oppositional behaviors. They are passive and tolerate medical procedures. The older children and adolescents grow to cooperate with their parents' deceptions and begin to fabricate their own history of symptoms. The child victims of Munchausen Syndrome by Proxy become Munchausen Syndrome patients. It is very difficult to stop this cycle of learned behavior because of the extreme denial and manipulation that occurs in both generations (McGuire & Feldman, 1989).

## LANGUAGE DELAY

Most maltreated children demonstrate some degree of language delay. The more securely attached infants with better infant-mother attachment, however, consistently demonstrate better linguistic output and general language development (Martinez-Roig et al., 1983; Cicchetti, 1989).

## DELAYED COGNITIVE FUNCTIONING

Maltreated children are delayed in their cognitive functioning. Children who have been verbally assaulted are less persistent in exploring their environment and have increased difficulty with problem solving and task completion. These skills are necessary for learning to occur (Zajonc, 1980; Egeland et al., 1983). The abusive environment appears to encourage the development of aggressive behavior as an adaptive coping strategy. Cognitive-affective imbalance in maltreated children can cause them to interpret ambiguous stimuli as being threatening and aggressive. Maltreated children are more likely than normal children to interpret behavior as aggressive and respond in a like manner. This results in difficulty when interacting with their peers. Perhaps this can explain why maltreated children have more negative expectations of interpersonal relations (Cicchetti, 1989).

## ATTACHMENT DISORDERS

Bowlby (1977) believed that parental threats to abandon the child and commit suicide are forms of emotional abuse by rejection and would have pathogenic effects on the child's attachment mechanism. These pathological conditions can emerge as early as the preschool years and are manifested as childhood borderline disorders, attention deficit disorders, dissociative disorders, and childhood depression (Bemporad et al., 1982; American Psychiatric Association, 1987). Children of psychologically unavailable mothers, as compared to a control group of children 4 to 6 years old, were more aggressive, less involved with peers, unpopular with peers, nervous, overactive, and lower overall in academic performance. Emotional abuse to children as a result of mothers being psychologically unavailable appears to impair both socioemotional and cognitive development of the children (Erickson et al., 1986). Interaction with their mothers was characterized by negativity, noncompliance, lack of affection, and a high degree of avoidance.

## ◆ SUMMARY

Following all types of psychological abuse, children experience impairment in all areas of development. The impairment can be minimized when the child is securely attached, when the abuse is not combined with other forms of maltreatment, and when the abuse is mild or over a short period of time. However, in all cases, some impairment occurs in all areas of development. The child's self-esteem is lowered. The child enjoys life less and either becomes withdrawn and passive or aggressive and hostile. Cognitive and language ability are also delayed. Physically the child's growth and motor abilities may be delayed. Ritualistic or multiple-victim multiple-perpetrator abuse leaves the most profound impairment because it is systematically planned, is continuous, and involves multiple types of maltreatment including "brain-washing" of the child.

## ◆ BIBLIOGRAPHY

Achenbach, TM: The child behavior profiles. I: Boys aged 6-11, *J Consult Clin Psychol* 46:478-488, 1978.

Achenbach, TM, and Edelbrock, CS: The child behavior profiles. II: Boys aged 12-16 and girls aged 6-11 and 12-16, *J Consult Clin Psychol* 47:223-233, 1979.

Ainsworth, MD: Attachment in child abuse. In G Gerber, CJ Ross, and E Ziglers (eds): *Child Abuse Reconsidered: An Agenda for Action,* Oxford University Press, New York, 1980.

American Psychiatric Association Committee on Nomenclature: *Diagnostic and Statistical Manual of Mental Disorders III (Revised)*, American Psychiatric Association, Washington, DC, 1987.

Baily, TF, and Baily, WH: *Operational Definitions of Child Emotional Maltreatment*, Maine Department of Human Services, Augusta, ME, 1983.

Balla, DA, and Zigler, E: Preinstitutional social deprivation, responsiveness to social reinforcement, and IQ change in institutionalized retarded individuals: A 6 year follow-up study, *Am J Ment Defic* 80:228-230, 1975.

Bayley, N: *Manual for the Bayley Scales of Infant Development*, Psychological Corporation, New York, 1969, pp. 201-210.

Bemporad, J, Smith, H, Hanson, C, and Cicchetti, D: Borderline syndromes in childhood: Criteria for diagnosis, *Am J Psychiatry* 139:596-602, 1982.

Bowlby, J: The making and breaking of affectional bonds, *Br J Psychiatry* 130:201-210, 1977.

Brassard, MR, Stuart, NH, and Hardy, DB: The psychological maltreatment rating scales, *Child Abuse* 17:715-729, 1993.

Brothers, L: A biological perspective on empathy, *Am J Psychiatry* 146(1):10-19, 1989.

Bullard, DM, Glaser, HH, Hagarty, MC, and Pivchik, EC: Failure-to-thrive in the "neglected" child, *Am J Orthopsychiatry* 37(1):680-690, 1967.

Burgess, AW, Hartman, CR, and Kelly, SJ: Assessing child abuse: The TRIADS Checklist, *J Psychosoc Nurs* 28(4):7-14, 1990.

Burgress, R, and Conger, R: Family interaction in abusive, neglectful, and normal families, *Child Dev* 49:1163-1173, 1978.

Caffo, E, Guaraldi, GP, Magnani, G, and Tassi, R: Prevention of child abuse and neglect through early diagnosis and serious disturbances in the mother-child relationship in Italy, *Child Abuse Negl* 6(4)453-463, 1982.

Casanova, GM, Domanic, J, McCanne, TR, and Milner, JS: Physiological responses to non-child-related stressors in mothers at risk for child abuse, *Child Abuse Negl* 16(1):31-44, 1992.

Cerce, D, Rokouus, F, Diamond, D, Knight, R, and Prentky, R: Predicting criminal outcome from early developmental history. A paper presented at the National Symposium on Child Victimization, Anaheim, CA, April 27-30, 1988.

Cicchetti, D: How research on child maltreatment has informed the study of child development: Perspectives from developmental psycho pathology. In D Cicchetti and V Carlson, eds: *Child Maltreatment: Theory and Research on the Causes and Consequences of Child Abuse and Neglect*, Jossey-Bass Publishers, San Francisco, 1989.

Claussen, AH, and Crittenden, PM: Physical and psychological maltreatment: Relations among types of maltreatment, *Child Abuse Negl* 15(3):5-18, 1991.

Crittenden, PM: Internal representation models of attachment relationships, *J Infant Ment Health* 11:259-277, 1990.

Crittenden, PM, and Ainsworth, MD: Child maltreatment and attachment theory. In D Cicchetti & V Carson (eds): *Child Maltreatment: Theory and Research on the Causes and Consequences of Child Abuse and Neglect*, Cambridge University Press, New York, 1989.

Dean, D: Emotional abuse of children, *Child Today* 8(4):18-20, 1979.

Devereux, EC, Bronfenbrenner, U, and Suci, GJ: Patterns of parent behavior in the USA and the Federal Republic of Germany: A cross national comparison, *Int Soc Sci J* 14:488-506, 1962.

Edmundson, SE, and Collier, P: Child protection and emotional abuse: Definition, identification and usefulness within an educational setting, *Educational Psychol Practice* 8:4, 1993.

Egeland, B, and Erickson, M: Psychological unavailable caregiving. In MR Brassard, R Germain, and SN Hart (eds): *Psychological Maltreatment of Children and Youth,* Pergamon, New York, 1987.

Egeland, B, Stroufe, A, and Erickson, M: The developmental consequences of different patterns of maltreatment, *Child Abuse Negl* 7:459-469, 1983.

Elkind, D: *The Hurried Child: Growing Up Too Fast Too Soon*, Addison-Wesley Publishing Co, Reading, MA, 1982.

Erickson, MF, Egeland, B, and Pianta, R: Effects of maltreatment on the development of young children. In D Cicchetti and V Carlson, eds: *Child Maltreatment: Theory and Research on the Causes and Consequences of Child Abuse and Neglect*, Jossey-Bass Publishers, San Francisco, 1986.

Finkelhor, D: *Child Sexual Abuse*, Free Press, New York, 1984.

Fitts, WH: Manual: *Tennessee Self-Concept Scale*, Counselor Recording and Tests, Nashville, 1965.

Fontana, VJ: *Somewhere a Child is Crying: Maltreatment—Causes and Prevention*, Macmillan, New York, 1973.

Fortin, PJ, and Reed, SR: Diagnosing and responding to emotional abuse within the helping system, *Child Abuse Negl* 8:117-119, 1984.

Furnell, JRG: Emotional abuse of children: A psychologist's contribution to legal establishment, *Med Sci Law* 26(2):179-184, 1986.

Gamble, T, and Zigler, E: The effects of infant day-care, *The Network* 6(4):4, 1985.

Garbarino, J: The human ecology of child maltreatment, *J Marriage Fam* 39: 721-736, 1977.

Garbarino, J: The elusive 'crime' of emotional abuse, *Child Abuse Negl* 2:89-99, 1978.

Garbarino, J, Guttmann, E, and Seeley, JW: *The Psychologically Battered Child*, Jossey-Bass Publishers, San Francisco, 1986.

Gardner, LI: Deprivation dwarfism, *Sci Am* 227(1):76-82, 1972.

Gil, D: *Violence Against Children: Physical Child Abuse in the United States*, Harvard University Press, Cambridge, MA, 1970.

Giovannoni, JM, and Becerra, RM: *Defining Child Abuse*, Free Press, New York, 1979.

Green, A: Psychopathology of abused children, *J Am Acad Child Psychiatry* 17:92-103, 1978.

Harter, S, and Zigler, E: The assessment of effectance motivation in normal and retarded children, *Dev Psychol* 10:169-180, 1974.

Hartman, CR, and Burgess, AW: Sexual abuse of children. In D Cicchetti and V Carlson, eds: *Child Maltreatment: Theory and Research on the Causes and Consequences of Child Abuse and Neglect*, Jossey-Bass Publishers, San Francisco, 1989.

Helfer, RE, Schneider, CJ, and Hoffmeister, JK: *Report on Research on Using the Michigan Screening Profile of Parenting (MSPP): A 12-Year Study to Develop and Test a Predictive Questionnaire*, Office of Child Development, Department of Education, Washington, DC, 1978.

Hickox, A, and Furnell, JR: Psychosocial and background factors in emotional abuse of children, *Child Care Health Dev* 15(4):227-240, 1989.

Hodges, KK: The Child Assessment Schedule (CAS) diagnostic interview: A report on reliability and validity, *J Am Acad Child Psychiatry* 21:468-473, 1982.

James, B: The dissociatively disordered child, *The Advisor* 3(4):8-10, 1990.

Kelley, SJ: Ritualistic abuse of children: dynamics and impact, *Cult Studies J* 5(2):228-236, 1988.

Kempe, CH, and Kempe, R: *Child Abuse*, Harvard University Press, Cambridge, MA, 1978.

MacCarthy, D: Recognition of signs of emotional deprivation: A form of child abuse, *Child Abuse Negl* 3:423-428, 1979.

Martinez-Roig, A, Domingo-Salvany, F, Llorens-Terol, J, and Ibanez-Cacho, JM: Psychologic implications of the maltreated-child syndrome, *Child Abuse Negl* 7(3):261-263, 1983.

McGuire, TT, and Feldman, KW: Psychological morbidity of children subjected to Munchausen Syndrome by Proxy, *Pediatrics* 82(2):289-292, 1989.

Moos, RH: *Evaluating Correctional and Community Settings*, John Wiley and Sons, New York, 1975.

Mullen, PE, Martin, JC, Anderson, Romans, SE, & Herbison, GP: The long-term impact of physical, emotional, and sexual abuse of children: A community study. *Child Abuse Negl 20*(1):7-21, 1996.

Newberger, CM, and Cook, S: Parental awareness and child abuse: A cognitive-developmental analysis of urban and rural samples, *Am J Orthopsychiatry* 53:512-524, 1983.

Newberger, CM, and Newberger, E: Prevention of child abuse: Theory, myth and practice, *J Prevent Psychiatry* 1:443-451, 1982.

Ney, PG, Fung, T, and Wickett, AR: Child neglect: The precursor to child abuse, *Pre-Perinatal Psychol J* 8(2):95-112, 1993.

O'Hagan, KP: Emotional and psychological abuse: Problems of definition, *Child Abuse Negl* 19(4):449-461, 1995.

Olson, DH, Russell, DH, and Sprenkle, CS: Circumplex model of marital and family system. VI: Theoretical update, *Fam Process* 22:69-83, 1979.

Pemberton, DA, and Benady, DR: Consciously rejected children, *Br J Psychiatry* 123:575-578, 1973.

Polanky, N, Chalmers, M, Butterweiser, E, and Williams, D: *Damaged Parents*, University of Chicago Press, Chicago, 1981.

Polanky, NA, Borgman, RD, and De Saix, C: *Roots of Futility*, Jossey-Bass Publishers, San Francisco, 1972.

Powell, GF, Brasel, JA, and Blizzard, RM: Emotional abuse deprivation and growth retardation simulating idiopathic hypopituitarism, *N Engl J Med* 276(23):1271-1278, 1967.

Rand, DC: Munchausen Syndrome by Proxy: A complex type of emotional abuse responsible for some false allegations of child abuse in divorce, *Issues Child Abuse Accusations* 5(3):135-155, 1993.

Rohner, RP: Worldwide test of parental acceptance-rejection theory: An overview, *Beh Sci Res* 15:1-21, 1980.

Rohner, RP, and Rohner, EC: Antecedents and consequences of parental rejection: A theory of emotional abuse, *Child Abuse Negl* 4(3):189-198, 1980.

Rohner, RH, Saavedra, JM, and Granum, EO: *Development and Validation of the Personality Assessment Questionnaire*: Test Manual, ERIC Clearinghouse on Counseling and Personnel Services, Ann Arbor, MI, 1978.

Sackette, GP: Monkeys reared in isolation with pictures of visual input: Evidence for an innate reasoning, 5(4):1468-1473, 1966.

Schaefer, ES: Children's reports of parental behavior: An inventory, *Child Dev* 36(2):412-424, 1965.

Schwartz, JC, and Zuroff, DC: Family structure and depression in female college students: Effects of parental conflict, decision making power, and inconsistency of love, *J Abnorm Psychol* 88:398-406, 1979.

Snow, B, and Sorensen, T: Ritualistic child abuse in a neighborhood setting, *J Interpersonal Violence* 5(4):474-487, 1990.

Spielberger, CD: Trait-state anxiety and motor behavior, *J Motor Beh* 3:265-279, 1971.

Spielberger, CD, Gorsuch, RL, and Wishene, RE: *The Trait Anxiety Inventory*, Consulting Psychologists' Press, Palo Alto, CA, 1970.

Spitz, RA: Hospitalism: An inquiry into the genesis of psychiatric conditions in early childhood, *Psychoanal Study Child* 1:53-74, 1945.

Spitz, RA: Hospitalism: A follow-up report, *Psychoanal Study Child* 2:113-117, 1946.

Straus, MA, and Kantor, GK: Stress and child abuse. In RE Helfer and RS Kempe, eds: *The Battered Child*, ed 4, University of Chicago Press, Chicago, 1987.

Trowell, J: Emotional abuse of children, *Home Visitor* 56(7):252-255, 1983.

Vissing, YM, Straus, MA, Gelles, RJ, and Harrop, JW: Verbal aggression by parents and psychosocial problems of children, *Child Abuse Negl* 15(3)223-238, 1991.

Watkins, HD, and Bradbard, MR: Child maltreatment: An overview with suggestions for intervention and research, *Fam Relations* 31:323-333, 1982.

Wright, SA: Physical and emotional abuse and neglect of preschool children: A literature review, *Australian Occupa Ther J* 41:55-63, 1994.

Yates, A: Legal issues in psychological abuse of children, *Clin Pediatr* 21(10)587-590, 1982.

Young, WC, Sachs, RC, Bruan, BG, and Watkins, RT: Patients reporting ritual abuse in childhood: A clinical syndrome. Report of 37 cases, *Child Abuse Negl* 15(3):181-189, 1991.

Zajonc, RB: Feeling and thinking: Preferences need no inferences, *Am Psychol* 35:151-175, 1980.

Zigler, E, and Hall, NW: Child abuse in America. In D Cicchetti and V Carlson, eds: Child Maltreatment: Theory and Research on the Causes and Consequences of Child Abuse and Neglect, Jossey-Bass, San Francisco, 1989.

## Appendix: Instruments for Assessing Characteristics of the Maltreating Family and Parents and the Maltreated Child

| | Instrument | Purpose | Theoretical Basis | Examples of What Is Measured | Filled Out By |
|---|---|---|---|---|---|
| **Family Context** | Family Environment Scale | Assess social climate in family | Ecological approach to human systems | Interpersonal relationships Personal growth Family structure | Each family member |
| | Family Adaptability and Cohesion Scale | Assess family's level of cohesion and adaptability | Systems framework of family relationships | Emotional bonds Sharing Roles Feedback | Each family member |
| | Interparental Conflict and Influence Scales | Assess content and frequency of arguments, relative power in decision making | Parental conflict and decision making power | Finance Spouse characteristics Child-rearing practices Joint family activities | Each family member |
| **Parental Factors and Parent-Child Interactions** | Parental Acceptance-Rejection Questionnaire | Assess degree of parental acceptance or rejection | Parental acceptance-rejection theory | Warmth/affection Hostility Indifference Undifferentiated rejection | Each family member |
| | Children's Reports of Parental Behavior Inventory | Assess degree of parental love/hostility, autonomy/control, firm control/lax control | Relation of child's adjustment level to perception of parents | Sharing Affection Ignoring Intrusiveness Strictness | Each family member; mainly the child |
| | Bronfenbrenner's Parental Behavior Questionnaire | Assess parental loving, punishing, demanding | Relation of child's adjustment level to perception of parents | Nurturance Companionship Power Indulgence | Each family member; mainly the child |
| | Michigan Screening Profile of Parenting | Assess degree of existing maltreatment and predict further maltreatment | Child maltreatment is related to parental maltreatment as a child | Relationship with parents Expectations of children Coping skills | Parents |
| | Maternal Characteristics Scale | Assess how mother's personality affects maternal competence | Polansky's studies of neglectful mothers | Apathy-futility Childlike impulsivity | Practitioner |
| | Childhood Level of Living Scale | Assess quality of mother's child-rearing practices | Polansky's studies of neglectful mothers | Physical care of child Emotional-cognitive care of child | Practitioner |
| **Children's Behavior and Personality** | Bayley Scales of Infant Development | Assess infant's development of motor, mental, and social skills | Infant development and the interrelatedness of motor, mental, and social abilities | Verbal communication Coordination of muscles Tendency to approach stimulation | Trained practitioner, rating the child |
| | Tennessee Self-Concept Scale | Assess self-concept, self-acceptance, perception of own behavior | Theories of self-concept as influence on behavioral patterns | Self-criticism Positive self-perception Integrity across topics | Each family member; mainly the child |
| | State-Trait Anxiety Inventory | Assess extent to which child is tensed overall and at specific situations | State and trait theory of anxiety | Calmness Unhappiness Worry Fright | Each family member; mainly the child |
| | Personality Assessment Questionnaire | Assess personality and behavioral dispositions | Rohner's acceptance-rejection theory | Hostility Dependence Self-esteem Emotional stability | Each family member |
| | Child Behavior Checklist | Evaluate behavioral problems and competencies of child | General classifications of behavior problems | Participation in sports or activities Membership in organizations Grades in school Somatic complaints Hyperactivity | Each family member |
| | Child Assessment Schedule | Assess child's personality and personality disorders | Standard psychiatric diagnostic criteria and general classifications of behavior problems | Fears Moods Thought disorders Self-understanding | Practitioner |

*Garbarino, J., Guttmann, E. and Seeley, J.W.: Assessing the Causes and Effects of Maltreatment. In The Psychologically Battered Child: Strategies for Identification, Assessment, and Intervention, Jossey-Bass, San Francisco, 1986, pp. 101-102.*

# THE CYCLE OF ABUSE

JAMES J. WILLIAMS, M.D.

Relatively scant societal attention and resources have been directed to the study of human violence. While societal awareness of interpersonal violence has been raised by various groups who have come forward and identified it in their own lives, children are largely a silent group. To this list of sufferers must be added children who are themselves abusers. Our ideas about human violence are flawed when they ignore child maltreatment and its links to human violence. Abusive children have probably always existed, and they are a manifestation of a number of tragic circumstances. Family violence and neglect should be among the most preventable of situations. This chapter will deal with that particular cause, describing the cycle of abuse.

## ◆FAMILY VIOLENCE

Family violence is not entirely mysterious. To a large degree, it is predictable and understandable. When unchecked, its costs reach far beyond the tragedy of individual families. To the immediate costs of therapy are added the social costs of school failure, substance abuse, impaired parenting, psychiatric hospitalization, and criminal violence. These costs are more substantial for the victims but ultimately affect us all. Child protection has always varied with the value society has placed on the lives of its children. Successful intervention first requires recognition that abusive children exist and then a social commitment to respond to their suffering.

Though victims of family violence now receive increased public attention, the medical, legal, and social professions are still largely unaware of children who abuse other children. Revelations that children are battered or denied the necessities of life evoke contradictory and complex mixtures of denial and horror, disgust and fascination from the professions, media, and the public. It is even more incredible and unpleasant to contemplate that small children are the aggressors in situations of physical and sexual abuse. The response of the protective service system to young child perpetrators has been nearly nonexistent. The children remain essentially invisible, and society has great difficulty acknowledging them.

Historically, the widespread recognition of violence between family intimates is a modern phenomenon. Certain family functions, such as how children are disciplined and how spouses react to anger and frustration, have been addressed in western societies, exposing problems that have probably always existed. Paradoxically, the increased recognition has come in the same social context that minimizes spouse abuse. Child abuse exploded into public awareness in the 1960s (Caffey, 1946; Silverman, 1953; Kempe et al., 1962) and was championed by the child protection movement. In the 1970s, society became more aware of spouse abuse (e.g., Martin, 1976). Apart from the obvious physical differences between the sexes, social inequality explains why women and children remain the most vulnerable targets for men in family violence. Women and children continue to be viewed as *owned* by the male head of the household.

Sexual abuse was brought into the open as incest survivors told their stories of unacknowledged pain. With the additional recognition of elder abuse, violence is now seen to span the generations, making the family itself the center of concern. Despite the progress in recognizing these problems, major concerns remain. We need to consider the violence instigated by children as a marker for assessing family violence. Ignoring the violence impedes efforts to protect children and to understand family functioning.

The home retains its aura of privacy for citizens in our society, making well-designed studies of family violence difficult to pursue. Yet the home is where aggressive interactions begin.

Reliable information on the levels of violence by children is particularly difficult to find. Nationwide surveys suggest that several factors allow this violence to be overlooked (Straus et al., 1980). Many parents in the survey by Steinmetz (1977) exhibited poor recall of their children's violence. When social norms minimize rivalry and sibling abuse, parents often regard sibling conflicts as a routine part of family relations, not as particularly violent. Many parents expect their children to engage in minor acts of violence as an inevitable part of growing up, and only intervene to discourage more serious conflicts. Parents may believe that rivalry and aggression prepare the child for the competitive world outside the home and enhance self-image and social competence (Stark & McEvoy, 1970; Bank & Kahn, 1982).

Corporal punishment is another overlooked factor in children's violence. Parents who strongly believe in the utility of corporal punishment often do not recognize their children's violence as such or tend to dismiss it as normal and routine. In homes characterized by spouse abuse and high levels of corporal punishment, young males may receive a double message that their bodies are not safe from stronger males' violence and that it is part of their identity to be aggressive toward more vulnerable family members.

## ◆ PHYSICALLY ABUSIVE CHILDREN

Despite the limited literature on abusive children, research has shown that they have a common background of family violence and/or neglect. Many have experienced coercive parenting, witnessed spouse abuse, suffered severe abuse or neglect, or seen other family members being abused or neglected.

At the core of child maltreatment is a breakdown in the parent-child interaction (Dietrich et al., 1983). Parents may promote childhood antisocial behavior through poor monitoring of the child's activities; little or no parental empathy with the child; and harsh and inconsistent discipline (Bahr, 1979; Patterson et al.,

1989). No variable alone can be traced to the development of abusive behavior, but each factor influences the course of the parent-child relationship (Belsky, 1980), which the child considers as normative in applying to interactions with other people.

Victimization is a leading pathway to human violence. The child's experiences may develop into a persistent and dynamic state of post-traumatic pain, which is central to the pursuit of aggressive behaviors. This is internalized "victimization." The rules of violence learned by the victim become crucial to the perpetuation of violence from one generation to the next (**Table 21-1**). At the time of the abuse, confusion, fear, anger, and sometimes arousal are too intense for the child to feel safely. Victimization becomes a part of the child's self-image. To survive the repeated episodes of abuse, the child gives up any expression of distress and learns how not to feel. The child learns to alter thoughts and feelings about the abuse (Rieker & Carmen, 1986) and to accept the judgment of care providers concerning the experience of abuse. "My mother told me that nothing was really happening," one incest victim said, "so I remembered that my older brother teased me but I forgot the terrible things he did to me." Other survivors minimize the abuse they experienced. "My father hit me a few times, but I deserved it," a physical abuse victim said, "and I'm grateful that I was never allowed to get away with being bad." The thought patterns of the child survivor remain stable and firmly embedded in the personality long after the abuse has ceased.

Brutalized by experiences with family members, the severely abused child incorporates these personal interactions into a deranged schema of the self and the world. An adult who learned as a child to blame herself for abusive treatment said, "Even after years of therapy, there's a part of me that still blames myself for what happened." This forgetfulness or blocking of the events, denial of one's true feelings, and acceptance of the intrusion of others' judgments is called "victimization."

With increasing repetition and severity of abuse the child's emotional numbness develops into habitual cognitive and behavioral patterns that some have described as "soul murder" (Shengold, 1979). Harmful care providers are then reinterpreted, delusionally, as good. The delusions protect the child and allow him or her to survive the abuse and the loss of self-image. The delusion can persist and lead to destructive behaviors directed at self and others later. The family system perpetuates and reinforces the child's negative self-image, leading to possibly higher levels of violence.

| Table 21-1. Social and Family Factors Involved with an Increased Likelihood of Child Abuse |
| --- |
| History of abusive experience |
| Corporal punishment in the home |
| Being a witness to family violence |
| Lower educational status |
| Poor quality primary attachment with the parent |
| Poor parental supervision |
| Single parenthood and unwanted pregnancy |
| Other sources of family disruption: <br>    Spouse abuse <br>    Drug/alcohol addiction <br>    Child neglect |

## ◆ DEFINITIONS

Like abuse by adults, which has been studied for more than a generation, there is no adequate definition of what constitutes abuse by children (Giovanni, 1989). Despite the lack of precision, child abuse has been addressed from various directions—medicine, law, education, social work, sociology, and research—which greatly contributes to its recognition and treatment (Newberger & Bourne, 1978).

## ◆ PREVALENCE AND EARLY STUDIES

The Biblical story of Cain slaying his brother Abel (Genesis, Chapter 4) has been cited as the earliest recorded instance of sibling abuse. Throughout the ages, many children have died as the result of adult brutality or neglect (Langer, 1973; DeMause, 1974; English, 1984; Radbill, 1987). However, little attention has yet been paid to sibling abuse. Many jurisdictions in the United States do not even recognize sibling abuse as grounds for an investigation.

Several national surveys illustrate the problem, showing that children have many opportunities to learn and practice aggressive behaviors within the privacy of the home. Straus and Gelles (Straus et al., 1980; Straus & Gelles, 1986) found that conflict between children is the most prevalent single form of family violence. While 80% of the children engaged in some form of violence against their siblings, more than 50% employed at least one act of "severe violence" during the year studied. Nearly 5% of the children had, at some time in their lives, used or threatened to use a knife or gun against a sibling. Additionally, 1% of the children were beaten by their parents and 1% of parents beat each other, but 16% of the children had beaten a sibling. Males were only slightly more violent than females. This retrospective study depended on parents' ability to recall information and thus is limited in its predictive power and description. The actual extent of violence may have been much greater if single-parent households had been included and the data gathered directly from the children themselves.

Developmentally, all but the most severe violence decreases as children age, but aggression by older children may be more purposeful and severe than that among younger children. Studies of primary school children found that conflicts occur most frequently when the only children in the home are male who are less than 4 years apart in age (Furman & Buhrmester, 1985). Despite the bias of retrospective studies, the high rate of sibling conflict leads to the conclusion that childhood aggression is learned within the family and may be a characteristic of *normal* children, not only those referred for behavior problems.

## ♦CHILD MALTREATMENT AND AGGRESSION

Various concepts in child development and psychology provide a background from which to review childhood aggression. Perspectives on human aggression range from biologically based psychoanalytic theory (Freud, 1920/1955), ethologic theory (Lorenz, 1966), drive theory (Berkowitz, 1962), and ego psychology (Horney, 1950), to social learning theory (Bandura, 1973, 1978), attachment theory (Bowlby, 1969/1982), and social network theory (Lewis, 1982). Fundamental to most formulations is the conviction that a person's early experiences are foundational and become internalized to influence later life experiences.

### ATTACHMENT

The attachment model of human development (Bowlby, 1969/1982) is particularly germane to this study, since failure to recognize behavioral cues and personal boundaries are commonly found in physically and sexually abusive persons. Humans depend strongly on social supports for continued growth and development, which begins with the initiation of an affective bond with a parent (Ainsworth et al., 1978). By the end of the first year of life the child uses the parent as a base from which to explore the environment and then return during need; later, the parent is the child's base for developing social skills (Sroufe & Waters, 1977). Children who receive consistent and positive nurturing from the parent internalize these dimensions and will act similarly in future caregiving roles. During periods of stress and frustration, secure children can then remember empathetic attachment figures to regulate and label their emotional states (Matas et al., 1978; Bretherton et al., 1986). Conversely, research suggests that insecurely attached children have an impaired sense of self and are vulnerable to recurrent failure in relationships (Olweus, 1980; Egeland & Sroufe, 1981). Such a child may become an insecure adult parent who believes that the physical protection of his or her children is impossible. To protect this insecurity, the parent may prefer to withdraw from perceived threats rather than face them.

## SOCIAL LEARNING

Learning by modeling the self on others is crucial in human development. The social learning concept posits a link between cognition and aggression (Bandura, 1978). The abuser's modeling, reinforcement, punishment, and threats mediate a great deal of what the child learns from maltreatment or neglect. Accordingly, children resort to violence after they have witnessed or experienced abuse or neglect and internalized its negative messages (Mischel, 1973; Parke & Slaby, 1983). A schema of retaliatory norms and strategies develops before they are able to reject what they have learned.

The basis for children's relationships is through attachment and interaction with the parent (Bowlby, 1969/1982) and later with persons they associate with who model and reinforce behaviors (Bandura, 1973). In a sense, sibling aggression reflects what children see parents doing or neglecting to do for them and what they see parents doing to each other. Children at a pre-operational level of cognition perceive aggression and punishment to be the same. Parents, who may seek to curtail misbehaviors by severe corporal punishment one time and by ignoring them at another time, only add to the child's confusion about when aggressive behavior may be proper. Parental inconsistency and intrusiveness have disorganizing effects on children. In an observational and prospective study, Jacobvitz and Sroufe (1987) found, for example, that inconsistent maternal styles made it difficult for children to internalize self-control. The aggressive child evokes punitive behavior from the parent who, in turn, elicits a negative and frustrated emotional state in the child, further contributing to his high level of assertiveness. The pathologic quality in the parent-child relationship must be discovered long before the child begins to abuse other children.

Neglectful parents can be unaware of what is happening between siblings. Children have felt murderous rage at younger siblings who displace them in the mother's affections. Unable to grasp the permanence of death, children have even killed younger siblings. Neglectful parents tend to disbelieve their child when he or she complains of being hurt or dismiss it as sibling rivalry, saying in effect, "You must have deserved it." Parental interventions, even in severe situations, are often ineffectual or nonexistent if their attention is diverted, for example, by an unwanted pregnancy, mental illness, substance abuse, or spouse abuse. Parents can be immature, be disinterested in raising children, or feel trapped in their current situation.

Modern family life presents a less protective environment for children than has been previously assumed. The changing composition of the American family, with increasing numbers of nonrelated children living in the same household, gives new meaning to sibling rivalry and child protection. The vulnerability of children is increased when the parents expect the child to take over some or all of the care of younger children in the home during the parent's absence. Tragic instances have occurred when children, acting as caregivers, are too immature to understand how to parent. The older children may refer to their own experiences of violence and engage in destructive behavior.

Children's attachments and modeling progress during school age into peer group relationships. These contribute to the child's learning about empathy and social cooperation (Lewis, 1982). Children in the third year of life typically begin to describe their negative feeling states through increasingly complex language. They are more and more able to discern another's inner psychological state concurrent with their maturing ability to read social cues (Eisenberg & Mussen, 1989). However, abusive children have an inadequate basis on which to develop empathy, since they have learned not to label and share their distress (Wheeler & Berliner,

1988). Instead, their distressing experiences have been kept out of conscious awareness. The victimization remains alive, however, possibly to erupt inexplicably in future situations of stress. Eventually, aggressive children's behaviors increase the likelihood of rejection by less aggressive peers, association with antisocial peers, and academic failure in school (Patterson et al., 1989).

Aggressiveness is a stable personality trait over time. Critical contributions to the development of empathy and interpersonal cooperation are not made in an environment of parental and peer rejection. Aggression becomes a more likely outcome. Rejected male children tend to try to lessen their painful feelings by identifying with the aggressor. As victims who have become victimizers, the children are even less able to express feeling for the victim's distress.

The commonsense belief that "violence breeds violence" has been used by professionals to explain the origins of child abuse. Child abuse and adult violence are said to form an intergenerational continuum. Child victims carry their inner- or outer-directed distress into relationships with other children and, as adults, into the lives of their own children. There is conceptual support for this in several studies. Steinmetz (1977) found striking parallels between the methods used by parents and those used by their children to resolve conflicts. Adults who resolve disputes by verbal or physical methods tend to use these methods in disciplining their children. Their children tend to use similar behaviors in relationships with siblings and peers. Straus et al. (1980) found that parents who were punished severely as children were more than twice as likely to be violent with their own children. Male gender, being poorly socialized, and coming from a physically punitive family are factors associated with a higher likelihood of child violent action after witnessing or experiencing victimization. Yet recent reviewers have found the violence breeds violence hypothesis to be limited in its predictive power. Possibly its conclusion has been overgeneralized from retrospective and uncontrolled data.

## ◆ EFFECTS OF PHYSICAL ABUSE

The age and developmental level of the child at the time of the abuse have an important bearing on its lasting effects. The child's response is determined by how the experience is perceived (Finkelhor & Browne, 1985). Equally important is how the abuse affects family functioning and the parent-child interaction. Violent intrusions challenge the child's most basic assumptions about personal safety and the world as a predictable place. Emotional exploitation, the background of all child maltreatment and neglect, attacks the child's basic sense of self as lovable and worthy of care. Abuse at an early level of cognitive development is more likely to be internalized to mean that the child is *bad* (Piaget, 1965; Kohlberg, 1981), a feeling that is carried into future relationships. From current clinical research, severe maltreatment leads to impaired emotional development, poor social competence, and deviations in cognitive development and character formation (Dietrich et al., 1983). Gelles and Straus (1988) report that children from violent homes are more than twice as likely to experience personal troubles. These include having few friends, receiving failing grades in school, and engaging in aggressive fights with family members and persons outside the home. As they grow older, aggressive male children tend to report that their negative behaviors are often directed toward restoring a low self-image (Perry et al., 1986). As adolescents, severely abused children may be institutionalized for psychiatric illnesses or have antisocial, delinquent, or self-destructive behaviors. As adults, abuse victims are at risk for abusing their own children, being abused by others, or having emotional disorders, criminal records, and substance abuse problems.

The early case literature on abusive children reported only the most violent examples. A prior history of victimization and family disorganization were common denominators in most of the reports. The children were negativistic, lacked impulse control (Elmer, 1967), were angry (Fontana, 1973), and exhibited overly hostile behavior (Morse et al., 1970). Some committed homicide (Bender, 1940; Adelson, 1972; Tooley, 1977). In their study, Easson and Steinhilber (1961) found confirmed or suggestive past histories of parental maltreatment in five of eight boys who had committed murder. Some were encouraged by their care provider to be violent (Easson & Steinhilber, 1961; Sargent, 1972; Tooley, 1975; Rosenthal & Doherty, 1984) or were identified as *dangerous* by the parent because they took the place of a hated ex-spouse or boyfriend (Rosenthal & Doherty, 1984). Other studies speculated that poor primary bonding and negative role modeling were factors in children's murderous assaults (Bender, 1953). Adelson's study (1972) of five children, all of whom were under 8 years of age at the time they committed homicide, postulated that many felt jealousy and rage at the infant sibling's presence in the home.

Later studies on maltreatment outcomes support the social learning and attachment perspectives on aggression. As violent behavior becomes accepted as "normal" by the victimized child, it is more available to him to employ against siblings and peers. When he gains greater physical strength, such violence is more readily available in confrontations with parents and other adults. The level of violence between children seems directly related to the amount of violence between their care providers. Straus et al. (1980), for example, found that severe sibling violence occurred in 100% of the 2,143 homes where parents frequently attacked each other and their children, compared to 20% of nonviolent homes.

Controlled empirical studies have increased our understanding of victimization's effects. Thus abused infants, 14 months old, were more likely to turn away from their parent's attentions than controls (Wasserman et al., 1983). Abused toddlers, 1 to 3 years of age, avoided peers four times more often than controls. They hit peers, verbally or physically assaulted care providers, and were less likely to approach care providers in response to friendly gestures (George & Main, 1979) than nonabused children. Abused children, 4 years old, were more likely than controls to engage in aggressive behaviors with peers (Hoffman-Plotkin & Twentyman, 1984). Abused children, 6 to 7 years old, were more aggressive than controls in fantasy, free play, and the school environment (Reidy, 1977). Abused children, 5 to 12 years old, were more likely to depict themselves as sad, unpopular, poorly behaved, and outwardly aggressive toward others than nonabused controls (Kinard, 1980).

Available data concerning the effects on children who witness violent spouse abuse also suggest a similar development (Hershorn & Rosenbaum, 1985; Wolfe et al., 1985; Jaffe et al., 1990). This work consistently shows the lasting negative effects of domestic violence as evidenced by the emergence of increased aggression in children who witness such instances.

## SELF-DESTRUCTIVENESS

Studies show that child abuse also leads to withdrawal and self-destructive behaviors. Martin and Beezley (1977) noted the development of these behaviors in 12 of the 50 abused children they studied. Carmen et al. (1984) and Mills et al. (1984) studied children who were both sexually and physically abused and noted that they were more likely to be physically harmful to themselves compared to subjects who were only physically abused. Hendin (1969) found a history of physical abuse in many case histories of suicidal black adults.

## THE CENTRALITY OF VIOLENCE

Prospective controlled studies have established the central place of violence and neglect in the maldevelopment of the child. Earlier studies were unable to predict which children who had been maltreated subsequently became abusive or violent. Prospective studies surpassed the earlier ones and developed baseline data on violent behavior in various demographic groups. Widom (1989a), in well-designed research on a group of 319 abused children, matched and controlled for age, sex, and race, found that maltreatment increased the risk of delinquency and subsequent violent criminal behavior by as much as 42% over controls.

Dodge et al. (1990), in a study of 309 children age 4 to kindergarten, concluded that early abuse increased the risk of developing deviantly aggressive behavior by nearly threefold. This increase was unexplained by the relative contributions made by poverty, divorce, marital violence, and the child's health and temperament. Abused children comprised 15% of the sample and were identified through interviews with mothers, visible bruises, and a medical history. Behaviors were assessed by teacher evaluations, peer ratings, and direct observation. Dodge's study has benefitted others by establishing a baseline rate for abuse in children who do not come to official attention.

Aggression develops at a cognitive-emotional as well as a behavioral level. Research has been interested in not only specific behaviors, but also in psychological processes that underlie, proceed, and follow aggression. Dodge and Somberg (1987), for example, found that young aggressive children, compared to their peers, have biased and deficient patterns of processing social cues. They overattribute hostile intent to their playmates, even when it is unwarranted, and they become less accurate in their attributions when they are under stress. They display far more aggression than they receive. Their bias leads peers to expect greater hostility from them. Given the series of inevitable negative interactions, their perceptions perpetuate a cycle of hostile attributions, aggressive behavior, school failure, and peer rejection.

Nevertheless, cognitive biases only partially explain the origin of aggressive behavior. It has been suggested that abused and aggressive children's deficits are conceptually similar to the inhibition deficit found in impulsive children (Dodge & Frame, 1982), who fail to inhibit inappropriate behaviors that are more readily available (Camp, 1977; Dodge & Neuman, 1981). Abused and aggressive children can not only be cognitively delayed, but also develop along a deranged path resulting from early relationships and socialization.

## ◆ SEXUALLY ABUSIVE CHILDREN

Sexually abusive prepubertal children have been greatly understudied and are poorly recognized in the constellation of family violence. Yet the increasing numbers of reports of severe outcomes of sexual assault have forced clinicians to reconsider the nature of sexual activity between children (e.g., Johnson, 1988, 1989). The position taken here is that children's abusive behaviors arise from severe prior sexual or physical victimization. Sexual abuse by children is the sexual expression of aggression, not the aggressive expression of sexuality. When these problem behaviors are present, they are among the few specific indicators that sexual abuse has occurred (Friedrich et al., 1987; Corwin, 1988; Friedrich & Luecke, 1988). Younger children who manifest extreme sexual aggression were likely to have been victimized in a preexisting abusive family context.

There are several reasons why sexual abuse by children has remained unnoticed. In western culture, sexuality is not usually ascribed to children. There is little empirical knowledge of what is typical sexual behavior between children despite clinical impressions by many that it is common. Society has assumed that sexually abusive behaviors are perpetrated by adults so that what occurs between children is often dismissed as "just a phase." When adolescent perpetrators were identified in high numbers in the 1980s (Scherzer & Lala, 1980; Ryan et al., 1987), clinicians came to realize that children may also be sexual abusers. Sexually abused children have similar adverse outcomes despite the age level of the perpetrator. Also, "sex play" has been misused as a cover for behaviors as diverse as "you show me yours and I'll show you mine" to forced oral, genital, or rectal penetration. Next, it has been assumed that sexual activity between children in the home is less serious than with contacts outside the home. Increasing numbers of sexual abuse cases have been reported in which biologically and nonbiologically related children living in the same home have been the identified perpetrators. The former distinction between inside and outside the home cannot be made a discriminator for abuse.

## ♦ EXPERIMENTATION OR ABUSE?

The clinician is often called upon to distinguish between consensual sexual play of nonabused children and reenactment behavior of sexually abused children. Children's typical sexual behaviors are age, activity, and culturally dependent. Sexual behaviors may appear shortly after birth. Genital self-stimulation occurs in the first year of life as infants develop motor coordination and awareness of the penis or clitoris (Litt & Martin, 1981). By 3 years of age, most children have identified themselves as either boys or girls. Between 3 and 6 years of age, children become increasingly aware of anatomical genital differences, and genital play is common during this time (Rutter, 1971). Usually the play involves age-mates in some degree of undressing and touching in games, such as "doctor" or "house." This has sometimes been misinterpreted as a sign of earlier sexual abuse. The current understanding, however, is that typical childhood behavior is mutual and noncoercive in nature and in keeping with the child's developmental level (**Table 21-2**). Simulated intercourse will sometimes occur after viewing overt sexuality in motion pictures or in the home. More invasive acts, such as penetration of the genitalia or rectum, with or without coercion, are not typical and require investigation. During latency, sexual exploration continues to increase, although more covertly, within the peer group. With the onset of puberty, peer and family-related exploration diminishes and interest in sexual roles and sexual identity is added to curiosity and pleasure in motivating sexual contacts. In doubtful cases, an interview with the child may be most helpful in distinguishing the motivation.

| Table 21-2. Consequences of Sexual Abuse |
| --- |
| Age-inappropriate sexual behavior |
| Adult sexual adjustment problems |
| Being at increased risk for sexual victimization |
| Sexually victimizing others |
| Physical aggressiveness |
| Acting out |
| Conduct disorders |
| Self-destructive behaviors |
| Marked anxiety, fear, withdrawal, depression |
| Guilt, low self-esteem |
| Overly compliant, anxious to please |
| Dissociative disorders, split personality |

## ♦ PREVALENCE

While the data on the prevalence of child sexual abuse by adults are sparse and unreliable, there are no data on the extent of child sexual offenders. Rates of child sexual victimization vary greatly in surveys. Finkelhor (1979) found that 9% of the men and 19% of the women, in a survey of 796 college students, had experienced either contact or noncontact sexual abuse during childhood. Fritz et al. (1981) found that 5% of the males and 8% of the females, in a sample of 952 students, had been sexually abused. Russell (1983, 1984) reported that 28% of 903 women had experienced some form of unwanted sexual contact before 14 years of age. Wyatt (1985) reported that 45% of the 248 women surveyed had experienced some form of sexually abusive contact. Kinsey et al. (1953), in the earliest U.S. estimate, found that 9% of 4,441 nonrandomly selected women had sexual contacts with an adult before the age of 14. Variations in the samples make the results difficult to compare, but the figures establish that sexual abuse occurs in the lives of many children.

Abusive sexual activity among siblings, cousins, and nonrelated children who are age-mates is considered to be common but is infrequently documented. In a sample of 831 abused children referred to a university hospital, De Jong (1989) found that 10% of the sexual abuse was by siblings or cousins, in which a majority described attempted vaginal or rectal penetration. Finkelhor's (1979, 1980b) student survey found that sibling incest occurred among 15% of the abused females and 10% of the abused males. Russell (1983) found that 2.5% of the women had been victimized by a sibling and that 15% of all incest was by siblings. Wyatt (1985) found that 3% of 248 randomly selected women reported sibling incest, or 12% of all incest. Cousin incest, which is at least as common as sibling incest, accounted for 15% (De Jong, 1989) to 28% (Finkelhor, 1979, 1984) of incest in various surveys. While most perpetrators in these surveys were adolescents, we have no idea of the frequency of incestuous sexual abuse by children under 12 years of age.

## ◆ THE IMPACT OF SEXUAL ABUSE

To understand children with sexual behavior problems, we must first try to conceptualize the negative impact of sexual abuse itself. Sexual victimization can be understood as a combination of post-traumatic stress responses and socially learned cognitive and behavioral adaptations.

### TRAUMATIZING FAMILY PRECURSORS

Sexual abuse often results from complex, pathological family interactions. Children become involved in sexual activity for a variety of reasons. Many children acquiesce to the abuser's sexual advances because the love, care, and approval they need are otherwise lacking in their lives. Their care providers may be physically or emotionally absent, neglectful, distracted by other needs and/or substance abuse, or sexually punitive; they offer little protection to the child and may have a history of being victimized themselves.

### TRAUMATIZING ABUSE

The impact of abuse varies with the child's perceptions of it as stigmatizing, sexualizing, and whether it is marked by powerlessness and betrayal (Finkelhor & Browne, 1985). Traumatic powerlessness occurs when the child perceives that his or her personal boundaries have been invaded and damaged. This can lead to severe post-traumatic pain and to later significant impairment of the ability to modulate aggressive behavior. Feeling in control of oneself is a foundational element of social development that is missing from the abused child's self-image. Male victims of abuse are more likely to turn outward in anger with antisocial and aggressive behaviors. They may define themselves as the abuser. "I wanted it," one male child victim said, "and I seduced him, not the other way around." Stigmatization is experienced when the child feels internally disfigured and shamed by the abuse. Betrayal is experienced when an emotionally significant person, on whom the child depended for his or her identity, care, and safety, is perceived to have caused harm. Traumatic sexualization occurs when the child's emotional growth is thwarted by the introduction of developmentally inappropriate behaviors. These factors result in an acceleration of sexual knowledge but at the cost of distorting the child's sense of intimate friendship. The victim can feel that the abuser owns his or her body. Male victims may become confused over sexual identity or attempt to master their pain by repeating the victimization on younger children (Finkelhor, 1981). Finkelhor's *traumagenesis model* explains the multiplicity of symptoms found in sexual abuse. It points out that more severe symptoms occur in situations (1) where the perpetrator is closely related or emotionally significant to the child, (2) where the abuse is repetitive or of long duration, (3) when physical force is used, (4) when the victim is older and can understand what happened, and (5) when the experience involves oral, genital, or rectal penetration.

## Traumatizing Family Responses

The coping abilities of the child and the family have a great influence on recovery. Greater damage occurs to the child who lives in a family environment that is itself abusive. Such families are characterized by exploitation, coerciveness, invasiveness of physical and emotional boundaries, and betrayal of trust. Care providers can engage in coercive sexual or physical behavior toward each other, the child, or others, and they often lack empathy and functional interpersonal skills. Maintaining family secrecy is central to this family's value system (Rush, 1980). It is not surprising, therefore, that if the child discloses abuse, his or her revelations are likely to be delayed, unconvincing, and often followed by their retraction and denial (Summit, 1983).

## ◆The Effects of Sexual Abuse

Children who sexually abuse other children are likely to have suffered prior sexual or physical victimization. Empirical studies find sexual abuse to be associated with a wide range of psychological and behavioral effects (**Table 21-3**). Some abused children are described as "wild" and "out of control," with their distress channeled outward into aggressiveness and inappropriate sexual activity. As with physical abuse, child sexual abuse victims are at risk for compulsive repetition of the abuse and loss of conscious memory of the trauma (Terr, 1988). Symptoms may also be directed inwardly and include somatic complaints, sleep problems, academic failure, running away, substance abuse, self-hatred, disturbed relationships with others, and inability to trust others and protect oneself. With severe victimization, self-destructive behaviors can occur (Wyatt & Powell, 1988). In studying the traumatic precursors of borderline personality, van der Kolk et al. (1988) found significant associations between child sexual abuse and later development of self-harm, particularly starving and cutting oneself.

---

**Table 21-3. Criteria for Defining Sexual Abuse Between Children**

*Sexual contact between children may be considered inappropriate or abusive in the presence of any of these conditions:*

1. Sexual activity between children who are not of a similar age (not within 5 years) or developmental level.

2. Sexual activity that is not consistent with the developmental level of the child.

3. Sexual activity in which force or threats are used.

4. Sexual activity between children in which there is outside coercive influence from another, older individual.

5. Sexual activity that results in documented injury or predominantly negative feelings in the victim.

---

## Sexual Behavior Problems

Researchers have attempted to distinguish sexually abused from nonsexually abused children based on problematic sexualized behaviors (Mannarino & Cohen, 1986; Mian et al., 1986; Friedrich et al., 1987; Corwin, 1988; Friedrich & Luecke, 1988; Gale et al., 1988; Kolko et al., 1988). It is not clear whether these behaviors represent reenactment of the victimization or premature and distorted activation of sexual capacities. Still, there are no reliably predictive profiles of who will become a sexual abuser. Not all sexually abused children will develop problem behaviors. However, it should be assumed that the abusive experience is so potentially toxic to developing sexuality that therapeutic measures should be taken accordingly.

## SEXUALLY REACTIVE CHILDREN

Children with sexual behavior problems have been tentatively described as either sexually reactive or sexually aggressive (Friedrich, 1990). The sexually reactive child exhibits physically or sexually inappropriate behaviors reflecting the acute issues of recent abuse. The symptoms may result from confusion about self-boundaries. He may be a toddler, for example, who engages in increased masturbation, sexual exploration, exposure of genitals, sexualized play, or inviting others to become inappropriately sexually involved. These behaviors may have elements of aggressiveness but they are noncoercive in nature. Generally, they reflect a sexualization of activities only and do not imply an underlying psychopathology. The frequency of these behaviors is not known because care providers may minimize them as transitory or "sex play."

## SEXUALLY ABUSIVE CHILDREN

Other children are referred to therapy because of behaviors that far exceed those typical of sex play. These behaviors involve overt and often coercive sexual activity. The child's aggressiveness has been firmly entrenched for some time. It has been maintained by ongoing abuse, by caregivers who treat the child like a scapegoat, and by a neglectful family environment. Children whose sexual behavior is driven by anger, depression, and anxiety are often male, and their history of sexual abuse is severe and prolonged. Typically, they have been victimized repeatedly, often by multiple perpetrators. Often they also have a preexisting physical abuse history. Less severe behavior problems, rejection by peers, and failure in school may occur before the sexually coercive behaviors toward other children become obvious.

The psychotherapeutic literature detailing the condition of these children is very sparse. Data come from case reports and small groups of children who are referred for treatment after their problem behaviors were discovered. Fehrenbach et al. (1986) report that 22% of the sample of youthful sex offenders were between 11 and 13 years old. Poor academic achievement, behavior problems, social isolation, and a background of sexual or physical abuse were common. In two studies, Johnson described 47 boys (1988) and 13 girls (1989), 4 to 13 years old, who overtly and coercively molested other children. Nearly half of the molested children were siblings. The behaviors included fondling and oral copulation with anal and/or vaginal penetration. Nearly 50% of the boys were victims of prior sexual abuse and 19% had been physically abused. All of the girls had been previously sexually abused, and 31% had been physically abused. A family history of substance abuse was also found in many cases.

The proportion of male to female sexually abusive children parallels that of adult sex abusers. Most of the reported offenders are boys. Girls, however, seem to suffer more abuse or neglect before becoming sexually abusive themselves. However, girls are less likely to follow the path toward abusing other children.

Friedrich and Luecke (1988) studied 16 sexually aggressive children (12 were males), 4 to 11 years old, and compared them to a group of sexually abused children who did not have problem behaviors. All the problem behavior children had prior sexual abuse of greater severity and duration than was found in earlier surveys (e.g., Finkelhor, 1979, 1984; Gomes-Schwartz et al., 1986). Most of the problem children were sexually preoccupied, and their behaviors paralleled their abuse experiences. All experienced oral, anal, or vaginal penetration, and many were also exposed to physical violence. In the study by Fehrenbach et al. (1986), in contrast, only 23% of the sexually offending children were involved in the sexual coercion of other children, but a majority were so involved in Friedrich's sample.

A high degree of personal and parental psychopathology, predating their abuse of other children, was found in Friedrich's group. All the children had a concurrent DSM-III (APA, 1980) diagnosis of a conduct or oppositional disorder, indicating extreme aggression. Their nonabusive parents had a high rate of depression and substance abuse and often covertly reinforced the children's aggressive behavior by labeling them as *bad*, categorizing them as being the same as offending adults. Family issues centered on inconsistent and neglectful parenting and lack of empathy.

## ◆ ABUSED-TO-ABUSER CYCLE

Research is leading clinicians to speculate on the possibility that there exists a cycle of violence for victims of physical and sexual abuse. Although limited in scope and predictive power, available studies suggest that sexual abuse in childhood appears to increase the risk for later sexual aggression, probably for the more severely traumatized children (Longo, 1982; Gaffney et al., 1984; Becker, 1988). The greater the trauma of the abuse, the more likely the experience will be deflected from awareness, perhaps to reappear as abusive activity in the future. Studies of sex offenders have revealed that many began their activities in mid-childhood after being sexually molested. Sexual abuse as a child and the later development of juvenile delinquency and/or adult criminality have been associated in several studies. Lewis et al. (1988), in a study of 14 juveniles condemned to death for murder in 1987, showed that 12 young people had been brutally physically abused and five had been severely sexually abused by relatives. Burgess et al. (1987), in a prospective study of 34 sexually abused boys, found an association between drug abuse, delinquency, and criminality 6 to 8 years later. Boys who were physically and sexually abused, unsupported in disclosing the abuse, and socially rejected were more likely to become delinquent or criminal than boys from supportive families.

Information has also come from adolescent sex offenders. In a review of the literature, Peters et al. (1986) discovered prior child sexual abuse in 3% to 30% of male and in 8% to 38% of female offenders interviewed. Adolescent sex offender treatment programs have reported prior sexual abuse in 19% to 47% of their clients (Longo, 1982; Becker, 1988). Many adult sex offenders may have been sexually abused in adolescence even before puberty.

Although the limited research cannot reliably predict who will become abusive, there is ample evidence of the damaging influence of abuse. While little direct evidence exists for an intergenerational transmission of sexual abuse, the complex traumatic components of child maltreatment are clearly associated with the behavioral symptoms, especially the physical and sexual aggressiveness of abused children (Finkelhor & Browne, 1985; Dodge et al., 1990).

## ◆ FACTORS IN ALTERING THE CYCLE OF ABUSE

Maltreated or neglected children are not necessarily predestined to develop into sexually or physically offending adults. In 1987 Kaufman and Zigler reviewed the extant literature and estimated that the actual transmission rate of physical abuse was 30% to 50%. Subsequent reviews (Widom, 1988, 1989a,b) have generally supported this conclusion. Although 30% is six times the rate of abuse in the general population (Parke & Collmer, 1975; Gelles & Straus, 1988a,b), the implication is that most abused children escape at least the severe outcomes of the cycle and do not come to official attention.

Clinical research is not so naive as to attempt to prove direct causality in the cycle of violence. The child copes not only with the effects of victimization or witnessing family violence, but violence also results from the multiple family changes it sets in motion. These effects include (1) reduced maternal parenting effectiveness, (2) increased family dysfunction, and (3) increased (male) child aggressiveness as a result of modeling an abusive parent's behavior. As the child's efforts to cope with the violence place greater strain on the parents' relationship, a vicious cycle is set in motion. Similarly, mental health professionals' efforts at therapeutic interventions to correct a child's deviant aggressive behavior have often been undermined by continuing spouse abuse.

The relation between trauma and an aggressive outcome is not linear, for clinical experience has shown that variables serve to modify and buffer its impact. These variables have been found within individuals, the family, and the social environment. They include good cognitive abilities, absence of major psychopathology, and available nonabusing adults and peers.

A negative self-image, derived from early abusive relationships, is carried forward as the persistence of abusive behaviors in the abuse cycle unless it is interrupted. Children who are given a chance to make sense of their abuse with a nonabusing adult are less likely to repeat the patterns of victimization in their later lives. The same is true in abuse prevention for adults who have a high risk of abusing their children (Kempe, 1976; Olds et al., 1986; Olds & Kitzman, 1990). Egeland et al. (1988), in a controlled sample of 44 mothers who had been abused as children, found that those who did not maltreat or neglect their children had either a supportive adult available during childhood or extensive psychological counseling at some time in their lives. Parents who became abusive had neither. Therefore the availability of alternate relationships is important in interrupting the cycle of abuse.

## ◆ TREATMENT PERSPECTIVES

The family's response to the physically or sexually aggressive child is critical for the success of treatment. Parent training in how to respond to the child's sexual behaviors and a peer support group may be all that is needed for the child who is reactive to abuse. Parents who deal in a consistent and caring manner with the recently molested child, who is acting with increased masturbation, for example, will go far in eliminating the behavior by helping him to understand the proper boundaries regarding touching. On the other hand, parents who view the child as a scapegoat or as *damaged goods* add to his or her trauma.

Sexually or physically abusive children present far greater challenges. Their behaviors are more firmly established than those who have been abused but do not act aggressively. Typically, their families possess few, if any, mitigating resources. While therapy may start with small and easily achievable goals, there are larger patterns of failure requiring attention, including parent training, social competence and peer relations, and academic performance. Both parents and child need intense behavioral, cognitive, and affective therapy (Azar & Siegel, 1990). Therapy must be based on such factors as the child's developmental age at the onset of the abuse, the age at which the child's aggressions began, the duration of the behaviors, and prior efforts at intervention. It is also necessary to evaluate all siblings for collateral abuse and their need for treatment.

Foster home placement, while sometimes necessary, is insufficient to treat the emotional damage of abusive children. In Reidy's study (1977), abused children in foster placement displayed as much physical aggression as abused children in their natural homes. Foster care was inadequate to reduce their level of aggression and problems at school.

Family system failure must also be addressed. The families of sexually aggressive children often have a long history of coercive interactions and inconsistent parenting. Their response to the child's aggressive behaviors has often been inappropriate or even encouraging. Greater assistance from local protective service agencies is needed to involve the parents in the treatment of their abusive children. Many are wary of or indifferent to professional involvement. Without an official agency's firm support, the parents often do not follow through and bring the child to treatment. Therapy will take a long period of time. Parents do not realize the length of the commitment nor do they have the energy or interest to invest in it.

Therapeutic intervention involves alternate adult and peer models of social interaction for the children and their parents. Integrating abused children into programs with normal peers and parents into support groups helps with more appropriate behavior models. Research is greatly needed in this area.

## ♦ BIBLIOGRAPHY

Abel, GG, Mittelman, MS, and Becker, JV: Sexual offenders: Results of assessment and recommendations for treatment. In MH Ben-Aron, SJ Hucker, and CD Webster, eds: *Clinical Criminology: Current Concepts*, M&M Graphics, Toronto, 1985, pp. 191-205.

Abramaovitch, R, Corter, C, and Landro, B: Sibling interaction in the home, *Child Dev* 50:997-1003, 1979.

Abramovitch, R, Corter, C, and Pepler, D: Observations of mixed-sex sibling dyads, *Child Dev* 51:1268-1271, 1980.

Abramovitch, R, Corter, C, Pepler, JF, and Stanhope, L: Sibling and peer interaction: A final follow-up and a comparison, *Child Dev* 57:217-229, 1986.

Adelson, L: The battering child, *JAMA* 222:159-161, 1972.

Ainsworth, MDS, Blehar, M, Waters, E, and Wall, S: *Patterns of Attachment: Observations in the Strange Situation at Home*, Erlbaum, Hillsdale, NY, 1978.

Azar, ST, and Siegel, BR: Behavioral treatment of child abuse: A developmental perspective, *Behav Mod* 14:279-300, 1990.

Bahr, SJ: Family determinants and effects of deviance. In WR Burr, R Hill, FI Nye, and IL Reiss, eds: *Contemporary Theories About the Family, Volume 1*, Free Press, New York, 1979, pp. 615-643.

Bandura, A: *Aggression: A Social Learning Analysis*, Prentice Hall, Englewood Cliffs, NJ, 1973.

Bandura, A: Social learning theory of aggression, *J Commun* 28:12-29, 1978.

Bank, SP, and Kahn, MD: *The Sibling Bond*, Basic Books, New York, 1982.

Bays, J: Substance abuse and child abuse: Impact of addiction on the child, *Pediatr Clin North Am* 37:881-904, 1990.

Becker, JV: The effects of child sexual abuse on adolescent sexual offenders. In GE Wyatt and GJ Powell, eds: *The Lasting Effects of Child Sexual Abuse*, Sage Publications, Newbury Park, CA, 1988, pp. 193-207.

Belsky, J: Child maltreatment: An ecological integration, *Am Psychol* 35:320-355, 1980.

Bender, L: Children and adolescents who kill, *J Crim Psychopathol* 1:297-322, 1940.

Bender, L: Children with homicidal aggression. In L Bender, ed: *Aggression, Hostility, and Anxiety in Children*, Charles C Thomas, Springfield, IL, 1953, pp. 91-115.

Bender, L: Children and adolescents who have killed, *Am J Psychiatry* 116:510-513, 1959.

Berkowitz, L: *Aggression: A Social Psychological Analysis*, McGraw-Hill, New York, 1962.

Black, R, and Mayer, J: Parents with special problems: Alcoholism and opiate addiction, *Child Abuse Negl* 4:45-54, 1980.

Blumberg, ML: Psychopathology of the abusing parent, *Am J Psychother* 28:21-29, 1974.

Bowlby, J: *Attachment and Loss: Volume 1. Attachment*, Basic Books, New York, 1969/1982.

Bowlby, J: *Attachment and Loss: Volume 3. Loss, Sadness, and Depression*, Basic Books, New York, 1980.

Bretherton, I, Fritz, J, Zahn-Waxler, C, and Ridgeway, D: Learning to talk about emotions: A functionalist perspective, *Child Dev* 57:530-548, 1986.

Burgess, AW, ed: *Child Pornography and Sex Rings*, Lexington Books, Lexington, MA, 1984.

Burgess, AW, Hartman, CR, and McCormack, A: Abused to abuser: Antecedents of socially deviant behavior, *Am J Psychiatry* 144:1431-1436, 1987.

Caffey, J: Multiple fractures in the long bones of infants suffering from chronic subdural hematoma, *AJR* 56:163-173, 1946.

Camp, B: Verbal mediation in young aggressive boys, *J Abnorm Psychol* 86:145-153, 1977.

Carmen, E, Reiker, PP, and Mills, T: Victims of violence and psychiatric illness, *Am J Psychiatry* 141:378-383, 1984.

Chasnoff, IJ, Burns, WJ, Schnoll, SH, Burns, SH, et al: Maternal-neonatal incest, *Am J Orthopsychiatry* 56:577-580, 1986.

Conte, JR, and Schuerman, JR: The effects of sexual abuse on children: A multidimensional view. In GE Wyatt and GJ Powell, eds: *Lasting Effects of Child Sexual Abuse*, Sage Publications, Newbury Park, CA, 1988, pp. 157-170.

Coons, PM, Bowman, ES, Pellow, TA, and Schneider, P: Post-traumatic aspects of the treatment of victims of sexual abuse and incest, *Psychiatr Clin North Am* 12:325-335, 1990.

Corwin, D: Early diagnosis of child sexual abuse: Diminishing the lasting effects. In GE Wyatt and GJ Powell, eds: *Lasting Effects of Child Sexual Abuse*, Sage Publications, Newbury Park, CA, 1988, pp. 251-269.

Curtis, GC: Violence breeds violence-perhaps? *Am J Psychiatry* 120:386-387, 1963.

Cummings, EM, Iannotti, RJ, and Zahn-Waxler, C: Aggression between peers in early childhood: Individual continuity and developmental change, *Child Dev* 60:887-895, 1989.

De Jong, AR: Sexual interactions among siblings and cousins: Experimentation or exploitation? *Child Abuse Negl* 13:271-279, 1989.

DeMause, L: *The History of Childhood*, Harper & Row, Publishers, New York, 1974.

Dietrich, KN, Starr, RH, and Wiesfeld, GE: Infant maltreatment: Caretaker-infant interaction and developmental consequences at differing levels of parenting failure, *Pediatrics* 72:532-540, 1983.

Dodge, KA, Bates, JE, and Pettit, GS: Mechanisms in the cycle of violence, *Science* 250:1678-1683, 1990.

Dodge, KA, and Frame, CL: Social cognitive biases and deficits in aggressive boys, *Child Dev* 53:620-635, 1982.

Dodge, KA, and Neuman, JP: Biased decision making processes in aggressive boys, *J Abnorm Psychol* 90:375-379, 1981.

Dodge, KA, and Somberg, DR: Hostile attributional biases among aggressive boys are exacerbated under conditions of threats to the self, *Child Dev* 58:213-224, 1987.

Dubowitz, H: Prevention of child maltreatment: What is known, *Pediatrics* 83:570-577, 1989.

Easson, WM, and Steinhilber, RM: Murderous aggression by children and adolescents, *Arch Gen Psychiatry* 4:27-35, 1961.

Egeland, B, Jacobvitz, D, and Sroufe, LA: Breaking the cycle of abuse, *Child Dev* 59:1080-1088, 1988.

Egeland, B, and Sroufe, LA: Attachment and early maltreatment, *Child Dev* 52:44-52, 1981.

Eisenberg, N, and Mussen, P: *The Roots of Prosocial Behavior in Children*, Cambridge University Press, Cambridge, 1989.

Elmer, E: *Children in Jeopardy*, University of Pittsburgh Press, Pittsburgh, PA, 1967.

English, PC: Pediatrics and the unwanted child in history: Foundling homes, disease, and the origins of foster care in New York City, 1860-1920, *Pediatrics* 73:699-711, 1984.

Famularo, R, Kinscherff, R, Fenton, T, and Bolduc, SM: Child maltreatment among runaway and delinquent children, *Clin Pediatr* 29:713-718, 1990.

Famularo, R, Stone, K, Barnum, R, and Wharton, R: Alcoholism and severe child maltreatment, *Am J Orthopsychiatry* 56:481-485, 1986.

Fehrenbach, PA, Smith, W, Monastersky, C, and Deisher, RW: Adolescent sexual offenders, *Am J Orthopsychiatry* 56:225-233, 1986.

Finkelhor, D: Psychological, cultural and family factors in incest and sexual abuse, *J Marriage Fam Counseling* 4:41-49, 1978.

Finkelhor, D: *Sexually Victimized Children*, Free Press, New York, 1979.

Finkelhor, D: Risk factors in the sexual victimization of children, *Child Abuse Negl* 4:265-273, 1980a.

Finkelhor, D: Sex among siblings: A survey of prevalence, variety, and effects, *Arch Sex Behav* 9:171-194, 1980b.

Finkelhor, D: The sexual abuse of boys, *Victimization* 6:76-84, 1981.

Finkelhor, D: *Child Sexual Abuse: New Theory and Research*, Free Press, New York, 1984.

Finkelhor, D: The trauma of child sexual abuse: Two models. In GE Wyatt and GJ Powell, eds: *The Lasting Effects of Child Sexual Abuse*, Sage Publications, Newbury Park, CA, 1988, pp. 61-82.

Finkelhor, D, and Browne, A: The traumatic impact of child sexual abuse: A conceptualization, *Am J Orthopsychiatry* 55:530-541, 1985.

Finkelhor, D, Williams, L, and Burns, N: *Nursery Crimes: Sexual Abuse in Day Care*, Sage Publications, Newbury Park, CA, 1988.

Fisher, M: Adolescent adjustment after incest, *Sch Psychol Int* 4:217-222, 1983.

Fontana, V: *Somewhere a Child is Crying*, Macmillan, New York, 1973.

Freud, S: *Beyond the Pleasure Principle*, Volume 18 (Strachey, J, ed and translator), Hogarth, London, 1920/1955.

Friedrich, WN: Behavior problems in sexually abused children: An adaptational perspective. In GE Wyatt and GJ Powell, eds: *The Lasting Effects of Child Sexual Abuse*, Sage Publications, Newbury Park, CA, 1988, pp. 171-191.

Friedrich, WN: *Psychotherapy of Sexually Abused Children and Their Families*, WW Norton, New York, 1990.

Friedrich, WN, Beilke, RL, and Urquiza, AJ: Sexually abusive families: A behavioral comparison, *J Interpersonal Violence* 2:391-402, 1987.

Friedrich, WN, Beilke, RL, and Urquiza, AJ: Behavior problems in young sexually abused boys, *J Interpersonal Violence* 3:21-28, 1988.

Friedrich, WN, and Luecke, WJ: Young school-age sexually aggressive children, *Prof Psychol Res Pract* 19:155-164, 1988.

Friedrich, WN, Urquiza, A, and Beilke, R: Behavior problems in sexually abused young children, *J Pediatr Psychol* 11:47-57, 1986.

Fritz, G, Stoll, K, and Wagner, A: A comparison of males and females who were sexually molested as children, *J Sex Marital Ther* 7:54-59, 1981.

Furman, W, and Buhrmester, D: Children's perceptions of the qualities of sibling relationships, *Child Dev* 56:448-461, 1985.

Gabarino, J: What kind of society permits child abuse? *Infant Ment Health J* 1:270-280, 1980.

Gabarino, J: An ecological approach to child maltreatment. In LH Pelton, ed: *The Social Context of Child Abuse and Neglect*, Human Sciences Press, New York, 1981, pp. 228-267.

Gaffney, GR, Laurie, SF, and Berlin, FS: Is there familial transmission of pedophilia? *J Nerv Ment Dis* 172:546-548, 1984.

Gale, J, Thompson, RJ, Moran, T, and Sack, WH: Sexual abuse in young children: Its clinical presentation and characteristic patterns, *Child Abuse Negl* 12:163-170, 1988.

Gelinas, D: The persisting negative effects of incest, *Psychiatry* 46:312-332, 1983.

Gelles, RJ: Violence in the family: A review of research in the seventies, *J Marriage Fam* 42:873-885, 1980.

Gelles, RJ, and Straus, MA: How violent are American families? In GT Hotaling, D Finkelhor, JT Kirkpatrick, and MA Straus, eds: *Family Abuse and Its Consequences*, Sage Publications, Newbury Park, CA, 1988a, pp. 14-36.

Gelles, RJ, and Straus, MA: *Intimate Violence*, Simon and Schuster, New York, 1988b.

George, C, and Main, M: Social interactions of young abused children: Approach, avoidance, and aggression, *Child Dev* 50:306-318, 1979.

Gil, D: *Violence Against Children: Physical Child Abuse in the United States*, Harvard University Press, Cambridge, MA, 1973.

Giovanni, J: Definitional issues in child maltreatment. In D Cicchetti and V Carlson, eds: *Child Maltreatment: Theory and Research on the Causes and Consequences of Child Abuse and Neglect*, Cambridge University Press, Cambridge, UK, 1989, pp. 3-37.

Gold, ER: Long-term effects of sexual victimization in childhood: An attributional approach, *J Consult Clin Psychol* 54:471-475, 1986.

Gomes-Schwartz, B, Horowitz, J, and Sauzier, M: Severity of emotional distress among sexually abused preschool, school age, and adolescent children, *Hosp Community Psychiatry* 36:503-508, 1986.

Hendin, H: Black suicide, *Arch Gen Psychiatry* 21:407-422, 1969.

Hershorn, M, and Rosenbaum, A: Children of marital violence: A closer look at the unintended victims, *Am J Orthopsychiatry* 55:260-266, 1985.

Hoffman-Plotkin, D, and Twentyman, C: A multimodal assessment of behavioral and cognitive deficits in abused and neglected preschoolers, *Child Dev* 55: 794-802, 1984.

Horney, K: *Neurosis and Human Growth*, WW Norton, New York, 1950.

Hotaling, G, and Sugarman, D: An analysis of risk markers in husband to wife violence: The current state of knowledge, *Violence Victims* 1:101-124, 1986.

Hunter, RS, and Kilstrom, N: Breaking the cycle in abusive families, *Am J Psychiatry* 136:1320-1322, 1979.

Jacobvitz, D, and Sroufe, LA: The early caregiver-child relationship and attention-deficit disorder with hyperactivity in kindergarten: A prospective study, *Child Dev* 58:1496-1504, 1987.

Jaffe, PG, Wolfe, DA, and Wilson, SK: *Children of Battered Women*, Sage Publications, Newbury Park, CA, 1990.

Johnson, CF, and Showers, J: Injury variables in child abuse, *Child Abuse Negl* 9:205-215, 1985.

Johnson, TC: Child perpetrators: Children who molest other children: Preliminary findings, *Child Abuse Negl* 12:219-229, 1988.

Johnson, TC: Female child perpetrators: Children who molest other children, *Child Abuse Negl* 13:571-585, 1989.

Kaplan, PJ, Waters, J, and White, G, et al: Toronto multi-agency research project: The abused and the abuser, *Child Abuse Negl* 8:343-351, 1984.

Kaufman, J, and Zigler, E: Do abused children become abusive parents? *Am J Orthopsychiatry* 57:186-192, 1987.

Kempe, CH: Approaches to preventing child abuse: The health visitor's concept, *Am J Dis Child* 130:941-947, 1976.

Kempe, CH, Silverman, FN, Steele, BF, Drogemueller, W, and Silver, HK: The battered child syndrome, *JAMA* 181:17-24, 1962.

Kinard, EM: Emotional development in physically abused children, *Am J Orthopsychiatry* 50:686-696, 1980.

Kinsey, AC, Pomeroy, WB, Martin, CE, and Gebhard, PH: *Sexual Behavior in the Human Female*, WB Saunders Co, Philadelphia, 1953.

Kohan, MJ, Pothier, P, and Norbeck, JS: Hospitalized children with history of sexual abuse: Incidence and care issues, *Am J Orthopsychiatry* 67:258-264, 1987.

Kohlberg, L: *The Philosophy of Moral Development, Volume 1*, Harper & Row, Publishers, San Francisco, 1981.

Kolko, DJ, Moser, TM, and Weldy, SR: Behavioral/emotional indicators of sexual abuse in child psychiatric inpatients: A controlled comparison with physical abuse, *Child Abuse Negl* 12:529-541, 1988.

Langer, WL: Infanticide: An historical survey, *History Child Q* 1:353-365, 1973.

Lewis, D, Pincus, J, Bard, B, et al: Neuropsychiatric, psychoeducational and family characteristics of 14 juveniles condemned to death in the United States, *Am J Psychiatry* 145:584-589, 1988.

Lewis, JO, Shanok, SS, Grant, M, and Ritvo, E: Homicidally aggressive young children: Neuropsychiatric and experiential correlates, *Am J Psychiatry* 140:148-153, 1983.

Lewis, M: The social networks systems model. In T Field, ed: *Review of Human Development*, Plenum Press, New York, 1982.

Litt, IF, and Martin, JA: Development of sexuality and its problems. In M Levine, WD Carey, AC Crocker, and RT Gross, eds: *Developmental-Behavioral Pediatrics*, WB Saunders, Philadelphia, 1981, pp. 633-649.

Longo, RE: Sexual learning and experiences among adolescent sexual offenders, *Int J Offender Ther Comparative Criminology* 26:235-241, 1982.

Lorenz, K (Wilson, MK, translator): *On Aggression*, Harcourt, Brace & World, New York, 1966.

Mannarino, AP, and Cohen, JA: A clinical-demographic study of sexually abused children, *Child Abuse Negl* 10:17-23, 1986.

Martin, D: *Battered Wives*, Simon and Schuster, New York, 1976.

Martin, HP, and Beezley, P: Behavioral observations in abused children, *Dev Med Child Neurol* 19:373-387, 1977.

Martin, HP, Beezley, P, Conway, E, and Kempe, CH: The development of abused children, *Adv Pediatr* 21:25-73, 1974.

Matas, L, Arend, R, and Sroufe, L: Continuity of adaptation in the second year: The relationship between the quality of attachment and later competence, *Child Dev* 49:547-556, 1978.

Mian, M, Wehrspann, W, Klanjner-Diamond, H, et al: Review of 125 children 6 years of age and under who were sexually abused, *Child Abuse Negl* 10:223-229, 1986.

Mills, T, Reiker, PP, and Carmen, E: Hospitalization experiences of victims of abuse, *Victimology* 9:436-449, 1984.

Mischel, W: Toward a cognitive social learning reconceptualization of personality, *Psychol Rev* 80:252-283, 1973.

Morse, C, Sahleer, O, and Friedman, S: A three-year follow-up study of abused and neglected children, *Am J Ment Defic* 79:327-330, 1981.

Morse, CW, Sahleer, OJZ, and Friedman, SB: A follow-up study of abused and neglected children, *Am J Dis Child* 120:439-446, 1970.

Murphy, S, Orkow, B, and Niola, RN: Prenatal prediction of child abuse and neglect: A prospective study, *Child Abuse Negl* 9:225-235, 1985.

Newberger, EH, and Bourne, R: The medicalization and legalization of child abuse, *Am J Orthopsychiatry* 48:593-607, 1978.

Nielsen, T: Sexual abuse of boys: Current perspectives, *Personnel Guidance J* 62:139-142, 1983.

Olds, DL, Henderson, CR, Chamberlin, R, and Tatelbaum, R: Preventing child abuse and neglect: A randomized trial of nurse home visitation, *Pediatrics* 78:65-78, 1986.

Olds, DL, and Kitzman, H: Can home visitation improve the health of women and children at environmental risk? *Pediatrics* 86:108-116, 1990.

Olweus, D: Familial and temperamental determinants of aggressive behavior in adolescent boys: A causal analysis, *Dev Psychol* 16:644-660, 1980.

Parke, R, and Collmer, C: Child abuse: An interdisciplinary analysis. In EM Hetherington, ed: *Review of Child Development Research*, Volume 5, University of Chicago Press, Chicago, 1975.

Parke, RD, and Slaby, RG: The development of aggression. In PH Mussen and EM Hetherington, eds: *Handbook of Child Psychology*, Volume IV, John Wiley and Sons, New York, 1983, pp. 547-641.

Patterson, GR: Performance models for antisocial boys, *Am Psychol* 41:432-444, 1986.

Patterson, GR, DeBarysche, BD, and Ramsey, E: A developmental perspective on antisocial behavior, *Am Psychol* 44:329-335, 1989.

Perry, DG, Perry, LC, and Rasmussen, P: Cognitive social learning mediators of aggression, *Child Dev* 57:700-711, 1986.

Peters, SD, Wyatt, GE, and Finkelhor, D: Prevalence. In D Finkelhor, ed: *A Sourcebook on Child Sexual Abuse*, Sage Publications, Newbury Park, CA, 1986, pp. 15-59.

Piaget, J: *The Moral Judgement of the Child*, Free Press, New York, 1965.

Radbill, SX: Children in a world of violence: A history of child abuse. In RE Helfer and RS Kempe, eds: *The Battered Child*, ed 4, University of Chicago Press, Chicago, 1987, pp. 3-22.

Reidy, TJ: The aggressive characteristics of abused and neglected children, *J Clin Psychol* 33:1140-1145, 1977.

Rieker, PP, and Carmen, E: The victim-to-patient process: The disconfirmation and transformation of abuse, *Am J Orthopsychiatry* 56:360-370, 1986.

Roscoe, B, Goodwin, MP, and Kennedy, D: Sibling violence and agonistic interactions experienced by early adolescents, *J Fam Violence* 2:121-137, 1987.

Rosenthal, PA, and Doherty, MB: Serious sibling abuse by preschool children, *J Am Acad Child Psychiatry* 23:186-190, 1984.

Rush, F: *The Best Kept Secret: Sexual Abuse of Children*, McGraw-Hill Book Co, New York, 1980.

Russell, DEH: The prevalence and incidence of intrafamilial and extrafamilial sexual abuse of female children, *Child Abuse Negl* 7:133-146, 1983.

Russell, DEH: *Sexual Exploitation*, Sage Publications, Newbury Park, CA, 1984.

Rutter, M: Normal psychosexual development, *J Child Psychol Psychiatry* 11:259-283, 1971.

Ryan, G, Lane, S, Davis, J, and Isaac, C: Juvenile sexual offenders: Development and correction, *Child Abuse Negl* 11:385-395, 1987.

Sargent, DA: The lethal situation: Translation of the urge to kill from parent to child. In J Fawcett, ed: *Dynamics of Violence*, American Medical Association, Chicago, 1972, pp. 105-114.

Scherzer, LN, and Lala, P: Sexual offenses committed against children, *Clin Pediatr* 19:679-685, 1980.

Shengold, LL: Child abuse and deprivation: Soul murder, *J Am Psychoanal Assoc* 27:533-559, 1979.

Showers, J, and Johnson, CF: Child development, child health and child rearing knowledge among urban adolescents: Are they adequately prepared for the challenges of parenthood? *Health Educ* 16:37-41, 1985.

Silverman, FN: The roentgen manifestations of unrecognized skeletal trauma in infants, *AJR* 69:413-426, 1953.

Snow, B, and Sorenson, T: Ritualistic child abuse in a neighborhood setting, *J Interpersonal Violence* 5:474-487, 1990.

Sonsonnet-Hayden, H, Haley, G, Marraige, K, and Fine, S: Sexual abuse and psychopathology in hospitalized adolescents, *J Am Acad Child Adolescent Psychiatry* 26:753-757, 1987.

Spinetta, JJ, and Rigler, D: The child-abusing parent: A psychological review, *Psychol Bull* 77:296-304, 1972.

Sroufe, LA, and Waters, E: Attachment as an organizational construct, *Child Dev* 48:1184-1199, 1977.

Stark, R, and McEvoy, J, III: Middle class violence, *Psychol Today* 4:52-65, 1970.

Steinmetz, S: *The Cycle of Violence: Assertive, Aggressive, and Abusive Family Interaction*, Prager, New York, 1977.

Straus, MA: Ordinary violence, child abuse, and wife beating: What do they have in common? In D Finkelhor, RJ Gelles, GT Hotaling, and MA Straus: *The Dark Side of Families: Current Family Violence Research*, Sage Publications, Newbury Park, CA, 1983, pp. 213-234.

Straus, MA, and Gelles, RJ: Societal change and change in family violence from 1975 to 1985 as revealed by two national surveys, *J Marriage Fam* 48:465-479, 1986.

Straus, MA, Gelles, RJ, and Steinmetz, S: *Behind Closed Doors: Violence in the American Family*, Doubleday, Garden City, NY, 1980.

Summit, RC: The child sexual abuse accommodation syndrome, *Child Abuse Negl* 7:177-193, 1983.

Terr, L: What happens to early memories of trauma? *J Am Acad Child Adolescent Psychiatry* 1:96-104, 1988.

Tooley, KM: The small assassins: Clinical notes on a subgroup of murderous children, *J Am Acad Child Psychiatry* 14:306-318, 1975.

Tooley, KM: The young child as victim of sibling attack, *Soc Casework* 58:25-28, 1977.

van der Kolk, B, Herman, J, and Perry, J: Childhood trauma and self-destructive behavior in adulthood. Unpublished data. In B van der Kolk: Compulsion to repeat the trauma, *Psychiatr Clin North Am* 12:398-411, 1988.

Wasserman, GA, Green, A, and Allen, R: Going beyond abuse: Maladaptive patterns of interaction in abusing mother-infant pairs, *J Am Acad Child Psychiatry* 22:254, 1983.

Wheeler, JR, and Berliner, L: Treating the effects of sexual abuse on children. In GE Wyatt and GJ Powell: *Lasting Effects of Child Sexual Abuse*, Sage Publications, Newbury Park, CA, 1988, pp. 227-247.

Widom, CS: The intergenerational transmission of violence. In NA Weiner and ME Wolfgang, eds: *Pathways to Criminal Violence*, Sage Publications, Newbury Park, CA, 1988, pp. 137-201.

Widom, CS: The cycle of violence, *Science* 244:160-166, 1989a.

Widom, CS: Child abuse, neglect, and adult behavior: Research design and findings on criminality, violence, and child abuse, *Am J Orthopsychiatry* 59:355-367, 1989b.

Widom, CS: Does violence beget violence? A critical examination of the literature, *Psychol Bull* 106:3-28, 1989c.

Wolfe, DA, Jaffe, P, Wilson, SK, and Zak, L: Children of battered women: The relation of child behavior to family violence and maternal stress, *J Consult Clin Psychol* 53:657-665, 1985.

Wright, K: Sociocultural factors in child abuse. In BA Bass, GE Wyatt, and GJ Powell: *The Afro-American Family Assessment: Treatment and Research Issues*, Grune & Stratton, New York, 1982, pp. 237-261.

Wyatt, GE: The sexual abuse of Afro-American and white American women in childhood, *Child Abuse Negl* 9:507-519, 1985.

Wyatt, GE, and Powell, GJ, eds: *The Lasting Effects of Child Sexual Abuse*, Sage Publications, Newbury Park, CA, 1988.

Zuravain, SJ: Unplanned pregnancies, family planning problems and child maltreatment, *Fam Relations* 36:135-139, 1987.

# The Role of Law Enforcement in the Investigation of Child Maltreatment

Gus H. Kolilis, B.S.
Richard P. Easter

Technically, the role of law enforcement in the investigation of child maltreatment is clear. The abuse, neglect, and exploitation of children is a crime. Police officers report and investigate crime; however, the investigation of crimes involving children and families is only a sliver of law enforcement's overall responsibilities. Other than in the largest departments, there are very few police officers dedicated to the investigation of children's events. The lack of specialized training and experience in very difficult and complicated cases contributes to the ongoing dilemma of how to prove or disprove allegations or suspicions of child maltreatment. Formal multidisciplinary teams of police officers, medical personnel, and social workers provide an efficient and effective approach to these very complex and emotional cases.

All investigations begin with a suspicion or allegation. Most reports of crime to police departments are by victims eager to provide details and information. Adult reporters generally hope that the investigation of the event reported will be successful. The police officers taking these reports usually can initiate effective and appropriate actions with a reasonable expectation of solving the crime. However, crimes against children are considerably different from crimes involving adult victims. The report or disclosure of the event is seldom deliberate. As a rule, children do not report being abused. Depending on the child's age and developmental level, he or she may not understand what has happened or even the fact that they were abused. Many child victims are confused, afraid, and intimidated. Infants and very young children may lack the ability to comprehend or communicate what has occurred. In addition, in many cases the systems which are in place to protect children and investigate and prosecute offenders are complicated and ineffective. Child abuse investigations are among the most difficult cases handled by law enforcement agencies. *In fact, children can be perfect victims, for the following reasons:*

1. Because of their physical, mental, and emotional development, children are usually unable to "protect" themselves from abuse, neglect, and exploitation.

2. The crimes are usually conducted in a private place, in a one-on-one setting, meaning there are no witnesses and no accomplices.

3. Defendants in such cases usually do not brag about their crimes, so, unlike with other criminal activity, they are unlikely to be informed on by others.

4. Children are often viewed as less credible or competent than the suspected adult offender.

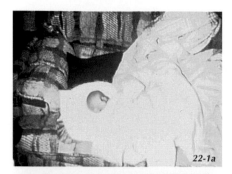

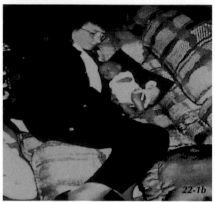

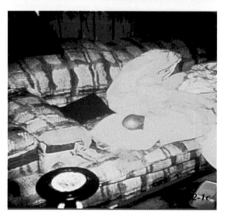

**Figure 22-1a-c.** *This is an investigation following the death of a baby. The mother initially stated that she found the child laying motionless and not breathing. She placed the doll in the position she found the child (a). With the help of the DFS worker she placed the doll in the position taken when they were sleeping together (b). She finally admitted that when she woke up, the baby was at her feet, face down in the bedding (c). The mother had been taking drugs. The cause of death was determined to be a laying-over by the mother.*

5. Communities are in denial of the problem. People do not want to get involved, or they want to avoid the negative publicity concerning their community.

6. Interviews of children require special training, understanding, and patience.

7. For many reasons, children do not tell about abuse or the disclosure is delayed and/or delivered piecemeal over an extended period of time.

8. Children often do not want the offender punished; they may only want the abuse to stop. They may not even understand that they are being abused.

9. Most crimes against children are not isolated incidents. They take place over a period of time and may involve multiple victims.

10. Crimes of abuse often have no physical or medical evidence. If such evidence does exist, it does not necessarily prove who the suspect is.

11. Child maltreatment cases often involve concurrent civil, criminal, and sometimes administrative investigations that result in investigative conflicts and obstructions.

12. Cases often cross jurisdictional and political boundaries, making determination of venue difficult.

13. The criminal justice system was not designed with the special needs of children considered. Children may be frightened and intimidated by the court room/trial process.

14. Child abuse and neglect crimes are often investigated by personnel with little specialized training or experience in dealing with children's events.

Initiating an investigation of suspected child maltreatment begins with a clear allegation. The abuse may be physical, sexual, or emotional, or it may involve some form of neglect. The investigator(s) is responsible for using every legal means to validate the allegation by collecting verifiable evidence and information to prove or disprove that the crime has occurred. The majority of information is collected by interviewing the victim(s), witness(es), expert(s), and suspect(s). How these interviews and interrogations are conducted will, in large part, determine the ultimate outcome of the investigation, which will, in turn, determine what interventions are needed to protect the interests of the child victim. It may also identify other children at risk, as well as crimes not directly associated with the allegation.

## ♦ INTERVIEW GUIDELINES

### GENERAL INTERVIEW PREPARATION

An interview is simply the process of one person obtaining information from another by a question-and-answer method. It is important to gather all available case and background information pertinent to the nature of the interview. If necessary, the scene can be revisited and photographs reviewed. Dolls can be useful in investigating a death scene and determining the cause of death **(Figures 22-1 to 22-3)**. The investigator should make sure he or she understands the offense and what happened to the victim. Neither guilt nor innocence should be assumed. Every event should be evaluated and investigated on its own merit.

All persons interviewed must be properly identified in notes and reports. *The following must be documented:*

*—Correct spelling of person's name*

*—Date of birth and Social Security number*

*—Home address—apartment number, floor, and location (front or rear)*

*—Telephone number—both home and work*

*—Secondary contact person—name, address, telephone numbers, both home and work*

The interview(s) should be conducted away from other victims, witnesses, or suspected perpetrator(s). *Suggested sites include the following:*

—*A place convenient and familiar to the subject.*

—*A neutral setting—the two most undesirable places for a victim or witness interview are where the alleged abuse took place (especially for the victim) and at the police station. However, the police station is an appropriate place to interview the suspected perpetrator(s).*

—*With a child interview, any place that is child friendly, where privacy is assured, is appropriate.*

Interviews should take place as soon as possible after the event has occurred so the witness' statements are not affected by memory loss, by talking to others, etc. One person should conduct all interviews, if possible. Thoughts should be communicated clearly and accurately, avoiding any display of bias in nonverbal communications. Above all, the investigator must be professional.

First, the interviewer determines what information is to be obtained from the person being interviewed. Questions are focused on the injury/event being investigated, keeping in mind the alleged offense. *When formulating questions, the following guidelines are appropriate:*

—*Keep questions short, clear, and easily understood.*

—*Confine questions to one topic at a time.*

—*Avoid "yes," "no," and leading questions that begin with "did" or "does."*

—*Use comparison-type questions to pinpoint details.*

Even though each interview is unique, there are seven general steps to conducting any interview:

1. Develop interview objectives (what needs to be known).
2. Use an introduction and warm-up.
3. Use the opening statement to set the tone of the interview.
4. Ask what happened and then **listen**.
5. Start over and get specific details (including what occurred before, during, and after the injury/event).
6. Obtain any other information required for the investigation.
7. Bring the interview to a conclusion.

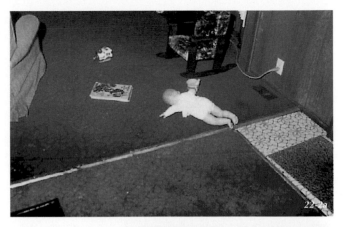
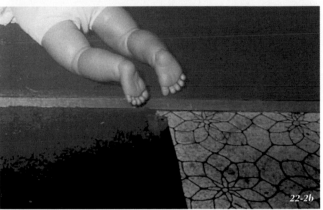

**Figure 22-2a,b.** *An 11 month-old boy died with a closed head injury, due to shaken infant syndrome. The mother's live-in boyfriend stated the child had tripped over the carpet edge and struck his head. He placed the doll in the position of the fall (a and b).*

## ◆ THE VICTIM INTERVIEW

When interviewing a child, the investigator must remember both the developmental level and the communicative abilities of the child, as well as the circumstances surrounding the interview. He or she must also be aware of young children's eating and sleep schedules, avoiding interviews when they are hungry, sleepy, or otherwise physically uncomfortable. To minimize the size differential between the interviewer and the child, the investigator must get on the same physical level. Interviewing tools (such as dolls, drawings, paper, crayons, doll house, etc.) may be used, but should not detract from the interview and should only be used if the investigator has received proper training. Sufficient time must be allotted to conduct the interview. The child must be assured that he or she is not in trouble or at fault.

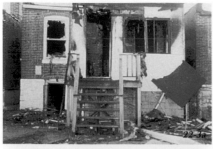

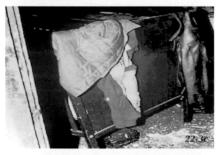

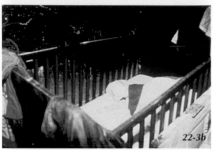

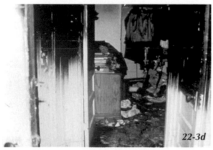

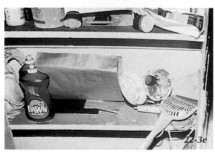

**Figure 22-3a-e.** *A child died in this fire (a to d). The fire broke out on the porch, next to the baby's room. Note the smoke line. The child was asleep below the smoke line. The bedding was clean. He died of breathing other noxious gases. The tragedy could have been avoided. The smoke detector was in a closet with the door closed and had the battery removed (e).*

Information gained before the interview can help in relating to the child on his developmental level. Questions and sentences should be kept simple, using words that are familiar to the child. The interviewer should use the child's words for body parts and not assume that his or her meaning of a word is the same as the child's. Pronouns (like he or she) and words like "there" and "that" should be used carefully. The child may be unable to follow the meaning. The child should be told that it is okay to answer "I don't know" or "I don't understand" rather than guess.

As already noted, questions should be asked that encourage the child to give more than a "yes" or "no" answer. Leading questions that start with "did" or "does" should be avoided, as should "why" questions; they imply blame or identify a specific person. The child must be reassured that she is believed and that she is not at fault for what happened.

The investigator should be aware of the child's nonverbal communication and allow him plenty of time to respond to any question asked. In addition, the investigator should be careful of his or her own nonverbal communication (i.e., touching, facial expressions, eye contact, body posturing, hand gesturing, body distance) because it can affect the child's responsiveness during the interview. Neither the child's nor the investigator's body parts should be used to evaluate the child's knowledge of anatomy.

## CONDUCTING THE INTERVIEW

At the beginning of the interview, introductions should be made and a simple explanation given of the job of an interviewer. The investigator must take time to establish rapport with the child. *Some sample questions that can assist in establishing rapport are as follows:*

—*What is your name? How old are you?*

—*Where do you live? Who lives with you? Who visits you?*

—*What are your mother's and father's names?*

—*What school do you go to? What grade are you in?*

—*What is your favorite subject? Your least favorite?*

—*What is your teacher's name? Who was your teacher last year?*

—*What makes you happy? Sad? Mad? Scared?*

—*What do you like best about the people you live with? Least?*

—*What kind of things do you like to do alone?*

—*Why are you here today?*

The investigator should ask as few direct questions as possible, but attempt to obtain the what, who, how, where, and when of the allegation (**Table 22-1**).

## CONCLUDING THE INTERVIEW

On completing the interview, the child should be asked if he has any questions. Then the investigator should answer them honestly. The child should be comforted, but the investigator must not make promises that may not be kept.

The investigator should ask the child what she expects will happen, then explain what is likely to happen. Then he or she should state whether there will be further contacts or interviews. If additional interviews are needed, it is less traumatic for the child to deal with the same interviewer.

If the child has not disclosed abuse but there are indicators that abuse did take place, it may be necessary to refer him to a qualified counselor. However, if

**Table 22-1. Questions That Can Be Asked of the Child Victim**

*What happened to you?*
This question allows the child to describe the event in his own words. Help the child expand on the information by asking the following:
—What were you wearing? What was the suspected perpetrator wearing?

—What happened to your clothes? Suspected perpetrator's clothes?

—What did he or she say? What did you say to him or her?

—Who did you tell this to?

*Are you hurt or sick now?*
Never delay emergency medical care. If the child indicates that she is hurt, ask where.

*What happened next?*
This question encourages more detail. When a child begins to disclose, you may prompt him with questions such as the following:
—What else do you remember? What else do I need to know?

—Could you tell me what you mean by _____? I need to understand a little more here.

—Were pictures taken? Of what? By whom? Where are the pictures?

—Were you asked not to tell anyone? Who asked you? What were you asked not to tell? Who were you not supposed to tell? This helps to determine the use of threats or bribes.

*Who did this to you?*
If information is not volunteered, it is important to ask the name and/or relationship of the abuser.
—Were you touched by anyone? Who? Where?

—How do you know him or her?

—Has anyone else done this to you? Who? Where?

*How did this happen?*
Asking this question will encourage an explanation of the event.
—What were you touched with (an object may have been used)?

*When did this happen?*
Determining when the event happened may require association with other dates, such as holidays, visits, day or night, etc.
—Time of day? Month? Year? With a younger child, you may need to link this with the clothes he was wearing, before or after a meal, during a television show, describing the weather, birthdays, anniversaries, holidays, etc.

—Has this happened before? When? Where? (If sexual abuse is alleged, look for grooming and events leading up to the act.)

*Who saw this happen?*
Asking this question corroborates witness information and addresses the possibility of multiple victims or suspected perpetrators.
—Was anyone else in the room when this happened? Who was there?

—Were you seen by anyone else? Who?

—Was there anyone else this happened to?

—Was anyone else touched? By whom? Where?

—Was anyone else at home? Where were they?

—Has anyone else done this to you?

prosecution is a possibility, counseling, therapy, or other abuse-related treatment (including hypnosis) could compromise the criminal case. Such treatment should be discussed with the prosecutor before arranging for these types of services.

# ◆ THE WITNESS INTERVIEW

## BASIC REQUIREMENTS OF WITNESSES

Some of the more important factors to be considered when conducting an interview are discussed here. However, before attempting to weigh their effect on the witness' story, the interviewer must first determine that the witness meets three essential requirements:

1. The witness was present during the event or a portion of it.
2. The witness was conscious (aware) of what was happening.
3. The witness was attentive to what was happening. (This final element is the most difficult to establish.)

## CONDUCTING THE INTERVIEW

When interviewing a witness, the investigator must first allow the person to tell what happened or what he or she observed in a narrative style. Specific questions can be asked later to gather more detail and to jog the witness' memory.

The investigator should be sure to (1) ask the witness for the correct spelling of names and for the addresses and phone numbers of other persons talked about; (2) ask if the victim disclosed the incident to the witness; (3) ask if there is anything he or she failed to ask; (4) ask if there is anything else the witness wants to discuss; and (5) obtain a written statement, if possible.

At the end of the interview, the witness is told that there are no further questions at this time, but as the investigation continues, he or she may be needed to talk about new information or clarify what has just been revealed. The witness should be encouraged to contact the law enforcement office with any additional information. A witness should never be told that by talking now he or she will not have to appear in court.

# ◆ INTERROGATING THE SUSPECTED PERPETRATOR

**The interviewer should always follow local dictates. Procedures or practices should be guided by the investigative agency's rules/procedures and applicable local, state, and federal laws.**

A background check on those involved can be invaluable. *It is important to gather as much background information as possible before interviewing the suspected perpetrator(s), including the following:*

*—Criminal history*

*—Social history*

*—Medical history*

*—Driving record*

*—Credit history*

*—Family, friends, hobbies, likes, dislikes, and personal history*

*—Evidence or previous report of domestic violence in residence*

In addition, original reports (e.g., police) should be read and other professionals (e.g., social worker) consulted.

If two interviewers are present, one should conduct the interview while the other one takes notes and shows support by displaying positive gestures.

## Conducting the Interview

First, introductions are made and an explanation given as to why the interview is being conducted. This will set the stage for the interview, so the interviewer must be candid, honest, and polite. For example, the interviewer should shake the person's hand.

*First impressions are lasting impressions.* Care should be taken to communicate on the same level as the person being interviewed. Using big, difficult words to impress or embarrass the other person should be avoided. The interviewer should be attentive at all times, maintain eye contact, and use reflective listening techniques–mirroring back to the person what is said to indicate real interest in what he or she has to say. In addition, the interviewer should be patient, making sure that sufficient time has been scheduled for the interview, and be empathetic.

If dealing with a person in custody, the interview is begun by reading the Miranda rights and having him or her sign and date a waiver. If a person not in custody starts making incriminating statements, he or she should be advised of the Miranda rights and sign and date a waiver before the interview continues. These steps should be guided by the investigative agency's policy and procedures.

During the interview process it should be the interviewer's goal to build rapport. Openness can be encouraged by sharing *noncritical* information. The interviewer should avoid being judgmental; exhibiting personal feelings and emotions, such as anger or disgust, can influence the interview. Instead, he or she should demonstrate interest in the suspected perpetrator as a person. It is essential to control your actions, reactions, and expressions. The suspected perpetrator is allowed to talk about himself or herself. The interviewer pays attention to the suspect's interests and fantasies, and appeals to the person's emotions. Photographs of the victim can be shown, but the suspected perpetrator must not be allowed to show disrespect for the victim.

To reduce any feelings of threat, the investigator can emphasize positive characteristics to bolster the suspected perpetrator's ego. He or she should remain open-minded and empathize with the weaknesses and defects of the suspected perpetrator. The suspected perpetrator should be helped to look at the problem with a lowered level of personal threat, perhaps with phrases such as, "I understand how these things can happen; sometimes we just lose control." The investigator may suggest that "There are always two sides to every story. This may be your last chance to tell exactly what happened and why. It's never as bad as you think." "It's better to put this behind you so you can start over."

Certain information must be obtained: who, what, when, where, why, and how, if possible. However, the investigator should avoid the direct question, "Did you do it?" If applicable, the suspected perpetrator may be asked if drugs or alcohol were used and whether they could be responsible for what happened. He or she can also ask if photographs were taken and/or videotapes made.

Verbal and nonverbal cues should be noted. It should be remembered that most of the time the person being interviewed is looking for help or a release from guilt. He or she may be remorseful if the correct emotional response can be triggered. Denials and objections should be differentiated. Guilty people often object; innocent people use denial or profess guilt. Objections should not be taken personally. A face-saving situation should be provided for the suspected perpetrator, if applicable. When appropriate, the interview is closed on a cooperative note, remembering that the suspect may have to be interviewed again.

The use of videotaped or audiotaped recordings during interviews and interrogations is becoming increasingly popular. They may be used as monitoring devices or to document interviews/interrogations. Investigative agency procedures should be followed and checked with the prosecutor. The best equipment available should be used by an investigator proficient in its use.

## ◆ PRELIMINARY INVESTIGATIVE CHECKLIST

To facilitate a more timely and comprehensive assessment of the case, checklists are an excellent investigative aid. They act as reminders to obtain specific information and provide a means to organize and measure the status of the investigation. Checklists can be adapted to meet most agency requirements. The checklist in **Table 22-2** outlines information essential to the investigation of suspected child maltreatment. Field investigators are encouraged to evaluate the list and make modifications appropriate to specific case needs and objectives. This checklist is

---

**Table 22-2.** Preliminary Investigative Checklist

**How was the allegation received?**

—By whom?

—Has a child abuse and neglect hotline report been made?

—Incident number?

—Date?

—Reporter? *(NOTE: In most states, the name of the child abuse and neglect reporters are, by law, confidential.)*

—County of incident?

**Nature of allegation(s)?**

—Who?

—What?

—When?

—Where? (What is the exact location and venue where the alleged event took place?)

—How?

—How many times?

**Victim(s)–full pedigree?**

—Name?

—Date of birth?

—Race?

—Social Security number?

—Child protective services client number?

—Home address, phone number, county?

—Where the child(ren) lived at the time of this report (foster care, etc.)?

—Is the victim(s) at risk?

—Protective custody taken?

—Has the victim(s) been injured? If so, is the victim(s) in need of medical treatment?

—Sibling(s) in the home?

—Sibling(s) at risk?

**Parent(s)–full pedigree?**

—Father and/or mother's name?

—Date of birth?

---

| **Table 22-2.** Preliminary Investigative Checklist—*Continued* |
| :--- |

—Race?

—Social Security number?

—Child protective services client number?

—Home address, phone number, county?

—Employer? Work phone number?

**Name of guardian/caretaker(s)–full pedigree (if other than parent)?**
—Their date of birth?

—Their race?

—Their Social Security number?

—Their child protective services client number?

—Their home address, phone number, county?

—Their employer? Their work phone number?

—Their relationship to the victim?

**Medical treatment–Was it needed?**
—Nature of the illness/injury?

—When?

—Where?

—By whom?

—Were photographs taken of injury? By whom?

**If sexual abuse is alleged, has a sexual assault forensic examination been completed on the victim?**
—When?

—Where?

—By whom?

—Findings?

—Colposcope or other image documentation used?

**Has the victim been interviewed?**
—By whom?

—When?

—Where?

—Recorded by audio or video?

—"Cool call" considered? (Is it appropriate for the victim to make a monitored and recorded phone call to the suspect? Is the child developmentally and emotionally able to make such a call?)

**Suspected perpetrator(s)–full pedigree?**
—Name(s)?

—Date of birth?

—Race?

—Social Security number?

—Child protective services client number?

—Home address, phone number, county?

—Employer? Work phone number?

—Relationship to victim?

**Table 22-2.** Preliminary Investigative Checklist—*Continued*

**Records checks completed?**
—Local?

—State?

—FBI?

—Other applicable state(s)?

—Social history?

—Child abuse and neglect hotline prior reports?

—Medical and health records?

**Is there physical evidence?**
—Description?

—Chain of custody?

—Present location?

**Are there witnesses?**
—Name(s)?

—Date of birth?

—Race?

—Social Security number?

—Child protective services client number?

—Home address, phone number, county?

—Employer? Work phone number?

—Relationship to victim?

**Have documented statements been taken from witnesses and others?**
—From whom?

—By whom?

**Child protective services/juvenile court actions taken to date?**
—What?

—When?

**Criminal justice action taken to date?**
—Investigation in progress?

—Charges pending?

—Charges filed?

—Arrest(s) made? If yes, is suspect still confined?

**What agencies and investigators are involved in the investigation?**
—What are their responsibilities?

only a reminder and guide. Every effort should be made to verify and expand on information as it becomes known. It is essential to a credible investigation to differentiate between *investigative leads* and *verified facts*.

## ◆SERIOUS CRIME/EVENT SCENE PROCEDURES

Child maltreatment often comes to the attention of law enforcement officers as they respond to a call for service. While the call may concern a report of child abuse, it may originate as a domestic disturbance or the report of an accidental injury. Based on what is seen and heard, the responding officer(s) may suspect abuse. In some cases, it may be necessary to immediately protect the child by removing him from the home. Regardless of how the call is received or what

**Table 22-3. Guide for Law Enforcement Officers Responding to the Scene of a Reported Event**

*Assignment or notification*
Record time of assignment and arrival at scene. Attempt to obtain all available information from reporter.

*Preserve and protect life*
Determine if there are injuries or imminent dangers that require immediate attention. If injuries are present and there is **any** possibility of life, seek medical help immediately (obtain names of medical personnel and other responders). Normally, the injured should not be moved before medical assistance arrives unless in immediate danger (fire, water, etc.). Call for other assistance as necessary (could include law enforcement, coroner/medical examiner, child protective services, juvenile court officer, fire department, utility company, etc.).

*Determine what crime and/or event has occurred*
Identify victim(s) and witness(es); make a preliminary determination of what has occurred and what actions are required.

*If appropriate, identify and/or arrest suspected perpetrator(s)*
If a suspected perpetrator is identified but is not on the scene, obtain and broadcast a complete description, including name/alias(es)/nickname (if available); race; sex; age and date of birth; address; physical description (height, weight, hair, eyes, complexion, scars, tattoos, etc.); clothing description, any other identifiers; vehicle; direction of flight; weapon description (if any). Broadcast the description and what the person is wanted for as soon as possible, and update with new information as it becomes available.

If the suspected perpetrator is on the scene and is believed to be armed or is concealed and/or barricaded, request assistance and follow the investigative agency's policy.

If an immediate arrest is required, secure and search the suspected perpetrator as quickly as possible. For officer protection, search for anything that could cause harm. While conducting this search of the suspected perpetrator, any weapons, evidence, or contraband is seizable and usually admissible as evidence.
*NOTE: Safety and the protection and preservation of life are paramount. DO NOT take unnecessary risks.*

*Establish and protect the crime/event scene*
Once identified, "freeze" the scene and everything in it. With the exception of assisting the injured, the crime/event scene should remain untouched pending appropriate processing and photographing. If possible, secure and protect the perimeters with rope, tape, or other markers. Within manpower limitations, identify, separate, and isolate witness(es) before interviewing.
*NOTE: In the case of an obvious death (no possibility of life), do not move the body or anything surrounding it before the coroner/medical examiner arrives. Photograph the body and scene before other processing. While conveying a body to the morgue or other facility, take necessary measures to protect the head and extremities from accidental damage (paper bags on hands and feet, etc.). If the body is in rigor mortise, do not attempt to move or force extremities before moving it.*

If the victim appears near death (and it does not interfere with medical assistance), attempt to obtain a dying declaration of what occurred.
*NOTE: The **sudden, unexplained death of an infant (1 week to 1 year of age)** is commonly referred to as sudden infant death syndrome (SIDS). The cause of SIDS remains unknown, but criteria for its diagnosis have been established by the National Institute of Child Health and Human Development. For the death of an infant to be diagnosed as SIDS, an **autopsy, clinical history review**, and a thorough **death scene investigation** must be performed. In conducting these very sensitive and complex investigations, obtain all information available concerning social and medical history of the infant, as well as the death scene and circumstances surrounding the death.*

*Process the scene*
When in doubt, "freeze" the scene and take no unnecessary actions until it can be processed correctly. Do not hesitate to ask for outside advice and assistance.

Develop investigative goals and objectives.

Determine the legal basis for any search and seizure, particularly beyond the immediate crime/event scene. Considering the investigative agency's policy and procedures, the prosecuting attorney should be consulted on specific legal questions, such as consent to search versus the need for a search warrant and other "search and seizure" issues.

Establish a chain-of-custody log (who found what and where) to be maintained by a single officer. Designate that person to receive and take charge of all physical evidence at the scene.
*NOTE: Prior to seizing, all evidence should be photographed and logged as found. Only designated persons should search the crime scene and handle evidence. All others, excluding emergency medical assistance personnel, should remain outside the protected area.*

**Table 22-3. Guide for Law Enforcement Officers Responding to the Scene of a Reported Event—*Continued***

Take measurements and make sketches that will relate directly to the photographs. Indicate "North" in all sketches.

Take a complete photographic sequence of the entire scene area, including a "landmark" photograph (front of the house, vehicle license plate, etc.). Complete and use photo cards with a measuring scale when appropriate, as in close-ups, specific objects, etc. Document every phase of evidence handling.

Photographs and corresponding sketches should be taken from the general to the specific, such as an overall room shot, to the bed, to a blood stain on the pillow. Body pictures should be taken from at least two views and be full-length. Close-up photographs of wounds and abnormalities, when possible, should be visible in the full-length pictures. If the body has been removed, use body silhouettes (paper body cutouts) to reconstruct the scene. In the case of an infant, a doll may be more appropriate.

Prior to seizure, if appropriate, evidence should be examined for latent fingerprints. Weapons and nontraditional surfaces (paper, cardboard, leather, masonry, etc.) are best processed at the laboratory. Such evidence should be handled with care and is usually best transported in a paper or cardboard container.
*NOTE: All recovered and seized weapons should be considered **loaded and dangerous** until examined and deemed safe by a qualified person familiar with firearms.*

All seized evidence should be properly marked, packaged, and placed in a secure evidence locker or conveyed to the appropriate laboratory for processing. A chain-of-custody log should track the handling of every piece of evidence. It is essential that evidence be handled and packaged in containers appropriate for the material. Some evidence should be sealed and frozen, while others require air drying or special containers. Consult a crime laboratory for specific evidence handling instructions.

*Interview/interrogation process*
If the person(s) to be interviewed is a child, consider requesting the assistance of someone experienced in interviewing children. Child protective services and juvenile court officers are mandated to participate in some investigations. Seek advice and help. Before the interview, make a checklist of information needs and objectives. The suspected perpetrator(s) and witnesses should be separated and interviewed individually.

The suspected perpetrator(s) should be interrogated relative to his/her part in the crime/event. Improbabilities and inconsistencies should be noted and used to enhance the questioning process. Contradicting statements can be an important part of the case. It is important for the interviewer to lock-in the suspects to an alibi or explanation so that it can be proven or disproven.
*NOTE: Follow the investigative agency's policy and procedures for advising suspected perpetrators of their Miranda rights and obtaining verbal and written waiver of those rights.*

Witnesses should be questioned regarding their first-hand knowledge of the event, that is, what they actually saw or heard. To obtain the most detail, **ask specific questions** concerning the event and the persons involved. Always ask for and look for more detail. As an investigative tool, second-hand information can be valuable if it leads to an unidentified witness or suspected perpetrator; by itself, the information has very limited value. Always attempt to obtain names and specific verifying facts. If appropriate, initiate a canvass of the entire neighborhood or area. Many people will divulge information if asked, but will not voluntarily come forward as a witness.

**Make note of spontaneous statements**. From the moment of arrival on the scene, be alert to spontaneous statements made by witness(es), family, and/or suspected perpetrator(s). **Unsolicited**, voluntary utterances usually do not require that the subject have prior warning of his or her Miranda rights. Initial statements can be a very important part of the investigation; for example, they may contradict a later statement, implicate a person or persons in a particular action, or indicate remorse for an act that is denied later.

actions are taken by officers, assignments involving the possibility of child maltreatment are potentially very dangerous. **Table 22-3** is a guide for officers responding to the scene of a reported event.

## ♦ PREPARING A REPORT

All of the information that has been obtained should be assembled into a logical sequence of events, accurately reflecting the results of the entire investigation. Observations, statements, evidence, sketches, photographs, and medical and technical findings should clearly portray all the known facts of the case. If new or additional information becomes available, a **supplemental** report is prepared and distributed to all participating agencies.

All investigative results (interviewing, disposition of evidence, names of responders and what they did, etc.) are recorded according to the policy and procedures of the investigative agency. The investigator may need to take handwritten notes, record electronically, videotape, or use a combination of all these methods. Whatever the means, every step of the investigation must be **recorded and documented**.

While the primary role of law enforcement in the investigation of child maltreatment is to investigate alleged crimes, the ultimate responsibility is to identify and protect children at risk. Beyond the case being investigated, law enforcement officers should be alert to any situation that puts a child in harm's way. The assessment and immediate actions taken by law enforcement may save a child's life and improve the opportunity to preserve the family.

## ♦ BIBLIOGRAPHY

Garbino, J, et al.: *What Children Can Tell Us*, Jossey-Bass, Inc., California, 1989.

Monteleone, JA: *Recognition of Child Abuse for the Mandated Reporter, Second Edition*, GW Medical Publishing, Inc., St. Louis, Missouri, 1996.

Pence, D, and Wilson, C: *Team Investigation of Child Sexual Abuse*, Sage Publications, California, 1994.

Walker, AG, Ph.D.: *Handbook on Questioning Children: A Linguistic Perspective*, ABA on Children and the Law, Washington, DC, 1994.

# REVIEW PROCESS

JAMES A. MONTELEONE, M.D.
RICHARD P. EASTER

*An 18-month-old boy was admitted to the hospital from a small downstate community. The child was first seen with symptoms of abdominal discomfort, anorexia, and vomiting. A chest film revealed old, healed, fractured ribs. Liver enzyme levels were elevated, and CT scan of the abdomen revealed a lacerated liver. With the diagnosis of blunt trauma to the abdomen and child abuse, the case was reported to the Division of Family Services via the abuse hotline. Social Services found that the mother, a 21-year-old, was single and living with a paramour.*

*The Division of Family Services substantiated abuse. On recovery the child was sent home with the mother with the understanding that the paramour was no longer in the home.*

*Two weeks later, the Child Protection Team was called by the physician who had initially referred the child to the hospital. She had learned that, shortly after the child returned home, he was taken to a different emergency room. The mother stated she had found him motionless in his crib. He was pronounced dead at that hospital. The coroner/undertaker was out of town and the sheriff was called to see the child. He declared the cause of death "crib death," and the child was buried.*

*Despite requests by the Child Protection Team, the local physician, and medical examiner, the local authorities refused to exhume the body or to open a case.*

## ◆THE DEATH REVIEW PROCESS

Society has a responsibility to protect those who cannot protect themselves, but it does not always do this. Research conducted by the National Committee for the Prevention of Child Abuse found that 25% to 50% of fatal child abuse victims had prior involvement with child protective services. The National Committee for the Prevention of Child Abuse (NCPCA) estimated that in 1991 1,383 children in the United States died from child abuse and neglect, or 2.15 per 100,000 children. This is almost four child fatalities per day. It has been estimated that an additional two deaths per day go undetected (Robinson & Stevens, 1992). In Missouri between 1983 and 1986, 334 children between birth and age 4 years died as a result of injury (Ewigman & Kivlahan, 1990). Twenty percent of these children (68) died of inflicted injuries: 48% inflicted by their mothers, 24% by their fathers, and 16% by the mother's boyfriend. The perpetrator was unknown for 11 of the children. More than 30% of the children in this study died because they were exposed to hazards, 5% from neglect, and 3% from unrecognized hazards. The records were not adequate to determine the cause of death in 39% of the cases. Several explanations exist for inaccurate records: inadequate death scene investigations, failure to order autopsies, limited coordination among agencies, inconsistency in the quality of medical records, and a lack of personnel with specialized training in the area of suspicious child fatalities.

Ewigman and Kivlahan assert that fatal child abuse is a threat to the health and welfare of our children. National data show a rise in the number of reported child abuse and neglect fatalities. According to data collected by the National Center for the Prevention of Child Abuse, in 1989 child maltreatment-related fatalities increased by 5% over the number reported in 1988. Since 1985, reported child fatalities have increased by 57% nationwide. The number of overall reports of child abuse and neglect grew to almost 2.7 million in 1991, a 31% increase since 1985. This increase may represent an actual increase in the number of fatalities or a more accurate count of the problem. These figures represent the lowest estimate of the problem. A number of studies show that many child abuse and neglect fatalities are not reported.

Homicide is the leading cause of injury death for children under age 1 year. The National Center of Health Statistics reported that the homicide rate for children under 1 year of age rose 55% between 1985 and 1988, climbing from 5.3 per 100,000 to 8.2 per 100,000.

In 1991 approximately 36% of the child fatality victims died from neglect and 64% from physical abuse. The average age of the victim of fatal abuse was under 5 years, with 54% of them under age 1 year. The average age of the victim of nonfatal child abuse was 7 years of age.

Victims of child abuse often fall through the cracks. Injuries are mistakenly declared accidental because they occur suddenly and are considered unpredictable and uncontrollable. But injuries do not just happen; they are caused, they are predictable, and they should be controllable.

Childhood deaths resulting from violence and unintentional injury occur more frequently in the United States than in any other industrialized country. Injuries caused by motor vehicle accidents are the leading cause of death. Homicide is second, suicide is third, and drowning, fourth. Minorities are disproportionately affected in most categories, especially homicide.

For homicide victims, there are patterns with respect to perpetrators and methods. The usual perpetrator in the newborn period is the mother and the cause of death is frequently suffocation or drowning. For infants, a parent is usually the perpetrator and bodily force is most often the cause. For adolescents, strangers and occasional acquaintances are frequent perpetrators. Adolescents are killed by guns, knives, and cars.

Many states have adopted procedures to review child fatalities. The development of child fatality review teams is a positive step toward accurate identification and future prevention of such deaths. These teams, generally multidisciplinary and interagency, review child deaths to gain insight into the actual cause of the death and, more importantly, to suggest actions that need to be taken in the future to prevent such deaths (see Chapter 24).

In 1978 Los Angeles County formed the nation's first interagency child death review team involving criminal justice and health and human service professionals. By the end of 1992, 33 states had some form of death review team, at the state level, throughout the state in counties or cities, or only in limited local areas. The number of review teams in a state is usually determined by whether such teams are statutorily mandated. In California, there is no California statute mandating review teams—it is up to each individual county to form a team. In Georgia and Missouri, laws were passed that mandate a team in each county, in addition to a state board with oversight responsibility. Most review teams are not authorized by state statute. As of 1992 only eight states had passed statutes mandating child abuse death review teams.

Georgia provides for local child abuse review committees to evaluate medical examiners' reports regarding the death of any child and make their own investigations and reports regarding those deaths. Georgia requires a medical examiner's inquiry of all unexpected or unexplained deaths of children under 7 years of age. Georgia has also established a state-wide Fatality Review Panel to evaluate child death reports delivered by child abuse protocol committees and make its own report and recommendations. The committees, after reviewing details surrounding the fatalities, provide information and recommendations for policy changes to prevent future fatalities.

Several states have implemented or are considering new policies as a result of review committee findings and recommendations. Because of the large number of its children dying in neglectful families, Maine has developed guidelines employing a broader definition of risk factors, with an emphasis on substance abuse. Connecticut, after a review committee report stressed the need for comprehensive, face-to-face investigations of all reports and a more critical evaluation of the child's extended family for placement, improved training for school, medical, and criminal justice personnel. New York responded by making efforts to better educate workers regarding substance abuse and domestic violence, among other areas, by including these topics in their child abuse training.

It is important to identify child abuse/neglect fatalities. Families in which these deaths occur often need services such as counseling and treatment, and the siblings in the home may be at risk of harm and need to be removed from the home. Also, criminal prosecution may be warranted.

The American Bar Association has stressed the need for accurate, systematic reviews of child deaths (Kaplan, 1992). *The reasons given are as follows:*

1. We do not know the number of children who die each year and the accurate causes of their deaths.

2. We do not know the number of children who die each year from child abuse and neglect.

3. There is an underreporting of deaths from abuse and neglect in state vital records systems, and there is a significant difference between the causes of death on children's death certificates and the causes of deaths indicated in police and child protective services records.

4. There are no nationwide accepted and used standards for child autopsies or death investigations.

5. In many states, child protective services have no involvement in a death suspected to result from child abuse or neglect unless there are surviving siblings. In other states, child protective services are not notified of the death even if there are surviving siblings.

6. Many states operate with a coroner system. Coroners are often elected officials who have no medical training or training in forensic pathology. Some medical examiners have no training in pathology or in evaluating child deaths resulting from abuse or neglect.

## ◆STUDIES OF CHILDHOOD DEATHS AND CATASTROPHIC INJURIES

A number of states have conducted studies of childhood fatalities *(see Bibliography at the end of the chapter)*. The author, because of his familiarity with the studies and procedures in his state and the availability of the results of these studies, has included some of the results of those studies. In the mid-1980s and early 1990s two studies of childhood fatalities and catastrophic injuries were conducted in Missouri. One study was done by the St. Louis Child Abuse Network and the other by Ewigman and Kivlahan.

The St. Louis Child Abuse Network study had two components. The first phase of the study reviewed the cases of 37 children who died or had catastrophic injuries believed to result from abuse. The second phase of the study compared these children to two matched control groups—one of children with histories of mild abuse and one group with no history of abuse (Dodson et al., 1988; Monteleone et al., 1988).

The Ewigman and Kivlahan study reviewed death certificates of children who had died as the result of injury.

### THE ST. LOUIS CHILD ABUSE NETWORK STUDY, PHASE ONE

In 1983 a group of child abuse professionals in St. Louis, represented by the state Division of Family Services (DFS), local juvenile court and law enforcement, and two pediatric hospitals, organized and initiated a review process to study severe child maltreatment in the area (referred to as the Board of Inquiry). The project was entitled the *St. Louis Board of Inquiry to Investigate Fatal and Catastrophic Injuries Due to Child Abuse and Neglect.* The purpose of the Board's review was to determine how to prevent severe child maltreatment. This study is particularly significant because it is one of few, if any, studies comparing abusive families with matched nonabusive families.

#### BACKGROUND STATISTICS

The association between child abuse and neglect and violent crime as reported in the literature was verified by the crime statistics in St. Louis in the years before the study; these trends were confirmed over time. Reports showed that 3.5% of Missouri's children have been reported as abused or neglected. Fifteen percent of these abuse reports originated in the St. Louis metropolitan area. Approximately 2.5% of the state's children receive services related to abuse and neglect. Deaths caused by abuse and neglect are estimated at more than 30 per year statewide. Over a 3-year period before the study, the number of deaths resulting from maltreatment known through St. Louis Children's Hospital ranged from 4 to 11 per year and totaled 22. Severe maltreatment with permanent intellectual handicaps occurred in at least 15 cases. The statistics concerning abused children seen at the second hospital, Cardinal Glennon Children's Hospital, were similar.

#### DATA SOURCE

The Board of Inquiry reviewed all available information about fatal or nearly fatal cases of child maltreatment available from DFS records and medical records, including the medical examiner's findings. They also heard testimony from case workers, hospital social service workers, and police.

## CRITERIA FOR CASE REVIEW

The cases reviewed included all those in which children either died, had burns over 50% of their body surface, or had objective medical evidence of severe head injury as noted on skull X-ray or CT brain scan. In the St. Louis metropolitan area, all children with severe injuries of these types were known to personnel at the hospitals of the medical examiner's office.

## APPROACH OF THE BOARD OF INQUIRY

When reviewing the cases, the Board of Inquiry asked several questions, which formed an outline of information to be collected for each case.

*Specific judgments that the board tried to render included the following:*

Was the case potentially preventable? If so, how?

Did the public and private agencies function as intended? If not, where did the malfunction occur?

In addition, the Board of Inquiry carefully examined family structures that contained paramours. It looked for evidence of other family violence and considered possible intervention for families who were isolated relative to community services in general and the child health delivery system specifically. The answers to all these questions were tabulated on summary forms and computerized for analysis and compilation of summary results.

The decision to include severe but nonfatal cases in the review process enhanced the project. There were no differences in demographic features between the survivors and those who died. However, by including the nonfatal cases the Board of Inquiry was able to define the extreme morbidity in the injuries that would have been fatal except for medical intervention. This approach also provided a sample allowing statistically meaningful comparisons of severely abusive families as compared to other groups. The Board of Inquiry was able to determine the degree of handicap among the survivors. The degree of handicap information allowed one to project the long-term dollar costs for the future care of the handicapped victims. Furthermore, the participation of the hospitals allowed retrospective tabulation of the acute medical costs.

## BOARD OF INQUIRY FINDINGS

Over a period of 18 months (October 1983 to May 1985), the Board of Inquiry reviewed 37 cases, the equivalent of 1 year's local experience. Four cases were judged not to be the result of abuse. Eleven were fatal cases and 22 nonfatal. The average age in the nonfatal cases was 10 months. The average age of the children who died was 1 year, 8 months. The major findings are summarized in **Table 23-1**.

The victims' ages, the type of abuse, and the injury are listed in **Table 23-2**. Whiplash shaking injuries were present in eight children and were concentrated among the very young. These injuries were associated with a high incidence of

| Table 23-1. Board of Inquiry Summary of Findings | |
|---|---|
| **Summary of Case Results** | |
| Number of cases reviewed | 37 |
| Judged nonabuse | 4 |
| **Died** | 11/33 |
| Average age | 10 months |
| Recovered | 1 year, 8 months |
| **Human Outcomes** | |
| Death | 11/33 |
| Recovered | 11/33 |
| Permanent severe handicap | 11/33 |
| **Children** | |
| Incomplete immunizations | 14/33 |
| Lack of routine medical care | 9/33 |
| Prior medical problems | 9/33 |
| "Shaken infant" injury | 8/33 |
| **Families** | |
| Family violence | 9/33 |
| Substance abuse | 8/33 |
| Hostile to DFS worker | 9/33 |
| Known to DFS | 16/33 |
| Paramour present | 15/33 |
| **Acute Fiscal Outcomes** | |
| Total acute costs | $550,000 |
| Average survivor costs | $22,391 |
| **Future Costs** | |
| Care for each impaired child | $2,000,000 |
| **Other Features** | |
| Judged "preventable" | 10/33 |
| Perinatal risk factors | 13/33 |

permanent injury. The most frequent perpetrators were live-in boyfriends, who were involved in 14 cases and were perpetrators or co-perpetrators in 10 cases. These boyfriends were involved in five of the fatal cases and usually injured toddlers and older children. Although they had fathered children, none had been married. Mothers were perpetrators in four fatal cases, and biological fathers were perpetrators in two cases.

| Victim Age | Case Number | Type of Abuse | Type of Injury |
|---|---|---|---|
| **Table 23-2. Description of Abuse and Neglect Cases, Type of Maltreatment, and Injuries** | | | |
| 0.12 | 35 | N | Skull FX/neglect/lack of supervision |
| 0.15 | 5 | A | Multiple injuries/strangulation |
| 0.21 | 17 | A | SIS |
| 0.21 | 28 | A | CNS, possible SIS |
| 0.23 | 26 | A | CNS |
| 0.24 | 6 | A | SIS |
| 0.25 | 37 | N | CNS |
| 0.31 | 9 | A | WSIS/broken ribs |
| 0.32 | 32 | A | Head injury/skull FX |
| 0.33 | 33 | A | SIS, beating/shaking |
| 0.35 | 20 | A | Neglect/hypoglycemia |
| 0.41 | 2 | N | Exposure/pneumonia |
| 0.45 | 6 | A | SIS/subdural |
| 0.46 | 21 | A | SIS/subdurals |
| 0.47 | 23 | A | Head injuries + |
| 0.51 | 10 | A | SIS/shaking/possible strangulation |
| 0.62 | 11 | A | Malnutrition/bilateral subdural hematomas |
| 0.80 | 14 | A | CNS/multiple injuries |
| 1.05 | 29 | A | CNS/new & old arm FX |
| 1.25 | 24 | A | Burns—immersion |
| 1.29 | 4 | A | Spinal cord/multiple bruises |
| 1.34 | 15 | A | Head injury/beating |
| 1.41 | 27 | A | Multiple injuries |
| 1.59 | 1 | N | Drowning |
| 1.72 | 19 | A | Beating/ruptured duodenum |
| 1.74 | 22 | A | CNS/liver |
| 1.75 | 3 | A | Skull FX/meningitis/multiple FX/malnutrition |
| 1.76 | 7 | A | Multiple injuries/beating SIS + |
| 1.97 | 13 | A | Trauma/unilateral skull FX |
| 2.30 | 8 | A | Beating/ruptured duodenum |
| 2.52 | 25 | A | CNS |
| 4.71 | 30 | A | CNS |
| 5.66 | 12 | A | Head injury/beating |

*(The four cases determined to be nonabusive are not listed.)*

***Abbreviations:*** *\* A, Abuse; N, neglect; SIS, shaken infant syndrome; CNS, central nervous system injury; FX, fracture.*

In 18 cases the panel judged that the overall system had malfunctioned. Recommendations for change were made in 20 of the 33 abuse cases (**Table 23-3**).

| Table 23-3. Recommendations |
| --- |

**General**

1. Education for prevention, parenting skills—coping mechanisms, discipline techniques, normal child behavior, toilet-training techniques, prevention of shaken infant syndrome, babysitter recommendations.

2. Delineate lay (nonmandated reporter) responsibility to report abuse. (3*)

**Juvenile Court**

1. Juvenile Courts should have participated in Board of Inquiry. (29)

2. More expeditious action by Juvenile Court in cases involving injured children. (9)

3. Change law regulating court agreements for custody. (25)

4. Juvenile Court investigation records should be available to DFS case workers responsible for family. (29)

5. Workers (DFS, medical) need clear understanding of Juvenile Court's requirements to protect children. (29)

6. Juvenile Court should be involved in cases with serious injuries other than those cases where the child is dead or dying. (29)

**State Social Services**

1. *Develop guidelines* for DFS workers to assess risk to child, other children in the household, and subsequent children when abuse has been substantiated. (29)

2. *Develop guidelines* for DFS workers dealing with families in which one of the parents is mentally ill. (29)

3. In those cases with a mentally ill parent, worker should be given proper psychiatric diagnosis and evaluation of parent and his or her potential to do harm to the child. (29)

4. Cases should be kept open longer in those families known to have been severely abusive. (32)

5. DFS should perform computer check of *babysitter* in all cases in which a sitter is involved. (32)

6. When multiple workers are involved with a family, there should be *continuity of care* and a presented plan and assurance that the plan will be carried out after the initial worker has changed. (33,34)

7. Adequate *respite care* should be provided. (33)

8. Workers should concentrate on and emphasize parenting skills and coping mechanisms. (33,34)

9. DFS should stay involved longer after the child is placed in foster care. (5)

10. Develop special foster care facilities for runaway, difficult adolescents. (37)

11. Adolescent mothers receiving state funds for child support should be carefully supervised to ensure that these funds are being spent as intended—for child support. (37)

**Medical**

1. Medical personnel should realize the necessity to report to the hot line fractures in infants that could not have been self-inflicted. (1)

2. Better tracking of medical neglect cases (missed appointments). (1,2)

3. Medical doctors need education to recognize abuse and willingness to report it. (8)

**Police**

1. Clarify and simplify jurisdictional problems involving police of different municipalities, cities, counties, etc. (28)

2. Better *coordination and cooperation* between police and DFS. (9)

*\* The number in parentheses refers to the specific case as noted in Table 23-2.*

The high medical costs for care were also a major finding. The total acute hospital care costs were more than $550,000. The acute care costs among survivors averaged more than $22,000 each. For each child who died, approximately one child was permanently and severely disabled. So, in addition to the personal tragedies, these cases were also expensive. A lifetime of custodial care costs $2,000,000 per child. The 10 disabled children found in this study will accrue $20,000,000 in future costs.

Eighteen of 33 cases were either judged preventable or had perinatal risk factors detectable by the High Risk Infant Follow-up Program of the St. Louis Regional Maternal and Child Health Council. In 1985 the network created a targeted prevention program, Project First Step, to link public health nurses who do high-risk newborn infant follow-up screening with social service case workers to help families deal with intense risk factors.

## RISK FACTORS IDENTIFIED BY CASE STUDIES

Risk factors identified by the study included health care, housing, family structure, and family violence.

## THE VICTIMS

Seven children had not received standard immunizations. Nine children had special medical problems before the injury. Among these, six had not received appropriate follow-up treatment. Eleven children had not received routine well-baby care. In total, 12 children lacked either immunizations or routine well-baby care. Growth was normal in 17 children, abnormal in three.

Only two of 33 victims were known to survive their injuries with no apparent physical sequelae, although the outcome was unknown in four. Twenty-one victims either died or suffered permanent severe neurological impairment, including mental retardation. Among these 21, the average age was 1.37 years, similar to the average age of the entire population, which was 1.17 years.

## CRIMINALITY

In 14 of 33 families with severe abuse or neglect, at least one of the primarily involved adults had a criminal record. This is exclusive of any criminal proceedings that occurred after the severe injury.

## PREVENTABILITY

The panel judged that 10 cases were preventable. Eighteen cases were either preventable or had perinatal risk factors that would have allowed early detection of risk. As already noted, recommendations were made for system change in 20 cases.

## CONCLUSIONS

*The conclusions drawn by the Board of Inquiry are as follows:*

1. Severe child maltreatment is expensive.
2. Severe child maltreatment is concentrated among very young children.
3. A large proportion of cases have detectable risk factors and even more should be preventable.
4. Live-in boyfriends are especially dangerous to toddlers.
5. The large number of families with criminal backgrounds indicates that preventive programs should be directed at criminal populations.
6. There is approximately one permanently handicapped survivor for each child who dies. Half of the survivors are permanently disabled and lost from the ranks of productive citizenship.
7. A large proportion of cases involve perinatal risk factors that could facilitate early recognition of risk for severe maltreatment.

8. If even a small number of severe but nonfatal cases were prevented, a preventive program would be highly cost-effective.

9. *Prevention programs should be targeted toward:*
   Newborns and very young children
   Newborns with perinatal risk factors
   Infants who are not receiving medical care
   Infants who are not brought for follow-up medical treatments
   Families with live-in boyfriends
   Families with criminal records

## THE ST. LOUIS CHILD ABUSE NETWORK STUDY, PHASE TWO

In addition to the first phase case review that was done by the Board of Inquiry, the second phase of the St. Louis Child Abuse Network Study was a case-control study of fatal versus mildly abusive versus nonabusive families.

### APPROACH

The cases evaluated by the Board of Inquiry were subjected to further analysis. This consisted of having the investigating case worker complete a lengthy family assessment questionnaire. Because this data form was designed before the Board of Inquiry's review, the lessons learned in that review were not incorporated. It was, however, based on modifications of a comprehensive family assessment data form developed at Brandeis University and considered as a means of computerizing social service information by the Missouri DFS.

Control subjects were selected as follows. The Missouri Division of Vital Statistics provided a list of birth-date–matched and zip-code–matched children and addresses for cases substantiated as mild abuse cases plus similarly matched cases with no record of abuse. There were three groups for comparison: severe abuse, mild abuse, and no abuse.

Investigations were done by off-duty investigators. They completed the same family assessment questionnaires used for severe abuse families. The nonabuse families were requested to give informed consent. The families were approached in sequential order according to their rank on the list. The nonabuse control families were paid for their time and were highly cooperative.

The data forms were subsequently entered into a computerized database (Dbase III) and analyzed with Abstat, a commercially available statistical package, using an IBM/AT personal computer.

### RESULTS

Overall, there were few differences found between the mild and severe abuse cases. However, the information regarding arrest records and the presence of paramours was incomplete. Among the severe cases, 15 of 33 families were known to contain a paramour from the Board of Inquiry's case review, whereas in the long data form, only two of 24 families had a paramour designated.

### SOCIAL CLASS

Even though the controls were matched by the child's date of birth and zip code, differences in social class were apparent in the early analyses. The parents' educational levels differed significantly ($p<0.0206$). The educational levels were 11.4, 9.7, and 13.8 years for the severe, mild, and nonabuse groups, respectively. The total income of control cases was also significantly higher than among abuse cases. There were no significant differences between mild and severe abuse cases. Food stamps were received by 16 of the severe abuse families, 17 of the mild abuse families, and only one of the nonabuse families. Medicaid distribution was similar, with 52% of severe families, 76% of mild families, but only 3% (1/34) of nonabuse families receiving this entitlement ($p<0.0000$). This raises the question of why more of the severely abusive families did not have Medicaid. Based on average income, they all should have qualified.

## PERINATAL ISSUES

The parents of the nonabuse controls were older than the abusive parents ($p<0.0008$). The ages of the parent groups were 24.40 years for the severe, 24.94 for the mild, and 30.18 for nonabuse groups, respectively. Even though teenage parents were rare among abusive parents, more abusive parents first became parents during their teens.

Only one mother who perpetrated severe abuse did not receive prenatal care. Although this variable did not achieve statistical significance, it should be retained for comparison with future studies. The prenatal care of nonabusive mothers typically began earlier in the pregnancy (mean = 1.9 months) than did the care of abusive mothers. The related variable length of prenatal care corroborated the findings from the month of onset of prenatal care.

## THE CHILDREN

The section that provided a problem scale for children revealed few differences. Significant differences were found in only two of 42 items.

## CAREGIVER PROBLEMS

Adult problems were readily detected and there were many significant differences. Items considered included childhood, isolation, anxiety, depression, somatic complaints, substance abuse, and history of arrest. Areas of job training and employment were also considered.

## Childhood

A surprising number of abusive caretakers reported living away from their parents during childhood. In fact, this was one of the most strongly significant findings ($p<0.0002$) with 4/20 of the severe, 9/15 of the mild, and 2/30 nonabusive caregivers living away from their parents during childhood.

## Isolation

Isolation of the caregiver was readily identified, but did not indicate the extent of risk. Significant differences were found for the question regarding membership in a church, social club, or similar organization. This differentiates between abusive and nonabusive families ($p<0.0008$), but not between mild and severe abusive situations.

The question "Have you requested help from an agency?" elicited a high frequency of *yes* responses from both severe (11/16) and mild (17/22) abusive groups versus nonabuse controls (7/30) and was highly significant ($p<0.0002$). Interestingly, 11 of the severe abuse group, 19 of the mild abuse group, and six of the nonabuse group answered *yes* to the question "Did you receive help from an agency?" ($p<0.0001$). This indicates inconsistency in the data collection, but it also raises the possibility that the severe abuse group was less successful in getting help than the mild abuse group.

## Substance Abuse

Inquiry regarding drinking problems for the primary caregiver had a unique pattern. There were no differences between the severely abusive group and nonabusive controls, but the mildly abusive families reported more problems than the other two groups. Confirmation is required to ensure that this discrepancy was not a statistical (random) artifact. The differences in reported drug use among primary caregivers did not reach statistical significance, but most of the severely abusive families indicated that this was a problem. There was no difference in the drug use inquiries among the primary caregivers.

## Employment

The item phrased "(Do you) have trouble getting or keeping a job?" revealed marked differences between abusive and nonabusive groups. For primary caregivers, no differences were seen between mild and severe abuse groups, but both groups reported much more difficulty than nonabusive primary caregivers. The mild abuse group reported the most trouble keeping a job, the severe abuse group was intermediate, and the nonabuse group had the least trouble.

## Arrests and Convictions

Questions regarding arrests for assault showed significant differences among primary but not secondary caregivers. *This item was the single major difference between severe and mildly abusive families.* Although there were no differences on *yes/no* items to the question "Have you ever been arrested for disturbing the peace?" there were differences in the number of times that individuals had been arrested for this problem ($p<0.0351$), with the severely abusive group having been arrested most often. Data on arrests for drunk and disorderly conduct did not differ, nor did the data for sex offenses. Combining the arrest variables added little. The variable "any arrest" was mildly significant ($p<0.0311$).

Total convictions among primary caregivers did not achieve statistical significance ($p<0.1249$) because several of the controls had been convicted. There were no differences among the secondary caregivers. Similarly, the factor "served time" was not significant ($p<0.1226$). A more discriminating item might be advisable.

*Family violence* in the caregiver's family was highly significant, even when "don't know" responses were excluded. Family violence was found in 4/14 of the severe, 6/10 of the mild, and 7/34 of the nonabusive groups. Caregivers' mothers had criminal records in one severe case and two mild cases but in none of the controls.

The item "physical fight" was based on the question "Have you ever had a physical fight with your mate?" This also generated significant differences ($p<0.0001$) between abusive and nonabusive families but not between mild and severe abuse groups. A majority of both mild and severe abusive couples reported having physical fights.

## CONCLUSIONS FROM CASE CONTROL STUDY

*The conclusions drawn by the Board of Inquiry from the control phase were as follows:*

1. Abusive families differ statistically from nonabusive families in many regards. Poverty-related, social class differences are most prevalent and obvious.

2. Severely abusive and mildly abusive families share the same demographic features and are largely indistinguishable. In fact, mildly abusive families often had more adverse scores than severely abusive families.

3. Currently, there are no criteria that allow one to differentiate degrees of risk for severe versus mild abuse. The most promising items seem to relate to caregivers' previous demonstrations of aggression and physical violence, especially arrests for assault. More items that reflect aggressive behaviors during the caregivers' childhood should amplify this set of factors.

## THE EWIGMAN AND KIVLAHAN STUDY

Ewigman and Kivlahan (1990) investigated the causes of death as a result of injury in children ages birth through 5 years in Missouri and suggested a new way to classify child injury fatalities and the childhood surveillance system. The study excluded occupant motor vehicle fatalities and children who were injured in other states and died in Missouri. They reviewed the records of 314 children whose deaths were attributed to injury as noted on death certificates and the deaths of 20 children who were determined to be victims of child abuse or neglect (substantiated by the Missouri DFS), but whose deaths were determined to be of natural causes on the death certificate. The study was to determine how children in Missouri die from injuries and whether child abuse was underreported or misclassified.

The study reviewed death certificates, birth certificates, DFS records, Federal Bureau of Investigation statistics, autopsy records, medical records, and legal records, as well as arrest, charge, or prosecution records.

"Accident" was listed as the manner of death on the death certificate of 222 of the 334 children in the study. Twenty cases had "natural" and 58 had "homicide" listed as the cause of death. Twenty-four cases had "undetermined" as the cause of death.

Ewigman and Kivlahan stated that death certificates do not provide the necessary information about child injuries or child abuse and cited two sample cases, as follows:

*A 4-year-old boy was struck by a motor vehicle on a residential street while riding his bicycle. He had a skull fracture and severe brain injury. The death was listed as an accident on the death certificate. The codes listed on the death certificate included skull fracture and motor vehicle traffic injury. No other information was on file with DFS or the State Bureau of Investigation, and there was no legal follow-up. Further investigation revealed that the 4-year-old had been allowed to ride his bicycle in the street, unsupervised, while the caregiver was several houses away from the event, drinking alcohol. This injury was not the result of an accident. The event was predictable, caused by neglect and lack of supervision.*

*A 2-year-old died from severe burns sustained in a residential fire. The manner of death listed on the death certificate was accidental, and the codes included house fire and burns. Further investigation revealed that the mother had left the child alone with a 6-year-old sibling while she went to the store for cigarettes. The trailer was heated by leaving the lit gas oven door open. The mother was convicted of endangering the welfare of a child and was sentenced to several years' probation. This event was also predictable and caused by neglect and lack of supervision.*

Ewigman and Kivlahan assigned a behavioral cause of death to all of the cases studied. The categories assigned were inflicted injuries, unmet needs, exposure to hazards, unrecognized hazards, and inadequate information. Forty percent of the cases could not be given a behavioral cause of death because they were inadequately investigated, inadequately documented, or both. The authors felt that this, alone, was an indictment of the system of investigating and classifying child fatalities.

About one-third of the cases fell under the category "exposure to hazards," which included electrocution by unsafe appliances, drownings, fire hazards, and gun hazards. Many of the children who died as a result of exposure to hazards were unsupervised or were supervised by caregivers who were influenced by mind- or mood-altering substances.

One-fifth of the deaths resulted from inflicted injuries or homicides. The injuries were inflicted by caregivers, 71% of whom were arrested. Two-thirds of those arrested were found guilty. Most were charged with murder, one with abuse of a child, and six with endangering the welfare of a child. One-third of the perpetrators were sentenced to 5 years or less, one-third 6 to 20 years, and one-third to more than 20 years.

Five percent of the deaths resulted from unmet needs, involving children left without food and protection. Three percent of the deaths resulted from unrecognizable hazards. The deaths were unpredictable and uncontrollable, even with adequate supervision.

This study demonstrated that many childhood deaths are inadequately investigated. Many children are dying from common household hazards resulting from inadequate supervision, and more are dying from child abuse and neglect.

*Ewigman and Kivlahan made three recommendations as a result of their study:*

1. All child fatalities must be reviewed to gain an understanding of child abuse-related deaths.

2. These reviews must arise at the state level so as to identify and correct systemic deterrents that failed to protect a child and to ensure a coordinated approach to the problem.

3. The review committee must have access to all relevant records, including social services reports, court documents, police records, autopsy records, mental health records, and hospital- or medical-related data.

## RECOMMENDATIONS OF TASK FORCE ON FATAL CHILD ABUSE

Based on the Ewigman and Kivlahan study, a task force was formed to make recommendations about what can be done to decrease the death rate from homicides and injuries caused by neglect of children in Missouri.

The Missouri Department of Social Services' Task Force on Fatal Child Abuse reviewed procedures followed by other states and heard testimony from numerous experts.

*As a result they made the following recommendations (Steinmetz, 1990):*

1. Establish child death review teams in every county of the state to determine the cause of suspicious deaths of children under 15 (now 17) years of age.

2. The cases investigated by the team are referred by the coroner/medical examiner.

3. A protocol defining suspicious circumstances is established by the Department of Social Services.

4. The county team includes the coroner/medical examiner, prosecutor, sheriff or police officer, and representatives of the DFS, the juvenile court, and the county health department. The prosecutor chairs the team.

5. Establish regional death review teams, with expertise in child death review, to aid local teams in detecting child abuse.

6. Establish a state death review team to review reports from the county teams, identify system problems, and suggest ways to prevent child abuse deaths. The state-wide team gathers data from the local and regional teams and submits an annual report to the governor.

7. Require autopsies of children in all deaths not attributed to well-documented accidents or to previously diagnosed fatal illnesses.

8. Require all health practitioners, law enforcement officials, social service personnel, and any other person with responsibility for the care of children to report the death of any child under the age of 15 (now 17) years to the coroner/medical examiner.

9. Allow unsubstantiated reports of abuse and neglect to remain available to the DFS and to law enforcement authorities for a period of 10 years. The records would be closed to all other persons.

10. Relax confidentiality restrictions between certain parties when it is in the best interests of the child.

11. Require the Department of Health to develop guidelines for physicians and hospitals to identify suspicious deaths.

## MISSOURI CHILD FATALITY REVIEW PROJECT

In 1991 Missouri legislators enacted House Bill #185, which created the Child Fatality Review Project. The bill mandates multidisciplinary investigations of deaths of children (**Table 23-4**). The aim of such legislation is to establish a multidisciplinary approach to investigating child fatalities. It provides for improved investigations of child deaths, which improves accuracy in reporting the cause of death, and offers advice regarding means of preventing childhood injuries and fatalities.

## Table 23-4. Mandated Activities for Child Fatalities

Every county must have a multidisciplinary child fatality review panel (114 counties and City of St. Louis).

The county panel must consist of at least the following six core members: prosecuting attorney, coroner/medical examiner, law enforcement representative, DFS representative, public health representative, and juvenile officer.

All deaths of children age birth to 14 years must be reported to the coroner/medical examiner.

Children age 1 week to 1 year who die in a sudden, unexplained manner must have an autopsy.

A state child fatality review panel must meet at least two times per year.

Panels must use uniform protocols and data collection forms.

Certified child-death pathologists must perform the autopsies.

## PROGRAM ACCOMPLISHMENTS

The program established, under the Department of Social Services, a State Technical Assistance Team (STAT) to coordinate activities, train panel members, develop protocols, collect data, and determine the criteria for child fatality review (**Table 23-5**). STAT developed a fatality data collection system that gathers detailed information not previously available regarding childhood deaths and links data from the county panels with birth and death certificates. In addition, STAT trained a large group of professionals to use a multidisciplinary approach to investigate children's deaths and trained selected panel members in skills such as forensic interviewing and death scene investigation. STAT developed tools for panel members to use during investigations. These included a crime scene checklist to ensure that pertinent aspects of an investigation are performed consistently, protocols to improve photography and sketches of the scene, and improved interviewing techniques to deal with victims, witnesses, and suspects.

## Table 23-5. Criteria for Child Fatality Review

| | |
|---|---|
| Possible inflicted injury. | Unexplained death or death in an undetermined manner. |
| Any firearm injury. | Suspected sexual assault. |
| Injury not witnessed by person in charge of child at time of the injury/event. | Other suspicious findings (describe). |
| Possible inadequate supervision. | Death due to confinement. |
| Sudden, unexplained death of a child under age 1 year. | Bathtub/bucket drowning. |
| Natural cause of death possibly due to malnutrition or to delay in seeking medical care. | Suffocation/strangulation. |
| Open DFS protection service case on victim. | Any poisoning. |
| Victim in DFS custody. | Severe unexplained injury. |
| Pedestrian driveway injury. | Prior DFS substantiation of child abuse or neglect of the victim or other children in the residence for similar circumstances. |

They improved the appropriate use and availability of autopsies. The Missouri Medicaid program paid for autopsies on eligible children and thereby assured that a county's financial status or a victim's socioeconomic status did not affect the quality or availability of this crucial component of the death investigation. In addition, program facilitators organized a state-wide group of pathologists specially trained to ensure the appropriate performance of autopsies. They arranged annual education programs to keep members informed of policies, provide current practice updates, and offer a forum for professional interchange.

Finally, the Department of Social Services appointed an eight-member state advisory panel to review all of the data and to recommend systemic improvements. The advisory group met every 6 months.

## CHILD FATALITY FINDINGS (JANUARY TO SEPTEMBER 1992)

The following is the first report from the DFS and the Commissioner of Health.

The Missouri Child Fatality Review Project has produced important information about the causes of childhood deaths and revealed details of child abuse deaths.

It has successfully addressed the problem of unreported childhood deaths caused by abuse or neglect. The panels reviewed 172 child deaths in the first 9 months of 1992. The number of deaths of children under 14 years of age in which officials have confirmed abuse or neglect nearly doubled since enactment of the bill. Investigators confirmed 84% more child deaths from abuse and neglect in 1992 than for the same period in 1989.

During the first 9 months of 1992, 765 Missouri children under the age of 15 years died. Most of the deaths (566) had nonsuspicious cause and were not referred for further review.

Seventy-nine percent of all deaths resulted from sudden infant death syndrome and other natural causes. A majority (335 infants) died in the first month of life, primarily of natural conditions such as premature birth. While approximately one-third of Missouri's children are less than 5 years old, 80% of those who died were in this age group. Among injury-related deaths for children less than 1 year of age, homicide was the leading cause of death (52%). For all children under the age of 15 years, motor vehicle accidents were the most common cause of injury-related deaths (39%).

Lack of supervision was a major factor leading to death in reviewed cases. For example, 41% (70) of children among reviewed cases were not supervised by adults at the time of injury leading to death.

Of the children who died, 40% were Medicaid eligible, while only 25% of all Missouri children are eligible for Medicaid.

Most of the children who died from injuries, homicide, and sudden unexplained death were living with unmarried parents, with mothers having less than a high school education, and in environments with conspicuous alcohol or drug abuse.

Homicide was the number one cause of injury deaths in children younger than 1 year. Homicide victims are more likely to be poor and racial minorities.

## CHILD ABUSE AND NEGLECT DEATHS

The program's most striking finding was the sharp increase in the number of child abuse and neglect fatalities confirmed by the DFS. The number of substantiated fatalities rose from 25 cases in 1989 to 46 cases in 1992, an 84% increase. This increase reflects more cases being brought to official attention through the panel review process. During this period the DFS did not change the investigative criteria for substantiation of abuse or neglect.

Of the fatal child abuse cases substantiated by the DFS, 36% of the children died of physical abuse, 53% died as a result of neglect, 9% were medically neglected, and 2% were sexually maltreated.

## AUTOPSIES

The autopsy is a critical component in determining the cause of death. For example, diagnosing sudden infant death syndrome (SIDS) requires an autopsy to exclude other causes of death, such as intracranial bleeding from shaken infant syndrome. Since the law mandated that all children 1 week to 1 year of age who died in a sudden, unexplained manner have an autopsy performed, for the first time, 100% of Missouri children dying from SIDS had an autopsy. In past years, as many as 13% of the deaths attributed to SIDS (in 1987) were not autopsied.

Although the law mandated autopsies in certain cases, the overall number of autopsies for children from birth through age 14 did not change significantly from 1989 to 1992. Rather than causing more autopsies to be performed, this legislation fostered more appropriate use of this procedure. The autopsy rate for SIDS, accidents, and reviewed deaths increased, while the rate for motor vehicle accidents decreased. The majority (81%) of cases requiring panel review were autopsied, while 40% of nonreviewed cases were autopsied.

The review process and the reimbursement incentive significantly increased the number of autopsies performed on Medicaid children. While Medicaid reimbursement for autopsies ensured that eligible children who die will receive autopsies when necessary, there is a need to fund autopsies for children not covered by Medicaid. Autopsy cost is a significant burden on counties with few financial resources. The performance of autopsies should be based on the needs in each specific case, not on county or family finances.

## OTHER BENEFITS OF THE PROJECT

Although the project was initiated to detect deaths caused by child abuse and neglect, the program has made the state aware of, and has precipitated interest in, other major causes of childhood mortality, such as SIDS, unintentional injuries, and infant deaths resulting from premature births.

As a result of this review, more than 2,500 county and state workers have better knowledge and skills for reviewing childhood deaths, hopefully increasing the likelihood that future children's deaths will be appropriately explained.

The number and quality of autopsies performed on children have improved through the organization of a group of specially trained pathologists.

The availability of autopsies for low-income children has increased through Medicaid reimbursement for eligible children. This ensures that economic status is no barrier to investigations of child deaths.

The Child Fatality Review Project links many data sources into a single comprehensive system, which depicts deaths caused by child abuse or neglect better than any previous system did.

## RECOMMENDATIONS

*The state advisory panel reviewed all of the data accumulated by the review panels and recommended the following improvements:*

1.  The state should continue allotting resources to facilitate community change.

    Consideration should be given to extending the comprehensive, multidisciplinary approach used for reviewing child deaths to other social and health problems such as cases of sexual abuse.

2.  Improve caregiver supervision through education and better access to child care services.

To prevent injuries and deaths resulting from lack of supervision, parents and caregivers need age-appropriate information on the behavior and needs of children, access to day care, and parent training.

3. Educate investigators about the importance of accurately recording the level of supervision and circumstances surrounding the death of the child.

   A significant number of children's deaths were investigated without determination of supervision status. Without this crucial knowledge, neglectful situations may be missed.

4. Monitor families at risk of a second preventable death or injury and provide them with services.

   Surviving children in the same family or household are often at risk for morbidity and mortality. Case coordinators should be trained to follow through on services recommended by county panels for high-risk families.

5. Fund autopsies for the highest risk children.

   Medicaid reimbursement for autopsies increased the utilization of this important procedure for eligible children. The state should provide additional funds to finance autopsies for children not covered by Medicaid.

6. Implement a strategy aimed at reducing injuries and preventable deaths.

   The data from this project define how and why children are dying in Missouri. The state should develop prevention strategies with the collaboration of hospitals, health departments, schools, social service agencies, and community organizations to reduce injuries and preventable deaths in children.

---

THE MANUAL ON THE FOLLOWING PAGES WAS PREPARED BY THE MISSOURI STATE TECHNICAL ASSISTANCE TEAM AS A GUIDE IN INVESTIGATION. THE ENCLOSED PROTOCOLS AND CHECKLISTS WERE DEVELOPED AS INVESTIGATIVE AIDS.

NOTE: The forms for Death-Scene Investigative Checklist for Child Fatalities, Child Fatality Review Panel Data Report, and Coroner/medical Examiner Data Report are reproduced in Chapter 24 on pages 516 to 530.

## ◆MISSOURI CHILD FATALITY REVIEW PROGRAM– PROTOCOLS & PROCEDURES

MISSOURI DEPARTMENT OF SOCIAL SERVICES
STATE TECHNICAL ASSISTANCE TEAM
*When a child dies...*

*The loss of a loved one...particularly a child...is perhaps the greatest loss an individual or family can experience. Many overwhelming feelings follow the death of a child—numbness, shock, pain, anger, guilt, loneliness, fear and more. This grief and sadness is a natural and normal reaction to an irreplaceable loss.*

*To better understand why and how our children die, the State of Missouri has implemented the Child Fatality Review Program. By reviewing child fatalities, we hope to identify causes and strategies that will ultimately lead to a reduction, in certain cases, of child fatalities. Missouri state law (RSMo 210.192) now requires that any child, birth through age 17, who dies from any cause, be reported to the coroner/medical examiner. The coroner/medical examiner is mandated to follow specific procedures concerning these fatalities. These include:*

- *All sudden, unexplained deaths of infants from one week to one year are required to be autopsied by a certified child-death pathologist. The most common question of parents, "Why did our baby die?" can really only be answered by having an autopsy performed. During an autopsy, the internal organs are examined. It is done in a professional manner so that the dignity of the child is maintained. The procedure will not prevent having an open casket at the funeral. Preliminary results may be available in a few days; however, the final report may take several weeks.*

- *In all other child deaths, the coroner/medical examiner is required to consult with a certified child-death pathologist regarding the circumstances of death. In some cases, an autopsy will be ordered.*

- *If the fatality meets certain criteria, the circumstances surrounding the death will be reviewed by the county child fatality review panel. Facts regarding the death are discussed by the professionals who serve on the panel. The represented agencies on the panel have a responsibility to contribute to a more accurate determination of the cause of death; they also try to identify ways to prevent future deaths from occurring. All information is kept confidential.*

*The Child Fatality Review Program is a true expression of child advocacy. Like you, we want to know why the death occurred. We will do everything we can to explain and help you understand why.*

## ◆ MISSOURI DEPARTMENT OF SOCIAL SERVICES STATE TECHNICAL ASSISTANCE TEAM (STAT)

### MISSION

Recognizing the importance of multi-disciplinary interaction in dealing with dysfunctional families, child abuse and neglect, the State Technical Assistance Team (STAT) facilitates cooperation and coordination among dissimilar organizations with shared responsibilities and mandates. (Department of Social Services [DSS], law enforcement, prosecutors, health, juvenile, coroners, medical professionals, educators, etc.). Recognizing that some agencies have dual roles and responsibilities (investigative/enforcement, protection, services, etc.), STAT acts as an intermediary to bring these purposes and groups together. By introducing these principles, STAT encourages communities to identify and address problems often avoided by those who lack the confidence to become involved. To build and maintain that confidence, STAT trains, supports and assists the field level investigative community that realistically converts policy into results. All evaluation/investigations are the responsibility of those disciplines mandated to be involved. As an integral part of the process, it is essential that Division of Family Services (DFS) form meaningful partnerships with other community services. STAT promotes this attitude of enhanced cooperation and coordination.

### RESPONSIBILITIES

■ Implement, support and institutionalize the Child Family Review Program (CFRP) (RSMo 210.192, 210.195, et al.).

— Develop and support an efficient and effective delivery system (regional coordinators, urban case coordinators, State CFRP panel, etc.).

— Train and maintain 115 county-based child fatality review panels.

— Provide services and assistance as necessary.

— Collect information and data that identifies patterns or risk.

— Encourage communities, organizations and agencies to develop deterrent and prevention strategies that reduce child injuries and fatalities.

■ Organize and develop multi-disciplinary teams to investigate serious sexual abuse involving children (RSMo 660.520, 660.526, 210.145, 210.180, et al.).

— Organize and train county-based child sexual abuse teams.

— Provide expertise and direct assistance in those cases that meet our criteria for involvement.

■ Be an accessible and responsive children's events informational resource (24 hours a day, 365 days a year, via 800 number) to the entire investigative community (DFS, law enforcement, coroner/medical examiners, prosecutors, juvenile court, health professionals, etc.).

— Answer specific procedural questions relative to the fatality and sexual abuse programs.

— Provide referral, technical and informational support concerning all child events (literature searches, medical consults, prosecution support, etc.) including physical abuse and other incidents outside the fatality and sexual abuse programs. We recognize that many child fatalities are the end result of uninterrupted patterns of abuse and neglect.

— Through its awareness programs, newsletter and injury prevention initiatives, STAT transforms field experience into data collection; data collection into useable information, and information into knowledge. Knowledge, along with experience, will help prevent future childhood injuries and fatalities.

Beyond the fatality and sexual abuse programs, STAT is perceived by many as an "omni-source" of information for the entire multi-disciplinary community of professionals dealing with child abuse and neglect events. All inquiries are addressed in some way.

## REFERRALS TO STAT

The Child Abuse and Neglect (CA/N) Hotline number, (800) 392-3738, should always be used to report incidents of suspected child abuse and neglect. If additional assistance is needed on specific cases, STAT is available as a resource for local multidisciplinary child fatality and child sexual abuse/assault investigations and training.

STAT has been designed to handle specific types of cases. Incoming phone calls will be screened based on the following criteria:

■ The investigation and review of child fatalities, birth through 17 years.

■ Child sexual abuse reports involving:

— Multiple victims/perpetrators

— Centers/homes for child care, at the request of the Out-of-Home Investigations (OHI) Unit

— Residential treatment facility, at the request of the OHI Unit

— Repeat offender/suspected perpetrator

— Complex issues (including but not limited to):

> Death or serious injury
> Suspected perpetrator is a law enforcement or city/county
>    official, or there is a potential conflict of interest
> Limited resources/expertise/manpower
> Cross-jurisdictional issues
> Ritualistic abuse

Cases meeting the above criteria and defined within RSMo 210.110 will be given priority over those that meet the above criteria but are not defined within RSMo 210.110.

It is recognized that child fatalities are often the result of uninterrupted patterns of abuse and neglect. As a prevention intervention, within the limits of its resources, STAT will provide the following services to multi-disciplinary teams or members:

- Technical information concerning any serious child event:

    — Medical consultations regarding injuries, illnesses or other maladies

    — Medical research/literature searches to substantiate or refute initial findings

All requests for technical medical consultation and/or research must be directed to STAT for authorization. Any costs incurred other than those specifically approved by STAT will be the responsibility of the requesting agency.

To assist prosecutors with complex child abuse and neglect cases, a PROSECUTORS PEER GROUP (made up of prosecutors experienced in children's events) has been formed to offer assistance and advice. This prosecutor-to-prosecutor support system may be accessed informally by phone. Every prosecutor will be made aware of this new service. Questions regarding this program should be directed to either STAT, (573) 751-5980; Division of Legal Services, (573) 751-3229 or the Missouri Office of Prosecution Services, (573) 751-2415.

A 24-hour toll-free number, (800) 487-1626, can be called if questions or investigative assistance is needed. From 8:00 a.m. to 5:00 p.m., Monday through Friday, all incoming phone calls will be received, screened and routed to an investigator if needed. After working hours, on holidays and weekends, calls will be directly received by an on-call investigator.

If requested by a local investigative team, STAT will arrange and provide training, phone consultation and, if necessary, direct assistance in an investigation. In the absence of a local team, individual disciplines may request STAT assistance by calling the toll-free number, (800) 487-1626.

> The State Technical Assistance Team's goal is to enhance the skills of the local investigative team. When STAT assistance is needed, it should be requested as soon as possible. The State Technical Assistance Team will respond in some way to all inquiries concerning the Child Fatality Review Program and child sexual abuse teams, as well as other serious abuse and neglect cases.

> County child fatality review panels are mandated by law (RSMo 210.192). Formation of a local multi-disciplinary team for the investigation of child sexual abuse is optional as is the adoption of the protocols. It is not necessary for a county to have a formal multi-disciplinary team to request assistance from the State Technical Assistance Team. However, it is preferred that a team be in place while the case is being worked. Requests may come from local multi-disciplinary teams, DFS, law enforcement agencies, prosecutors and other disciplines involved in children's events in any county.

## ◆ MISSOURI CHILD FATALITY REVIEW PROGRAM

### INTRODUCTION

In 1989 and 1990, a cooperative study by the Departments of Social Services and Health and the University of Missouri found that a significant number of child deaths (birth through age 5) were not being accurately reported. The study revealed the causes of death were also not being adequately investigated or identified. As a result of this study, a task force was appointed in August 1990 by Gary Stangler, Director of the Department of Social Services, to further study child fatalities. The task force made recommendations that became the basis for House Bill 185 (HB 185), which established a statewide county-based system of child fatality review panels. This bill was passed in May 1991 and signed into law by Governor John Ashcroft in June 1991. The law, RSMo 210.192, became effective August 28, 1991, and Missouri's Child Fatality Review Program (CFRP) was implemented on January 1, 1992.

RSMo 210.192, et al., require that every county in Missouri (114 counties and the City of St. Louis) establish a multi-disciplinary CFRP panel to examine the deaths of all children, birth through age 17, that occur in Missouri. Counties have been grouped into seven regions, and regional coordinators (who live and have primary jobs in the regions they represent) offer oversight, technical assistance and systemic evaluation to the counties in their region. The State Technical Assistance Team (STAT) assists the regions and individual panels with expert training and investigative assistance. A state-level panel provides oversight and makes recommendations for change and refinement to STAT.

RSMo 210.192, et al., provides a mechanism for the legal exchange of information between cooperating disciplines and agencies. Every child death is evaluated. If the death meets specific criteria, it is referred to the county's CFRP panel. Unlike an inquest, no vote or consensus of opinion is sought at the conclusion of the panel review. This is not an attempt to criminalize all child deaths, but to obtain a more accurate and timely determination of cause and appropriate response.

The CFRP panels consist of local community professionals who bring their own expertise and skills to the review and attempt to identify the cause and circumstances of child deaths. The value of the panel's work is measured by the improvement in the services provided by the individual participating disciplines. The collection and interpretation of resultant findings of a comprehensive review of child fatalities by each county can be used to determine trends, target prevention strategies, identify specific family/community needs or, when appropriate, support criminal justice intervention. The findings of each CFRP panel review are sent through established channels where they become valuable, retrievable statistics linked to Department of Health birth and death data. These statistics are reviewed by STAT and are used to identify issues, needs and prevention strategies on a statewide level.

While problem identification and resolution can be used for the public's benefit, specific case details are never divulged or discussed outside the panel meeting. Panel reviews are not open to the public. Each panel and its members are advocates for the health and welfare of every child in their community; this includes the reasonable preservation of privacy.

Training sessions for all panel members are held at different locations around the state. Regional in-service training is conducted annually. Individual panel training, both scheduled and upon county request, is provided as necessary. STAT also makes CFRP awareness and educational presentations to professional and community/civic organizations upon request.

Child fatality review panels, beginning with the coroner/medical examiner, shall evaluate all deaths of children, birth through age 17, that occur in Missouri. Those that meet the criteria established by RSMo 210.192 will be reviewed in detail by the panel in the county where the fatal illness/injury/event occurred.

## MISSION STATEMENT

We recognize that the responsibility for responding to and preventing child fatalities lies with the community, not with any single agency or entity. We recognize that promoting more accurate identification and reporting of childhood fatalities may result in the development of prevention strategies for all potentially fatal childhood events. Finally, we recognize that the implementation of child fatality review panels will lead to improved coordination of services for children and families.

## LONG-TERM GOALS

The long-term goals of this program include the development of a data base involving on-going surveillance of all childhood fatalities; continuous commitment to train each profession involved in the investigation of child fatalities; and initiation of state and local community prevention activities that respond to identified risks to children.

Questions concerning a particular investigation or Missouri's Child Fatality Review Program should be directed to STAT at (800) 487-1626. STAT is accessible and responsive 24 hours a day, via the 800 number, and all inquiries are addressed in some way.

## URBAN MODELS

Due to the volume and complexity of child death-related issues in the major urban areas (Jackson County, St. Louis County and St. Louis City), individual urban models have been created to address special requirements. While these panels do not have individual meetings for every reviewable death, they have information gathering and distribution systems that address the requirement for concurrent review. The review process begins with notification, not at the scheduled meeting.

Because the demands on the three major urban panels are so great, DFS provides full-time staffing to support their efforts. These Urban Case Coordinator (UCC) positions were created with the sole purpose of assisting the panels to meet their program objectives. Beyond offering staff assistance to the panels, the UCC coordinates community services and programs to benefit children and families and to reduce initial and repeat fatalities in the highest-risk settings. This follow-up and follow-through approach encourages the integration and coordination of services from the entire spectrum of community agencies.

## REGIONAL COORDINATORS

In order to help monitor and provide technical assistance to the statewide review system, the statute mandates the use of a regional coordinator network. For the purpose of implementing this network, the State of Missouri has been divided into seven regions, and each region has been assigned a regional coordinator. Other than the STAT managed urban areas, regional coordinators live in and have primary job responsibilities in the regions they represent.

The regional coordinators monitor, for completeness and consistency, the data generated from the local review panels in their region by:

- receiving and reviewing Data Form 1 (Coroner/Medical Examiner Data Report) and Data Form 2 (Child Fatality Review Panel Data Report) from the panel chairperson; signing and forwarding the forms to STAT.

- providing assistance to the local review panels, as needed, by collaborating with other panels in their areas; assisting front-line investigators and workers on the panel; and calling upon the services of the STAT chief investigator.

- when requested by local panels, attending review panel meetings within their region.

- identifying local panel training needs and communicating those needs to the STAT chief investigator.

- reviewing and analyzing data reports which reflect the comprehensiveness of each panel's reviews as compared with death certificate information.

## STAT Chief Investigator

The chief investigator is STAT's liaison with the regional coordinators. The chief investigator (based in Jefferson City) assists the regional coordinators and individual panels by providing expert training and investigative assistance. The chief investigator also makes recommendations to the STAT director concerning program issues.

## State Panel

Missouri statutes provide that a state-level child fatality review panel be appointed by the Department of Social Services. (The state CFRP panel is convened bi-annually to provide oversight, identify systemic problems and bring concerns to the attention of STAT.) The composition of the state panel mirrors that of the county panels; each multi-disciplinary profession is represented (including optional members).

- Coroner/Medical Examiner
- Law Enforcement
- Public Health
- Division of Family Services
- Juvenile Officer
- Prosecuting Attorney
- Emergency Medical Services
- Optional Member(s)

## Information Sharing

The panels are charged to evaluate and review all suspicious deaths of children who die in Missouri. This cannot be accomplished unless all information known to panel participants is shared during the review of a death, and it is each participant's legal obligation to do so fully.

Participants are expected to access all information related to the victim, victim's family, and/or persons and circumstances surrounding the death. This includes medical, hospital and Department of Mental Health records, except as provided in RSMo 630.167, which can be obtained by the coroner/medical examiner, public health and Division of Family Services (DFS) representatives. Concerning any reported death of a child (birth through age 17), the CFRP panel also has access to information that includes juvenile records, as provided in RSMo 211.321, and Division of Youth Services records, as provided in RSMo 219.061. Any legally recognized privileged communication, except that between attorney and client, shall not apply to situations involving the death of a child under the age of eighteen years, who is eligible to receive a certificate of live birth. (See "Excerpts from Missouri Laws," section 210.140.)

All information presented at the panel meeting should be considered lead information that needs to be confirmed by the individual discipline as true and factual before being included in any individual narrative reports. While reports and documents may be shared and reviewed at panel meetings, they should not be copied and distributed. Outside of the CFRP review, agencies may share reports consistent with their policies and other legal constraints. The only reports generated and maintained by the Child Fatality Review Program are Data Forms 1 and 2.

## CONFIDENTIALITY/MEETING CLOSURE POLICY

A proper panel review of a death requires a thorough examination of all relevant data, including historical information concerning the deceased child and his/her family. Much of this information is protected from disclosure by law, especially medical and child abuse/neglect information. Therefore, all meetings conducted, all reports and records made and maintained pursuant to sections 210.192 to 210.196 by the local child fatality review panel shall be confidential and not open to the general public. Panel members should also be aware that the legislation which established the child fatality review panels provides official immunity to all panel participants.

Each panel should appoint a media spokesperson. Requests or inquiries concerning panel meetings should be directed to the spokesperson. The spokesperson should limit his or her public statements to the fact that the panel met, and that each panel member was charged to implement their own professional mandates. In no case should any other information about the case or panel discussions be disclosed outside of the panel. Failure to observe this procedure may violate DFS regulations as well as confidentiality statutes that contain penalties.

Any panel member may make public statements about the general purpose or nature of the CFRP process as long as it is not identified to a specific case. The page at the beginning of the book, *"When a Child Dies..."* is an appropriate description for surviving parents and caregivers, as well as the media and public.

The following points may be useful in responding to more detailed inquiries concerning the Child Fatality Review Program:

- House Bill 185 was passed during the 1991 legislative session and implemented in January 1992. It requires that every county in Missouri (including the City of St. Louis) establish a multi-disciplinary panel to examine the deaths of all children, birth through age 17. If the death meets a specific criteria, it is referred to the county's multi-disciplinary CFRP panel. (Missouri is the only state that examines, or attempts to examine, every child death in every county–rural or urban.)

- The panels are not designed to criminalize all child deaths. Instead, the panels include local community professionals who attempt to identify the cause and circumstances of child deaths. The local community and state use the findings to determine trends, target prevention strategies, identify specific family and community needs or, when appropriate, support criminal justice interventions. Panel members may not disclose case-specific information obtained from the meeting.

- The CFRP panels do not act as investigative bodies. Their purpose is to enhance the knowledge base of the mandated investigators and to evaluate the potential service and preventive interventions for the family and community. But, in fulfilling their individual job requirements, certain panel members like the coroner, prosecuting attorney or Division of Family Services, may be directly involved in the investigation.

- Of all child deaths in Missouri in this age population (about 1,300-1,400 deaths annually), about one-third merit review. To come under review, the cause of the child's death must be unclear, unexplained or of a suspicious circumstance. All sudden, unexplained deaths of children, birth through age 1, are required to be reviewed by the CFRP panel.

- The CFRP expands and refines the traditional coroner/medical examiner system of reporting and investigating child deaths. The unique attribute of the CFRP is that all child deaths are evaluated, and those requiring it will be reviewed by a community panel. CFRP panels are made up of at least seven disciplines–each bringing his or her own expertise and skills to the case. The minimum core review panel membership for each county includes the following representatives:

— Coroner/medical examiner

— Law Enforcement

— Public Health

— Division of Family Services

— Juvenile Officer

— Prosecuting Attorney

— Emergency Medical Services

— Optional Member(s)

Each panel can call upon experts from the community on a per-case basis or to sit as permanent "optional" members of the panel. NOTE: The chairperson/media spokesperson for the panel may wish to mention the names of those who serve on the county's child fatality review panel.

■ The coroner/medical examiner of the county plays the key role in the initiation of the process for child fatality reviews. They must determine the need for an autopsy, fill out the appropriate forms and notify the child fatality review panel chairperson within 24 hours if the death meets certain criteria. The panel must then convene as soon as possible to review the information provided by its members.

■ The Department of Social Services, Division of Family Services' State Technical Assistance Team (STAT) based in Jefferson City serves as an information resource and technical-assistance provider for the 115 Missouri CFRP panels. The unit is accessible 24 hours a day, seven days a week to answer questions or provide on-site assistance.

■ If county-specific or statewide statistical data (such as leading causes of child death or number of substantiated child abuse and neglect deaths) is needed, you may wish to contact STAT at (800) 487-1626 to obtain current information.

## RECORD HANDLING

All official records generated by the county CFRP panel (CFRP Data Forms 1 and 2) will be forwarded through the regional coordinators to STAT, where they will be linked with Department of Health birth and death data. If the Child Fatality Review Program Worksheet is used, it should be destroyed by the coroner/medical examiner upon completion of the Data Form 1. No copies of completed CFRP Data Forms 1 and 2 should be maintained in local files.

## CERTIFIED CHILD-DEATH PATHOLOGIST NETWORK

Missouri's Certified Child-Death Pathologist Network ensures autopsies performed on children, birth through age 17, are performed by professionals with expertise in forensic pediatrics. Additionally, Network members are available to consult with coroners and others investigating child deaths. The pathologists in the Network are also eligible to be reimbursed for autopsies through STAT when the fatality is reviewed by the county CFRP panel. A description of the autopsy reimbursement procedure follows:

■ A signed contractual agreement between the certified child pathologist and the State of Missouri/Department of Social Services (DSS)/Child Fatality Review Program (CFRP) must be on file.

- For each autopsy performed by a certified child-death pathologist on a child, birth through age 17, the pathologist should complete the CFRP invoice and submit it and the full autopsy report, along with the death-scene investigative checklist, to the Child Fatality Review Program, P.O. Box 88, Jefferson City, MO 65103-0088.

- Upon receipt by STAT, the invoice, autopsy report and death-scene investigative checklist are matched with the appropriate Data Form 1. (Data Form 1's are required on all deaths in this age population and copies are maintained by STAT.) The Data Form 1 must be marked and signed as reviewable in order for the claim to be paid by DSS. A Data Form 2, containing information obtained from the review process, is to be completed and sent to the Regional Coordinator within 45 days.

- If the case meets program criteria, it will be paid by DSS. For each claim submitted, a form letter is generated and sent to the pathologist notifying him/her of the status of the claim; for example, the claim is being paid, the claim is not payable because the case was not reviewable, etc.

STAT notifies the Department of Health (DOH) of all suspected SIDS cases. Likewise, DOH informs STAT any time they receive a request for autopsy reimbursement on suspected SIDS cases. Communication between these offices ensures duplication of payment does not occur when the child is Medicaid eligible. DOH will pay for autopsies on suspected SIDS cases only when they are not Medicaid-eligible cases.

## MISSOURI CHILD FATALITY REVIEW PROGRAM COORDINATOR REGIONS

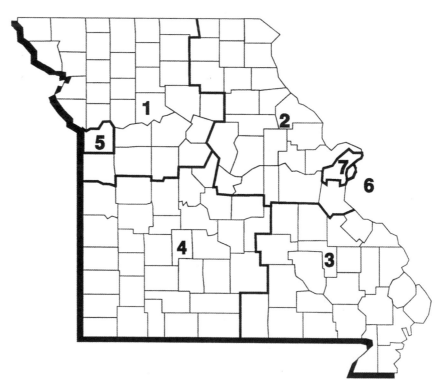

## ◆PANEL MEMBER ROLES

### CORE PANEL MEMBERS

The panel will be made up of a minimum of seven members. They will select their chairperson. When a panel vacancy occurs among non-elected officials, the panel chairperson should appoint a replacement with input and approval by the panel members. Should a chairperson vacancy occur, it should be filled as soon as possible by the panel. If not filled immediately, an interim chairperson should be elected by the panel.

Representatives of the following agencies are mandated to be members of this panel and may serve as long as they hold the position which made them eligible for appointment:

- Prosecuting attorney or circuit attorney
- Coroner or medical examiner
- Law enforcement personnel
- Representative from the Division of Family Services
- Representative of the Juvenile Court
- Provider of Public Health Care Services
- Emergency Medical Services representative

## OPTIONAL PANEL MEMBERS

Additional members may also be appointed to serve on the panel in a temporary or permanent capacity. An example of a case specific optional member might be a fire investigator who investigated a death by fire. In some cases, the involved DFS Children's Services worker may be required to appear and provide relevant information. A permanent optional member can be anyone that the panel believes brings value to the review process. It is the responsibility of the chairperson to notify and invite potential optional members. Optional members have full membership authority and rights.

Under certain circumstances, special investigation units (DFS Out-of-Home Investigative Unit, Department of Mental Health investigators, etc.) may be mandated to participate in child fatality investigations and may be valuable optional panel members. In all cases, their involvement should be coordinated with the primary investigators. It is the responsibility of the chairperson to make optional members aware of CFRP policies and procedures.

## PANEL RESPONSIBILITY

The purpose of bringing together this particular collection of professionals is to quickly gather the most comprehensive picture of the circumstances surrounding the child fatality/illness/injury/event. Each panel member is responsible for presenting any pertinent information their discipline has been able to gather on the case from their own system, asking questions to better understand the circumstances surrounding the death and making recommendations for further actions from the CFRP panel itself or other relevant parties. This enhanced information may draw different conclusions about the cause or circumstances of death than was indicated initially. The panel will also identify strategies (immediate and/or for the future through data collected from completion of Data Forms 1 and 2) which may prevent or reduce future fatalities.

The local review panels are encouraged to meet, at least annually, outside the normal review process for an evaluation of their progress. At this time, they may identify training needs, update protocols and seek technical assistance, if necessary. In addition, the panel should review local child fatalities to determine patterns and trends and develop prevention strategies.

## CHAIRPERSON ROLE

1. Accept the notification and report from the coroner/medical examiner of all deaths of children, birth through age 17.

2. Along with the coroner/medical examiner, make a determination on which cases should be reviewed by the local panel. Indicators for "reviewable deaths" are defined in Section B of Data Form 1. If ANY of these items are checked, the case is automatically reviewed by the panel.

3. The following factors may contribute to the decision to review the case:

- nature of death
- previous agency involvement
- insufficient information at initial review
- incompatibility of information regarding the death
- improvement in the recognition and prevention of child abuse
- recognition of a pattern of child abuse
- evaluation of system response

4. When appropriate, contact and invite potential optional members to panel meeting(s) and ensure that they, as well as new members, are aware of CFRP policies and procedures.

5. Co-sign **all** Coroner/Medical Examiner Data Reports (Data Form 1) and forward to the regional coordinator **within 48 hours** of death.

6. On reviewable deaths, ensure panel members are notified of the information regarding the child's death, and schedule a meeting as soon as practical after the death notification.

7. Make a courtesy call notifying the regional coordinator of the meeting time and location for the panel review.

8. Ensure information from investigative reports, medical records, autopsy reports and other relevant items is made available to panel members at the meeting.

9. Chair the meeting of the panel.

10. Sign **all** Child Fatality Review Panel Data Reports (Data Form 2) and send to the regional coordinator **within 45 days** of the date of death.

11. Identify strategies for the prevention of child deaths and serious injuries.

12. Observe local county patterns or trends in circumstances of death.

13. Oversee adherence to the panel review process.

14. At the annual evaluation meeting, review with members the types of child deaths the chairperson did not send for panel review.

## Prosecuting Attorney Role

1. Provide legal opinions, definitions and explanations.

2. Obtain criminal history as appropriate to the case.

3. Provide assistance/guidance to:

- initiate investigations
- determine if there is any pending criminal investigation
- provide assistance and communication between participating agencies as needed

4. Serve as liaison with prosecuting attorneys within the state and nationwide as needed.

5. Serve as liaison with other legal entities involved in the review of this fatality (e.g., city attorney, county counsel).

6. Provide feedback on cases that enter the criminal justice system. Track cases through the system.

7. Identify strategies for the prevention of child deaths and serious injuries.

## CORONER/MEDICAL EXAMINER ROLE

1. (PRIORITY) Go to the scene and conduct a death-scene evaluation/ investigation.

2. Refer all appropriate cases to the certified child-death pathologist to determine need for an autopsy. If an autopsy is required, ensure the Death-Scene Investigative Checklist is completed and accompanies the body to the certified child-death pathologist.

3. Obtain reports of all deaths of children, birth through age 17, that occur in their jurisdiction. Notify coroner/medical examiner in county of illness/ injury/event, if applicable. NOTE: Both of these may be accomplished by completing the Child Fatality Review Program Worksheet; however, some cases may require immediate notification.

4. Contact the DFS Central Registry Unit (CRU), Child Abuse and Neglect Hotline, (800) 392-3738, to:

   ■ notify the division of all deaths of children, birth through age 17

   ■ determine if there is a prior history of abuse and neglect

5. Complete the Coroner/Medical Examiner Data Report (Data Form 1) on all deaths of children, birth through age 17. Destroy Child Fatality Review Program Worksheet upon completion of Data Form 1 (if information was obtained from the Child Fatality Review Program Worksheet).

6. Refer Data Form 1 to chairperson of the CFRP panel for co-signature on all cases.

7. Provide forensic information to the panel including autopsy and investigative reports.

8. Provide interpretation for the panel of the cause and manner of death.

9. Assist law enforcement and other agencies involved with the death investigation.

10. Identify strategies for the prevention of child deaths and serious injuries.

## LAW ENFORCEMENT ROLE

1. As necessary, assist the coroner/medical examiner in conducting a death scene evaluation/investigation.

2. Provide reports containing witness information and witness statements.

3. Provide scene photographs, latent and physical evidence, measurements and sketches.

4. Provide background information on involved parties. Conduct further inquiry as suggested by panel (criminal history, prior complaints).

5. Provide suspect information.

6. Serve as a liaison with other law enforcement agencies locally, at the state level and across state lines.

7. Identify strategies for the prevention of child deaths and serious injuries.

The duties of the officer at the death scene are to interview, document and photograph the scene of death and assist the coroner in determining the cause, manner and mode of death. If other children are present, the officer should assess their safety and, if necessary, take immediate steps to protect them from imminent danger. As soon as possible, contact juvenile authorities and the Child Abuse/Neglect Hotline (800) 392-3738.

## DIVISION OF FAMILY SERVICES ROLE

1. Provide investigation and intervention as appropriate.

2. Provide records and information (past or present) involving the child or family.

3. Complete investigation of the child abuse and neglect report and assist law enforcement in its investigation for possible criminal action.

4. Interview siblings and children in the home, if there are any, and others as needed for protection of surviving siblings and children.

5. Provide follow up and support for surviving family members in abusive high-risk families with surviving children.

6. Serve as liaison with counterparts locally, in other counties and at the state level.

7. Identify strategies for the prevention of child deaths and serious injuries.

## JUVENILE OFFICER ROLE

1. As necessary, provide protection of siblings and other children in the home.

2. Assist in the investigation as appropriate.

3. Keep the juvenile court informed of developments affecting the family and children.

4. Provide background information and records on the family.

5. Identify strategies for the prevention of child deaths and serious injuries.

## PUBLIC HEALTH ROLE

1. Serve as a liaison with the medical community. Contact primary care provider (if known) regarding fatality review.

2. Assist in the discovery and review of previous health care/medical records from both public and private sources.

3. Assist in completing birth certificate forms (when applicable) and provide vital statistics data as appropriate.

4. Serve as a liaison and make referrals to health-based prevention/intervention systems (e.g., hospital teams, public health nursing).

5. Use data and case histories from the child fatality review to assist in the development of prevention programs with high risk populations.

6. As the designated CFRP prevention liaison, identify strategies for the prevention of child deaths and serious injuries and encourage implementation of these strategies.

**To assist the public health representative on the child fatality review panel, a physician's role, as an optional member, could include the following:**

1. Provide expertise regarding normal infant and childhood growth and development.

   ■ Interpret the findings of cases in the context of normal growth and development.

   ■ Assist in the identification of cases where findings are inconsistent with normal growth and development.

2. Provide expertise in the expected course of disease and medical conditions of infancy and childhood and assist in the interpretation of case findings in this context.

3. Provide expertise in the expected outcome and complications of various treatments and interpret case findings in this context.

4. Provide expertise in the area of community standards of medical care.

5. Serve as a liaison with the medical community. Contact the child's primary care provider (if known) to obtain appropriate medical history.

6. Assist in the discovery and review of other previous health care/medical records.

7. Provide the panel with current and pertinent medical information literature.

## EMERGENCY MEDICAL SERVICES ROLE

1. Assist in investigation by awareness of proper scene management of evidence, documentation of death scene observations and spontaneous statements.

2. Provide and verify information for the Death-Scene Investigative Checklist.

3. Notify coroner/medical examiner of deaths of children, birth through age 17. Complete the Child Fatality Review Program Worksheet or other checklists, if appropriate.

4. Serve as a liaison with hospitals and the medical community.

5. Assist in the discovery and review of previous health care/medical records relevant to the EMS function.

6. Identify strategies for the prevention of child deaths and serious injuries.

# ♦ORGANIZATIONAL PROCEDURES

## ELECTION OF CHAIRPERSON

The panel will elect its own chairperson who is responsible for convening the review panel. The chairperson can be elected from either the core or optional panel members. The chairperson will need to function in a neutral capacity on the panel. Should a chairperson vacancy occur, it should be filled as soon as possible by the panel. If not filled immediately, an interim chairperson should be elected. Local panels may choose to rotate the chairperson role by setting specific term limits. If the panel needs assistance in filling panel vacancies, contact STAT.

## TERMS OF OFFICE

The seven core panel members mandated by law may serve as long as they hold the position which made them eligible for an appointment to the local review panel. All subsequent appointments to the review panel will be made by the chairperson with input from the panel and the discipline in question and with the approval of the panel members.

## LENGTH OF TERM

The chairperson and all members may serve as long as they hold the position that made them eligible for an appointment and choose to remain a panel member.

## REMOVAL OF MEMBERS

If a panel member misses three consecutive meetings without good cause, or because of death, resignation, mental or physical incapacitation which limits the member from effectively serving, or for good cause as determined by a majority vote of the local review panel, they shall be removed from the child fatality review panel. The chairperson will notify the panel member of the action of the panel.

## AUTHORIZED DESIGNEES

If a panel member is unable to attend a review meeting, they may send an appropriate authorized designee in their place. The intention of this option is to accommodate the difficulties members may have in making every review meeting. It will not be useful to the panel to have a continually changing membership; when possible, a permanent designee should be selected.

An authorized designee will have full privileges and responsibilities of the panel member they represent.

## MEETING ATTENDANCE

**ALL** members should be notified and encouraged to attend scheduled CFRP panel meetings and reviews. If a member is unable to attend, when possible, the authorized designee should be substituted. In **ALL** cases, information concerning the review should be obtained from the non-attending member.

## ◆ THE REVIEW PROCESS

### DEFINING LIVE BIRTH

A birth is considered viable and "live" if the attending medical person determines that a birth certificate is appropriate. If a birth certificate is not issued and a determination of "stillbirth" is made, evaluation and review by the CFRP panel is not required.

Non-attended births under unusual or suspicious circumstances, where the **possibility** of a live birth exists, are appropriate for CFRP panel evaluation and review. The coroner/medical examiner should be notified and an autopsy considered. If an autopsy is performed and there are findings indicating a live birth, a birth certificate can be obtained.

**All questions concerning birth certification (unattended and/or in-home births) should be directed to the local health department representative or the Missouri Department of Health, Bureau of Vital Records (314) 751-6381.**

### PURPOSE OF THE REVIEW PROCESS

The following process is initiated on **all** deaths of children, from birth through age 17, that occur in Missouri. The purpose of this review process is to provide accurate information and consistent reporting on all deaths of children in this age group. Reviews will always be conducted by the CFRP panel in the county where the illness/injury/event occurred. (**NOTE:** CFRP panels may review out-of-state deaths, if the illness/injury/event that lead to the death occurred in Missouri, but it is not required.) In those situations when the death meets the criteria for review, the review process will effectively assemble the most comprehensive set of information surrounding the case for a more accurate determination of cause of death.

### FORMS INVOLVED

- Death-Scene Investigative Checklist for Child Fatalities (To accompany the body to the certified child-death pathologist)

- Child Fatality Review Program Worksheet (Optional)

- Coroner/Medical Examiner Data Report (Data Form 1)

- Child Fatality Review Panel Data Report (Data Form 2)

### PERSONS INVOLVED

The seven core panel members or their authorized designees and any optional panel members in the county where the illness/injury/event occurred review the case.

### NOTIFICATION OF DEATH

The process is initiated by the coroner/medical examiner in the county of death when he/she receives notification from a mandated reporter regarding any death of a child, birth through age 17, that occurs in Missouri. Mandated reporters include all persons described under RSMo Section 210.110 and any other person who becomes aware of a child's death within this age group. The mandated reporter may complete and include the Child Fatality Review Program Worksheet as part of the notification process, but this step is not mandatory.

In every death of a child, birth through age 17, the coroner/medical examiner shall contact the DFS Central Registry Unit (CRU) Child Abuse and Neglect Hotline (800) 392-3738 or the local DFS office to report the death. The coroner/medical examiner shall also obtain from CRU any prior child/family history to help determine if the case meets the criteria for review by the local panel.

The coroner/medical examiner should refer all appropriate cases to the certified child-death pathologist to determine the need for an autopsy. If an autopsy is required, the coroner/medical examiner should also ensure that the Death-Scene Investigative Checklist is completed and accompanies the body to the certified child-death pathologist.

**NOTE:** When a death occurs outside the county of illness/injury/event, the coroner/medical examiner is responsible for notifying the coroner/medical examiner in the county of illness/injury/event as soon as possible. Some cases may require immediate notification. All available information regarding the death should be completed on a Child Fatality Review Program Worksheet and forwarded to the coroner/medical examiner in the county of illness/injury/event, who is responsible for finalizing and submitting the Data Form 1.

## PREPARING THE CHILD FATALITY REVIEW PROGRAM WORKSHEET
The Child Fatality Review Program Worksheet provides the mandated reporter an additional means of notifying the coroner/medical examiner of preliminary information as to the cause and circumstances of the child's death. All applicable information should also be listed. It is not mandatory this form be completed. If used, the worksheet should be destroyed after the coroner/medical examiner has obtained appropriate information for completing the Data Form 1.

## PREPARING THE CORONER/MEDICAL EXAMINER DATA REPORT (DATA FORM 1)
Data Form 1 provides preliminary information as to the cause and circumstances of the child's death. It is the responsibility of the coroner/medical examiner to determine if the circumstances surrounding the death meet the criteria for review. This criteria does not necessarily mean "suspicious," but indicates that the cause of death is not clear.

The coroner/medical examiner is also asked to select the most accurate category from the form to identify the "cause" of death. All applicable "circumstance" codes should also be listed. In addition, Data Form 1 provides information from the death-scene investigation on the family of the child and information on those deaths resulting from injuries.

The law requires that the coroner/medical examiner have the chairperson of the child fatality review panel co-sign the form.

## WITHIN 48 HOURS OF NOTIFICATION OF DEATH
The chairperson will send the signed Data Form 1 to the regional coordinator within 48 hours of the notification of death.

## AUTOPSIES
The statute mandates that an autopsy be conducted on any "sudden infant death" of a child between the ages of one week and one year. The autopsy must be conducted by a certified child-death pathologist. (If a pathologist referral is needed, call 1-800-487-1626.)

For all other deaths of children in this age group, the coroner/medical examiner is required to consult with a certified child death pathologist to determine the need for an autopsy. The pathologist, in conjunction with the coroner/medical examiner, shall determine the need for an autopsy.

## If There is a Disagreement Regarding the Need for the Autopsy

The certified child-death pathologist shall file a report with the CFRP panel chairperson indicating the basis for disagreement.

## Within 12 Hours

The certified child-death pathologist's decision prevails unless the CFRP panel overrides that decision within 12 hours of receiving the above-mentioned report.

## If an Autopsy is Determined Necessary, Within 24 Hours of Receipt of the Body

The certified child-death pathologist will conduct or agree to perform the autopsy (whichever is later).

## Non-Reviewable Deaths

When the chairperson co-signs the Data Form 1, they will review Section B to determine if any of the indicators for a "reviewable death" have been checked.

In general, if no indicators are checked in Section B, the chairperson will co-sign Data Form 1 and send it to the regional coordinator within 48 hours of the notification of death.

The case is closed.

## Reviewable Deaths

Within 24 hours of receipt of Data Form 1 by the chairperson from the coroner/medical examiner, if **ANY** of the indicators under Section B have been checked, the case meets the criteria for a reviewable death. The chairperson of the CFRP panel will activate the CFRP panel by notifying the individual panel members.

In addition, there may be other occasions when the chairperson determines that a case should be reviewed by the panel. Other members may request a review by contacting the panel chairperson.

The child fatality review panel in the county of illness/injury/event will be activated regardless of the county of residence or death.

CFRP panels may review out-of-state fatalities, but it is not required. Other states are not mandated to notify Missouri counties of such deaths even if the injury/illness/event occurred in Missouri.

## Notification of CFRP Panel Meeting

Within 24 hours of receiving the Data Form 1 that has been noted as reviewable, the chairperson will activate the panel by notifying all seven core members and other optional members of preliminary information and the date and time of the review.

Notification can be done by telephone and should include the case name and other identifiers so that members can gather relevant case information from their systems for discussion at the meeting. When appropriate, the regional coordinator may be notified of the scheduled review.

## CFRP Panel Meeting

The purpose of the review is to assemble the most comprehensive set of information available on the case to help in an assessment of the circumstances.

Therefore, the seven core panel members or their authorized designees and any optional members must be involved in order to conduct a review. If anyone is unable to attend, in **ALL** cases, information concerning the review should be obtained from the non-attending member. Formal case presentations may be made by representatives of the different disciplines using a format consistent with their own professional training and experience.

The panel will provide sufficient information to complete the Data Form 2. It is recommended that a panel member be designated to complete this form.

Because of the more comprehensive nature of the review process, the information on the Data Form 2 may expound upon or be different from the preliminary information gathered earlier on Data Form 1 as part of the coroner/medical examiner's data report.

Within 45 days of death, the chairperson signs, dates, and sends the Data Form 2 to the regional coordinator.

### ADDITIONAL PANEL CONSIDERATIONS

The review process gives CFRP panels the opportunity to identify needs and provide immediate services specific to families and community. Panels may wish to have in place pre-determined systems and resources to deal with complex fatalities and other serious children's events.

## ◆ PROCESS FOR CHILD FATALITY REVIEWS

Any child, birth through age 17, who dies will be reported to the coroner/medical examiner.

Coroner/medical examiner conducts a death-scene investigation, notifies the division and completes Data Form 1 on all deaths of children, birth through age 17. Coroner/medical examiner, with certified child-death pathologist determines need for autopsy.

If autopsy needed, it is performed by a certified child-death pathologist. Results brought to child fatality review panel by coroner/medical examiner if reviewable criteria are met.

If death is *not reviewable*, Data Form 1 completed by coroner/medical examiner. Coroner/medical examiner sends to chairperson of child fatality review panel for co-signature. Chairperson sends Data Form 1 to Regional Coordinator within 48 hours.

If death is *reviewable*, the coroner/medical examiner sends the Data Form 1 to chairperson of child fatality review panel for co-signature. Chairperson sends Data Form 1 to Regional Coordinator within 48 hours. The chairperson refers the death to child fatality review panel. (Panel notified within 24 hours.)

Regional Coordinator reviews for accuracy and completeness, signs and sends Data Form 1 to STAT; STAT links Data Form 1 to Department of Health birth and death data.

Panel meeting is scheduled by chairperson as soon as possible. Panel reviews circumstances surrounding death and takes appropriate actions. Data Form 2 is completed, co-signed by chairperson and sent to Regional Coordinator within 45 days.

Regional Coordinator signs and sends Data Forms 1 and 2 to STAT; STAT links Data Forms 1 and 2 to Department of Health birth and death data. Panel members pursue the mandates of their respective agencies.

## ◆DEATH-SCENE INVESTIGATIVE CHECKLIST FOR CHILD FATALITIES

The Death-Scene Investigative Checklist for Child Fatalities (see Chapter 24, pages 516 to 522) may be prepared as an attachment to the investigative report; however, its primary purpose is to enhance the outcome of the autopsy. Information obtained concerning the history and circumstances of death will contribute to a more accurate cause-of-death diagnosis. The Death-Scene Investigative Checklist should **accompany the body to the certified child-death pathologist.**

NOTE: Any section **not completed** should be marked accordingly in the left-hand column.

The Death-Scene Investigative Checklist may also be an evaluation/investigation aid to assist investigators. If a RECONSTRUCTION of the scene is appropriate, make every effort to obtain first-person information.

In interviewing parents, caregivers and witnesses, NEVER assume criminality or negligence. BE THOROUGH AND OBJECTIVE. An empathetic, non-confrontational approach is both appropriate and effective. Explain that the information is necessary to accurately determine the cause of death.

## ◆INSTRUCTIONS FOR COMPLETING FORMS

GRID FOR EXPECTATION OF PREPARED DATA FORM 1 BY COUNTY OF RESIDENCE AND OCCURRENCE OF INJURY/ILLNESS/EVENT

| County of Residence | County of Injury/Illness/Event | County of Death | Data Form 1 Expected |
|---------------------|-------------------------------|-----------------|----------------------|
| Dade | **Dade** | Greene | **Dade** |
| Dade | **Greene** | Greene | **Greene** |
| Dade | **Greene** | Dade | **Greene** |
| Greene | **Dade** | Greene | **Dade** |
| Greene | **Greene** | Greene | **Greene** |
| Dade | **Dade** | Dade | **Dade** |

## GRID FOR EXPECTATION OF PREPARED DATA FORM 1 BY COUNTY OF RESIDENCE AND OCCURRENCE OF BIRTH

| County of Residence | County of Birth | County of Death | Data Form 1 Expected |
|---------------------|-----------------|-----------------|----------------------|
| Dade | **Dade** | Greene | **Dade** |
| Dade | **Greene** | Greene | **Greene** |
| Dade | **Greene** | Dade | **Greene** |
| Greene | **Dade** | Greene | **Dade** |
| Greene | **Greene** | Greene | **Greene** |
| Dade | **Dade** | Dade | **Dade** |

When a death occurs in a county other than the county where the injury/illness/event **occurred,** the coroner/medical examiner should notify that county coroner/medical examiner of the death and known circumstances. This may be done by preparing a Child Fatality Review Program Worksheet with *available* information and circumstances, and forwarding it to the coroner/medical examiner in the county of injury/illness/event. The Data Form 1 will then be completed, signed and forwarded from that county.

**NOTE:  SOME CASES MAY REQUIRE IMMEDIATE NOTIFICATION OF THE CORONER/MEDICAL EXAMINER IN THE COUNTY OF INJURY/ILLNESS/EVENT.**

## GRID FOR EXPECTATION OF PREPARED DATA FORM 1 BY STATE OF RESIDENCE AND OCCURRENCE OF INJURY/ILLNESS/EVENT

| State of Residence | State of Injury/Illness/Event | State of Death | Data Form 1 Expected |
|--------------------|-------------------------------|----------------|----------------------|
| MO | MO | MO | Y |
| MO | MO | IL | N* |
| MO | IL | MO | Y Section A Only |
| MO | IL | IL | N |
| IL | MO | MO | Y |
| IL | MO | IL | N* |
| IL | IL | IL | N |
| IL | IL | MO | Y Section A Only |

## GRID FOR EXPECTATION OF PREPARED DATA FORM 1 BY STATE OF RESIDENCE AND OCCURRENCE OF BIRTH

| State of Residence | State of Birth | State of Death | Data Form 1 Expected |
|---|---|---|---|
| MO | MO | MO | Y |
| MO | MO | IL | N |
| MO | IL | IL | N |
| IL | IL | MO | Y Section A Only |
| IL | MO | MO | Y |

If an out-of-state resident gives birth to a baby in Missouri, that dies in Missouri, without leaving Missouri, a Data Form 1 is expected. If it meets the criteria for review, the review should take place in the county of birth or injury/illness/event.

* Other states are not mandated to notify Missouri counties of such deaths even if the injury/illness/event occurred in Missouri. However, these deaths may be reviewed and the forms submitted.

## CHILD FATALITY REVIEW PROGRAM WORKSHEET

### PURPOSE

The Child Fatality Review Program Worksheet is an additional means by which a mandated reporter can notify the coroner/medical examiner of the death of a child, birth through age 17. The coroner/medical examiner can complete the Data Form 1 based on the information available from the worksheet. It is recognized that this information is preliminary and will likely change in many cases. After the initial information is obtained by the coroner/medical examiner, this worksheet is destroyed.

### INSTRUCTIONS

Answer all applicable questions by checking the appropriate box(es) or printing information where requested. Forward the completed worksheet to the coroner/medical examiner in the county of death. If the event that caused the death occurred in another county, the coroner/medical examiner will ensure that the coroner/medical examiner in the county of event is notified. Questions concerning the completion of this form should be directed to the State Technical Assistance Team at (800) 487-1626.

### SECTION A: IDENTIFICATION INFORMATION

Answer all questions in this section. If the county of residence or illness/injury/event is not in Missouri, write "Out of State" in the appropriate box(es). Print the child's given name, date of birth and date of death. Do not use nicknames. If a newborn child is known as Baby Boy Jones, place Baby Boy in the First Name area and Jones in the Last Name area. In child fatalities involving same sex, newborn multiple births/deaths, complete a separate worksheet for each child. When completing name information place the letter in the Middle Initial area; i.e., First Name - Baby Boy, Middle Initial - A, Last Name - Jones and First Name - Baby Boy, Middle Initial - B, Last Name - Jones.

The mother's name and date of birth are important in matching birth and death certificate information. However, do not let the lack of this information delay the notification/review process.

## Section B: Indications for Review

Check all indicators in this section that apply to this child's death. When the coroner/medical examiner receives the worksheet with one of the indicators in Section B checked, the coroner/medical examiner will contact the CFRP panel chairperson about activating the CFRP panel.

## Section C: Child Abuse/Neglect Hotline

The Division of Family Services, Child Abuse/Neglect Hotline will accept all notifications of death for any child birth through age 17. Circumstances surrounding the death will determine if the notification is handled as information only, a referral for service or a case for investigation.

Complete this section by checking the appropriate box(es) based on information received from the DFS Child Abuse/Neglect Hotline.

## Section D: Social Information

Complete this section by checking the appropriate box(es) based on available household data. Check only one head of household for the person responsible for the residence in which the child resides.

On the corresponding line, write the letter for the appropriate age range of the checked individual(s), i.e., if the person checked is 30 years of age, write the letter "E".

## Section E: Death/Scene Information

Complete this section by checking the appropriate boxes and, if applicable, filling in the applicable information based on available death/scene data. Complete time information using standard time and check AM or PM. **Do not use military time.**

If applicable, complete the CFRP Pathologist information by writing the last name only.

## Section F: Supervision

Complete this section by checking the appropriate boxes based on available supervision data.

## Section G: Cause of Death

Check the appropriate category ("Injury," "Illness or Other Natural Cause" or "Unknown Cause") which, based on preliminary information available at that time, most accurately describes the cause of death.

If the "Injury" category is checked and the death is due to a vehicular accident which does not meet indications for review as listed in Section B, complete questions 1 through 9. If the death is from another type of injury other than a non-reviewable vehicular accident, complete questions 1 and 2, and continue to Section H.

If the "Illness or Other Natural Cause" category is checked and the child is over 1 year of age, complete questions 1 and 2. If the child is under 1 year of age, complete questions 1 through 8.

If the "Unknown Cause" category is checked, complete questions as applicable.

## Section H: Circumstances of Death

Check the most appropriate circumstances of death. If none apply to the death, continue to Section I.

## Section I: Narrative Description of Circumstances or Other Comments

This space allows the mandated reporter to make any additional comments on the data.

MISSOURI DEPARTMENT OF SOCIAL SERVICES
DIVISION OF FAMILY SERVICES
## CHILD FATALITY REVIEW PROGRAM WORKSHEET
FOR USE IN REPORTING DEATHS OF CHILDREN < 18 YEARS OF AGE TO CORONER/MEDICAL EXAMINER

### INSTRUCTIONS:

Complete Child Fatality Review Program Worksheet with as much detail and accuracy as possible by interviewing available members of the decedent's family or reviewing medical records. The preliminary information is important and sometimes remains the only information describing circumstances of the child's death. Upon completing the worksheet, send it to the county coroner/medical examiner. State law requires the county coroner/medical examiner be notified of **EVERY** child's death (birth through age 17).

### A. IDENTIFICATION OF THE DECEDENT

1.
   a. ☐ Illness/injury/event is in Missouri.
   b. ☐ Illness/injury/event occurred ouf-of-state, but death occurred in Missouri.

| 1. COUNTY OF RESIDENCE | STATE USE ONLY | 2. COUNTY OF ILLNESS/INJURY/EVENT | STATE USE ONLY | 2. COUNTY OF DEATH | STATE USE ONLY |
|---|---|---|---|---|---|
| | | | | | |

| 5. DECEDENT'S NAME (FIRST, MI, LAST) | 6. DATE OF BIRTH (MM/DD/YY) | 7. DATE OF DEATH (MM/DD/YY) |
|---|---|---|
| / / | __ __ / __ __ / __ __ | __ __ / __ __ / __ __ |

| 8. SEX | 9.RACE | | 10. IS DECEDENT OF HISPANIC ORIGIN? |
|---|---|---|---|
| a. ☐ MALE | a. ☐ WHITE    c. ☐ ASIAN/PACIFIC ISLANDER    e. ☐ UNKNOWN | | a. ☐ YES |
| b. ☐ FEMALE | b. ☐ BLACK    d. ☐ AMERICAN INDIAN/ALASKAN NATIVE | | b. ☐ NO |

| 11. MOTHER'S NAME (FIRST, MAIDEN, LAST) | 11. MOTHER'S DATE OF BIRTH |
|---|---|
| / / | __ __ / __ __ / __ __ |

### B. INDICATIONS FOR REVIEW— (ALL DEATHS)

1. Mark all that apply to this fatality.

   a. ☐ Sudden, unexplained death, age <1 year
   b. ☐ Unexplained/undetermined manner
   c. ☐ DFS reports on decedent or other persons in the residence
   d. ☐ Decedent in DFS custody
   e. ☐ Possible inadequate supervision
   f. ☐ Possible malnutrition or delay in seeking medical care
   g. ☐ Possible suicide
   h. ☐ Possible inflicted injury
   i. ☐ Firearm injury
   j. ☐ Injury not witnessed by person in charge at time of injury
   k. ☐ Confinement
   l. ☐ Suspicious /criminal activity

   m. ☐ Drowning
   n. ☐ Suffocation or strangulation
   o. ☐ Poison/chemical/drug ingestion
   p. ☐ Severe unexplained injury
   q. ☐ Pedestrian/bicycle/driveway injury
   r. ☐ Drug/alcohol-related vehicular injury
   s. ☐ Suspected sexual assault
   t. ☐ Fire injury
   u. ☐ Autopsy by certified child death pathologist
   v. ☐ Panel discretion
   w. ☐ Other suspicious findings (injuries such as electrocution, crush or fall)

### C. CHILD ABUSE/NEGLECT HOTLINE (800-392-3738)

**Notify Child Abuse/Neglect Hotline of all deaths of children <18 years of age.**

1. Was the Child Abuse/Neglect Hotline notified of this death?    a. ☐ Yes    b. ☐ No

2. Current notification to Child Abuse/Neglect Hotline was accepted as:
   a. ☐ Information/Referral only    b. ☐ Report for investigation    c. ☐ Unknown

## D. SOCIAL INFORMATION

1. For all persons living in the residence of the decedent, indicate their relationship to the decedent, their age range, and who is head of household. (Select only one head of household)

Use corresponding letter for appropriate age range:

**A** = 0-5 yrs.  **B** = 6-9 yrs.  **C** = 10-14 yrs.  **D** = 15-18 yrs.  **E** = 19-40 yrs.  **F** = >40 yrs.

| | | Age Range | Head of Household | | | Age Range | Head of Household |
|---|---|---|---|---|---|---|---|
| a. ☐ | Natural father | ____ | ☐ | i. ☐ | Other relative | ____ | ☐ |
| b. ☐ | Natural mother | ____ | ☐ | j. ☐ | Other relative | ____ | ☐ |
| c. ☐ | Adoptive father | ____ | ☐ | k. ☐ | Mother's paramour | ____ | ☐ |
| d. ☐ | Adoptive mother | ____ | ☐ | l. ☐ | Father's paramour | ____ | ☐ |
| e. ☐ | Stepfather | ____ | ☐ | m. ☐ | Other non-relative | ____ | ☐ |
| f. ☐ | Stepmother | ____ | ☐ | n. ☐ | Another child | ____ | ☐ |
| g. ☐ | Foster father | ____ | ☐ | o. ☐ | Another child | ____ | ☐ |
| h. ☐ | Foster mother | ____ | ☐ | p. ☐ | More than two children (list in narrative) | | |

2. Current marital status of head of household?

a. ☐ Married    c. ☐ Divorced    e. ☐ Unknown
b. ☐ Widowed    d. ☐ Never married

## E. DEATH/SCENE INFORMATION

1. Place of death?

a. ☐ Decedent's home    e. ☐ Public drive    i. ☐ Other private property    m. ☐ Body of water
b. ☐ Other home    f. ☐ Street    j. ☐ Licensed child care facility    o. ☐ Work place
c. ☐ Rural road    g. ☐ Private drive    k. ☐ Unlicensed child care facility    p. ☐ Hospital
d. ☐ Highway    h. ☐ Farm    l. ☐ Child care residential facility    q. ☐ Other: _____

2. Date of injury/event?    a. ☐ __ __ / __ __ / __ __ (MM/DD/YY)    b. ☐ Unknown

3. Time of injury/event?    a. ☐ __ __ : __ __ (Hour:Minute) ☐ AM ☐ PM    b. ☐ Unknown

4. Time pronounced dead?    a. ☐ __ __ : __ __ (Hour:Minute) ☐ AM ☐ PM    b. ☐ Unknown

5. Was an autopsy performed?    a. ☐ Yes    b. ☐ No    c. ☐ Unknown

If yes:
1. ☐ By CFRP pathologist?    (NOTE: Autopsies performed by non-certified child pathologists are limited to
2. ☐ By hospital physician?    hospital deaths resulting from a **known** medical condition/illness.)

3. ☐ Name of CFRP pathologist? (Last name only) _____

## F. SUPERVISION

1. Who was in charge of watching the decedent at the time of injury/event?

a. ☐ Natural father    g. ☐ Foster father    m. ☐ Unlicensed babysitter/child care worker
b. ☐ Natural mother    h. ☐ Foster mother    n. ☐ Child, age: _____
c. ☐ Adoptive father    i. ☐ Other relative    o. ☐ Hospital staff
d. ☐ Adoptive mother    j. ☐ Parent's male paramour    p. ☐ Other non-relative
e. ☐ Stepfather    k. ☐ Parent's female paramour    q. ☐ No one in charge of watching
f. ☐ Stepmother    l. ☐ Licensed babysitter/child care worker    r. ☐ Due to age, no one in charge

2. Was the decedent adequately supervised?    a. ☐ Yes    b. ☐ No    c. ☐ Unknown    d. ☐ Not applicable

If no:
1. Did the person(s) in charge appear to be intoxicated, under influence of drugs, mentally ill or limited, or otherwise impaired at time of injury/event?
a. ☐ Yes    b. ☐ No    c. ☐ Unknown

2. Was the person(s) preoccupied, distracted or asleep at the time of the injury/event?
a. ☐ Yes    b. ☐ No    c. ☐ Unknown

3. Was injury/event witnessed by at least one person?    a. ☐ Yes    b. ☐ No    c. ☐ Unknown

## G. CAUSE OF DEATH
**(Select most appropriate cause of death and if applicable, complete Section H)**

**1. ☐ INJURY (Complete questions 1 and 2 for all injuries)**

1. Was the injury inflicted?  a. ☐ Yes   b. ☐ No   c. ☐ Unknown
   (Inflicted - defined as assaultive or aggressive action)

2. Was the injury intentional?  a. ☐ Yes   b. ☐ No   c. ☐ Unknown

**If vehicle accident, non-reviewable, answer questions 3 through 9.  If reviewable vehicle accident (pedestrian/bicycle/driveway injury, drug/alcohol related or other suspicious/criminal activity), skip the following questions and complete Section H.**

3. Position of decedent?
   a. ☐ Operator   b. ☐ Passenger   c. ☐ Other   d. ☐ Unknown

4. Vehicle in which decedent was occupant?
   a. ☐ Car   c. ☐ Motorcycle/ATV   e. ☐ Semi/Tractor trailer unit
   b. ☐ Truck/RV/Van   d. ☐ Farm vehicle   f. ☐ Other

5. Was another vehicle involved in accident?   a. ☐ Yes   b. ☐ No

6. Condition of road?
   a. ☐ Normal   c. ☐ Wet   e. ☐ Other
   b. ☐ Loose gravel   d. ☐ Ice or snow   f. ☐ Unknown

7. Restraint used by decedent?
   a. ☐ Present, not used   c. ☐ Used correctly   e. ☐ Unknown
   b. ☐ None in vehicle   d. ☐ Used incorrectly   f. ☐ Not applicable

8. Helmet used by decedent?
   a. ☐ Helmet worn   b. ☐ Helmet not worn   c. ☐ Not applicable

9. Primary cause of accident?
   a. ☐ Speeding   c. ☐ Mechanical failure   e. ☐ Driver error
   b. ☐ Carelessness   d. ☐ Weather conditions   f. ☐ Other

**2. ☐ ILLNESS OR OTHER NATURAL CAUSE**

1. Known condition _____

2. Was inadequate care or neglect involved in death?   a. ☐ Yes   b. ☐ No
   **(If yes, mark Section H, Number 2)**

**Complete questions 3 - 8 if death in infant <1 year of age.**

3. History information provided by?   a. ☐ Parent   b. ☐ Physician/Medical facility   c. ☐ Other

4. Age at death?
   a. ☐ 0 - 24 hours after birth   c. ☐ 48 hours - 6 weeks   e. ☐ 6 months - 1 year
   b. ☐ 24 - 48 hours   d. ☐ 6 weeks - 6 months

5. Gestational age?
   a. ☐ <25 weeks   b. ☐ 25 - 30 weeks   c. ☐ 30 - 37 weeks   d. ☐ >37 weeks   e. ☐ Unknown

6. Birth weight in grams (approximate lbs./oz.)?
   a. ☐ <750 (<1 lb. 10 oz.)   c. ☐ 1,500 - 2,499 (3 lbs. 6 oz. to 5 lbs. 5 oz.)   e. ☐ Unknown
   b. ☐ 750 - 1,499 (1 lb. 10 oz. to 3 lbs. 5 oz.)   d. ☐ >2,500 (>5 lbs. 6 oz.)

7. Multiple birth?   a. ☐ Yes   b. ☐ No

8. Have there been other infant deaths in the immediate family?   a. ☐ Yes   b. ☐ No   c. ☐ Unknown

**3. ☐ UNKNOWN CAUSE (Describe in narrative)**

1. Was death sudden and unexplained in infant < 1 year of age?   a. ☐ Yes   b. ☐ No
   **If yes, also complete Section G, Number 2, question 3 - 8 and mark Section H, Number 1.**

**H. CIRCUMSTANCES OF DEATH**
**(Mark circumstances most applicable to death)**

1. ☐ Sudden Unexplained Death of Infant <1 Year
2. ☐ Inadequate Care or Neglect
3. ☐ Vehicular
   (Includes pedestrian/bicycle/driveway injury, drug/alcohol
   related, or other suspicious/criminal activity)
4. ☐ Drowning
5. ☐ Firearm
6. ☐ Suffocation/Strangulation
7. ☐ Electrocution

8. ☐ Fall Injury
9. ☐ Poisoning/Overdose
10. ☐ Fire/Burn
11. ☐ Crush
12. ☐ Confinement
13. ☐ Shaken/Impact Syndrome
14. ☐ Other Inflicted Injury
    (Describe in narrative)
15. ☐ Other Circumstances
    (Describe in narrative)

**I. NARRATIVE DESCRIPTION OF CIRCUMSTANCES OR OTHER COMMENTS**

| WORKSHEET COMPLETED BY | TITLE | TELEPHONE NUMBER | DATE (MM/DD/YY) |
|---|---|---|---|
| | | ( ) | __ __ / __ __ / __ __ |

**CORONER/MEDICAL EXAMINER SHOULD DESTROY WORKSHEET AFTER COMPLETING DATA FORM 1**

MO 886-3071 (12-96)

PAGE 4

## 1997 Data Form 1
## Coroner/medical Examiner Data Report

### Purpose

The Data Form 1 is completed by the coroner/medical examiner on ALL deaths of children, birth though age 17. This form initiates the process by which the coroner/medical examiner notifies the chairperson. If the child's death meets the indications for review, the CFRP panel shall be convened to more closely examine the case. The coroner/medical examiner completes this data form based on information available within the first 48 hours following the death. Death-scene investigations and autopsy information may not be available and should not delay completion of this form.

### Instructions

Answer all applicable questions by checking the appropriate box(es) of printing information where requested. Forward the completed data form to the chairperson. Do not mark in areas indicated "STATE USE ONLY." If the event that caused the death occurred in another county, ensure that the coroner/medical examiner in the county of event is notified. Questions concerning completion of this data form should be directed to the State Technical Assistance Team at (800) 487-1626.

### Section A: Identification Information

Answer all questions in this section. If the county of residence or illness/injury/event is not in Missouri, write "Out of State" in the appropriate box(es).

Print the child's given name, date of birth and date of death. Do not use nicknames. If a newborn child is known as Baby Boy Jones, place Baby Boy in the First Name area and Jones in the Last Name area. In child fatalities involving same sex, newborn multiple births/deaths, complete a separate worksheet for each child. When completing name information place the letter in the Middle Initial area; i.e., First Name - Baby Boy, Middle Initial - A, Last Name - Jones and First Name - Baby Boy, Middle Initial - B, Last Name - Jones. The mother's name and date of birth are important in matching birth and death certificate information. However, do not let the lack of this information delay the notification/review process.

### Section B: Indications for Review

If any indicator found in this section applies and is checked, the case has, by definition, met the criteria for review and will be referred to the chairperson of the local CFRP panel. When the chairperson receives a Data Form 1 with one of the indicators in Section B checked, the CFRP panel shall be activated within 24 hours of receipt of the data form.

### Section C: Child Abuse/Neglect Hotline

The Division of Family Services, Child Abuse/Neglect Hotline will accept all notifications of death for any child birth through age 17 and respond to the coroner/medical examiner's inquiry about prior Hotline reports. Circumstances surrounding the death will determine if the notification is handled as information only, a referral for service or a case for investigation. Complete this section by checking the appropriate box(es) based on information received from the DFS Child Abuse/Neglect Hotline.

### Section D: Social Information

Complete this section by checking the appropriate box(es) based on available household data. Check only one head of household for the person responsible for the residence in which the child resides. On the corresponding line, write the letter for the appropriate age range of the checked individual(s), i.e., if the person checked is 30 years of age, write the letter "E".

## SECTION E: DEATH/SCENE INFORMATION

Complete this section by checking the appropriate boxes and, if applicable, filling in the applicable information based on available death/scene data. Complete time information using standard time and check AM or PM. **Do not use military time.** If applicable, complete the CFRP Pathologist information by writing the last name only.

## SECTION F: SUPERVISION

Complete this section by checking the appropriate boxes based on available supervision data.

## SECTION G: CAUSE OF DEATH

Check the appropriate category ("Injury," "Illness or Other Natural Cause" or "Unknown Cause") which, based on preliminary information available at that time, most accurately describes the cause of death.

If the "Injury" category is checked and the death is due to a vehicular accident which does not meet indications for review as listed in Section B, complete questions 1 through 9. If the death is from another type of injury other than a non-reviewable vehicular accident, complete questions 1 and 2, and continue to Section H.

If the "Illness or Other Natural Cause" category is checked and the child is over 1 year of age, complete questions 1 and 2. If the child is under 1 year of age, complete questions 1 through 8.

If the "Unknown Cause" category is checked, complete questions as applicable and describe known circumstances in Section I.

## SECTION H: CIRCUMSTANCES OF DEATH

Check the most appropriate circumstances of death. If none apply to the death, continue to Section I.

## SECTION I: NARRATIVE DESCRIPTION OF CIRCUMSTANCES OR OTHER COMMENTS

This space allows for any additional comments concerning the death.

## SECTION J: PREVENTION

Complete this section by checking the appropriate box(es) based on prevention-related community actions prompted by the child's death.

NOTE: See the forms for the Coroner/Medical Examiner Data Report in Chapter 24, on pages 527-530.

# 1997 DATA FORM 2
## CHILD FATALITY REVIEW PANEL DATA REPORT

### PURPOSE

The Data Form 2 is completed by the local CFRP panel after they have conducted a review of the child's death. Information for completion of Data Form 2 should be gathered and reported independently of data reported on Data Form 1.

### INSTRUCTIONS

After the review panel has met and discussed the case, all sections of the Data Form 2 are completed. The chairperson signs, dates and forwards the data form to the regional coordinator within 45 days of the date of death. Do not mark in areas indicated "STATE USE ONLY." Questions concerning the completion of this data form should be directed to the State Technical Assistance Team (STAT) at (800) 487-1626.

## Section A: Identification Information

Answer all questions in this section. If the county of residence is not in Missouri, write "Out of State" in the corresponding box.

Print the child's given name, date of birth and date of death. Do not use nicknames. If a newborn child is known as Baby Boy Jones, place Baby Boy in the First Name area and Jones in the Last Name area. In child fatalities involving same sex, newborn multiple births/deaths, complete a separate worksheet for each child. When completing name information place the letter in the Middle Initial area; i.e., First Name - Baby Boy, Middle Initial - A, Last Name - Jones and First Name - Baby Boy, Middle Initial - B, Last Name - Jones. The mother's name and date of birth are important in matching birth and death certificate information. However, do not let the lack of this information delay the data form completion.

## Section B: Child Abuse/Neglect Hotline

Complete this section by checking the appropriate box(es) based on information received from the DFS Child Abuse/Neglect Hotline by either the coroner/medical examiner or the DFS Representative.

## Section C: Social Information

Complete this section by checking the appropriate box(es) based on available household data. Check only one head of household for the person responsible for the residence in which the child resides. On the corresponding line, write the letter for the appropriate age range of the checked individual(s), i.e., if the person checked is 30 years of age, write the letter "E".

## Section D: Death/Scene Information

Complete this section by checking the appropriate boxes and, if applicable, filling in the applicable information based on available death/scene data. Complete time information using standard time and check AM or PM. **Do not use military time**. If applicable, complete the CFRP Pathologist information by writing the last name only.

## Section E: Supervision

Complete this section by checking the appropriate boxes based on available supervision data.

## Section F: Panel Findings

Complete this section by checking the appropriate boxes and printing information based on panel review information.

## Section G: Person(s) Arrested/Charged

Complete this section only if someone was arrested or charged in relation to this child's death. If no one was arrested or charged, skip this section and continue to Section H.

## Section H: Cause of Death

Check the appropriate category ("Injury," "Illness or Other Natural Cause" or "Unknown Cause") which, based on information available at that time, most accurately describes the cause of death.

If the "Injury" category is checked complete all questions and continue to Section I.

If the "Illness or Other Natural Cause" category is checked and the child is over 1 year of age, complete question 1 only. If the child is under 1 year of age, complete questions 1 through 11.

If the "Unknown Cause" category is checked, continue to Section J and describe the circumstances.

## Section I: Circumstances of Death

Check the most appropriate circumstances of death and answer the corresponding questions for the circumstances.  If none apply to the death, continue to Section J.

Section J: Narrative Description of Circumstances or Other Comments
This space allows for any additional comments concerning the death.

Section K: Services Provided
Check all services provided as a result of this child's death.

Section L: Prevention
Complete this section by checking the appropriate box(es) based on prevention-related community actions prompted by the child's death.

MISSOURI DEPARTMENT OF SOCIAL SERVICES
DIVISION OF FAMILY SERVICES

## CHILD FATALITY REVIEW PANEL DATA REPORT

TO BE COMPLETED FOR ALL REVIEWABLE CHILD DEATHS < 18 YEARS OF AGE

| STATE USE ONLY | | DATA FORM |
|---|---|---|
| DEATH CERT. NO. | BIRTH CERT. NO. | **2** |
| CFRP CASE NO. | DECEDENT DCN | |
| ☐ MEDICAID | CA/N INCIDENT NO. | |

DEATH CERTIFICATE MANNER OF DEATH

| a. | NATURAL | d. | HOMICIDE |
|---|---|---|---|
| b. | ACCIDENT | e. | UNDETERMINED |
| c. | SUICIDE | f. | PENDING |

### INSTRUCTIONS:

Notify Child Abuse/Neglect Hotline (800-392-3738) of all deaths of children <18 years of age.

Complete the form with all known information and forward to the regional coordinator within forty-five days of the death.

### A. IDENTIFICATION OF THE DECEDENT

| 1. COUNTY OF RESIDENCE | STATE USE ONLY | 2. COUNTY OF ILLNESS/INJURY/EVENT | STATE USE ONLY | 3. COUNTY OF DEATH | STATE USE ONLY |
|---|---|---|---|---|---|

| 4. DECEDENT'S NAME (FIRST, MI, LAST) | 5. DATE OF BIRTH (MM/DD/YY) | 6. DATE OF DEATH (MM/DD/YY) |
|---|---|---|
| /        / | __ __ / __ __ / __ __ | __ __ / __ __ / __ __ |

| 7. SEX | 8. RACE | | | 9. IS DECEDENT OF HISPANIC ORIGIN? |
|---|---|---|---|---|
| a. ☐ MALE | a. ☐ WHITE | c. ☐ ASIAN/PACIFIC ISLANDER | e. ☐ UNKNOWN | a. ☐ YES    b. ☐ NO |
| b. ☐ FEMALE | b. ☐ BLACK | d. ☐ AMERICAN INDIAN/ALASKAN NATIVE | | |

| 10. MOTHER'S NAME (FIRST, MAIDEN, LAST) | 11. MOTHER'S DATE OF BIRTH (MM/DD/TT) |
|---|---|
| /                          / | |

### B. CHILD ABUSE/NEGLECT HOTLINE (800-392-3738)

1. Were there prior reports to the Child Abuse/Neglect Hotline?    a. ☐ Yes    b. ☐ No

If yes, mark all that apply:

1. ☐ Involving child
2. ☐ Involving anyone else in family
3. ☐ Involving caretaker (other than family)
4. ☐ Total number of DNS reports

2. Current notification to Child Abuse/Neglect Hotline was accepted as:

a. ☐ Information/Referral only          b. ☐ Report for investigation

### C. SOCIAL INFORMATION

1. For all people living in residence of the decedent, indicate their relationship to the decedent, their age range and who is head of household. (Select only one head of household)

Use of corresponding letter for appropriate age range:

**A** = 0-5 yrs.     **B** = 6-9 yrs.     **C** = 10-14 yrs.     **D** =15-18 yrs.     **E** = 19-40 yrs.     **F** = >40 yrs.

| | Age Range | Head of Household | | | Age Range | Head of Household |
|---|---|---|---|---|---|---|
| a. ☐ Natural father | ___ | ☐ | i. ☐ Other relative | | ___ | ☐ |
| b. ☐ Natural mother | ___ | ☐ | j. ☐ Other relative | | ___ | ☐ |
| c. ☐ Adoptive father | ___ | ☐ | k. ☐ Mother's paramour | | ___ | ☐ |
| d. ☐ Adoptive mother | ___ | ☐ | l. ☐ Father's paramour | | ___ | ☐ |
| e. ☐ Stepfather | ___ | ☐ | m. ☐ Other non-relative | | ___ | ☐ |
| f. ☐ Stepmother | ___ | ☐ | n. ☐ Another child | | ___ | ☐ |
| g. ☐ Foster father | ___ | ☐ | o. ☐ Another child | | ___ | ☐ |
| h. ☐ Foster mother | ___ | ☐ | p. ☐ More than two children (list in narrative) | | | |

1. Current marital status of head of household?

a. ☐ Married          c. ☐ Divorced          e. ☐ Unknown
b. ☐ Widowed          d. ☐ Never married

## D. DEATH/SCENE INFORMATION

1. Place of death

| | | | |
|---|---|---|---|
| a. ☐ Decedent's home | e. ☐ Public drive | i. ☐ Other private property | m. ☐ Body of water |
| b. ☐ Other home | f. ☐ Street | j. ☐ Licenced child care facility | n. ☐ Work place |
| c. ☐ Rural road | g. ☐ Private drive | k. ☐ Unlicenced child care facility | o. ☐ Hospital |
| d. ☐ Highway | f. ☐ Farm | l. ☐ Child care residential facility | p. ☐ Other |

2. Date of injury/event?    a. ☐ __ __ / __ __ / __ __ (MM/DD/YY)    b. ☐ Unknown

3. Time of injury/event?    a. ☐ __ __ : __ __ (Hour:Minute) ☐ AM ☐ PM    b. ☐ Unknown

4. Time pronounced dead?    a. ☐ __ __ : __ __ (Hour:Minute) ☐ AM ☐ PM    b. ☐ Unknown

5. Autopsy performed by?    a.  CFRP Pathologist (Last Name Only)_____

    b.  Not performed

## E. SUPERVISION

1. Who was in charge of waching the decedent at the time of injury/event?

| | | |
|---|---|---|
| a. ☐ Natural father | g. ☐ Foster father | m. ☐ Unlicenced babysitter/child care worker |
| b. ☐ Natural mother | h. ☐ Foster mother | n. ☐ Child, age: _____ |
| c. ☐ Adoptive father | i. ☐ Other relative | o. ☐ Hospital staff |
| d. ☐ Adoptive mother | j. ☐ Parent's male paramour | p. ☐ Other non-relative |
| e. ☐ Stepfather | k. ☐ Parent's female paramour | q. ☐ No one in charge of watching |
| f. ☐ Stepmother | l. ☐ Licenced babysitter/child care worker | r. ☐ Due to age, no one in charge |

2. Was the decedent adequatly supervised?    a. ☐ Yes    b. ☐ No    c. ☐ Unknown    d. ☐ Not applicable

If no:

1. Did the person(s) in charge appear to be intoxicated, under influence of drugs, mentally ill or limited, or otherwise impaired at time of injury/event?
   a. ☐ Yes    b. ☐ No    c. ☐ Unknown

2. Was the person(s) preocuppied, distracted or asleep at the time of the injury/event?
   a. ☐ Yes    b. ☐ No    c. ☐ Unknown

3. Was injury/event witnesssed by at least one person?    a. ☐ Yes    b. ☐ No    c. ☐ Unknown

## F. PANEL FINDINGS

1. Date of first panel meeting    a. ☐ __ / __ / __ (MM/DD/YY)

2. Panel members participating?

| | | |
|---|---|---|
| a. ☐ Coroner | e. ☐ EMS | h. ☐ Juvenile officer |
| b. ☐ Prosecutor | f. ☐ Medical examiner | i. ☐ Optional member |
| c. ☐ DFS worker | g. ☐ Law enforcement officer | j. ☐ Optional member |
| d. ☐ Public health/Physician | | |

3. Total number of meetings held?    a. ☐ One    b. ☐ Two    c. ☐ Three or more

4. Death scene investigation conducted?    (Mark all that apply)

   a. ☐ By law enforcement    c. ☐ By medical examiner    e. ☐ By fire investigator    g. ☐ Not conducted

   b. ☐ By coroner    d. ☐ By EMS    f. ☐ By other agency

5. Investigation by law enforcement?

   a. ☐ Conducted, no arrest    b. ☐ Conducted, arrest for: _____    c. ☐ Pending    d. ☐ Not conducted

6. Investigation/evaluation by juvenile officer?

   a. ☐ Conducted, no action    b. ☐ Conducted, juvenile court action    c. ☐ Pending    d. ☐ Not conducted

7. Reveiw of records by Department of Health?

   a. ☐ Conducted, no action    b. ☐ Conducted, services provided    c. ☐ Pending    d. ☐ Not conducted

8. Review of history by Division of Family Services?

   a. ☐ Conducted, no action     c. ☐ Conducted, case investigation     e. ☐ Not conducted

   b. ☐ Conducted, services provided     d. ☐ Pending

9. Action by prosecutor?

   a. ☐ Suspended perpetrator, no charge filed     c. ☐ Pending or in progress

   b. ☐ Charge filed for: _____     d. ☐ No action

10. Review of medical/trip records by EMS?

   a. ☐ Conducted, no action    b. ☐ Conducted, services provided    c. ☐ Pending    d. ☐ Not conducted

11. Did the review lead to additional investigation?    a. ☐ Yes    b. ☐ No

12. Were additional services provided as a result of the review?    a. ☐ Yes    b. ☐ No

13. Were changes in agency policies or practices recommended as a result of the review?    a. ☐ Yes    b. ☐ No

## G. PERSON(S) ARRESTED/CHARGED
**If no arrest or charge, go to Section H**

1. Number of person(s) arrested/charged?    a. ☐ One    b. ☐ Two    c. ☐ Three or more

2. Number of persons arrested or charged responsible for supervision of the child at time of fatal illness/injury/event ?

   a. ☐ One    b. ☐ Two    c. ☐ Three or more    d. ☐ Not applicable

3. Review of medical/trip records by EMS?

   a. ☐ Yes    b. ☐ No

4. Indicate the relationship of person(s) arrested or charged to the decedent.

   a. ☐ Natural father     g. ☐ Foster father     m. ☐ Babysitter/child care worker
   b. ☐ Natural mother     h. ☐ Foster mother     n. ☐ Friend
   c. ☐ Adoptive father     i. ☐ Other relative     o. ☐ Acquaintance
   d. ☐ Adoptive mother     j. ☐ Sibling     p. ☐ Other non-relative
   e. ☐ Stepfather     k. ☐ Parent's male paramour     q. ☐ No one in charge of watching
   f. ☐ Stepmother     l. ☐ Parent's female paramour     r. ☐ Stranger

## H. CAUSE OF DEATH
**Complete section appropriate to death**

1. ☐ **INJURY (If marked, also complete Section 1)**

   1. Was the injury inflicted?    a. ☐ Yes    b. ☐ No    c. ☐ Unknown

      (Inflicted - defined as assaultive or aggressive action)

   2. Was the injury intentional?    a. ☐ Intentional    b. ☐ Unintentional/Accidental    c. ☐ Unknown

   3. If intentional, was decedent?    a. ☐ Intended victim    b. ☐ Random victim

   4. Person(s) inflicting injury? (Mark all that apply)

      a. ☐ Self     e. ☐ Stepfather     i. ☐ Other relative     m. ☐ Sibling
      b. ☐ Mother     f. ☐ Mother's paramour     j. ☐ Acquaintance     n. ☐ Other Child
      c. ☐ Father     g. ☐ Father's paramour     k. ☐ Friend     o. ☐ Stranger
      d. ☐ Stepmother     h. ☐ Foster parent     l. ☐ Child care worker     p. ☐ Unknown

   5. Age of primary person inflicting injury?    a. ☐ _____    b. ☐ Unknown

   6. Race of primary person inflicting injury?

      a. ☐ White     c. ☐ Asian/Pacific Islander     e. ☐ Unable to determine
      b. ☐ Black     d. ☐ American Indian/Alaskan Native     f. ☐ Unknown

9. Was the injury drug related?    a. ☐ Yes    b. ☐ No    c. ☐ Unknown

10. Was the injury gang related?    a. ☐ Yes    b. ☐ No    c. ☐ Unknown

11. Did the injury occur during the commission of a crime?    a. ☐ Yes    b. ☐ No    c. ☐ Unknown

12. If suicide: (Mark all that apply)

  a. ☐ Prior attempts            c. ☐ Had previously received mental health services

  b. ☐ Talked of suicide           d. ☐ Suicide completely unexpected

  c. ☐ Prior mental health problems

**2. ☐ ILLNESS OR OTHER NATURAL CAUSE**
**(If applicable, complete Inadequate Care or Neglect in Section 1)**

  1. ☐ Known Condition _____

**Complete questions 2 - 11 if natural cause death in infant <1 year of age (INCLUDING SIDS)**

2. Age at death?

  a. ☐ 0 - 24 hours after birth    c. ☐ 48 hours - 6 weeks    e. ☐ 6 months - 1 year

  b. ☐ 24 - 48 hours    d. ☐ 6 weeks - 6 months

3. Gestational age at birth?

  a. ☐ <25 weeks  b. ☐ 25 - 30 weeks  c. ☐ 30 - 37 weeks  d. ☐ <37 weeks  e. ☐ Unknown

4. Birth weight in grams (approximate lbs./oz.)?

  a. ☐ <750 (<1 lb. 10 oz.)    c. ☐ 1,500 - 2,400 ( 3lbs. 6 oz. to 5 lbs. 5 oz.)  e. ☐ Unknown

  b. ☐ 750 - 1,499 ( 1lb. 10 oz. to 3lbs. 5 oz.)  d. ☐ >2500 (>5 lbs. 6 oz.)

5. Multiple birth?    a. ☐ Yes    b. ☐ No

6. Total number of prenatal visits?

  a. ☐ None    b. ☐ 1 - 3    c. ☐ 4 - 6    d. ☐ 7 - 10    e. ☐ Unknown

7. First prenatal visit occurred during?

  a. ☐ First trimester    b. ☐ Second trimester    c. ☐ Third trimester    d. ☐ Unknown

8. Medical complications during pregnancy?    a. ☐ Yes    b. ☐ No    c. ☐ Unknown

9. Smoking during pregnancy?    a. ☐ Yes    b. ☐ No    c. ☐ Unknown

10. Drug use during pregnancy?    a. ☐ Yes    b. ☐ No    c. ☐ Unknown

11. Alcohol use during pregnancy?    a. ☐ Yes    b. ☐ No    c. ☐ Unknown

**3. ☐ UNKNOWN CAUSE (Describe in narrative)**

**I. CIRCUMSTANCES OF DEATH**

**1. ☐ SUDDEN INFANT DEATH SYNDROME (Also complete Section H-2, questions 2-11)**

1. Position of decedent at discovery?

  a. ☐ On stomach, face down  c. ☐ On stomach, face position unknown  e. ☐ On side

  b. ☐ On stomach, face to side  d. ☐ On back  f. ☐ Unknown

2. Normal sleeping position?

  a. ☐ On back    b. ☐ On stomach    c. ☐ On side    d. ☐ Varies    e. ☐ Unknown

3. Location of decedent when found?

  a. ☐ Crib    b. ☐ Playpen    c. ☐ Bed    d. ☐ Couch    e. ☐ Floor    f. ☐ Other    g. ☐ Unknown

4. Was decedent sleeping alone?

  a. ☐ Yes    b. ☐ No    c. ☐ Unknown

**2.** ☐ **INADEQUATE CARE OR NEGLECT** (Mark all that apply)

- a. ☐ Apparent lack of supervision
- b. ☐ Apparent lack of medical care
- c. ☐ Munchausen Syndrome by Proxy
- d. ☐ Failure to Thrive (non-organic)
- e. ☐ Malnutrition
- f. ☐ Dehydration
- g. ☐ Oral water intoxication
- h. ☐ Delayed medical care
- i. ☐ Inadequate medical attention
- j. ☐ Out-of-hospital birth
- k. ☐ Other

**3.** ☐ **VEHICLE ACCIDENT**

1. Position of decedent?

- a. ☐ Operator
- b. ☐ Pedestrian
- c. ☐ Passenger
- d. ☐ Bicyclist
- e. ☐ Other
- f. ☐ Unknown

2. Vehicle in which decedent was occupant?

- a. ☐ Car
- b. ☐ Truck/RV/Van
- c. ☐ Motorcycle
- d. ☐ Bicycle
- e. ☐ Riding mower
- f. ☐ Farm tractor
- g. ☐ Other farm vehicle
- h. ☐ All-terrain vehicle
- i ☐ Semi/Tractor trailer unit
- j. ☐ Other
- k. ☐ Not applicable

3. Vehicle in which decedent was not occupant?

- a. ☐ Car
- b. ☐ Truck/RV/Van
- c. ☐ Motorcycle
- d. ☐ Bicycle
- e. ☐ Riding mower
- f. ☐ Farm tractor
- g. ☐ Other farm vehicle
- h. ☐ All-terrain vehicle
- i ☐ Semi/Tractor trailer unit
- j. ☐ Other
- k. ☐ Not applicable

4. Condition of road?

- a. ☐ Normal  b. ☐ Loose gravel  c. ☐ Wet  d. ☐ Ice or snow  e. ☐ Other  f. ☐ Unknown

5. Restraint used?

- a. ☐ Present, not used
- b. ☐ None in vehicle
- c. ☐ Used correctly
- d. ☐ Used incorrectly
- e. ☐ Unknown
- f. ☐ Not applicable

6. Helmet used?

- a. ☐ Helmet worn
- b. ☐ Helmet not worn
- c. ☐ Not applicable

7. Alcohol and/or other drug use?

- a. ☐ Decedent impaired
- b. ☐ Driver of decedent's vehicle impaired
- c. ☐ Driver of other vehicle impaired
- d. ☐ Not applicable

8. Primary cause of accident?

- a. ☐ Speeding
- b. ☐ Carelessness
- c. ☐ Mechanical failure
- d. ☐ Weather conditions
- e. ☐ Driver error
- f. ☐ Other
- g. ☐ Unknown

**4.** ☐ **DROWNING**

1. Place of drowning?

- a. ☐ Lake, river, pond or creek
- b. ☐ Bathtub
- c. ☐ Swimming pool
- d. ☐ Well/Cistern
- e. ☐ Bucket
- f. ☐ Wading pool
- g. ☐ Other
- h. ☐ Unknown

2. Activity at time of drowning?

- a. ☐ Boating
- b. ☐ Playing at water's edge
- c. ☐ Swimming
- d. ☐ Playing
- e. ☐ Other
- f. ☐ Unknown

3. Was decedent wearing a floatation device?  a. ☐ Yes  b. ☐ No

4. Did decedent enter area of water unattended?  a. ☐ Yes  b. ☐ No  c. ☐ Unknown  d. ☐ Not applicable

5. Could decedent swim?  a. ☐ Yes  b. ☐ No  c. ☐ Unknown  d. ☐ Not applicable

6. Were alcohol or drugs a factor?  a. ☐ Yes  b. ☐ No

**5.** ☐ **FIREARM**

    1. Person handling the firearm?

        a. ☐ Decedent     b. ☐ Family member     c. ☐ Acquaintance     d. ☐ Stranger     e. ☐ Unknown

    2. Type of firearm?

        a. ☐ Handgun     b. ☐ Rifle     c. ☐ Shotgun     d. ☐ Other     e. ☐ Unknown

    3. Age of person handling firearm?     a. ☐ _____     b. ☐ Unknown

    4. Use of firearm at time of injury?

        a. ☐ Shooting at other person     d. ☐ Target shooting     g. ☐ Playing
        b. ☐ Shooting at self     e. ☐ Loading firearm     h. ☐ Other
        c. ☐ Cleaning firearm     f. ☐ Hunting     i. ☐ Unknown

    5. Did person handling firearm attend safety classes?     a. ☐ Yes     b. ☐ No     c. ☐ Unknown

**6.** ☐ **SUFFOCATION/STRANGULATION**

    1. Cause of suffocation/strangulation?

        a. ☐ Other person overlaying or rolling over decedent     f. ☐ Object exerting pressure on victim's neck/chest
        b. ☐ Wedging     g. ☐ Small object or toy in mouth
        c. ☐ Food     i. ☐ Other
        d. ☐ Other person's hand(s)     j. ☐ Unknown
        e. ☐ Object covering decedent's mouth/nose

    2. If sleeping, location of decedent at the time?

        a. ☐ In crib     c. ☐ In couch/chair     e. ☐ In infant car seat     g. ☐ Other
        b. ☐ In bed     d. ☐ Being held     f. ☐ On floor     h. ☐ Unknown

    3. If sleeping, was decedent sleeping alone?

        a. ☐ Yes     b. ☐ No     c. ☐ Unknown

    4. If bedding was involved:

        1. Was the design of the bed hazardous?
            a. ☐ Yes     b. ☐ No     c. ☐ Unknown

        2. Was decedent placed on soft bedding?
            a. ☐ Yes     b. ☐ No     c. ☐ Unknown

        3. Was there improper use of bedding?
            a. ☐ Yes     b. ☐ No     c. ☐ Unknown

**7.** ☐ **ELECTROCUTION**

    1. Source of electricity?

        a. ☐ Water contact     c. ☐ Electrical outlet     e. ☐ Tool     g. ☐ Other
        b. ☐ Electrical wire     d. ☐ Appliance     f. ☐ Lightening     h. ☐ Unknown

**8.** ☐ **FALL INJURY**

    1. Fall was from?

        a. ☐ Open window     c. ☐ Natural elevation     e. ☐ Man-made elevation
        b. ☐ Furniture     d. ☐ Stairs or steps     f. ☐ Other

    2. Height of fall?     a. ☐ # feet _____     b. ☐ Unknown

    3. Landing surface composition/hardness?     a. ☐ Carpet     b. ☐ Concrete     c. ☐ Ground     d. ☐ Other

    4. Was decedent in a baby walker?     a. ☐ Yes     b. ☐ No     c. ☐ Not applicable

    5. Was decedent thrown or pushed down?     a. ☐ Yes     b. ☐ No     c. ☐ Unknown

**9. ☐ POISONING/OVERDOSE**

1. Type of poisoning?

   a. ☐ Prescription medicine   d. ☐ Illegal drug   g. ☐ Food product
   b. ☐ Over-the-counter medicine   e. ☐ Alcohol   h. ☐ Other
   c. ☐ Chemical   f. ☐ Carbon monoxide or other gas inhalation   i. ☐ unknown

2. Was substance in safety package?

   a. ☐ Yes   b. ☐ No   c. ☐ Unknown   d. ☐ Not applicable

3. Location of drug or chemical?

   a. ☐ In closed, secured area   b. ☐ In closed, unsecured area   c. ☐ In open area

**10. ☐ FIRE/BURN**

1. If fire, the source?

   a. ☐ Matches   c. ☐ Cigarette   e. ☐ Explosives   g. ☐ Space heater   i. ☐ Other
   b. ☐ Lighter   d. ☐ Combustibles   f. ☐ Fireworks   h. ☐ Faulty wiring   j. ☐ Unknown

2. Smoke alarm present?   a. ☐ Yes   b. ☐ No   c. ☐ Unknown   d. ☐ Not applicable

3. Smoke alarm in working order?   a. ☐ Yes   b. ☐ No   c. ☐ Unknown   d. ☐ Not applicable

4. Fire started by?   a. ☐ Decedent   b. ☐ Other   c. ☐ No one   d. ☐ Unknown

5. Activity of person starting the fire?

   a. ☐ Playing   c. ☐ Cooking   e. ☐ Other   g. ☐ Not applicable
   b. ☐ Smoking   d. ☐ Suspected arson   f. ☐ Unknown

6. Construction of fire site?

   a. ☐ Wood frame   b. ☐ Brick/stone   c. ☐ Metal   d. ☐ Trailer   e. ☐ Other   f. ☐ Not applicable

7. Multiple fire injuries or deaths?   a. ☐ Yes   b. ☐ No

8. For structure fire, where was decedent found?

   a. ☐ Hiding   b. ☐ In bed   c. ☐ Stairway   d. ☐ Close to exit   e. ☐ Other

9. Did decedent know of a fire escape plan?

   a. ☐ Yes   b. ☐ No   c. ☐ Unknown   d. ☐ Not applicable

10. If burn, the source?

   a. ☐ Hot Water   b. ☐ Appliance   c. ☐ Cigarettes   d. ☐ Heater   e. ☐ Chemical   f. ☐ Other

**11. ☐ CRUSH (Non-vehicle)** (Describe in narrative)

1. Where did crush occur?   a. ☐ Indoors   b. ☐ Outdoors

**12. ☐ CONFINEMENT**

1. Place of confinement?

   a. ☐ Refrigerator/Appliance   c. ☐ Chest/Box/Locker   e. ☐ Other
   b. ☐ Motor vehicle   d. ☐ Room/Building

**13. ☐ SHAKEN/IMPACT SYNDROME**

1. Prior history of abuse?

   a. ☐ Yes   b. ☐ No

2. Suspected cause?

   a. ☐ Crying   b. ☐ Disobedience   c. ☐ Feeding difficulty   d. ☐ Toilet training   e. ☐ Other   f. ☐ Unknown

**14.** ☐ **OTHER INFLICTED INJURY**

   1. Manner of injury?

      a. ☐ Cut/stabbed    b. ☐ Struck    c. ☐ Thrown    d. ☐ Other    e. ☐ Unknown

   2. Injury inflicted with?
      a. ☐ Sharp object (e.g., knife, scissors)    c. ☐ Hands/feet    e. ☐ Unknown
      b. ☐ Blunt object (e.g., hammer, bat)    d. ☐ Other

**15.** ☐ **OTHER CAUSE** (Describe in narrative)

## J. NARRATIVE DESCRIPTION OF CIRCUMSTANCES OR OTHER COMMENTS

 

 

 

 

 

## K. SERVICES PROVIDED

   1. List services provided by agencies as a result of the death. (Mark all that apply)

      a. ☐ Bereavement counseling    d. ☐ Emergency shelter    g. ☐ Health care    j. ☐ No services
      b. ☐ Economic support    e. ☐ Mental health services    h. ☐ Legal services
      c. ☐ Funeral arrangements    f. ☐ Social services    i. ☐ Other

## L. PREVENTION

   1. To what degree was this death believed to be preventable?

      a. ☐ Not at all    b. ☐ Possibly    c. ☐ Definitely

   2. Primary risk factors involved in the child's death? (Mark all that apply)

      a. ☐ Medical    c. ☐ Economic    e. ☐ Environmental    f. ☐ Drugs or alcohol
      b. ☐ Social    d. ☐ Behavioral    f. ☐ Product safety    h. ☐ Other

   3. Were these risk factors identified in your community prior to the death?    a. ☐ Yes    b. ☐ No

   4. Was any action taken in your community to address the risk factors prior to the death?    a. ☐ Yes    b. ☐ No

   5. Could the family or child have taken any actions to reduce the risk?    a. ☐ Yes    b. ☐ No    c. ☐ Unknown

   6. What prevention activities have been proposed since the death? (Mark all that apply)

      a. ☐ Legislation, law or ordinance    f. ☐ Consumer product safety action (800-638-8095)
      b. ☐ Community safety project    g. ☐ News services
      c. ☐ Public forums    h. ☐ Changes in agency practice
      d. ☐ Educational activities in school    i. ☐ Other programs or activities
      e. ☐ Educational activities in the media    j. ☐ None

   7. Target populations for prevention activities? (Mark all that apply)

      a. ☐ Children    c. ☐ Parents/Care givers    e. ☐ Others
      b. ☐ General public    d. ☐ Child protection professionals

   8. Estimated costs for prevention?

      a. ☐ No cost involved    c. ☐ <$100    e. ☐ >$500
      b. ☐ All services donated    d. ☐ $100-$500    f. ☐ Unknown

   9. Lead organization?

      a. ☐ Health/Medical services    d. ☐ Schools    g. ☐ Other
      b. ☐ Social services    e. ☐ Mental health services
      c. ☐ Law enforcement    f. ☐ Local community group

CFRP CHAIR SIGNATURE           DATE (MM/DD/YY)
▶                                    __ __ / __ __ / __ __

REGIONAL COORDINATOR SIGNATURE        DATE (MM/DD/YY)
▶                                    __ __ / __ __ / __ __

## ♦SUDDEN UNEXPLAINED DEATH OF INFANTS

### SUDDEN INFANT DEATH SYNDROME (SIDS)

SIDS is the **sudden, unexplained** death of an infant less than one year of age. While research continues, to date, it has failed to find a specific cause for SIDS. Instead of a single finding, many researchers now believe that several risk factors may contribute to SIDS:

- sleep position
- rebreathing
- prematurity/low birth weight
- young mothers
- smoking, alcohol and chemical use during pregnancy

Not all sudden, unexplained infant deaths are SIDS related. In a small number of cases, these fatalities can be attributed to a specific cause:

- accidental injury/suffocation
- undiagnosed congenital defects
- inflicted injury/event

To help the certified child-death pathologist make an accurate causal determination, there must be a complete evaluation of the history and circumstances surrounding the death. According to the National Institute of Child Health and Human Development, for an infant death to be classified as SIDS, the evaluation must include three components:

- thorough death-scene investigation
- clinical and social history
- complete autopsy

STAT's Death-Scene Investigative Checklist will ensure that the most appropriate information is obtained. This checklist and instructions for its use can be found on page 516. The completed checklist should accompany the body to the certified child-death pathologist or be forwarded to the pathologist as soon as possible.

Completing the checklist requires inspection of the death scene and interviewing family and/or caregivers as soon as possible. Evaluations/investigations which are thorough, objective and empathetic result in better autopsy and causal determination.

### SIDS RESOURCES, INC.

When a baby dies of SIDS, the immediate and extended families of that child need medical information and support. The most effective way to provide this help is through a well-informed and consistent network of health professionals and volunteers. SIDS Resources, Inc., a not-for-profit organization, initiates these services and coordinates the information and support network. SIDS Resources, Inc. is a partnership among SIDS families, health professionals, emergency responders and business and corporate representatives from throughout the state. This statewide organization is committed to:

- providing services for families who lose infants to SIDS
- providing professional education for members of the SIDS service delivery network
- providing community education to heighten factual understanding of SIDS and to focus attention on Sudden Infant Death Syndrome as a research/medical problem

SIDS Resources works with families, friends and child care providers to offer support and supply current, pertinent, medical information about SIDS. Ongoing support is available to families and friends through individual counseling, support group sessions, home visits and research update meetings.

SIDS Resources initiates programs designed to educate and inform the community about SIDS. They also serve as a source of information and support for health professionals (physicians, nurses, emergency room staffs) and first responders (police, firemen, paramedics).

One of the future goals of SIDS Resources is to help find the answers to the mystery of SIDS in conjunction with existing local and national research programs. Until such answers are found, SIDS Resources is dedicated to serving those who are touched by the tragedy of Sudden Infant Death Syndrome.

## YOU CAN HELP

All services, programs and activities are planned by SIDS Resources with the specific purposes of commemorating the children whose lives have been taken by this tragedy, informing the community about SIDS and enlisting public support in the fight against Sudden Infant Death Syndrome. **SIDS Resources provides all services at no charge.**

If additional information is needed call or write:

SIDS Resources, Inc.
143 Grand
St. Louis, MO 63122
(314) 822-2323
(800) 421-3511
FAX: (314) 822-2098

## ◆ PREVENTION

### PREVENTION–WHAT CAN WE DO?

STAT facilitates prevention efforts by channeling injury prevention education materials and ideas with effective, proven interventions to the county child fatality review panels. Materials will be provided based on ongoing data collection that permits the identification of specific injuries causing the highest mortality and morbidity in the program's target population.

- **Invest resources to facilitate community change.**

    To continue this intensive process of community education and professional skill development, consideration should be given to extending the comprehensive, multi-disciplinary approach used for reviewing children's deaths to other complex social and health problems. STAT and its network is being used to evaluate and provide investigative assistance on the complex cases of abuse/neglect.

- **Improve parental/caregiver supervision through education and better access to child care services.**

    Far too many children were unsupervised at the time of their deaths. To prevent injuries and deaths because of lack of supervision, parents and caregivers need age-appropriate information on the behavior and needs of children, access to child care and parent training.

- **Educate the multi-disciplinary investigative community and child fatality review panel members about the importance of accurately recording the level of supervision and circumstances immediately surrounding the death of the child.**

- **Closely monitor families at risk of a second preventable death or injury and provide them with appropriate services.**

Too often, surviving children in the same family or household are at risk for significant morbidity and mortality. In the urban areas, urban case coordinators will be responsible for managing agency and community services and programs to benefit the siblings, their families and the community and to reduce further fatalities in these high-risk families. The urban case coordinator will integrate agency and community services for immediate intervention and have ongoing contact with the family to ensure positive outcomes.

- **Implement a coordinated strategy aimed at reducing injuries and preventable deaths.**

    It is clear that the data from this program will more accurately define how and why children are dying in Missouri. By designating a member of each child fatality review panel to serve as a "prevention" liaison, STAT will encourage using the data to focus resources on interventions and prevention strategies. Panels will be encouraged to collaborate with hospitals, health departments, schools, social services agencies and community organizations in order to improve the success of programs and projects selected.

## PREVENTION–WHAT CAN I DO?

As professionals committed to the prevention of child injuries, we have a responsibility to help keep children and families safe. Opportunities to observe family behaviors and environment are available to us as we interact and spend time in clients' homes.

As child and family advocates, we can intervene without intrusion, when we identify risks to children and families. An opportunity to educate parents and care-givers on interventions that could save a child's life should never be missed. When visiting clients' homes, we recommend that you:

- **Promote back or side sleep position for healthy infants.**

    Researchers have yet to find the answer to what causes Sudden Infant Death Syndrome (SIDS). It appears there is no single cause, but rather, SIDS may be the result of multiple risk factors. Several groups, including the American Academy of Pediatrics and the SIDS Alliance, believe parents can reduce their baby's risk of SIDS by simply placing the infant on its back to sleep.

- **Educate parents and caregivers about proper sleeping arrangements and soft bedding products.**

    Parents and caregivers should be made aware that it is dangerous to sleep with an infant. Infants die from accidental suffocation due to overlying every year.

    The U.S. Consumer Product Safety Commission has recommended that parents not put infants to sleep on soft bedding, including those products intended for use by infants. Some infants placed on fluffy, plush products such as sheepskins, quilts, comforters and pillows have been found on their stomach (the prone position) with their face, nose and mouth covered by the soft bedding. Such soft products may cause infants to rebreath exhaled air and suffocate.

    Ensure infants are put to sleep in a crib with a firm, flat infant mattress. Cribs should meet safety standards and not contain pillows, toys or other inappropriate materials.

■ **Discuss fire safety.**

Ensure working smoke detectors are installed in the home and that fire escape routes are in place. Family, caregivers and babysitters should know how to access emergency services (fire, police, ambulance, etc.).

■ **Discuss appropriate disciplinary methods. If others care for the child, ensure they have similar disciplinary techniques.**

It is never appropriate to hit a child. Alternatives to physical punishment include removing privileges, time-outs, and isolating or sending a child to his or her room. The methods of discipline should be adapted as the child grows older.

■ **Discuss age-appropriate behaviors for children and unrealistic expectations of parents.**

Beginning to toilet train at an inappropriate age causes stress and anxiety for the child and the parent. When children can't meet unrealistic demands, parents may become abusive to the child. There is no hard and fast rule for when children are developmentally ready to accomplish such activities. Remind parents to be patient and understanding.

■ **Never shake an infant.**

Shaken Baby Syndrome, or more accurately, Shaken/Impact Syndrome, refers to possible brain, spinal and eye trauma resulting from shaking or impacting a baby's head. It is important that parents, child care providers and other caregivers understand the serious risks associated with shaking, striking or throwing an infant or young child. The violent whiplash of shaking or the sudden deceleration of being thrown into a crib or bed can cause irreversible or fatal injuries.

■ **Discuss supervision.**

Parents should never leave a child home alone or with another child, even for a minute. While parents should be encouraged to have time to relax away from their children, babies and young children cannot take care of themselves and should not be left home alone. If they leave the house, even for a minute, encourage parents to take their child with them or get a responsible person to watch the child. Another child—even a brother or sister—should not be left to take care of a baby until that child is old enough to do so. Never leave children alone in a car.

## ◆DEFINITIONS

**CARETAKER:** A person who is responsible for the care of the child at the time of the injury or death event.

**CERTIFIED DEATH:** Death reported by death certificate.

**CFRP AUTOPSY:** As reported on Data Forms 1 or 2, that decedent was autopsied. If an autopsy was completed, the name of the certified child-death pathologist should also be listed on the form.

**CFRP CAUSE OF DEATH:** As reported on Data Forms 1 and 2, includes categories for natural cause, SIDS, sudden unexplained death, and injuries classified by the type of agent or force which caused the injury.

**CFRP COUNTY OF DEATH:** The county, reported by the Data Forms 1 and 2, in which the death occurred. If the county of death is in Missouri, but the county of incidence is not, only identifying information (Section A of Data Form 1) is required.

**CFRP COUNTY OF INJURY/ILLNESS/EVENT:** The county, reported by Data Forms 1 or 2, in which the fatal illness, injury or event occurred. If the child is a newborn and never leaves the hospital, the county of death is also the county of injury/illness/event.

**CFRP COUNTY OF RESIDENCE:** The county, reported by Data Forms 1 or 2, as the county of decedent's residence. If the child is a newborn, the newborn's county of residence is the mother's county of residence.

**CFRP DATA BASE:** Data system maintained within the Missouri Department of Social Services to collect, analyze and report data on child fatalities. The system uses data from Data Forms 1 and 2, as well as death and birth certificates, Medicaid eligibility and substantiated child abuse and neglect deaths.

**CFRP REGION:** Seven geographic regions defined for the CFRP program (see map).

**CHILD ABUSE/NEGLECT (CA/N) FATALITY:** Death determined by DFS to be the result of child abuse or neglect. Determination may result from DFS investigation or court adjudication. As a cause of death, abuse refers to any physical injury, sexual abuse or emotional abuse inflicted on a child other than by accidental means by those responsible for the child's care, custody or control, except that discipline including spanking, administered in a reasonable manner, shall not be construed to be abuse. Neglect refers to failure to provide, by those responsible for the care, custody and control of the child, the proper or necessary support, education as required by law, nutrition or medical, surgical, or any other care necessary for the child's welfare.

**CHILDREN IN THE RESIDENCE:** Children in the residence may include natural brothers and sisters, legally adopted children, stepbrothers and stepsisters, half brothers and sisters, foster children and other unrelated children whose primary residence is the same as the victim's.

**DEATH-SCENE INVESTIGATION:** An attempt by any person functioning in their official capacity to gather information or evidence at the site where the fatal illness/injury/event occurred or where the child was ill prior to the death for the purpose of determining the causes and circumstances of the death.

**DRIVER:** The person who is operating or intending to operate the vehicle.

**EXPOSURE:** An injury resulting from allowing exposure of a child at inappropriate age to agents or circumstances known to be hazardous.

**INFLICTED INJURIES:** Inflicted injuries occur as a direct result of a person transferring force or energy, resulting in injury, to another person without regard to intent or purpose of the action. Examples include: shaking, throwing or striking, shooting with a gun, cutting with a knife, burning, poisoning, and immersing under water. Although intent to injure or kill may be present, persons inflicting injuries sometimes do so without full recognition of the consequences of their behavior; i.e., a frustrated caretaker shaking or striking a crying infant in an attempt to quiet them is an inflicted injury, even if no harm was meant.

**MALTREATMENT DEATH:** Death operationally defined as being due either to homicide or to substantiated child abuse/neglect as reported by DFS.

**MISSOURI INCIDENCE DEATHS:** Those deaths of children, birth through 17 years of age, which occur within the State of Missouri. Excluded are those deaths resulting from injury or other causes which occurred or originated outside the state. Although by law all child deaths occurring in Missouri are reported, the Missouri-incidence deaths are of primary interest. The most complete data are collected on these cases. Deaths where the illness/injury/event occurred in Missouri, but the child died in another state, may not be reported to Missouri officials. Review and forms preparation in these cases is optional.

**MORTALITY FILE CAUSE OF DEATH:** Cause of death as reported on Missouri death certificates.

**MORTALITY FILE MANNER OF DEATH:** Cause of death reported on death certificate formatted to conform to "Manner of Death" variables. This includes six categories: natural, accident (unintentional injury), suicide, homicide, undetermined and pending investigation.

**NON-OCCUPANT VEHICLE:** Any vehicle involved in the incident that the victim was not riding in or on.

**OCCUPANT VEHICLE:** The vehicle that the victim was in or on when injured.

**PEDESTRIAN:** A child not riding in a motor vehicle when struck by a vehicle.

**PERSON IN CHARGE OF OR PROVIDING IMMEDIATE CARE OF VICTIM:** In addition to the parents or other legal custodians, the following are included: babysitters, daycare personnel, school teachers, youth leaders, siblings or other relatives, paramours, or persons left in charge of watching the child at the time of the fatality, illness, injury or event.

**PROBABLE CAUSE:** Available facts when viewed in the light of surrounding circumstances which would cause a reasonable person to believe a child was abused or neglected.

**REVIEWABLE DEATH:** Death which has been reported by Data Form 1 as having met criteria for review by the CFRP panel, whether or not the review has yet been completed and reported.

**REVIEWED DEATH:** Death which has been reviewed by a local CFRP panel and reported on Data Form 2.

**SUDDEN INFANT DEATH SYNDROME (SIDS):** Sudden unexplained death of an infant, less than one year of age, which is unexplained by clinical history review, death-scene investigation and in which a thorough postmortem examination, including autopsy, fails to demonstrate an adequate cause of death. For an infant death to be classified as SIDS, all three components must be completed.

**SUDDEN UNEXPLAINED DEATH:** Sudden death of an infant, less than one year of age, due to an unexplained cause; a thorough investigation and postmortem examination are still needed.

**UNSUPERVISED DEATH:** Death for which data from Data Forms 1 and 2 suggest that the decedent may not have had adequate supervision at the time of the fatal injury or death event. Defining variables include reports that the event was unwitnessed, that the caretaker was asleep at the time (except during normal sleeping hours), or that there was no adult caretaker.

**WITNESS:** A witness is a person who has first-hand knowledge of the illness/injury/event leading to death. This excludes information obtained from other persons. A person inflicting injury on a child or identified as a perpetrator is NOT considered a witness. The witness may or may not be in charge of or providing immediate care for the child and may or may not have custody of the child. First-hand knowledge usually includes seeing or hearing the fatal illness/injury/event occur.

## ♦EXCERPTS FROM MISSOURI LAWS RELATING TO CHILD FATALITY REVIEWS

REFER TO LATEST EDITION OF THE MISSOURI REVISED STATUTES CUMULATIVE SUPPLEMENTS FOR COMPLETE STATUTE REVIEW

### CHILD FATALITY REVIEW PANELS

**210.192. Child fatality review panel to investigate deaths–qualifications–prosecutors and circuit attorneys to organize–report on investigations–immunity from civil liability–program for prevention.** –1. The prosecuting attorney or the circuit attorney shall impanel a child fatality review panel for the county or city not within a county in which he serves to investigate the deaths of children under the age of eighteen years, who are eligible to receive a certificate of live birth. The panel shall be formed and shall operate according to the rules, guidelines and protocols provided by the department of social services.

2. The panel shall include, but shall not be limited to, the following:

(1) The prosecuting or circuit attorney;

(2) The coroner or medical examiner for the county or city not within a county;

(3) Law enforcement personnel in the county or city not within a county;

(4) A representative from the division of family services;

(5) A provider of public health care services;

(6) A representative of the juvenile court;

(7) A provider of emergency medical services.

3. The prosecuting or circuit attorney shall organize the panel and shall call the first organizational meeting of the panel. The panel shall elect a chairman who shall convene the panel to meet to review suspicious deaths of children under the age of eighteen years, who are eligible to receive a certificate of live birth, in accordance with the rules, guidelines and protocols developed by the department of social services. The panel shall issue a final report of each investigation to the department of social services, state technical assistance team and to the director of the department of health. The final report shall include a completed summary report form. The form shall be developed by the director of the department of social services in consultation with the director of the department of health. The department of health shall analyze the child fatality review panel reports and periodically prepare epidemiological reports which describe the incidence, causes, location and other factors pertaining to childhood deaths. The department of health and department of social services shall make recommendations and develop programs to prevent childhood injuries and deaths.

4. The child fatality review panel shall enjoy such official immunity as exists at common law.

(L. 1991 H.B. 185 § 1, A.L. 1991 S.B. 190 § 12, A.L. 1994 S.B. 595)

**210.194. Panels, coroners and medical examiners–rules authorized for protocol and identifying suspicious deaths.** –1. The director of the department of social services, in consultation with the director of the department of health, shall promulgate rules, guidelines and protocols for child fatality review panels established pursuant to section 210.192 and for state child fatality review panels.

2. The director shall promulgate guidelines and protocols for coroners and medical examiners to use to help them to identify suspicious deaths of children under the age of eighteen years, who are eligible to receive a certificate of live birth.

10. All meetings conducted, all reports and records made and maintained pursuant to sections 210.192 to 210.196 by the department of social services and department of health and its divisions, including the state technical assistance team, or other appropriate persons, officials, or state child fatality review panel and local child fatality review panel shall be confidential and shall not be open to the general public except for the annual report pursuant to section 210.195.

(L. 1991 H.B. 185 § 2, A.L. 1993 S.B. 52, A.L. 1994 S.B. 595)

**210.195. State technical assistance team, duties–regional coordinators, appointment, duties–state child fatality review panel, appointment, duties, annual report, content.** –1. The director of the department of social services shall establish a special team which shall:

(1) Develop and implement protocols for the evaluation and review of child fatalities;

(2) Provide training, expertise and assistance to the county child fatality review panels for the review of child fatalities;

(3) When required and unanimously requested by the county fatality review panel, assist in the review and prosecution of specific child fatalities; and

(4) The special team may be known as the department of social services, state technical assistance team.

2. The director of the department of social services shall appoint regional coordinators to serve as resources to child fatality review panels established pursuant to section 210.192.

3. The director of the department of social services shall appoint a state child fatality review panel which shall meet biannually to provide oversight and make recommendations to the department of social services, state technical assistance team. The department of social services, state technical assistance team shall gather data from local child fatality review panels to identify systemic problems and shall submit an annual report to the director of the department of social services, the governor, the speaker of the house of representatives, the president pro tempore of the senate, and the children's services commission on ways to prevent further child abuse deaths.

(L. 1991 H.B. 185 § 3, A.L. 1994 S.B. 595)

**210.196. Hospitals and physicians, rules authorized for protocol and identifying suspicious deaths–child death pathologist, qualifications, certification–rules, procedure.** –1. The director of the department of health, in consultation with the director of the department of social services, shall promulgate rules, guidelines and protocols for hospitals and physicians to use to help them to identify suspicious deaths of children under the age of eighteen years, who are eligible to receive a certificate of live birth.

2. The director of the department of health shall promulgate rules for the certification of child death pathologists and shall develop protocols for such pathologists. A certified child death pathologist shall be a board-certified forensic pathologist or a board-certified pathologist who through special training or experience is deemed qualified in the area of child fatalities by the department of health.

10. Except as provided in section 630.167, RSMo, any hospital, physician, medical professional, mental health professional, or department of mental health facility shall disclose upon request all records, medical or social, of any child eligible to receive a certificate of live birth under the age of eighteen who has died to the coroner or medical examiner, division of family services representative, or public health representative who is a member of the local child fatality review panel

established pursuant to section 210.192 to investigate the child's death. Any legally recognized privileged communication, except that between attorney and client, shall not apply to situations involving the death of a child under the age of eighteen years, who is eligible to receive a certificate of live birth.

(L. 1991 H.B. 185 § 4, A.L. 1993 S.B. 52, A.L. 1994 S.B. 595)

**210.115. Reports of abuse, neglect, and under age eighteen deaths–who required to report–deaths required to be reported to child fatality review panel, when.** –1. When any physician, medical examiner, coroner, dentist, chiropractor, optometrist, podiatrist, resident, intern, nurse, hospital or clinic personnel that are engaged in the examination, care, treatment or research of persons, and any other health practitioner, psychologist, mental health professional, social worker, day care center worker or other child care worker, juvenile officer, probation or parole officer, teacher, principal or other school official, Christian Science practitioner, peace officer or law enforcement official, or other person with responsibility for the care of children has reasonable cause to suspect that a child has been or may be subjected to abuse or neglect or observes a child being subjected to conditions or circumstances which would reasonably result in abuse or neglect, that person shall immediately report or cause a report to be made to the division in accordance with the provisions of sections 210.109 to 210.183. **As used in this section, the term "abuse" is not limited to abuse inflicted by a person responsible for the child's care, custody and control as specified in section 210.110, but shall also include abuse inflicted by any other person.**

2. Whenever such person is required to report under sections 210.109 to 210.183 in an official capacity as a staff member of a medical institution, school facility, or other agency, whether public or private, the person in charge or a designated agent shall be notified immediately. The person in charge or a designated agent shall then become responsible for immediately making or causing such report to be made to the division. Nothing in this section, however, is meant to preclude any person from reporting abuse or neglect.

3. Notwithstanding any other provision of sections 210.109 to 210.183, any child who does not receive specified medical treatment by reason of the legitimate practice of the religious belief of the child's parents, guardian, or others legally responsible for the child, for that reason alone, shall not be found to be an abused or neglected child, and said parents, guardian or other persons legally responsible for the child shall not be entered into the central registry. However, the division may accept reports concerning such a child and may subsequently investigate or conduct a family assessment as a result of that report. Such an exception shall not limit the administrative or judicial authority of the state to ensure that medical services are provided to the child when the child's health requires it.

4. In addition to those persons and officials required to report actual or suspected abuse or neglect, any other person may report in accordance with sections 210.109 to 210.183 if such person has reasonable cause to suspect that a child has been or may be subjected to abuse or neglect or observes a child being subjected to conditions or circumstances which would reasonably result in abuse or neglect.

5. Any person or official required to report under this section, including employees of the division, who has probable cause to suspect that a child who is or may be under the age of eighteen, who is eligible to receive a certificate of live birth, has died shall report that fact to the appropriate medical examiner or coroner. The medical examiner or coroner shall accept the report for investigation, shall in a timely manner notify the division of the child's death pursuant to this

section and shall report the findings to the child fatality review panel established pursuant to section 210.192.

6. Any person or individual required to report **may also report the suspicion of abuse or neglect to any law enforcement agency or juvenile office.** Such report shall not, however, take the place of reporting or causing a report to be made to the division. **(CA/N HOTLINE CALL)**

(L. 1975 H.B. 578 § 2, A.L. 1980 S.B. 574, A.L. 1982 H.B. 1171, et al., A.L. 1991 H.B. 185, A.L. 1993, S.B. 253 & S.B. 394, A.L. 1994 S.B. 595)

**210.140. Privileged communications not recognized, exception.** –Any legally recognized privileged communication, except that between attorney and client, shall not apply to situations involving known or suspected child abuse or neglect and shall not constitute grounds for failure to report as required or permitted by sections 210.110 to 210.165, to cooperate with the division in any of its activities pursuant to sections 210.110 to 210.165, or to give or accept evidence in any judicial proceeding relating to child abuse or neglect.

(L. 1975 H.B. 578 § 7, A.L. 1980 S.B. 574)

**210.145. Telephone hot line and central registry for reports on child abuse–division of family services, duties, investigation within twenty-four hours, exception–training program–admissibility of reports in custody cases.** –1. The division shall establish and maintain an information system operating at all times, capable of receiving and maintaining reports. This information system shall have the ability to receive reports over a single, statewide toll-free number. Such information system shall maintain the results of all investigations, family assessments and services, and other relevant information.

2. The division shall maintain a central registry

3. Although reports may be made anonymously, the division shall in all cases, after obtaining relevant information regarding the alleged abuse or neglect, attempt to obtain the name and address of any person making a report.

4. Upon receipt of a report, the division shall immediately communicate such report to its appropriate local office, after a check has been made with the information system to determine whether previous reports have been made regarding actual or suspected abuse or neglect of the subject child, of any siblings, and the perpetrator, and relevant dispositional information regarding such previous reports. Such relevant information as may be contained in the information system shall be also reported to the local office of the division.

5. Upon receipt of a report, which, if true, would constitute violation of section 565.020, 565.021, 565.023, 565.024 or 565.050, RSMo, if the victim is a child less than eighteen years of age, section 566.030 or 566.060, RSMo, if the victim is a child less than eighteen years of age, or other crime under chapter 566, RSMo, if the victim is a child less than eighteen years of age and the perpetrator is twenty-one years of age or older, section 567.050, RSMo, if the victim is a child less than eighteen years of age, section 568.020, 568.030, 568.045, 568.050, 568.060, 568.080, or 568.090, RSMo, section 573.024 or 573.035, RSMo, or an attempt to commit any such crimes, the local office shall contact the appropriate law enforcement agency and provide such agency with a detailed description of the report received. In such cases the local division office shall request the assistance of the local law enforcement agency in all aspects of the investigation of the complaint. The appropriate law enforcement agency shall assist the division in the investigation or provide the division, within a reasonable time, an explanation in writing detailing the reasons why it is unable to assist.

6. The local office of the division shall cause a thorough investigation to be initiated immediately or no later than within twenty-four hours of receipt of the report from the division, except in cases where the sole basis for the report is educational neglect. If the report indicates that educational neglect is the only complaint and there is no suspicion of other neglect or abuse, the investigation shall be initiated within seventy-two hours of receipt of the report. If the report indicates the child is in danger of serious physical harm or threat to life, an investigation shall include direct observation of the subject child within twenty-four hours of the receipt of the report.

7. The investigation shall include but not be limited to the nature, extent, and cause of the abuse or neglect; the identity and age of the person responsible therefor; the names and conditions of other children in the home, if any; the home environment and the relationship of subject child to the parents or other persons responsible for the child's care; any indication of incidents of physical violence against any other household or family member; and other pertinent data.

8. When a report has been made by a person required to report under section 210.115, the division shall contact the person who made such report within forty-eight hours of the receipt of the report in order to ensure that full information has been received and to obtain any additional information or medical records, or both, that may be pertinent.

9. Upon completion of the investigation if the division suspects that the report was made maliciously or for the purpose of harassment, the division shall refer the report and any evidence of malice or harassment to the local prosecuting or circuit attorney.

10. Protective or preventive social services shall be provided by the division to the family and subject child and to others in the home to prevent abuse or neglect, to safeguard their health and welfare, and to help preserve and stabilize the family whenever possible. The juvenile court shall cooperate with the division in providing such services.

11. Multidisciplinary services shall be used whenever possible in conducting the investigation and in providing protective or preventive social services, including the services of law enforcement, the juvenile officer, the juvenile court, and other agencies, both public and private. The division shall cooperate with law enforcement agencies and juvenile courts to develop training programs to increase the ability of division personnel, juvenile officers and law enforcement officers to investigate suspected cases of abuse and neglect. The division, with input from the department of health, shall assist in identifying pertinent training on child abuse and neglect in order for law enforcement to meet the requirements of section 590.105, RSMo.

12. Within thirty days of an oral report of abuse or neglect, the local office shall update the information in the information system. The information system shall contain, at a minimum, the determination made by the division as a result of the investigation, identifying information on the subjects of the report, those responsible for the care of the subject child and other relevant dispositional information. The division shall complete all investigations within thirty days, unless good cause for the failure to complete the investigation is documented in the information system. If the investigation is not completed within thirty days the information system shall be updated at regular intervals and upon the completion of the investigation. The information in the information system shall be updated to reflect any subsequent findings, including any changes to the findings based on an administrative or judicial hearing on the matter.

13. The division shall maintain a record which contains the facts ascertained which support the determination as well as the facts that do not support the determination.

14. A person required to report under section 210.115 to the division shall be informed by the division of his right to obtain information concerning the disposition of his report. Such person shall receive, from the local office, if requested, information on the general disposition of his report. The local office shall respond to the request within forty-five days.

15. In any judicial proceeding involving the custody of a child the fact that a report may have been made pursuant to sections 210.109 to 210.183 shall not be admissible. However, nothing in this subsection shall prohibit the introduction of evidence from independent sources to support the allegations that may have caused a report to have been made.

16. The division of family service is hereby granted the authority to promulgate rules and regulations pursuant to the provisions of section 207.201, RSMo, and chapter 536, RSMo, to carry out the provisions of sections 210.109 to 210.183.

(L. 1975 H.B. 578 § 8, A.L. 1980 S.B. 574, A.L. 1982 H.B. 1171, et al., A.L. 1986 S.B. 470, A.L. 1990 H.B. 1370 et al., A.L. 1993 S.B. 52, A.L. 1994 S.B. 595)

**210.150. Confidentiality of reports and records exceptions–violation, penalty.** –1. The division of family services shall ensure the confidentiality of all reports and records made pursuant to sections 210.109 to 210.183 and maintained by the division, its local offices, the central registry, and other appropriate persons, officials, and institutions pursuant to sections 210.109 to 210.183. To protect the rights of the family and the child named in the report as a victim, the division of family services shall establish guidelines, which will ensure that any disclosure of information concerning the abuse and neglect involving that child is made only to person or agencies that have a right to such information. The division may require persons to make written requests for access to records maintained by the division. The division shall only release information to persons who have a right to such information. The division shall notify persons receiving information pursuant to subdivisions (2), (7), (8) and (9) of subsection 2 of this section of the purpose for which the information is released and of the penalties for unauthorized dissemination of information. Such information shall be used only for the purpose for which the information is released.

2. Only the following persons shall have access to investigation records contained in the central registry:

(1) Appropriate federal, state or local criminal justice agency personnel, or any agent of such entity, with a need for such information under the law to protect children from abuse or neglect;

(2) A physician or a designated agent who reasonably believes that the child being examined may be abused or neglected;

(3) Appropriate staff of the division and of its local offices, including interdisciplinary teams which are formed to assist the division in investigation, evaluation and treatment of child abuse and neglect cases or a multidisciplinary provider of professional treatment services for a child referred to the provider;

(4) Any child named in the report as a victim, or a legal representative, or the parent, if not the alleged perpetrator, or guardian of such person when such person is a minor, or is mentally ill or otherwise incompetent, but the names of reporters shall not be furnished to persons in this category. Prior to release of any identifying information, the division of family services shall determine if the release of such identifying information may place a person's life or safety in danger. If the division makes the determination that a person's life or safety may be in danger, the identifying information shall not be released. The division shall provide a method for confirming or certifying that a designee is acting on behalf of a subject;

(5) Any alleged perpetrator named in the report, but the names of reporters shall not be furnished to persons in this category. Prior to the release of any identifying information, the division of family services shall determine if the release of such identifying information may place a person's life or safety in danger. If the division makes the determination that a person's life or safety may be in danger, the identifying information shall not be released. However, the investigation reports will not be released to any alleged perpetrator with pending criminal charges arising out of the facts and circumstances named in the investigation records until an indictment is returned or an information filed;

(6) A grand jury, juvenile officer, prosecuting attorney, law enforcement officer involved in the investigation of child abuse or neglect, juvenile court or other court conducting abuse or neglect or child protective proceedings, and other federal, state and local government entities, or any agent of such entity, with a need for such information in order to carry out its responsibilities under the law to protect children from abuse or neglect;

(7) Any person engaged in a bona fide research purpose, with the permission of the director; provided, however, that no information identifying the child named in the report as a victim or the reporters shall be made available to the researcher, unless the identifying information is essential to the research or evaluation and the child named in the report as a victim or, if the child is less than eighteen years of age, through the child's parent, or guardian provides written permission;

(8) Any child care facility; child placing agency; residential care facility, including group homes; juvenile courts; public or private elementary schools; public or private secondary schools; or any other public or private agency exercising temporary supervision over a child or providing or having care or custody of a child who may request an examination of the central registry from the division for all employees and volunteers or prospective employees and volunteers, who do or will provide services or care to children. Any agency or business recognized by the division of family services or business which provides training and places or recommends people for employment or for volunteers in positions where they will provide services or care to children may request the division to provide an examination of the central registry. Such agency or business shall provide verification of its status as a recognized agency. Requests for examinations shall be made to the division director or the director's designee in writing by the chief administrative officer of the above homes, centers, public and private elementary schools, public and private secondary schools, agencies or courts. The division shall respond in writing to that officer. The response shall include information pertaining to the nature and disposition of any report or reports of abuse or neglect revealed by the examination of the central registry. This response shall not include any identifying information regarding any person other than the alleged perpetrator of the abuse or neglect;

(9) Any person who inquires about a child abuse or neglect report involving a specific child care facility, child placing agency, residential care facility, public and private elementary schools, public and private secondary schools, juvenile court or other state agency. The information available to these persons is limited to the nature and disposition of any report contained in the central registry and shall not include any identifying information pertaining to any person mentioned in the report.

(10) Any state agency acting pursuant to statutes regarding a license of any person, institution, or agency which provides care for or services to children;

(11) Any child fatality review panel established pursuant to section 210.192 or any state child fatality review panel established pursuant to section 210.195.

3. Only the following persons shall have access to records maintained by the division pursuant to section 210.152 for which the division has received a report of child abuse and neglect and which the division has determined that there is insufficient evidence or in which the division proceeded with the family assessment and services approach:

(1) Appropriate staff of the division;

(2) Any child named in the report as a victim, or a legal representative, or the parent or guardian of such person when such person is a minor, or is mentally ill or otherwise incompetent. The names or other identifying information of reporters shall not be furnished to persons in this category. Prior to the release of any identifying information, the division of family services shall determine if the release of such identifying information may place a person's life or safety in danger. If the division makes the determination that a person's life or safety may be in danger, the identifying information shall not be released. The division shall provide for a method for confirming or certifying that a designee is acting on behalf of a subject.

(3) Any alleged perpetrator named in the report, but the names of reporters shall not be furnished to persons in this category. Prior to the release of any identifying information, the division of family services shall determine if the release of such identifying information may place a person's life or safety in danger. If the division makes the determination that a person's life or safety may be in danger, the identifying information shall not be released. However, the investigation reports will not be released to any alleged perpetrator with pending criminal charges arising out of the facts and circumstances named in the investigation records until an indictment is returned or an information filed;

(4) Any child fatality review panel established pursuant to section 210.192 or any state child fatality review panel established pursuant to section 210.195;

(5) Appropriate criminal justice agency personnel or juvenile officer;

(6) Multidisciplinary agency or individual including a physician or physician's designee who is providing services to the child or family, with the consent of the parent or guardian of the child or legal representative of the child;

(7) Any person engaged in bona fide research purpose, with the permission of the director; provided, however, that no information identifying the subjects of the reports or the reporters shall be made available to the researcher, unless the identifying information is essential to the research or evaluation and the subject, or if a child, through the child's parent or guardian, provides written permission.

4. After a period of not less than one year following a finding by the division, any person who is the subject of a report where there is insufficient evidence of abuse or neglect, may petition the circuit court to order the records removed from the division and destroyed. The division shall be named as respondent. Venue shall be in the county where the person resides, or in circuits with split venue in the venue in which the alleged perpetrator resides. If the alleged perpetrator is not a resident of the state, proper venue shall be in Cole County, naming the division of family services as respondent.

5. Any person who knowingly violates the provisions of this section, or who permits or encourages the unauthorized dissemination of information contained in the information system or the central registry and in reports and records made pursuant to sections 210.109 to 210.183, shall be guilty of a class A misdemeanor.

(L. 1975 H.B. 578 § 9, A.L. 1980 S.B. 574, A.L. 1982 H.B. 1171, et al., A.L. 1985 S.B. 401, A.L. 1986 H.B. 953, A.L. 1988 S.B. 719, A.L. 1991 H.B. 185, A.L. 1994 S.B. 595)

**211.321. Juvenile court records–records of peace officers, destruction, exceptions, release of certain information to victim.** –6. Records of juvenile court proceedings as well as all information obtained and social records prepared in the discharge of official duty for the court shall be disclosed to the child fatality review panel reviewing the child's death pursuant to section 210.192, RSMo, unless the juvenile court on its own motion, or upon application by the juvenile officer, enters an order to seal the records of the victim child.

(L. 1957 p. 642 § 2110.310, A.L. 1969 H.B. 227, A.L. 1980 S.B. 512, A.L. 1989 H.B. 502, et al., A.L. 1993 H.B. 562, A.L. 1994 S.B. 595)

**219.061. Aiding runaways–peace officers, duty of–records confidential, exceptions, penalty for divulging–division may sue for damages.** –3. Disclosure of any information contained in the records of the division relating to any child committed to it shall be made only in accordance with regulations prescribed by the division, provided that such regulations shall provide for full disclosure of such information to the parents or guardians, or if they be out of this state to the nearest immediate relative of such child, upon reasonable notice and demand and to the child fatality review panel reviewing the death of a child pursuant to section 210.192, RSMo. Any employee or officer of the division who shall communicate any such information in violation of any such regulations may be subject to immediate discharge.

(L. 1975 S.B. 170 § 12, A.L. 1994 S.B. 595)

**58.452. Child's death under age eighteen, notice to coroner by persons having knowledge–referral to child fatality review panel, when–procedure for nonsuspicious death, form, duties–autopsy, child death pathologist, when–disagreement on need for autopsy, procedure–violation by coroner, penalty.** –1. When any person in any county in which a coroner is required by section 58.010, dies and there are reasonable grounds to believe that such person was less than eighteen years of age, who is eligible to receive a certificate of live birth, the police, sheriff, law enforcement officer or official, health practitioner or hospital or any person having knowledge of such a death shall immediately notify the coroner of the known facts concerning the time, place, manner and circumstances of the death. The coroner shall notify the division of the child's death pursuant to section 210.115, RSMo. The coroner shall immediately evaluate the necessity for child fatality review and shall immediately notify the chairman of the child fatality review panel. The child fatality review panel shall be activated within twenty-four hours of such notice to review any death which includes one or more of the suspicious circumstances described in the protocol developed by the department of social services state technical assistance team pursuant to section 210.194, RSMo.

2. If the coroner determines that the death of the person under age eighteen years, who is eligible to receive a certificate of live birth, does not include any suspicious circumstances listed in the protocol, the coroner shall complete a nonsuspicious death form provided by the department of social services, state technical assistance team and have the form cosigned by the chairman of the child fatality review panel and forward the original to the department of social services, state technical assistance team within forty-eight hours of receiving notice of the child's death.

3. When a child under the age of eighteen years, who is eligible to receive a certificate of live birth dies, the coroner shall notify a certified child death pathologist to determine the need for an autopsy. The certified child death pathologist, in conjunction with the coroner, shall determine the need for an autopsy. If there is disagreement concerning the need for the autopsy, the certified child death pathologist shall make the determination unless the child fatality review panel, within twelve hours, decides against the certified child death pathologist.

4. When there is a disagreement regarding the necessity for an autopsy, the certified child death pathologist shall file a report with the chairman of the child fatality review panel indicating the basis for the disagreement. The pathologist's report on the disagreement shall be included in the report to the department of social services, state technical assistance team. If an autopsy is determined necessary, the autopsy shall be performed by a certified child death pathologist within twenty-four hours of receipt of the body by the pathologist or within twenty-four hours of the agreement by the pathologist to perform the autopsy, whichever occurs later.

5. Knowing failure by a coroner to refer a suspicious death of a child under the age of eighteen years, who is eligible to receive a certificate of live birth, to a child fatality review panel or to a certified child death pathologist is a class A misdemeanor.

(L. 1991 H.B. 185, A.L. 1994 S.B. 595)

**58.722. Child's death under age eighteen, notice to medical examiner by persons having knowledge–referral to child fatality review panel, when–procedure for nonsuspicious death, form, duties–autopsy, child death pathologist, when–disagreement on need for autopsy, procedure–violation by medical examiner, penalty.** –1. When any person dies within a county having a medical examiner and there are reasonable grounds to believe that such person was less than eighteen years of age, who was eligible to receive a certificate of live birth, the police, sheriff, law enforcement officer or official, or any person having knowledge of such a death shall immediately notify the medical examiner of the known facts concerning the time, place, manner and circumstances of the death. The medical examiner shall notify the division of the child's death pursuant to section 210.115, RSMo. The medical examiner shall immediately evaluate the necessity for child fatality review and shall immediately notify the chairman of the child fatality review panel. The child fatality review panel shall be activated within twenty-four hours of such notice to review any death which includes one or more of the suspicious circumstances described in the protocol developed by the department of social services state technical assistance team pursuant to section 210.194, RSMo.

2. If the medical examiner determines that the death of the person under age eighteen years, who is eligible to receive a certificate of live birth, does not include any suspicious circumstances listed in the protocol, the medical examiner shall complete a nonsuspicious child death form provided by the department of social services, state technical assistance team and have the form cosigned by the chairman of the child fatality review panel and forward the original to the department of social services, state technical assistance team within forty-eight hours of receiving notice of the child's death.

3. When a child under the age of eighteen years, who is eligible to receive a certificate of live birth dies, the medical examiner shall notify a certified child death pathologist to determine the need for an autopsy. The certified child death pathologist, in conjunction with the medical examiner, shall determine the need for an autopsy. If there is disagreement concerning the need for the autopsy, the certified child death pathologist shall make the determination unless the child fatality review panel, within twelve hours, decides against the certified child death pathologist.

4. When there is a disagreement regarding the necessity for an autopsy, the certified child death pathologist shall file a report with the chairman of the child fatality review panel indicating the basis for the disagreement. The pathologist's report on the disagreement shall be included in the report to the department of social services, state technical assistance team. If an autopsy is determined necessary, the autopsy shall be performed by a certified child death pathologist

within twenty-four hours of receipt of the body by the pathologist or within twenty-four hours of the agreement by the pathologist to perform the autopsy, whichever occurs later.

5. Knowing failure by a medical examiner to refer a suspicious death of a child under the age of eighteen years, who is eligible to receive a certificate of live birth, to a child fatality review panel or to a certified child death pathologist is a class A misdemeanor.

(L. 1991 H.B. 185, A.L. 1994 S.B. 595)

**194.117. Sudden infant death–notification–autopsy by certified child death pathologist required, procedure–cost, how paid–department of health, duties–rules and regulations.** –Any person who discovers the dead body of, or acquires the first knowledge of the death of, any child under the age of one year and over the age of one week, where the child died suddenly when in apparent good health, shall immediately notify the county coroner or medical examiner of the known facts concerning the time, place, manner, and circumstances of the death. All such deaths shall be autopsied by a certified child death pathologist. The coroner or medical examiner shall notify the parent or guardian of the child that an autopsy shall be performed at the expense of the state. The department of health shall receive prompt notification of such autopsy results. The results from the autopsy shall be reduced to writing and delivered to the state department of health. The term "sudden infant death syndrome" shall be entered on the death certificate as the principal cause of death where the term is appropriately descriptive of the circumstances surrounding the death of the child. The cost of the autopsy and transportation of the body shall be paid by the department of health, and the department shall pay, out of appropriations made for that purpose, as a reimbursement to the certified child death pathologist such costs that are within the limitation of maximum rates established by the rules and regulations of the department. Autopsies under this section shall be performed by pathologists deemed qualified to perform autopsies by the department of health and who agree to perform the autopsy according to protocols developed pursuant to section 210.196, RSMo. The department of health shall ensure that autopsy results are shared with the parents or guardian of the child and shall provide informational material on the subject of sudden infant death syndrome to the family. The coroner or medical examiner, certified child-death pathologist or family physician may release autopsy results to the parent or guardian of the child in cases of suspected sudden infant death syndrome. The director of the department of health shall prescribe reasonable rules and regulations necessary to carry out the provisions of this section, including the establishment of a cost schedule and standards for reimbursement of costs of autopsies performed pursuant to the provisions of this section. The provisions of this section shall not be construed so as to limit, restrict or otherwise affect any power, authority, duty or responsibility imposed by any other provision of law upon any coroner or medical examiner. The department of health may receive grants of money or other aid from federal and other public and private agencies or individuals for the administration or funding of this section or any portion thereof or for research to determine the cause and prevention of deaths caused by sudden infant death syndrome.

(L. 1978 S.B. 765 § 1, A.L. 1991 H.B. 185, A.L. 1993 S.B. 253 & S.B. 394)

## Child Sexual Abuse Cases
### Training–Investigation–Treatment

**590.105.** 6. Beginning on August 28, 1996, the peace officer standards and training commission with input from the department of health and the division of family services shall provide a minimum of thirty hours of initial education to all prospective law enforcement officers, except for agents of the conservation commission, concerning domestic and family violence.

7. The course of instruction and the objectives in learning and performance for the education of law enforcement officers required pursuant to subsection 6 of this section shall be developed and presented in consultation with public and private providers of programs for victims of domestic and family violence, persons who have demonstrated expertise in training and education concerning domestic and family violence, and the Missouri coalition against domestic violence. The peace officers standards and training commission shall consider the expertise and grant money of the national council of juvenile and family court judges, with their domestic and family violence project, as well as other federal funds and grant moneys available for training.

8. The course of instruction shall include, but is not limited to:

(1) The investigation and management of cases involving domestic and family violence and writing of reports in such cases, including:

(a) Physical abuse;

(b) Sexual abuse;

(c) Child fatalities;

(d) Child neglect;

(e) Interviewing children and alleged perpetrators;

(2) The nature, extent and causes of domestic and family violence;

(3) The safety of officers investigating incidents of domestic and family violence;

(4) The safety of the victims of domestic and family violence and other family and household members;

(5) The legal rights and remedies available to victims of domestic and family violence, including but not limited to rights and compensation of victims of crime, and enforcement of civil and criminal remedies;

(6) The services available to victims of domestic and family violence and their children;

(7) Sensitivity to cultural, racial and sexual issues and the effect of cultural, racial, and gender bias on the response of law enforcement officers and the enforcement of laws relating to domestic and family violence; and

(8) The provisions of applicable state statutes concerning domestic and family violence.

**660.520. Special team for child sexual abuse cases, assist in training, investigation, and prosecution–counties may develop team, members–division of family service duties.** –1. There is hereby established in the department of social services a special team which shall:

(1) Provide training, expertise and assistance to county multidisciplinary teams for the investigation and prosecution of child sexual abuse cases;

(2) Assist in the investigation of child sexual abuse cases, upon the request of local law enforcement agencies, prosecutors, or division of family services staff;

(3) Assist county multidisciplinary teams to develop and implement protocols for the investigation and prosecution of child sexual abuse cases.

(L. 1990 H.B. 1370 et al. § 1)

**660.523. Uniform rules for investigation of child sexual abuse cases–training provided for division of family services staff.** –2. The department of social services shall develop separate protocols for multiple-suspect and multiple-victim cases.

(L. 1990 H.B. 1370 et al. § 2)

**660.526. Child sexual abuse cases, annual training provided by division of family services.** –The division of family services shall ensure that all employees and persons with contracts with the division and who specialize in either the treatment, prosecution, or investigation of child sexual abuse receive a minimum of fifteen hours of annual training. Such training shall be in the investigation, prosecution, treatment, nature, extent and causes of sexual abuse.

(L. 1994 S.B. 595)

## ◆BIBLIOGRAPHY

Block, S, and Tilton, D: ICAN multi-agency child death review team, Report for 1992, ICAN, 1992.

Children's Services, State of Oregon: A report of Oregon child fatalities due to abuse and neglect, 1985-1989.

Colorado Department of Health, Colorado Department of Social Services, March 1993.

Dodson, WE, Monteleone, JA and Edwards, D: The St. Louis Case Control Study of Severe Child Abuse, VII International Congress on Child Abuse and Neglect, Sept. 25-28, 1988, Rio de Janeiro, Brazil.

Durfee, M: Fatal child abuse: Intervention and prevention, *Protecting Child* Spring:9-12, 1989.

Durfee, MJ, Gellert, GA, and Tilton-Durfee, D: Origins and clinical relevance of child death review teams, *JAMA* 267:3172-3175.

Ewigman, B, and Kivlahan, C: Final Recommendations of the Department of Social Services Task Force on Fatal Child Abuse, 1990.

Kaplan, SR: Child fatalities and child fatality review teams, unpublished document, ABA Center on Children and the Law.

Monteleone JA, Edwards, D, and Dodson, WE: The St. Louis Board of Inquiry Into Severe Child Abuse, VII International Congress on Child Abuse and Neglect, Sept. 25-28, 1988, Rio de Janeiro, Brazil.

Robinson, DH, and Stevens, GM: Child abuse and neglect fatalities: Federal and state issues and responses, CRS Report for Congress, Congressional Research Service, The Library of Congress, April 16, 1992.

Smith, P, and Durfee, MJ: Child death review: A review of unpublished reports by states, stabstract/NEWSTAT 1/10/92.

Stangler, G, and Kivlahan, C: Missouri Child Fatality Review Project, interim progress report, Missouri Departments of Social Services and Health, April 1993.

Witherspoon, D: Organizing a multi-agency child death review team (draft).

# CHILD FATALITY REVIEW TEAMS

DONNA M. (PRENGER) KOLILIS, B.S.

Multi-agency child fatality review teams now exist across the country. They were formed because of concern about the lack of detection and reporting of child deaths caused by abuse or neglect. Several models exist, including state-level-only teams, states with selected urban city or regional teams, local teams, and those with both local and state-level teams. A state team is helpful if the primary purpose is to study and implement agency-discipline policies statewide. Local teams can facilitate and enhance the investigation of child deaths.

Just as there are various models for teams, there are also various populations served. Ideally, teams evaluate all deaths of children under age 18 years. However, because of limited resources, teams often restrict their reviews to deaths from certain causes, unexplained deaths, suspicious deaths, or deaths of children known to the child protective service agency. Some teams review deaths of children in specific age categories, for example, 1 year, under 5 years, or under 14 years of age.

In Missouri, the county coroner/medical examiner plays a key role in initiating the child fatality review process. He or she must determine the need for any autopsy, fill out appropriate data collection forms, and notify the child fatality review chairperson if the death meets certain criteria. The review team then convenes as soon as possible to review the information provided by its members. This "concurrent" review process differs from others that are more retrospective, meaning that cases are reviewed only monthly or quarterly.

## ◆HISTORY

The first multi-agency child death review team began in Los Angeles County in 1978. Dr. Michael Durfee, concerned that child homicide victims were being missed, set up a system to retrieve cases from coroners' records. He was later joined in his efforts by a public health nurse with a background in working child abuse cases. Together they established a protocol for reviewing potentially suspicious deaths (Durfee, 1994). Other California counties established similar teams. In 1985-1986 Oregon and South Carolina formed the first state teams. By 1990 fatality review teams were operating in 12 states. Presently, 48 states have some type of review process; there are also review teams in Washington, D.C., two Canadian provinces, and Sidney, Australia.

## ◆COMPOSITION AND FUNCTIONS OF THE TEAM

The review team can be an internal one that reviews deaths from a particular agency or an external team that considers the activities of all agencies. The panels are not designed to criminalize or find fault in all child deaths. Instead the review teams, which comprise child protection professionals, attempt to identify the cause and circumstances of child deaths. The data collected from such findings are used to determine trends, target prevention strategies, identify specific family and community needs, or, when appropriate, support criminal justice interventions.

Local review teams do not act as investigative bodies. Their purpose is to enhance the knowledge base of the mandated investigators and service providers and to evaluate the potential needs and prevention interventions for the family and community. However, in fulfilling their individual job requirements, certain team members, like the coroner, prosecuting attorney and child protective service worker, may be directly involved in the evaluation or investigation process.

Review teams expand and refine traditional coroner/medical examiner systems of reporting and investigating child deaths. However, the unique attribute of the review team system is that all deaths can be evaluated, and those requiring it can be reviewed more extensively by local or state teams. Systems can be developed to assist in the initial death evaluation or investigation as well as to collect specific data. Information gathering, checklists, and uniform data collection forms document what is learned during the review process. The Missouri model has a standardized death scene checklist and data collection forms to maximize information gathering and documentation (**see pp. 516 to 526, Death-Scene Investigative Checklist for Child Fatalities and Child Fatality Review Panel Data Report**).

Local teams typically bring together anyone who had prior contact with the child. Various disciplines explore why a child died and attempt to determine if the death could have been prevented. Members include representatives from law enforcement, child protective services, coroner/medical examiners, prosecutors, public health, juvenile court system, pediatricians, and emergency medical services. Additional or optional members can attend reviews on a case-by-case basis and might include fire department personnel or teachers.

## ♦ INFANT AND CHILD PATHOLOGY

In many cases, the review of a child's death requires the services of a pathologist. The decision to autopsy is often a local one and is based on the availability of funds as opposed to need. Child fatality review programs are best served by specially trained child pathologists who follow a prescribed protocol specific to infants and children (**see pp. 527 to 530, Coroner/Medical Examiner Data Report**).

Missouri's certified Child-Death Pathologist Network ensures autopsies performed on children, birth through age 17 years, are performed by professionals with expertise in forensic pediatrics. Additionally, Network members are available to consult with coroners and others investigating child deaths. The pathologists in the Network are also eligible to be reimbursed for autopsies through the state's technical assistance team when the fatality is reviewed by the local/county child fatality review team. A description of the autopsy reimbursement procedures is as follows:

1. A signed contractual agreement between the pathologist and the State of Missouri, Department of Social Services (DSS), Child Fatality Review Program must be on file.

2. For each autopsy performed by a certified child pathologist on a child, birth through age 17 years, the pathologist invoices the State of Missouri, DSS. Accompanying the invoice is a complete autopsy report and a copy of the death-scene checklist.

3. Upon receipt, the invoice, autopsy report, and death-scene checklist are matched with the corresponding data collection Form 1. (A Data Form 1 is required for each death in this age population, and files are maintained by the DSS, Division of Family Services [DFS], State Technical Assistance Team [STAT]. The Data Form 1 must be completed and signed as reviewable for the claim to be paid by STAT.)

4. If the case meets program criteria, the autopsy invoice will be paid by STAT. For each claim submitted, a notification letter is generated and sent to the pathologist, notifying him or her of the status of the claim.

510

5. STAT notifies the Department of Health (DOH) of all suspected sudden infant death (SIDS) cases. Likewise, DOH informs STAT any time they receive a request for autopsy reimbursement on suspected SIDS cases. Communication between these offices ensures no duplication of payment occurs when the child is Medicaid-eligible. DOH pays for autopsies on suspected SIDS cases only when they are not Medicaid-eligible.

The Pathologist Network and reimbursement mechanism have ensured that those children requiring an autopsy receive one. Since the autopsy is one of the critical components needed to determine cause of death, we believe the Pathologist Network has contributed significantly to the child fatality review program in Missouri. More accurate determinations of all causes of deaths, in particular SIDS-type deaths, are being made. Other causes such as undiagnosed natural causes and accidental suffocations had previously been diagnosed as SIDS.

## GOALS

The goals of child death review teams appropriately are different, based on identified problems at the state and local level. Generally, they included the following:

1. The accurate identification and uniform reporting of the cause and manner of every child death

2. Enhanced coordination of efforts among participating agencies and improved individual agency responses to child death

3. Improved criminal investigations and improved response of the criminal justice system to child homicides

4. The design and implementation of cooperative, standardized protocols for the investigation of certain categories of child deaths

5. Improved communication and linkages among agencies and more timely notification of agencies when a child dies

6. The identification of needed changes in legislation, policy, and practices and expanded efforts in child health and safety to prevent child deaths.

## FUNDING

The federal government encourages cooperative child abuse investigations, including fatality investigations. The Child Abuse Prevention and Treatment Act of 1974 requires states that receive federal funds through the act to establish multidisciplinary teams. The Children's Justice Act of 1986 also offers funds to states for establishing task forces composed of child advocates, child protective services, health, judicial, law enforcement, legal, mental health, and parent participants to review and evaluate the handling of child abuse cases and fatalities. With this funding, many states have developed their multidisciplinary child death review teams, provided technical assistance to child protection professionals, prepared protocols for teams, and conducted joint training with the various child protection disciplines.

## PROTOCOLS AND TRAINING

The American Bar Association and the American Academy of Pediatrics have created model documents for laws, policies, and protocols for use in implementing teams. Teams should use such materials in developing localized procedures and protocols for child fatality investigations.

It is particularly important that joint training be provided to members of the team. Coroners/medical examiners, law enforcement, and other first responders should be adequately trained in death scene investigation and skilled in interviewing. Investigative aids such as death-scene checklists are particularly useful and ensure consistency in investigative efforts (**see pp. 516 through 522**).

A *technical assistance* team that serves as a centralized resource for local child fatality review teams is beneficial and can be key to the success of such teams. The investigation of child deaths is emotional, complex, and difficult, especially in rural counties where there are few deaths and limited resources. Consequently, when questions arise in the field, the technical assistance team can provide the help needed to ensure proper investigative techniques are used. The assistance team serves as a training opportunity, building confidence and increasing skill levels.

## CASE REVIEWS

The chronology of an actual "review" addressed the following events:

1. The death and the scene: Description of the child and the death scene.

2. The investigation and evaluation of circumstances: Actions being taken and information gathered that helps the team understand the cause and manner of death.

3. Interviews: With family members, witnesses, others.

4. Prior histories: Pertinent social, medical, and criminal backgrounds of the child, family, and others.

5. Agency-initiated actions that are being taken in the investigation, delivery of service, and prevention.

6. Team-initiated actions that should be taken by individual agencies and any collective response.

7. Need for follow-up: Additional meetings, if required.

Generally, this chronology of events is best achieved when the chairperson of the team calls on team members in the following order:

1. Coroner/medical examiner

2. Emergency medical services

3. Law enforcement

4. Child protective services

5. Public health

6. Juvenile court officers

7. Prosecuting attorney

8. Optional or other members, as appropriate.

Team members give a verbal report reflecting the information they have collected. (Teams with statutory authority usually have been given authority to access any and all records needed to investigate the death. However, all such records as well as the review itself are confidential and not available to the public.) Written reports and records from the various members may be reviewed by the team; however, copies of written reports and records are not made or distributed.

## FOLLOW-UP AND FOLLOW-THROUGH

Continued communication between panel members and additional meetings may be necessary. The review process gives teams the opportunity to enhance the evaluation and investigation process (if the review occurs concurrent with agency investigation) to identify risks and needs that require immediate community response and to monitor high-risk situations that remain after the death of a child. At the end of each review, teams should answer the following questions:

1. Is the fatality review complete and comprehensive? What more does the team need to do? Which team member(s) can provide this information?

2. Are there services that should be provided to surviving family and community members? Who on the panel can ensure these services are provided?

3. Does a potentially fatal risk still exist; if so, who should respond?

4. Are there children at immediate risk of harm?

5. Was the death preventable, and what actions should be taken individually and collectively, both short-term and long-term, to prevent similar deaths?

Determining the causes and circumstances of all child deaths–understanding how children die–is how we ultimately assist them in living.

*Most, but not all, parents love their children to the best of their ability. Some abilities are very poor; therefore, it is dangerous to be loved by some people.*

*Margaret Grant, MD*
*Psychiatric Consultant*
*Center for Trauma and Dissociation*

## ◆ WHAT IS BEING LEARNED FROM CHILD FATALITY REVIEW TEAMS

By reviewing child deaths, communities and agencies are improving their understanding of how and why children die. The collected data are identifying educational needs for professionals and caregivers and challenging and strengthening the practices of agencies–all in an effort to make communities healthier and safer for children across the country.

### INTERVENTIONS

While originally formed to address concerns about child deaths due to abuse or neglect, many fatality review teams have expanded their focus from suspicious deaths to all preventable deaths in an attempt to identify potentially fatal injuries and risks to children. Many child deaths are predictable and preventable. As child and family advocates, child protection professionals, who interact with parents and caregivers on a daily basis, can intervene without intrusion when risks to children and families are identified. What better time to observe family behaviors, identify environmental risks, and educate caregivers than when "making house calls." Opportunities to educate the community concerning the following interventions could save a child's life:

1. **Promote back or side sleep position for healthy infants.**

   Researchers have yet to find the answer to what causes SIDS. It appears there is no single cause, but rather SIDS may be a result from multiple risk factors. Several groups, including the American Academy of Pediatrics and SIDS Alliance, believe caregivers can reduce their baby's risk of SIDS by simply placing the infant on his or her back to sleep.

2. **Educate parents and caregivers about proper sleeping arrangements and soft bedding products.**

   Parents and caregivers should be made aware that it is dangerous to sleep with an infant. Infants die from accidental suffocation due to overlying every year. The U.S. Consumer Products Safety Commission has recommended that parents not put infants to sleep on soft bedding, including some products intended for use by infants. Some infants placed on fluffy, plush products such as sheepskins, quilts, comforters, and pillows have been found on their stomach (the prone position) with their face, nose, and mouth covered by the soft bedding. Such soft products may cause infants to rebreathe exhaled air and suffocate.

3. **Discuss fire safety.**

   Ensure working smoke detectors are installed in the home and that fire escape routes are in place. Family, caregivers, and babysitters should know how to access emergency services (fire, police, ambulance, etc.).

4. **Discuss appropriate disciplinary methods. If others care for the child, ensure they have similar disciplinary techniques.**

   The primary motive for infant and child homicides is an impulsive act of violence (with no fatal planned intent). Precipitating circumstances include crying or irritability; inappropriate toilet training, unreasonable developmental expectations, and physical punishment as a situational response. Parental education should include alternatives to physical punishment (removing privileges, time-outs, isolating or sending the child to his or her room). The methods of discipline should be adapted as the child grows older.

5. **Discuss age-appropriate behaviors for children and unrealistic expectations of parents.**

   Beginning to toilet-train at an inappropriate age causes stress and anxiety for the child and the parent. When children cannot meet unrealistic demands, parents may become abusive to the child. There is no hard and fast rule for when children are developmentally ready to accomplish such activities. Parents must be reminded to be patient and understanding.

6. **Discuss the risks associated with shaking an infant.**

   Shaken baby syndrome, or more accurately, shaken/impact syndrome, refers to possible brain, spinal, and eye trauma resulting from shaking or impacting a baby's head. It is important that parents, child care providers, and other caregivers understand the serious risks associated with shaking, striking, or throwing an infant or young child. The violent whiplash of shaking or the sudden deceleration of being thrown into a crib or bed can cause irreversible or fatal injuries.

7. **Discuss supervision.**

   Parents should not leave a child home alone or with another child, even for a few minutes. While parents should be encouraged to have time to relax away from their children, babies and young children cannot take care of themselves and should not be left home alone. Even responsible teens need to have "house" rules if they are left unsupervised, especially when identified hazards are present in or around the home (e.g., swimming pool, unsecured guns, medications, etc.). If parents need to leave the house, even for a minute, they should take the child with them or get a responsible person they trust to watch the child. Another child–even a brother or sister–should not be left to take care of a baby until that child is responsible enough to do so.

## BEYOND REVIEW: PREVENTION

Preventing child deaths is the ultimate goal of child fatality review teams. Prevention is simply thinking ahead and identifying injury risks to children, as illustrated by this list:

1. Do you put your infant (under age 1 year) in a safe crib for sleep?
2. Do you put your child in a seat belt or safety seat?
3. Do you hit your child or let anyone else hit him?
4. Can your children find matches or lighters in your house?
5. Do you leave your child under 10 years old alone near a body of water?
6. Are your window guards or screens in good condition?
7. Do you have any guns or air rifles in your house?
8. Do you know how to prevent your child from choking?
9. Are any of your babysitters under age 13 years?
10. Do you leave your child under age 5 years alone in the house, car, or yard?

The responsibility for responding to and preventing child fatalities lies with the community, not with any single agency or entity. By promoting more accurate identification and reporting of childhood fatalities, prevention strategies for all potentially fatal childhood events can be developed. Such strategies may include the following:

1.  Closely monitor families at risk for a second preventable death or injury and provide them with appropriate services.

2.  Improve parental/caregiver supervision through education and better access to child care services.

3.  Educate the multidisciplinary investigation community and child fatality review teams about the importance of accurately recording the level of supervision and circumstances immediately surrounding the death of a child.

4.  Implement coordinated, community-based strategies aimed at reducing injuries and preventable deaths. Use data collected by local child fatality review teams to document needs and focus resources.

## RED FLAGS FOR ABUSE

Abusive situations can occur when parental or caregiver stresses reach unhealthy levels. Often individuals who have not developed appropriate coping mechanisms end up inflicting injuries on children and family members. Professionals must consider the "red flag" characteristics of a potentially abusive parent listed in **Table 24-1**.

---

**Table 24-1. "Red Flag" Characteristics of Potentially Abusive Parents**

Considered abortion or giving child up for adoption
Excessively irritated by baby's crying
Repulsed and irritated at having to change diapers
Describes the child in negative terms–ugly, deformed, makes repulsive sounds
Passive, unconcerned about child's needs
Disciplines–spanks, slaps, yells at–infant under 6 months old for bad behavior
Does not talk to child
Tells others of disappointments with appearance or sex of infant
States that the infant "does things on purpose" to irritate or get even with parent(s)
Not involved with child
Plays very little with child
Very concerned about how soon infant will have control of bowel and bladder
Calls the child derogatory names
History of family or interpersonal violence and hostility

---

Deanne Tilton Durfee, Chair of the US Advisory Board on Child Abuse and Neglect and Executive Director of the Los Angeles Interagency Council on Child Abuse and Neglect, reflects that while fatal abuse "cannot always be predicted or prevented, we can improve our recognition, communication and accountability to reduce fatal risks to children, most of whom are too young to walk, talk, feed themselves, or resist a bottle of pills, an unfenced pool, or an unprepared or violent caretaker. The lessons we learn will hopefully provide valuable assistance in our nation's efforts to protect children, hold ourselves accountable for what we do in the name of child protection, reduce family isolation, and promote expertise, collaboration and support services that represent children's hope for a healthy future and, indeed, survival."

MISSOURI DEPARTMENT OF SOCIAL SERVICES
DIVISION OF FAMILY SERVICES
MISSOURI CHILD FATALITY REVIEW PROGRAM
**DEATH-SCENE INVESTIGATIVE CHECKLIST FOR CHILD FATALITIES**

615 HOWERTON COURT
JEFFERSON CITY, MO 65109
(314) 751-5980
(800) 487-1626

**(CORNER/MEDICAL EXAMINER SHOULD PREPARE AND SUBMIT TO CERTIFIED CHILD DEATH PATHOLOGIST PRIOR TO AUTOPSY.)**

## INSTRUCTIONS:
Complete each numbered item by providing the appropriate response and by marking the completed or not completed box in the left-hand margin. Make every attempt to obtain as much information as possible. For assistance, call (800) 487-1626.

COMPLETED   NOT COMPLETED

1. ☐ ☐

NAME OF DECEDENT _____ / (MI) _____ / (LAST)

RACE ☐ W = WHITE / B = BLACK / O = OTHER / U = UNKNOWN    SEX ☐ M ☐ F

DATE OF BIRTH (MM/DD/YY) _____   DATE OF DEATH (MM/DD/YY) _____   TIME OF DEATH: _____ ☐ AM ☐ PM

SCENE/EVENT ADDRESS (STREET, CITY, ZIP) _____   COUNTY OF SCENE/EVENT: _____

DECEDENT DISCOVERED BY (NAME): _____   DATE DISCOVERED (MM/DD/YY): _____ TIME: _____ ☐ AM ☐ PM

RELATIONSHIP TO DECEDENT: _____   DATE SCENE INVESTIGATION CONDUCTED (MM/DD/YY): _____ TIME: _____ ☐ AM ☐ PM

DEATH SCENE PHOTOGRAPHS OF DECEDENT OR SILHOUETTE TAKEN BY (NAME & TITLE): _____

DATE PHOTOS TAKEN (MM/DD/YY)? _____   TIME _____ ☐ AM ☐ PM   PRESENT LOCATION OF FILM/NEGATIVES/PRINTS: _____

WHO PRONOUNCED DECEDENT DEAD (NAME & TITLE)? _____   WHERE PRONOUNCED (HOME, MEDICAL FACILITY, ETC.) ADDRESS: _____

DFS HISTORY CHECKED BY (NAME & TITLE)? _____   DATE (MM/DD/YY): _____ TIME _____ ☐ AM ☐ PM   CFRP CRITERIA PREVIEWED? ☐ NO ☐ YES ☐ UNKNOWN

CERTIFIED CHILD-DEATH PATHOLOGIST CONSULTED (NAME)? _____   AUTOPSY REQUESTED? ☐ NO ☐ YES ☐ UNKNOWN

BODY DELIVERED TO PATHOLOGIST BY (NAME & TITLE): _____   DATE DELIVERED (MM/DD/YY) _____ TIME _____ ☐ AM ☐ PM

INVESTIGATOR(S) (NAME & TITLE): _____

INVESTIGATING AGENCY/DEPARTMENT _____   REPORT NUMBER _____

## ASSESSMENT OF HISTORY AND CIRCUMSTANCES

2. ☐ ☐

MEDICAL ASSISTANCE SUMMONED? ☐ NO ☐ YES ☐ UNKNOWN   IF YES, WHO WAS SUMMONDED? _____

WHO PLACED THE CALL (NAME & RELATIONSHIP)? _____   DATE (MM/DD/YY): _____ TIME: _____ ☐ AM ☐ PM

3. ☐ ☐

CONVEYED TO MEDICAL FACILITY? ☐ NO ☐ YES ☐ UNKNOWN

NAME AND ADDRESS OF MEDICAL FACILITY? _____

4. ☐ ☐

WAS DECEDENT PHOTOGRAPHED AT MEDICAL FACILITY? ☐ NO ☐ YES ☐ UNKNOWN

PHOTOS TAKEN BY (NAME & TITLE): _____

TIME: _____ ☐ AM ☐ PM   DATE (MM/DD/YY): _____   PRESENT LOCATION OF FILM/NEGATIVES/PRINTS: _____

5. ☐ ☐

RESUSCITATION BY EMS? ☐ NO ☐ YES ☐ UNKNOWN   ANYONE ELSE (NAME & RELATIONSHIP)? _____

IF NOT EMS, WAS PERSON CPR CERTIFIED? ☐ NO ☐ YES ☐ UNKNOWN

WHERE WAS RESUSCITATION INITIATED (HOME, NEIGHBOR'S HOME, HOSPITAL, ETC.)? _____   FOR HOW LONG? _____

6. ☐ ☐

DESCRIBE IN DETAIL, LOCATION WHERE DECEDENT WAS FOUND (BED, FLOOR, HOUSE, YARD, VEHICLE, TRASH CONTAINER, ETC.): _____

MO 886-3228 (3-95)   PAGE 1

**7.** ☐ ☐ | Describe anything unusual found on or around the body, especially anything that may have influenced the death (medicine, baby bottle, cleaning agent, bed clothing, etc.).

| SEIZED?<br>☐ NO  ☐ YES  ☐ UNKNOWN | IF YES, BY WHOM (NAME & TITLE)? | PRESENT LOCATION OF EVIDENCE: |
|---|---|---|

**8.** ☐ ☐

| WAS DECEDENT MOVED FROM ORIGINAL POSITION?<br>☐ NO  ☐ YES  ☐ UNKNOWN | MOVED BY WHOM (NAME AND RELATIONSHIP)? |
|---|---|

WHY MOVED?

**9.** ☐ ☐

| RIGOR MORTIS (RIGIDITY)<br>☐ NO  ☐ YES  ☐ UNKNOWN | WHERE OBSERVED ON DECEDENT? | DATE OBSERVED (MM/DD/YY): | TIME OBSERVED:<br>_____ ☐ AM ☐ PM |
|---|---|---|---|

(DO NOT ATTEMPT TO MOVE OR STRAIGHTEN FIXED EXTREMITIES)

**10.** ☐ ☐

| LIVOR MORTIS (SETTLING OF BLOOD)?<br>☐ NO  ☐ YES  ☐ UNKNOWN | WHERE OBSERVED ON DECEDENT? |
|---|---|
| TIME OBSERVED:<br>_____ ☐ AM  ☐ PM | CONSISTENT WITH POSITION WHEN FOUND?<br>☐ NO  ☐ YES  ☐ UNKNOWN |

**11.** ☐ ☐

| APPROXIMATE ENVIRONMENTAL TEMPERATURE AT LOCATION OF DEATH (IN FAHRENHEIT DEGREES)? _____ ° | TIME OBSERVED: _____ ☐ AM ☐ PM | DATE OBSERVED (MM/DD/YY): |
|---|---|---|

IF OUTSIDE, GENERAL WEATHER CONDITIONS:<br>☐ RAINING  ☐ SNOWING  ☐ SUNNY  ☐ OTHER: (DESCRIBE)_____

**12.** ☐ ☐

| TO THE TOUCH, APPARENT BODY TEMPERATURE OF DECEDENT AT LOCATION OF DEATH?<br>☐ WARM  ☐ SWEATY  ☐ COLD | DATE OBSERVED (MM/DD/YY): | TIME OBSERVED:<br>_____ ☐ AM ☐ PM |
|---|---|---|

**13.** ☐ ☐

| DATE DECEDENT LAST SEEN ALIVE (MM/DD/YY)? | TIME: _____ ☐ AM ☐ PM | BY WHOM (NAME & RELATIONSHIP)? |
|---|---|---|

WHAT WAS THE CONDITION OF THE DECEDENT WHEN LAST SEEN ALIVE?

**14.** ☐ ☐

| WAS DEATH WITNESSED?<br>☐ NO  ☐ YES  ☐ UNKNOWN | IF YES, BY WHOM (NAME & RELATIONSHIP)? DESCRIBE DETAILS IN NARRATIVE SECTION. |
|---|---|

**15.** ☐ ☐  WHAT WAS THE DECEDENT'S ACTIVITY PRIOR TO DEATH (e.g., SLEEPING, PLAYING, ETC.)?

**16.** ☐ ☐

APPEARANCE OF DECEDENT WHEN OBSERVED:<br>☐ CLEAN  ☐ DIRTY  ☐ OTHER:

DESCRIBE:

**17.** ☐ ☐

CLOTHING WORN?<br>☐ CLEAN  ☐ DIRTY  ☐ TORN OR DAMAGED    APPROPRIATE? ☐ NO  ☐ YES

DESCRIBE:

**18.** ☐ ☐

| CLOTHING SEIZED AND PACKAGED?<br>☐ NO  ☐ YES  ☐ UNKNOWN | IF YES, BY WHOM (NAME & TITLE)? |
|---|---|

PRESENT LOCATION OF EVIDENCE:

**19.** ☐ ☐

| BODY POSITION WHEN DISCOVERED:<br>☐ ON STOMACH  ☐ ON BACK  ☐ SEATED UPRIGHT  ☐ LEFT SIDE  ☐ RIGHT SIDE | IF APPLICABLE, BODY WAS:<br>☐ VERTICALLY PINNED  ☐ HORIZONTALLY PINNED  ☐ OTHER WEDGING  ☐ N/A |
|---|---|

PINNED OR WEDGED BY WHAT?

**20.** ☐ ☐

USUAL SLEEPING POSITION?<br>☐ ON STOMACH  ☐ ON BACK  ☐ SEATED UPRIGHT  ☐ LEFT SIDE  ☐ RIGHT SIDE

**21.** ☐ ☐

| POSITION OF FACE (NOSE/MOUTH) WHEN DISCOVERED:<br>☐ FACE DIRECTLY UP    ☐ FACE TO RIGHT<br>☐ FACE DIRECTLY DOWN    ☐ FACE TO LEFT | WERE PHOTOS TAKEN?<br>☐ NO  ☐ YES  ☐ UNKNOWN |
|---|---|
| IF PHOTOS TAKEN, WHO TOOK THEM (NAME & TITLE)? | DATE (MM/DD/YY): | TIME: _____ ☐ AM ☐ PM | PRESENT LOCATION OF FILM/NEGATIVES/PRINTS: |

**22.** ☐ ☐

| WAS DECEDENT'S FACE IN CONTACT WITH WET SUBSTANCE?<br>☐ NO  ☐ YES  ☐ UNKNOWN | SUBSTANCE APPEARED TO BE:<br>☐ MUCUS    ☐ VOMIT    ☐ BLOODY FROTH<br>☐ FOOD    ☐ SALIVA    ☐ DRIED SECRETION<br>☐ FORMULA    ☐ FROTH    ☐ BLOOD TINGED SECRETION<br>OTHER: _____ |
|---|---|

MO 886-3228 (3-95)

**23.** ☐ ☐ SUBSTANCE OBSERVED IN NOSE?
☐ NO ☐ YES ☐ UNKNOWN

SUBSTANCE APPEARED TO BE:
☐ MUCUS ☐ VOMIT ☐ BLOODY FROTH OTHER: _____
☐ FOOD ☐ SALIVA ☐ DRIED SECRETION
☐ FORMULA ☐ FROTH ☐ BLOOD TINGED SECRETION

**24.** ☐ ☐ SUBSTANCE OBSERVED IN MOUTH?
☐ NO ☐ YES ☐ UNKNOWN

SUBSTANCE APPEARED TO BE:
☐ MUCUS ☐ VOMIT ☐ BLOODY FROTH
☐ FOOD ☐ SALIVA ☐ DRIED SECRETION
☐ FORMULA ☐ FROTH ☐ BLOOD TINGED SECRETION

**25.** ☐ ☐ ANYTHING OBSTRUCTING FACE, NOSE OR MOUTH?
☐ NO ☐ YES ☐ IF YES, DESCRIBE

**26.** ☐ ☐ SECRETIONS FOUND ON:
☐ ☐ ☐ ☐ ☐ ☐

APPEARED TO BE:
☐ MUCUS ☐ VOMIT ☐ BLOODY FROTH OTHER: _____
☐ FOOD ☐ SALIVA ☐ DRIED SECRETION
☐ FORMULA ☐ FROTH ☐ BLOOD TINGED SECRETION

**27.** ☐ ☐ HEMORRHAGE OF EYES?  |  HEMORRHAGE OF EARS?
☐ NO ☐ YES ☐ UNKNOWN  |  ☐ NO ☐ YES ☐ UNKNOWN

DESCRIBE:

**28.** ☐ ☐ IS THERE A VISIBLE CREASE ON FACE, NECK OR HEAD FROM PILLOWS, CLOTHING, BEDDING, OR OTHER OBJECT?
☐ NO ☐ YES ☐ UNKNOWN

EXPLAIN:

**29.** ☐ ☐ SKETCH POSITION OF DECEDENT AS FOUND, AND IDENTIFY IF IN BED OR OTHER IDENTIFIABLE LOCATION. (INDICATE DIRECTION OF DECEDENT'S HEAD; CIRCLE DIRECTION INDICATOR.)

N
W — E
S

**30.** ☐ ☐ If appropriate, describe bed/crib/bassinet/couch/floor/water mattress/bean bag or other sleeping arrangement including all sheets, pillows, plastic covers, blankets, defects of miscellaneous objects in or near bedding where decedent was found. NOTE: If a crib, describe any defects, damage and/or inappropriate mattress size.

**31.** ☐ ☐ WAS ANYTHING SEIZED? DESCRIBE: _____ | BY WHOM (NAME & TITLE)? | PRESENT LOCATION OF ITEM(S):
☐ NO ☐ YES ☐ UNKNOWN

**32.** ☐ ☐ IF SLEEPING, WAS THE DECEDENT SLEEPING ALONE?
☐ NO ☐ YES ☐ UNKNOWN

IF NO, WHO WAS DECEDENT SLEEPING WITH? (NAME(S), RELATIONSHIP(S), AND AGE(S) NEEDED.)

| | |
|---|---|
| 33. ☐ ☐ | ANY POSSIBILITY OF OVERLAYING?<br>☐ NO  ☐ YES  ☐ UNKNOWN<br><br>IF YES, REPORTED RECENT ALCOHOL CONSUMPTION OR DRUG/MEDICINE USAGE BY PERSON SLEEPING WITH CHILD?<br>☐ NO  ☐ YES  ☐ UNKNOWN |
| 34. ☐ ☐ | IN GENERAL, DO LIVING CONDITIONS APPEAR OVERCROWDED?<br>☐ NO  ☐ YES  ☐ UNKNOWN<br>EXPLAIN: |
| 35. ☐ ☐ | IF ANY INJURY IS NOTED, HOW IS IT ALLEGED TO HAVE OCCURRED? |
| 36. ☐ ☐ | Fully describe any indications of trauma or injury including bruises, scrapes, cuts, rashes, burn marks, swelling, etc. Include colors, shapes, sizes and locations on body. (If not at scene, indicate location where body viewed?) |

| | | |
|---|---|---|
| 37. ☐ ☐ | IF INJURY WAS INFLICTED, APPARENT OBJECT OR WEAPON USED? | WHO INFLICTED INJURY (NAME & RELATIONSHIP)? |
| | WAS OBJECT SEIZED?<br>☐ NO  ☐ YES  ☐ UNKNOWN | SEIZED BY WHOM (NAME & TITLE)? |
| | PRESENT LOCATION OF OBJECT/WEAPON: | |

| | |
|---|---|
| 38. ☐ ☐ | IF INJURY RESULTED FROM A FALL, DESCRIBE WHAT DECEDENT FELL FROM, THE DISTANCE OF THE FALL AND SURFACE DECEDENT FELL ON (CARPET, CONCRETE, GROUND, ETC.). USE NARRATIVE SECTION, IF NECESSARY. |
| 39. ☐ ☐ | IF INJURY RESULTED FROM A BURN, DESCRIBE APPARENT CAUSE (HOT WATER, CIGARETTE, CHEMICAL, ETC.): |
| 40. ☐ ☐ | HAS DECEDENT HAD OTHER SERIOUS INJURIES DURING THE LAST YEAR?<br>☐ NO  ☐ YES  ☐ UNKNOWN<br>EXPLAIN: |
| 41. ☐ ☐ | HAS DECEDENT HAD A RECENT ILLNESS?<br>☐ NO  ☐ YES  ☐ UNKNOWN<br>EXPLAIN: |

MO 886-3228 (3-95)

PAGE 4

**42.** ☐ ☐ Has decedent been exposed to any contagious disease recently? ☐ NO ☐ YES ☐ UNKNOWN
If yes, explain: _____

_____

Symptoms Noted:

☐ Appetite change    ☐ Wheezes        ☐ Fussy
☐ Sniffles           ☐ Cough          ☐ Diarrhea
☐ Cold               ☐ Irritability   ☐ Runny nose
☐ Congestion         ☐ Other: _____    ☐ None noted
☐ Fever              ☐ How high? _____

**43.** ☐ ☐ WAS DECEDENT TAKEN FOR TREATMENT FOR PREVIOUS SYMPTOMS?
☐ NO ☐ YES ☐ UNKNOWN

| WHERE WAS TREATMENT RECEIVED (NAME OF FACILITY)? | WHO PROVIDED TREATMENT (NAME & TITLE)? |
|---|---|

IF YES, WHAT DIAGNOSIS WAS RENDERED?

**44.** ☐ ☐

| HAS DECEDENT BEEN ON MEDICATION? | IF YES, NAME OF MEDICATION: |
|---|---|
| ☐ NO ☐ YES ☐ UNKNOWN | |
| HAS DECEDENT RECEIVED RECENT IMMUNIZATION? | IF YES, WHAT TYPE? |
| ☐ NO ☐ YES ☐ UNKNOWN | |

IF YES, NAME OF MEDICAL PRACTITIONER/CLINIC:

**45.** ☐ ☐ ANY KNOWN ALLERGIES OR PREVIOUS REACTIONS TO SHOTS OR MEDICATIONS?
☐ NO ☐ YES ☐ UNKNOWN

IF YES, EXPLAIN:

**46.** ☐ ☐

| WHEN HAD DECEDENT LAST EATEN? DATE (MM/DD/YY): | TIME: _____ | ☐ AM ☐ PM | WHAT WAS EATEN OR INGESTED? |
|---|---|---|---|
| QUANTITY EATEN? | ANY FEEDING/EATING DIFFICULTIES (PAST OR RECENT)? Describe: _____ | | |

**47.** ☐ ☐ ANY KNOWN FOOD INTOLERANCE?
☐ NO ☐ YES ☐ UNKNOWN

IF YES, WHAT FOODS?

**48.** ☐ ☐

| IF INFANT, WAS DECEDENT BREAST FED? | FORMULA FED? | IF YES: |
|---|---|---|
| ☐ NO ☐ YES ☐ UNKNOWN | ☐ NO ☐ YES ☐ UNKNOWN | FORMULA BRAND:_____ |

**49.** ☐ ☐ HAD DECEDENT RECEIVED ANY OF THE FOLLOWING WITHIN THE LAST 48 HOURS?

☐ COW'S MILK           ☐ GOAT'S MILK       ☐ HONEY
☐ WATERED DOWN FORMULA ☐ UNKNOWN           OTHER: _____

**50.** ☐ ☐ HAS DECEDENT BEEN UNDER ROUTINE CARE OF A MEDICAL PRACTITIONER?
☐ NO ☐ YES ☐ UNKNOWN

IF YES, PRACTITIONER'S NAME/CLINIC:

DESCRIBE CHILD'S GENERAL TEMPERAMENT (e.g., COLICKY, FUSSY, HYPERACTIVE, QUIET, ETC.):

**51.** ☐ ☐ Name, age, and any known serious medical conditions of natural parents:

Mother (include maiden name):

Father:

| | |
|---|---|
| 52. ☐ ☐ | WHO DOES DECEDENT LIVE WITH IF DIFFERENT FROM PARENT(S) (NAME, ADDRESS & RELATIONSHIP)? |
| 53. ☐ ☐ | NAME, AGE, DOB AND ANY KNOWN SERIOUS HEALTH CONDITIONS OF SIBLINGS? |
| 54. ☐ ☐ | WHO ARE THE DECEDENT'S REGULAR PLAYMATES (NAMES & ADDRESSES)? |

**55. ☐ ☐**

IF PARENT(S) EMPLOYED, WHO ROUTINELY PROVIDED CHILD CARE FOR THE DECEDENT (NAME/ADDRESS/RELATIONSHIP)?

| WAS SIBLING RESPONSIBLE FOR CARING FOR THE DECEDENT AT TIME OF DEATH? <br> ☐ NO ☐ YES ☐ UNKNOWN | IF YES, WHICH SIBLING(S)? |
|---|---|

**56. ☐ ☐**

KNOWN MATERNAL PRE-NATAL HEALTH PROBLEMS (DIABETES, HYPERTENSION, ETC)?
☐ NO ☐ YES ☐ UNKNOWN

IF YES, DESCRIBE:

WAS MOTHER TAKING PRESCRIPTION MEDICATION FOR ABOVE MEDICAL CONDITION DURING PREGNANCY?
☐ NO ☐ YES ☐ UNKNOWN

IF YES, WHAT TYPE MEDICATION?

**57. ☐ ☐**

PRE-NATAL MATERNAL CIGARETTE, ALCOHOL OR DRUG USAGE?
☐ NO ☐ YES ☐ UNKNOWN

IF YES:    ☐ HEROIN    ☐ MARIJUANA    ☐ METHAMPHETAMINE
☐ ALCOHOL ☐ CIGARETTES ☐ COCAINE    OTHER: _____

**58. ☐ ☐**

KNOWN COMPLICATIONS OF PREGNANCY OR DELIVERY?
☐ NO ☐ YES ☐ UNKNOWN

IF YES, EXPLAIN:

LOCATION OF BIRTH AND NAME OF ATTENDING MEDICAL PRACTITIONER:

**59. ☐ ☐**

BIRTH DEFECTS OR OTHER ABNORMALITIES OF DECEDENT AT BIRTH; DESCRIBE:

**60. ☐ ☐**

ANY FAMILY HISTORY OF SIDS OR OTHER INFANT DEATH?
☐ NO ☐ YES ☐ UNKNOWN

IF YES, DESCRIBE DETAILS INCLUDING DATE OF DEATH & LOCATION OF OCCURRENCE:

FAMILY MEMBER OR OTHER CARE GIVER WITH KNOWN HISTORY OF AIDS?
☐ NO ☐ YES ☐ UNKNOWN

IF YES, PROVIDE NAME AND RELATIONSHIP:

## NARRATIVE

61. ☐ ☐    Provide additional comments (to include name(s) and pedigree(s) of all persons and responders at scene), continued answers to questions (include question number being responded to) or any other information pertinent to the death scene investigation. Use additional pages as needed.

_____

_____

_____

_____

_____

_____

_____

_____

_____

_____

_____

_____

_____

_____

_____

_____

_____

_____

_____

_____

_____

_____

_____

_____

_____

| SIGNATURE OF INVESTIGATOR: ▶ | PHONE NUMBER | DATE (MM/DD/YY): |
|---|---|---|

MO 886-3228 (3-95)

PAGE 7

MISSOURI DEPARTMENT OF SOCIAL SERVICES
DIVISION OF FAMILY SERVICES

## CHILD FATALITY REVIEW PANEL DATA REPORT
TO BE COMPLETED FOR ALL REVIEWABLE CHILD DEATHS < 18 YEARS OF AGE

| STATE USE ONLY | | FORM |
|---|---|---|
| DEATH CERT. NO. | BIRTH CERT. NO. | **2** |
| CFRP CASE NO. | DECEDENT DCN | |

☐ MEDICAID

**DIRECTIONS:**
Complete all sections of this form.
Place appropriate letter in box.

### A. IDENTIFICATION OF THE DECEDENT

1. DECEDENT'S NAME (FIRST) (MI) (LAST)

2. SEX ☐   M = MALE   F = FEMALE

3. DATE OF BIRTH (MM/DD/YY) __ __ / __ __ / __ __

4. DATE OF DEATH (MM/DD/YY) __ __ / __ __ / __ __

5. RACE ☐   W = WHITE   U = UNKNOWN   B = BLACK   O = OTHER

6. RESIDENCE (County)   STATE USE ONLY

7. ILLNESS/INJURY/EVENT (County)   STATE USE ONLY

8. DEATH RECORDED (County)   STATE USE ONLY

9. MOTHER'S NAME (FIRST) (MAIDEN) (LAST)

10. MOTHER'S DATE OF BIRTH (MM/DD/YY) __ __ / __ __ / __ __

11. MOTHER'S SOC. SEC. #

### B. SOCIAL INFORMATION (ALL DEATHS)

**MARK ALL THAT APPLY**

1. For all persons living in the residence of the decedent, indicate their relationship, their age and if they have legal custody of the child. (Use 0 if younger than 1 year.)

| | RELATIONSHIP TO DECEDENT ✔ | AGE | CUSTODY (CHECK) | | RELATIONSHIP TO DECEDENT ✔ | AGE | CUSTODY (CHECK) |
|---|---|---|---|---|---|---|---|
| a | Natural father | | | h | Foster mother | | |
| b | Natural mother | | | i | Other relative: _____ | | |
| c | Adoptive father | | | j | Parent's male paramour | | |
| d | Adoptive mother | | | k | Parent's female paramour | | |
| e | Step father | | | l | Another child | | |
| f | Step mother | | | m | Another child | | |
| g | Foster father | | | n | Other: _____ | | |

2. Current martial status of person(s) having legal custody of decedent?

☐   a. Married   c. Divorced   e. Unknown
    b. Widowed   d. Never married   f. Not Applicable

### C. TIME AND LOCATION (INJURY/UNEXPLAINED CAUSE OF DEATH)

**MARK ALL THAT APPLY**

1. Date of injury/event:
☐   a. __ / __ / __ (MM/DD/YY)   b. Unknown   c. Not Applicable

2. Time of injury/event:
☐   a. ____ : ____ (Hour/Minute) ☐ AM ☐ PM   b. Unknown
    c. Not Applicable

3. Time pronounced dead:
☐   a. ____ : ____ (Hour/Minute) ☐ AM ☐ PM   b. Unknown

4. Scene of injury/event
☐   a. Decedent's home          j. Other home
    b. Rural road               k. Highway
    c. Public drive             l. Street
    d. Private drive            m. Farm
    e. Other private property   n. Body of water
    f. Day child care facility  o. Hospital
    g. Residential child care facility
    h. Other _____
    i. Unknown

### D. CONTACT WITH DIVISION OF FAMILY SERVICES (ALL DEATHS)

**MARK ALL THAT APPLY**

1. Was Hotline call made?
☐   Y - Yes   N - No   If no, explain _____
_____

2. Was call accepted for investigation?
☐   Y - Yes   N - No   U - Unknown   I - Information/referral only

3. Incident Referral Number: _____

### E. WITNESSES (INJURY/UNEXPLAINED CAUSE OF DEATH)

**MARK ALL THAT APPLY**

1. Did the child lack adequate supervision?
☐   Y - Yes   N - No   U - Unknown   D - Does Not Apply

2. Who was in charge of watching the child at the time of injury/event? Give age (in years).

| | ✔ RELATIONSHIP TO DECEDENT | AGE | | ✔ RELATIONSHIP TO DECEDENT | AGE |
|---|---|---|---|---|---|
| a | Natural father | | i | Other relative: _____ | |
| b | Natural mother | | j | Parent's male paramour | |
| c | Adoptive father | | k | Parent's female paramour | |
| d | Adoptive mother | | l | Babysitter/child care worker | |
| e | Step father | | m | Another child | |
| f | Step mother | | n | Another child | |
| g | Foster father | | o | Other: _____ | |
| h | Foster mother | | p | No one in charge of watching | N/A |

3. Did any of the persons indicated in #2 appear to be intoxicated, under influence of drugs, mentally ill, retarded or otherwise impaired at the time of injury/event?
☐   Y - Yes   N - No   U - Unknown   D - Does Not Apply

4. Was the person(s) indicated in #2 asleep at time of the injury/event?
☐   a. All asleep    c. None asleep   e. Does not apply
    b. Some asleep   d. Unknown

MO 886-3218 (2-96)   **CONTINUE ON PAGE 2**   PAGE 1

## F. PANEL FINDINGS

**MARK ALL THAT APPLY**

☐ 1. Date of first panel meeting? a. ____ / ____ / ____ (MM/DD/YY)    b. Unknown

2. Panel members participating:
- a. ☐ Coroner
- b. ☐ Prosecutor
- c. ☐ DFS worker
- d. ☐ Physician/Public health
- e. ☐ Other(s)_____
- f. ☐ Medical Examiner
- g. ☐ Law enforcement officer
- h. ☐ Juvenile officer
- i. ☐ EMS

☐ 3. Total number of meetings held? a. #_____    b. Unknown

☐ 4. Autopsy? a. Performed by: _____    b. Not performed
Pathologist Name    c. Unknown

5. Death scene investigation conducted (mark all that apply)?
- a. ☐ Not conducted
- b. ☐ By law enforcement
- c. ☐ By fire investigator
- d. ☐ By Coroner
- e. ☐ By medical examiner
- f. ☐ By EMS
- g. ☐ By Other: _____

☐ 6. Investigation by law enforcement:
- a. Not conducted
- b. Conducted, arrested for: _____
- c. Unknown
- d. Conducted, no arrest
- e. Not applicable

☐ 7. Investigation/evaluation by juvenile officer:
- a. Not conducted
- b. Conducted, action taken: _____
- c. Unknown
- d. Conducted, no action
- e. Not applicable

☐ 8. Review of records by Department of Health:
- a. Not conducted
- b. Conducted, action taken: _____
- c. Unknown
- d. Conducted, no action
- e. Not applicable

☐ 9. Review of history by Division of Family Services:
- a. Not conducted
- b. Conducted, action taken: _____
- c. Unknown
- d. Conducted, no action
- e. Not applicable

☐ 10. Action by prosecutor:
- a. No action
- b. Suspected perpetrator, no arrest or charge filed
- c. Charge filed: _____
- d. Pending or in progress
- e. Unknown
- f. Not applicalble

☐ 11. Review of records by EMS:
- a. Not conducted
- b. Conducted, action taken: _____
- c. Unknown
- d. Conducted, no action
- e. Not applicable

## G. PERSON(S) ARRESTED/CHARGES (IF NO ARREST OR CHARGE, GO TO SECTION H)

☐ 1. Number of persons arrested?
- a. One
- b. Two
- c. Three or more

☐ 2. Was one or more of the person(s) arrested or charged responsible for care of the decedent at time of fatal illness/injury/event?

Y - Yes    N - No    U - Unknown

3. Indicate the relationship of the person(s) arrested or charged to the decedent, their age and race. (For race, enter W - White, B - Black, O - Other, U - Unknown.)

| | RELATIONSHIP | AGE | RACE | | | RELATIONSHIP | AGE | RACE |
|---|---|---|---|---|---|---|---|---|
| a | Natural father | | | | i | Other relative: _____ | | |
| b | Natural mother | | | | j | Parent's male paramour | | |
| c | Adoptive father | | | | k | Parent's female paramour | | |
| d | Adoptive mother | | | | l | Babysitter/child care worker | | |
| e | Step father | | | | m | Another child | | |
| f | Step mother | | | | n | Another child | | |
| g | Foster father | | | | o | Other: _____ | | |
| h | Foster mother | | | | | | | |

## H. CAUSE OF DEATH (COMPLETE SECTION APPROPRIATE TO DEATH)

☐ **1. INJURY (If yes, also complete Section I)**

☐ 1. Was the injury inflicted? Y - Yes    N - No
If yes, continue and answer the following questions:

☐ 2. Who inflicted the injury? a. Self-injured    b. Parent

c. Relative: _____    d. Other: _____    e. Unknown

☐ 3. Age of person inflicting injury: a. ____ years    b. Unknown
☐ Sex: M - Male  F - Female  U - Unknown

☐ Race: W - White  B - Black  O - Other  U - Unknown

☐ **2. ADEQUATE CARE**

☐ 1. Apparent lack of adequate care? Y - Yes    N - No

☐ 2. Apparent lack of medical care? Y - Yes    N - No

☐ 3. If yes,
- a. Malnutrition of dehydration
- b. Oral water intoxication
- c. Delayed medical care
- d. Inadequate medical attention
- e. Out-of-hospital birth
- f. Other: _____
- g. Unknown

☐ **3. SUDDEN INFANT DEATH SYNDROME (SIDS)**

☐ 1. Position of infant at discovery?
- a. On stomach, face down
- b. On stomach, face to side
- c. On stomach, face position unknown
- d. On back
- e. On side
- f. Unknown
- g. Other _____

☐ **4. ILLNESS OR OTHER NATURAL CAUSE**

☐ 1. Apparent illness or other condition?
- a. Known condition _____
- b. Prematurity

☐ **5. UNKNOWN CAUSE**
(If cause unknown, give any relevant known information.)

_____
_____
_____

## I. CIRCUMSTANCES OF THE INJURY DEATH (COMPLETE SECTION APPROPRIATE TO DEATH)

☐ **1. DROWNING**

☐ 1. Place of drowning?
- a. Creek, river, pond or lake
- b. Well, cistern, or septic tank
- c. Bathtub
- d. Swimming pool
- e. Bucket
- f. Wading pool
- g. Other _____
- h. Unknown

☐ 2. If creek, river, pond or lake, location prior to drowning?
- a. Boat
- b. Water edge
- c. Other _____
- d. Unknown

☐ 3. If creek, river, pond, lake or swimming pool, was decedent wearing flotation device?    Y - Yes    N - No    U - Unknown

☐ 4. U - Circumstances unknown

## I. CIRCUMSTANCES OF THE INJURY DEATH (COMPLETE SECTION APPROPRIATE TO DEATH)

### 2. VEHICULAR

1. Position of decedent?
   - a   Operator      d.   Other_____
   - b.   Pedestrian      e.   Unknown
   - c.   Passenger

2. Vehicle in which decedent was occupant?
   - a   Car      d.   Riding Mower      g.   Other Farm Vehicle
   - b.   Truck/R.V.      e.   Bicycleh.   All-terrain Vehicle
   - c.   Motorcycle      f.   Farm Tractor      i.   Other_____
   -              j.   Not Applicable

3. Vehicle in which decedent was not occupant?
   - a   Car      d.   Riding Mower      g.   Other Farm Vehicle
   - b.   Truck/R.V.      e.   Bicycleh.   All-terrain Vehicle
   - c.   Motorcycle      f.   Farm Tractor      i.   Other_____
   -              j.   Not Applicable

4. Condition of road?
   - a.   Normal      d.   Ice or snow      g.   Not Applicable
   - b.   Loose gravel      e.   Other _____
   - c.   Wet      f.   Unknown

5. If decedent was in vehicle, was safety belt or infant seat used?
   - a.   Present in vehicle, but not used      c.   Restraint used
   - b.   None in vehicle      d.   Unknown

6. If decedent was on bicycle, motorcycle or ATV, was decedent wearing helmet?      Y - Yes      N - No      U - Unknown

7. Vehicle in which decedent was occupant?
   - a.   Operator driving impaired (alcohol/drug)
   - b.   Speed/recklessness indicated:
     - (1) Approximate speed_____mph
     - (2) Speed limit_____ mph
   - c.   Other violation by operator      g.   Other_____
   - d.   No operator in vehicle      h.   Unknown
   - e.   Brake failure      i.   No violation
   - f.   Other mechanical failure      j.   Not applicable

8. Vehicle in which decedent was not occupant?
   - a.   Operator driving impaired (alcohol/drug)
   - b.   Speed/recklessness indicated:
     - (1) Approximate speed_____mph
     - (2) Speed limit_____ mph
   - c.   Other violation by operator      g.   Other_____
   - d.   No operator in vehicle      h.   Unknown
   - e.   Brake failure      i.   No violation
   - f.   Other mechanical failure      j.   Not applicable

9. U-Circumstances unknown

### 3. FIREARM

1. Person handling the firearm?
   - a.   Decedent.      c.   Unknown
   - b.   Other person      d.   Not Applicable

2. The firearm involved?
   - a.   Handgun      d.   Other_____
   - b.   Rifle      e.   Unknown
   - c.   Shotgun

3. Age of person handling firearm?
   - a. _____ years      b.   Unknown

4. Use of firearm at time of injury?
   - a.   Shooting at other person      e.   Loading   h.   Other
   - b.   Shooting at self      f.   Hunting   i.   Unknown
   - c.   Cleaning      g.   Playing
   - d.   Target shooting

5. Circumstances?
   - a.   Intentional      b.   Unintentional (accidental)      c.   Unknown

### 4. SUFFOCATION/STRANGULATION

1. Cause of suffocation/strangulation?
   - a.   Other person overlying or rolling over decedent
   - b.   Wedging
   - c.   Food
   - d.   Other person's hand(s)
   - e.   Object (eg., plastic bag) covering victim's mouth/nose
   - f.   Object (eg., rope) exerting pressure on victim's neck
   - g.   Small object or toy in mouth      i.   Other_____
   - h.   Carbon monoxide inhalation      j.   Unknown

2. Injury occurred in bed, crib, or other sleeping arrangement?
        Y - Yes      N - No      U - Unknown

3. If in bed/crib, due to?
   - a.   Hazardous design of crib/bed      e.   Unknown
   - b.   Malfunction/improper use of crib/bed      f.   Not Applicable
   - c.   Placement on soft sleeping surface (eg., waterbed)
   - d.   Other_____

4. U - Circumstances unknown

### 5. ELECTROCUTION

1. Cause of electrocution?
   - a.   Water contact      e.   Electrical tool
   - b.   Electrical wire      f.   Lightening
   - c.   Electrical outlet      g.   Other_____
   - d.   Electrical appliance      h.   Unknown

2. Electrical source defective?
        Y - Yes      N - No      U - Unknown

### 6. FALL INJURY

1. Fall was from?
   - a.   Open window      f.   Truck (eg., bed of truck)
   - b.   Furniture      g.   A man-made elevation (eg., bridge)
   - c.   A natural elevation      h.   Other_____
   - d.   Stairs, steps (in baby walker)   i.   Unknown
   - e.   Stairs, steps (other)

2. Height of fall?
   - a.   # feet _____      b.   Unknown

3. Landing surface composition/hardness?
   - a.   Carpet      c.   Ground
   - b.   Concrete      d.   Other_____

4. U - Circumstances unknown

### 7. POISONING/OVERDOSE

1. Name of drug or chemical?
   - a.   Name: _____      b.   Unknown

2. U - Circumstances unknown

### 8. FIRE/BURN

1. If non-fire burn, its source?
   - a.   Hot liquid      d.   Unknown
   - b.   Appliance      e.   Not Applicable
   - c.   Other_____

2. If ignition/fire, its source?
   - a.   Oven/stove      g.   Explosives
   - b.   Cooking appliance used as heat source      h.   Fireworks
   - c.   Matches      i.   Electrical wire
   - d.   Lit cigarette      j.   Other_____
   - e.   Lighter      k.   Unknown
   - f.   Space heater      l.   Not Applicable

3. If ignition/fire, was smoke alarm present at fire scene?
        Y - Yes   N - No      U - Unknown

4. If alarm present, did it sound?
        Y - Yes   N - No      U - Unknown

5. Was the fire started by a person?
        Y - Yes   N - No      U - Unknown

6. If started by a person, his/her age?
   - a. _____ years      b.   Unknown

7. If started by a person, his/her activity?
   - a.   Playing      e.   Other_____
   - b.   Smoking      f.   Unknown
   - c.   Cooking      g.   Not Applicable
   - d.   Suspected arson

8. If ignition/fire, type of construction of building burned?
   - a.   Wood frame      d.   Other_____
   - b.   Brick/stone      e.   Unknown
   - c.   Trailer      f.   Not Applicable

9. U - Circumstances unknown

**9. CRUSH (non-vehicle)**

    1. Describe circumstances:
       a. Description: _____
       b. Unknown

**10. CONFINEMENT**

    1. Place of confinement?
       a. Refrigerator/appliance    d. Room or building
       b. Motor vehicle           e. Other _____
       c. Chest, box, foot locker    f. Unknown

**11. SHAKEN (eg., Shaken Baby/Impact Syndrome)**

    1. Describe circumstances:
       a. Description: _____
       _____
       _____

       c. Unknown

**12. OTHER INFLICTED INJURY**

    1. Manner in which injury was inflicted?
       a. Cut/stabbed    c. Thrown  e. Unknown
       b. Struck    d. Other _____

    2. Injury inflicted with
       a. Sharp object (eg., knife, scissors)
       b. Blunt object (eg., hammer, bat)
       c. Hands/feet
       d. Other _____
       e. Unknown

**13. OTHER CAUSE**

Describe cause here only if not described elsewhere on this form.
_____
_____
_____
_____

**J. NARRATIVE DESCRIPTION OF CIRCUMSTANCES OR OTHER COMMENTS**

_____
_____
_____
_____
_____
_____
_____

**K. PREVENTION (TO BE COMPLETED BY CHAIRPERSON)**

1. WAS THIS DEATH PREVENTABLE?   [ ]  Y - YES  N - NO
A preventable death is defined as one in which awareness/education by an individual or the community may have changed the circumstances that led to death.

2. THIS CHILD'S DEATH PROMPTED THE PANEL/COMMUNITY TO TAKE THE FOLLOWING **PREVENTION-RELATED** ACTIONS (MARK ALL THAT APPLY):

    a. NEWSPAPER ARTICLE          d. TV/RADIO INTERVIEWS

    b. NEWSPAPER EDITORIAL       e. OTHER (LEGISLATION PROPOSED, LAW OR ORDINANCE PASSED,

    c. PRESS RELEASE             ETC.)

3. EDUCATIONAL/AWARENESS ACTIVITIES (MARK ALL THAT APPLY):

    TOPIC: _____

    a. DEVELOPMENT OF WRITTEN MATERIAL (SUCH AS BROCHURE, FLYER)    d. OTHER (EXPLAIN) _____

    b. DEVELOPMENT OF A RADIO OR TV PSA       e. PUBLIC PRESENTATIONS

    c. DEVELOPMENT OF AN EDUCATIONAL VIDEO

4. AUDIENCE OR POPULATION TARGETED (MARK ALL THAT APPLY):

    a. GENERAL PUBLIC          d. CHILDREN (DESCRIBE AGE GROUP, PRESCHOOLERS, TEENS, ETC.)

    b. CHILD PROTECTION PROFESSIONAL    _____

    c. PARENTS             e. OTHER (DESCRIBE) _____

5. ESTIMATED COST, IF ANY, OF PREVENTION MEASURES TAKEN:

    a. NO COST INVOLVED     c. < $100         e. > $500

    b. ALL SERVICES DONATED    d. $100-$500      f. UNKNOWN

6. DESCRIBE ACTIVITY, PARTICIPANTS AND RESULTS:

_____
_____
_____

| CFRP CHAIR SIGNATURE | DATE (MM/DD/YY) |
| --- | --- |
| ▶ | __ __ / __ __ / __ __ |
| REGIONAL COORDINATOR SIGNATURE | DATE (MM/DD/YY) |
| ▶ | __ __ / __ __ / __ __ |

MISSOURI DEPARTMENT OF SOCIAL SERVICES
DIVISION OF FAMILY SERVICES
## CORONER/MEDICAL EXAMINER DATA REPORT
TO BE COMPLETED FOR ALL REVIEWABLE CHILD DEATHS < 18 YEARS OF AGE

| STATE USE ONLY | | DATA FORM |
|---|---|---|
| DEATH CERT. NO. | BIRTH CERT. NO. | **1** |
| CFRP CASE NO. | DECEDENT DCN | |
| ☐ MEDICAID | CA/N INCIDENT NO. | |

DEATH CERTIFICATE MANNER OF DEATH

a. ☐ NATURAL    d. ☐ HOMICIDE
b. ☐ ACCIDENT    e. ☐ UNDETERMINED
c. ☐ SUICIDE    f. ☐ PENDING

### INSTRUCTIONS:

Notify Child Abuse/Neglect Hotline (800-392-3738) of all deaths of children <18 years of age.

If county of illness/injury/event is different from county of death, complete form with all known information before forwarding to coroner or medical examiner of county of illness/injury/event.

Notify the panel chairperson of the death.

Complete the form with all known information and forward to the panel chairperson for signature.

### A. IDENTIFICATION OF THE DECEDENT

1.
   a. ☐ Illness/injury/event is in Missouri. Complete all sections of Form 1.
   b. ☐ Illness/injury/event occurred ouf-of-state, but death occurred in Missouri. Complete Section A only.

2. COUNTY OF RESIDENCE    STATE USE ONLY    3. COUNTY OF ILLNESS/INJURY/EVENT    STATE USE ONLY    3. COUNTY OF DEATH    STATE USE ONLY

5. DECEDENT'S NAME (FIRST, MI, LAST)     5. DATE OF BIRTH (MM/DD/YY)     7. DATE OF DEATH (MM/DD/YY)

8. SEX
a. ☐ MALE
b. ☐ FEMALE

9. RACE
a. ☐ WHITE    c. ☐ ASIAN/PACIFIC ISLANDER    e. ☐ UNKNOWN
b. ☐ BLACK    d. ☐ AMERICAN INDIAN/ALASKAN NATIVE

10. IS DECEDENT OF HISPANIC ORIGIN?
a. ☐ YES    b. ☐ NO

11. MOTHER'S NAME (FIRST, MAIDEN, LAST)     12. MOTHER'S DATE OF BIRTH

### B. INDICATIONS FOR REVIEW— (ALL DEATHS)

1. Mark **all** that apply to this fatality. If one or more indicators are applicable, RSMo. 210.192 requires that the case **shall be referred** to the panel.

   a. ☐ Sudden, unexplained death, age <1 year
   b. ☐ Unexplained/undetermined manner
   c. ☐ DFS reports on decedent or other persons in the residence
   d. ☐ Decedent in DFS custody
   e. ☐ Possible inadequate supervision
   f. ☐ Possible malnutrition or delay in seeking medical care
   g. ☐ Possible suicide
   h. ☐ Possible inflicted injury
   i. ☐ Firearm injury
   j. ☐ Injury not witnessed by person in charge at time of injury
   k. ☐ Confinement
   l. ☐ Suspicious /criminal activity

   m. ☐ Drowning
   n. ☐ Suffocation or strangulation
   o. ☐ Poison/chemical/drug ingestion
   p. ☐ Severe unexplained injury
   q. ☐ Pedestrian/bicycle/driveway injury
   r. ☐ Drug/alcohol-related vehicular injury
   s. ☐ Suspected sexual assault
   t. ☐ Fire injury
   u. ☐ Autopsy by certified child death pathologist
   v. ☐ Panel discretion
   w. ☐ Other suspicious findings (injuries such as electrocution, crush or fall)

2. Referral to Panel (Mark one)

   a. ☐ One or more of the indicators marked above apply in this fatality. The case **shall be referred** to the review panel.
   b. ☐ None of the indicators listed apply in this fatality. The case is not referred to the panel.

### C. CHILD ABUSE/NEGLECT HOTLINE (800-392-3738)

**Notify Child Abuse/Neglect Hotline of all deaths of children <18 years of age.**

1. Were there prior reports to the Child Abuse/Neglect Hotline?    a. ☐ Yes    b. ☐ No
   If yes, mark all that apply:

   1. ☐ Involving child
   2. ☐ Involving anyone else in family
   3. ☐ Involving caretaker (other than family)
   4. ☐ Total number of DFS reports _____

2. Current notification to Child Abuse/Neglect Hotline was accepted as:

   a. ☐ Information/Referral only    b. ☐ Report for investigation    c. ☐ Unknown

MO 886-3219 (12-96)     **CONTINUE ON PAGE 2**     PAGE 1

## D. SOCIAL INFORMATION

1. For all persons living in the residence of the decedent, indicate their relationship to the decedent, their age range, and who is head of household. (Select only one head of household)

Use corresponding letter for appropriate age range:

**A** = 0-5 yrs.   **B** = 6-9 yrs.   **C** = 10-14 yrs.   **D** = 15-18 yrs.   **E** = 19-40 yrs.   **F** = >40 yrs.

| | | Age Range | Head of Household | | | | Age Range | Head of Household |
|---|---|---|---|---|---|---|---|---|
| a. ☐ | Natural father | ____ | ☐ | i. ☐ | Other relative | | ____ | ☐ |
| b. ☐ | Natural mother | ____ | ☐ | j. ☐ | Other relative | | ____ | ☐ |
| c. ☐ | Adoptive father | ____ | ☐ | k. ☐ | Mother's paramour | | ____ | ☐ |
| d. ☐ | Adoptive mother | ____ | ☐ | l. ☐ | Father's paramour | | ____ | ☐ |
| e. ☐ | Stepfather | ____ | ☐ | m. ☐ | Other non-relative | | ____ | ☐ |
| f. ☐ | Stepmother | ____ | ☐ | n. ☐ | Another child | | ____ | ☐ |
| g. ☐ | Foster father | ____ | ☐ | o. ☐ | Another child | | ____ | ☐ |
| h. ☐ | Foster mother | ____ | ☐ | p. ☐ | More than two children (list in narrative) | | | |

2. Current marital status of head of household?

   a. ☐ Married     c. ☐ Divorced     e. ☐ Unknown

   b. ☐ Widowed     d. ☐ Never married

## E. DEATH/SCENE INFORMATION

1. Place of death?

   a. ☐ Decedent's home    e. ☐ Public drive    i. ☐ Other private property    m. ☐ Body of water

   b. ☐ Other home    f. ☐ Street    j. ☐ Licensed child care facility    o. ☐ Work place

   c. ☐ Rural road    g. ☐ Private drive    k. ☐ Unlicensed child care facility    p. ☐ Hospital

   d. ☐ Highway    h. ☐ Farm    l. ☐ Child care residential facility    q. ☐ Other: _____

2. Date of injury/event?    a. ☐ __ __ / __ __ / __ __ (MM/DD/YY)     b. ☐ Unknown

3. Time of injury/event?    a. ☐ __ __ : __ __ (Hour:Minute) ☐ AM ☐ PM    b. ☐ Unknown

4. Time pronounced dead?    a. ☐ __ __ : __ __ (Hour:Minute) ☐ AM ☐ PM    b. ☐ Unknown

5. Was an autopsy performed?    a. ☐ Yes    b. ☐ No    c. ☐ Unknown

   If yes:

   1. ☐ By CFRP pathologist?       (NOTE: Autopsies performed by non-certified child pathologists are limited to

   2. ☐ By hospital physician?      hospital deaths resulting from a **known** medical condition/illness.)

   3. ☐ Name of CFRP pathologist? (Last name only) _____

## F. SUPERVISION

1. Who was in charge of watching decedent at the time of injury/event?

   a. ☐ Natural father     g. ☐ Foster father     m. ☐ Unlicensed babysitter/child care worker

   b. ☐ Natural mother     h. ☐ Foster mother     n. ☐ Child, age: _____

   c. ☐ Adoptive father     i. ☐ Other relative     o. ☐ Hospital staff

   d. ☐ Adoptive mother     j. ☐ Parent's male paramour     p. ☐ Other non-relative

   e. ☐ Stepfather     k. ☐ Parent's female paramour     q. ☐ No one in charge of watching

   f. ☐ Stepmother     l. ☐ Licensed babysitter/child care worker     r. ☐ Due to age, no one in charge

2. Was the decedent adequately supervised?    a. ☐ Yes    b. ☐ No    c. ☐ Unknown    d. ☐ Not applicable

   If no:

   1. Did the person(s) in charge appear to be intoxicated, under influence of drugs, mentally ill or limited, or otherwise impaired at time of injury/event?

     a. ☐ Yes    b. ☐ No    c. ☐ Unknown

   2. Was the person(s) preoccupied, distracted or asleep at the time of the injury/event?

     a. ☐ Yes    b. ☐ No    c. ☐ Unknown

3. Was injury/event witnessed by at least one person?    a. ☐ Yes    b. ☐ No    c. ☐ Unknown

## G. CAUSE OF DEATH
**(Select most appropriate cause of death and if applicable, complete Section H)**

**1. ☐ INJURY (Complete questions 1 and 2 for all injuries)**

   1. Was the injury inflicted?    a. ☐ Yes       b. ☐ No       c. ☐ Unknown
      (Inflicted - defined as assaultive or aggressive action)

   2. Was the injury intentional?    a. ☐ Yes       b. ☐ No       c. ☐ Unknown

**If vehicle accident, non-reviewable, answer questions 3 through 9. If reviewable vehicle accident (pedestrian/bicycle/driveway injury, drug/alcohol related or other suspicious/criminal activity), skip the following questions and complete Section H.**

   3. Position of decedent?
      a. ☐ Operator     b. ☐ Passenger     c. ☐ Other     d. ☐ Unknown

   4. Vehicle in which decedent was occupant?
      a. ☐ Car     c. ☐ Motorcycle/ATV     e. ☐ Semi/Tractor trailer unit
      b. ☐ Truck/RV/Van     d. ☐ Farm vehicle     f. ☐ Other

   5. Was another vehicle involved in accident?    a. ☐ Yes    b. ☐ No

   6. Condition of road?
      a. ☐ Normal     c. ☐ Wet     e. ☐ Other
      b. ☐ Loose gravel     d. ☐ Ice or snow     f. ☐ Unknown

   7. Restraint used by decedent?
      a. ☐ Present, not used     c. ☐ Used correctly     e. ☐ Unknown
      b. ☐ None in vehicle     d. ☐ Used incorrectly     f. ☐ Not applicable

   8. Helmet used by decedent?
      a. ☐ Helmet worn     b. ☐ Helmet not worn     c. ☐ Not applicable

   9. Primary cause of accident?
      a. ☐ Speeding     c. ☐ Mechanical failure     e. ☐ Driver error
      b. ☐ Carelessness     d. ☐ Weather conditions     f. ☐ Other

**2. ☐ ILLNESS OR OTHER NATURAL CAUSE**

   1. Known condition _____

   2. Was inadequate care or neglect involved in death?    a. ☐ Yes    b. ☐ No
      **(If yes, mark Section H, Number 2)**

**Complete questions 3 - 8 if death in infant <1 year of age.**

   3. History information provided by?    a. ☐ Parent    b. ☐ Physician/Medical facility    c. ☐ Other

   4. Age at death?
      a. ☐ 0 - 24 hours after birth     c. ☐ 48 hours - 6 weeks     e. ☐ 6 months - 1 year
      b. ☐ 24 - 48 hours     d. ☐ 6 weeks - 6 months

   5. Gestational age?
      a. ☐ <25 weeks    b. ☐ 25 - 30 weeks    c. ☐ 30 - 37 weeks    d. ☐ >37 weeks    e. ☐ Unknown

   6. Birth weight in grams (approximate lbs./oz.)?
      a. ☐ <750 (<1 lb. 10 oz.)     c. ☐ 1,500 - 2,499 (3 lbs. 6 oz. to 5 lbs. 5 oz.)     e. ☐ Unknown
      b. ☐ 750 - 1,499 (1 lb. 10 oz. to 3 lbs. 5 oz.)     d. ☐ >2,500 (>5 lbs. 6 oz.)

   7. Multiple birth?    a. ☐ Yes    b. ☐ No

   8. Have there been other infant deaths in the immediate family?    a. ☐ Yes    b. ☐ No    c. ☐ Unknown

**3. ☐ UNKNOWN CAUSE (Describe in narrative. <u>Death shall be reviewed.</u>)**

   1. Was death sudden and unexplained in infant < 1 year of age?    a. ☐ Yes    b. ☐ No
      **If yes, also complete Section G, Number 2, question 3 - 8 and mark Section H, Number 1.**

## H. CIRCUMSTANCES OF DEATH
**If any of the circumstances are applicable, <u>death shall be reviewed</u>.**

1. ☐ Sudden Unexplained Death of Infant <1 Year
2. ☐ Inadequate Care or Neglect
3. ☐ Vehicular
   (Includes pedestrian/bicycle/driveway injury, drug/alcohol related, or other suspicious/criminal activity)
4. ☐ Drowning
5. ☐ Firearm
6. ☐ Suffocation/Strangulation
7. ☐ Electrocution

8. ☐ Fall Injury
9. ☐ Poisoning/Overdose
10. ☐ Fire/Burn
11. ☐ Crush
12. ☐ Confinement
13. ☐ Shaken/Impact Syndrome
14. ☐ Other Inflicted Injury
    (Describe in narrative)
15. ☐ Other Circumstances
    (Describe in narrative)

## I. NARRATIVE DESCRIPTION OF CIRCUMSTANCES OR OTHER COMMENTS

_____
_____
_____
_____
_____
_____
_____
_____

## J. PREVENTION

1. To what degree was this death believed to be preventable?
   (Preventable death is defined as one in which awareness/education/action by an individual or the community may have changed the circumstances that led to death.)

   a. ☐ Not at all    b. ☐ Possibly    c. ☐ Definitely

2. Primary risk factors involved in the child's death? (Mark all that apply)

   a. ☐ Medical   c. ☐ Economic   e. ☐ Environmental   f. ☐ Drugs or alcohol
   b. ☐ Social   d. ☐ Behavioral   f. ☐ Product safety   h. ☐ Other

3. Were these risk factors identified in your community prior to the death?   a. ☐ Yes   b. ☐ No

4. Was any action taken in your community to address the risk factors prior to the death?   a. ☐ Yes   b. ☐ No

5. Could the family or child have taken actions to reduce the risk?

   a. ☐ Yes   b. ☐ No   c. ☐ Unknown

6. What actions can be taken by your community to prevent similar deaths?

   a. ☐ Legislation, law or ordinance
   b. ☐ Community safety project
   c. ☐ Product safety action
   d. ☐ Educational activities in school
   e. ☐ Educational activities in the media
   f. ☐ Public forums
   g. ☐ News services
   h. ☐ Changes in agency practice
   i. ☐ Other programs or activities
   j. ☐ None

| CORONER/MEDICAL EXAMINER SIGNATURE ▶ | REFER TO CFRP? a.☐YES b.☐NO | DATE (MM/DD/YY) __ __ / __ __ / __ __ |
| CFRP CHAIR SIGNATURE ▶ | REFER TO CFRP? a.☐YES b.☐NO | DATE (MM/DD/YY) __ __ / __ __ / __ __ |
| REGIONAL COORDINATOR SIGNATURE | | DATE (MM/DD/YY) __ __ / __ __ / __ __ |

# The Role of the Medical Examiner in Fatal Child Abuse

Michael Graham, M.D.

The medical examiner's role in deaths in which abuse or neglect may have played a part consists of (1) determining the cause and manner of death to a reasonable degree of certainty; (2) providing expert evaluation of the presence, absence, nature, and significance of injuries and disease; (3) collecting and preserving evidence; (4) correlating clinical and pathologic findings; and (5) presenting expert opinions in the proper forums. Modifications introduced by a changing society and by progressive medical technology, as in the area of transplantation, constantly redefine the extent and specifics of the medical examiner's role.

One area of expansion of the medical examiner's role involves evaluating the deaths of nonneonate, preteenage children who die because of nonaccidental injuries or neglect inflicted or permitted by their caretakers.

*It is convenient and practical to divide these deaths into two subgroups, recognizing that nonidentified episodes of previous injury result in some misclassification:*

1. Children who fall under the traditional definition of repeated episodes of abuse, exhibiting the results of these multiple episodes of intentionally inflicted harm. Approximately 20% of child abuse deaths fall into this category.

2. Currently a more common form of fatal abuse, children who die from injuries received during a single assaultive episode (Adelson, 1991).

Neonatal deaths (including infanticide) and deaths involving "adult" injuries, such as firearms and stabbings, are described by Adelson (1974) and DiMaio & DiMaio (1989).

The involvement of the medical examiner in child abuse and neglect traditionally begins at the time of death as specified by statute and modified by local custom. The particular statute or regulation governing each jurisdiction varies. In general, any sudden and unexpected death or one wherein an injury or "nonnatural" condition is suspected to have caused or contributed to the death must be reported to the medicolegal authority in whose jurisdiction it falls. By their very nature, all deaths suspected to involve abuse or neglect must be brought to the attention of the applicable medicolegal authority.

## ◆ Mortality Attributed to Physical Abuse

The incidence of deaths resulting from physical abuse is second only to the incidence of sudden infant death syndrome (SIDS) deaths in children under 1 year of age and is second only to accidents in children older than 1 year of age. An estimated 1,950 to 2,000 children ages birth to 17 years in the United States die each year as a direct result of physical abuse and neglect (McClain et al., 1993). Ninety percent of deaths occur among children less than 5 years old, with 41% of these deaths occurring during infancy (McClain et al., 1993). Although these children constitute only a small subgroup of abused children, it is this group that is traditionally most extensively evaluated by medical examiners in a formal medicolegal death investigation system.

In reporting the incidence of fatal abuse or neglect, the features and investigative problems depend somewhat on the age of the population and the definition of the term "child abuse or neglect." Any death that results from intentionally inflicted injuries can be categorized as abusive, but such broad usage of the term leads to confusion and blurring of the components traditionally referred to as "child abuse." This confusion makes it more difficult to study common features and establish diagnostic criteria than when a narrower definition is used. The modalities of injury and death involved in feticide and neonaticide (first 30 days of life) differ substantially from those of other children. They often involve issues (such as identification, viability, and live birth) not usually arising in deaths beyond this stage of life. Similarly, the deaths of teenagers differ significantly from those of pre-teen children. Findings in the teenage group approach those found in adults with regard to modalities and motives. Rarely does a child over the age of 10 years die of starvation or dehydration due to neglect or die of chronic battering, since children in this age group are generally able to avoid these lethal situations (Adelson, 1991).

## ◆ FACTORS IMPACTING INVESTIGATION

The extent and quality of the investigation into a particular death are influenced substantially by factors such as circumstances peculiar to the death, local custom, available expertise, and resources. Unfortunately, in many jurisdictions the offices charged with investigating these deaths operate under critical limitations of resources, both personnel and financial, and are being further strained by shrinking budgets and soaring costs. Resource considerations are increasingly significant in determining if the state-of-the-art evaluations that these types of deaths merit can, in fact, be carried out.

## ◆ DETERMINING CAUSE OF DEATH

Although the medical examiner's role is commonly perceived as being limited to determining the cause and manner of death, today his or her involvement is vastly more extensive and encompasses issues such as those listed in **Table 25-1**. Recent trends in child abuse investigation have also led the medical examiner into such areas as membership on multidisciplinary death review committees and evaluating cases involving nonlethally injured children when abuse is suspected. In this setting the medical examiner, usually a forensic pathologist, contributes expertise to aid clinicians and law enforcement authorities in evaluating the presence, nature, and mechanism of injuries sustained by these children.

The medical examiner must determine the cause of death as specifically as is reasonably possible. The cause of death can be defined as the disease or injury, or a combination of the two, that initiates the continuous series of events, however brief or prolonged, which culminates in death (Adelson, 1974). It is important not only to recognize the immediate cause of death (what killed the child now) but also to delineate any remote or underlying cause of death (the initiator of the series of events culminating in the immediate cause of death). For example, in a child dying of pneumonia as a result of a past head injury, the immediate cause of death is pneumonia and the underlying cause of death is the head injury. Establishing the causal connection between these two entities and properly recognizing the underlying cause of death have apparent and serious far-reaching implications, especially in the courtroom. There may also be coexistent conditions, those that may not be directly related to the "cause of death" but may contribute to death by enhancing or, occasionally, diminishing the lethality of another condition. They may affect the resistance or susceptibility of an individual to a particular process, such as the interaction between dehydration and sickle cell anemia to produce a fatal sickling crisis. Some deaths result from physiologic perturbations such as cardiac concussion (*commotio cordia*) from a blow to the chest and demonstrate no identifiable anatomic alterations, yet are still traumatic in nature. In some cases a

| Table 25-1. Medical Examiner's Role |
| --- |
| Establishing time of injury or injuries and death |
| Identifying the presence and nature of injuries |
| Evaluating modifying or contributing factors (injuries and diseases) |
| Documentation of pertinent findings (positive and negative) |
| Proper collection and preservation of evidence |
| Correlating findings with postinjury behavior |
| Presenting these issues in appropriate legal forums |

specific cause of death cannot be ascertained but other possible causes can be excluded; together with a consideration of the circumstances, the possibilities can be reduced to a single cause or category. An example of this is mechanical asphyxia. Successful resolution, including criminal prosecution, of these cases is possible even though no specific cause of death is identified if other causes have been excluded.

## ♦ DETERMINING MECHANISM OF DEATH

The cause of death should not be confused with the mechanism of death, which is the lethal physiologic derangement through which the cause of death acts (Adelson, 1974). Examples of mechanisms of death include hemorrhage, renal failure, anoxia, dehydration, and dysrhythmia. Multiple mechanisms can be operative in any particular case, especially in children who survive the initial injury only to die of multisystem failure after extensive therapeutic intervention. Recognition of the mechanism(s) of death is useful in establishing causal relationships and evaluating the clinical course of a process but should not be substituted for determination of the cause of death. For example, the recognition that disorders such as rhabdomyolysis (disintegration or dissolution of muscle associated with excretion of myoglobin in the urine), hyperkalemia (abnormally high potassium content of the blood), and soft tissue hemorrhage (mechanism) have led to death in the absence of visceral organ injury allows the death to be properly ascribed to soft tissue blunt trauma (cause of death) sustained in a beating.

## ♦ DETERMINING MANNER OF DEATH

The other major death certification issue facing the medical examiner is the manner of death, or the fashion in which the cause of death arises (Adelson, 1974). Deaths are traditionally classified as natural, homicide, accident, or suicide. If an opinion cannot be reached, the death is classified as undetermined. In some jurisdictions, deaths such as drug abuse or therapeutic misadventure are placed in a special "unclassified" category. The manner of death is an opinion separate from the cause of death.

All child abuse deaths are by their nature homicidal, the killing of one person by another. A ruling of homicide does not reflect the level or even the presence of criminal culpability—"homicide" does not equal "murder." Criminality is properly determined by the criminal justice system. "Natural" causes of death can occur homicidally (Davis, 1978). For example, sickle cell crisis can be precipitated by dehydration resulting from punitive withholding of water. Certain cases of neglect also fit into this category. It must also be recognized that a manner of death can be identified even in the absence of a known cause of death if the circumstances surrounding the death so warrant. The most common example of this is attributing death to SIDS. Although a thorough investigation and postmortem examination fail to establish a specific entity responsible for death in a child in a characteristic age group, the death is considered natural and its similarity to other unexpected, unexplained deaths in similar children allows it to be categorized in a well-defined specific category (SIDS) of unexplained natural deaths. Similarly, a witnessed death clearly arising from a cardiac rhythm disturbance of unknown cause (after thorough examination) may be certified as natural notwithstanding the lack of a demonstrable underlying precipitating disorder. Nonnatural manners of death can also be reasonably ascertained in some cases where the cause of death is not demonstrable. For example, the uninjured skeleton of an abducted 2-year-old child is recovered a year later in a shallow grave. The cause of death is not apparent, but the circumstances reasonably indicate the death is homicidal. The "cause of death" in such a case can be certified in a number of ways reflecting local custom, including "unable to be definitively established" or "homicidal violence of undefined nature." The manner of death is homicide.

In addition to the issues of cause and manner of death, questions arise about the nature, extent, and effects of injuries sustained by these children: How did the injuries occur? When did they occur? What effect did they have on the child? A comprehensive death investigation allows these issues to be evaluated and answered appropriately.

## ♦ MEDICOLEGAL EVALUATION OF DEATH

A common misconception is that the investigation of a death necessitates the performance of and is restricted to the findings obtained from an autopsy. The investigation of death has many components, of which autopsy is only one and not always a necessary one.

### INVESTIGATION PROCESS

The modern medicolegal evaluation of a death suspected to involve child abuse does not differ fundamentally from the evaluation of any other death, and indeed differs little from the approach to medical evaluation of any living patient. A history is obtained, the patient is examined, ancillary tests are performed, diagnoses are rendered, and a course of action is pursued. Medicolegal opinions, like working medical diagnoses, are based on interpretation of all available information at a given point in time and are subject to reevaluation and amendment as additional information surfaces.

### INVESTIGATION COMPONENTS

The components of a death investigation can be divided into examination of the history of pertinent past and present circumstances, physical evaluation of the scene and the body, and use of indicated ancillary studies such as radiography, toxicology, and other laboratory tests. Each component must be considered in the investigation, although some components can be more crucial than others.

### HISTORY

Knowledge of the circumstances before, during, and after the death is critical to interpreting findings derived from physical observations. The medical examiner must rely on others to provide this information when evaluating the death of a child. Informants include the parents and/or other caretakers, siblings, acquaintances, neighbors, witnesses, and medical and law enforcement personnel; added information can be gathered from prior health records. Because of potential criminal and civil liability associated with child abuse, a description of the events leading up to death and reference to past events is often intentionally vague, incomplete, or fallacious. Frequently these events involved only the perpetrator and the victim. The perpetrator commonly provides a "history" that exonerates him or her from any responsibility for the death. Other witnesses or knowledgeable persons are usually family members or family acquaintances. Some could have participated in the abusive act (Adelson, 1991), and others fear retribution or view the loss of the perpetrator as detrimental to their future well-being. Often the "history" provided is based on the actual events but altered to alleviate or shift responsibility from the perpetrator. Also, characteristically, the history will be inconsistent with the observed injuries and will change, sometimes radically, as the investigation proceeds. Explanations to account for the injuries often follow the general themes of the injuries being accidental, self-inflicted, or of unknown origin (Schmitt, 1984).

The history also allows documentation of prior injuries and diseases, gives an assessment of the child's health and development, and contains information about pre-existing conditions that can influence later events. A detailed, accurate history is crucial when evaluating deaths possibly related to nutritional neglect.

## Physical Examination

The second major component of the death investigation is examining, evaluating, and obtaining physical evidence. This is accomplished by assessing the alleged scene of injury and/or death and interpreting findings obtained from an autopsy.

Child abuse typically occurs in the privacy of the home. The nature of the act is reflected in the paucity of signs of environmental disturbance that accompany it. However, examination of the scene where the injuries were sustained can be rewarding in that the information derived can corroborate or refute the accuracy of the history presented to explain the child's condition. Instruments used to inflict injuries are usually typical household articles such as rods, belts, or brushes. Examination of the scene can verify the presence of instruments that could have inflicted specific injuries and may lead to the recovery of other evidence.

## Postmortem Examination

The postmortem examination of a child suspected to be abused includes a complete autopsy by a skilled pathologist with expertise in this area. A thorough gross examination coupled with microscopic evaluation as appropriate helps to determine and document the presence and absence of diseases or injuries as well as medical intervention. Appropriate photographic documentation is obtained for future review of the case as well as for use in legal proceedings.

A complete forensic postmortem examination should be performed when any child suffers a sudden and unexpected death or when the circumstances do not reasonably exclude an element indicative of abuse. A complete autopsy should be performed on the body of any child whose death could be attributed to abuse or neglect, either directly or indirectly. Although a detailed description of the postmortem examination of a potentially abused child is beyond the scope of this chapter, a brief overview of the procedure with particular reference to "special" techniques is presented.

### *Gross External Observation*

The first part of the examination includes documenting the general features and overall condition of the body. This includes describing the clothing as well as identifying and sealing evidentiary material. Detailed identification and documentation are performed of any external signs of injury, disease, or therapeutic intervention. In addition to a verbal description and photographic record of injuries, a diagrammatic record of injuries is often useful in identifying injury patterns, as often found in burns and scalds, where the distribution pattern is critical to the evaluation of how the injury was sustained.

### *Examination of Soft Tissues and Visceral Organs*

Most lethally abused children have external signs of injury, although a few children have only scant externally apparent injuries but extensive underlying damage. In up to 10% of all cases of fatal child abuse caused by blunt trauma, no marks are visible anywhere on the external body surface (DiMaio & DiMaio, 1989). To detect and evaluate injuries in fatally abused children requires a thorough examination of the soft tissues and visceral organs for indications of hemorrhage. In the soft tissues, the presence, amount, and depth of hemorrhage are noted.

Soft tissue hemorrhage is most accurately assessed by exposing the deep soft tissues via long incisions down the back and lower extremities. These incisions are needed because significant soft tissue hemorrhage can be externally inconspicuous or inapparent, especially in dark-skinned individuals, and only revealed by direct inspection of the tissues (**Figure 25-1a,b**). Hemorrhage in the deep soft tissues indicates the application of significant force. Care must be taken not to misinterpret areas of hyperpigmentation, such as Mongolian spots, as a sign of injury (**Figure 25-2**). If in doubt, an incision into such a mark will show no hemorrhage.

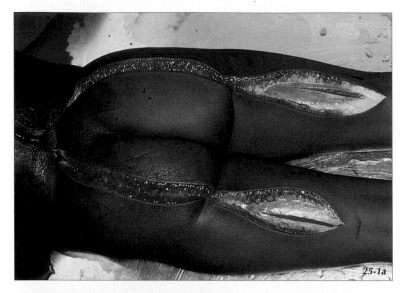

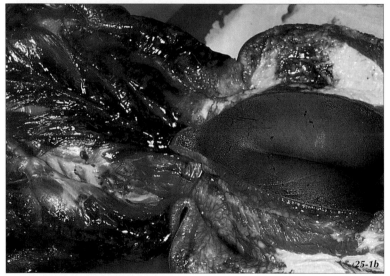

**Figure 25-1a,b.** *Soft tissue hemorrhage. The hemorrhage was not obvious before dissection.*

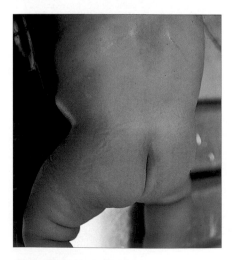

**Figure 25-2.** *Mongolian spot.*

The visceral organs are accessed using standard bitemporal and thoracoabdominal incisions. When indicated, notably in infant deaths, the eyes are removed and examined for retinal hemorrhage and separation. The cervical spine, soft tissues, and spinal cord can be examined via a vertical posterior neck incision. The gross examination is supplemented by microscopic evaluation of appropriate tissues. An extensive postmortem examination can be performed and the body subsequently shown at the funeral home with no apparent autopsy marks visible since the face is rarely altered during the autopsy.

## ANCILLARY STUDIES

The final data-yielding component of the death investigation process is the performance of appropriate ancillary studies, which can provide the key that unlocks the solution to a particular death. Routine ancillary studies in suspected child abuse deaths include radiography and toxicology. In some cases, postmortem microbiologic, chemical, and other laboratory determinations are required.

## RADIOGRAPHIC INPUT

The postmortem examination of the potentially abused or neglected child includes radiographic evaluation of the skeletal system using well-coned-down views of the head, trunk, spine, and extremities (Kleinman et al., 1989). The radiographic findings are useful in detecting, documenting, and detailing the presence or absence of injuries and disease, as well as determining when the injuries occurred and if the injuries reflect a series of episodes or a single incident. The radiographic studies also direct the removal and sampling of injured or diseased sites for histopathologic examination.

## LABORATORY INPUT

Samples of blood, urine, vitreous fluid, and other appropriate tissues are saved for indicated toxicologic, chemical, and microbiologic analysis. Trace evidence such as hairs, fibers, and particulate material is identified and collected. Smears and swabs for sexual assault evaluation are collected. Hair and blood samples to be used for future comparison studies are obtained when indicated. Transfer of blood, hair, and other body substances can occur between victim and assailant. The identification of the source of the substance can exclude some individuals as to its origination and, using DNA techniques, can often essentially identify the contributor. Samples of blood, hair, and other tissues serve as comparison standards for questioned samples. These samples can also be used to resolve parentage issues.

## ♦ DATA INTERPRETATION

After collecting all pertinent information, the data are correlated and interpreted by trained individuals. Credibility is essential to ensure that the expressed opinions are reasonable, are scientifically supportable, and can be offered with a reasonable degree of medical certainty as testimony. This process is dynamic, and opinions change as more data are accumulated, previously acquired data are refined, and all information is assessed according to current knowledge and experience.

The opinions formulated fall into two general categories: opinions related to what happened to the child and opinions related to what did not happen. In many cases a combination of these categories is used. It may not be possible to identify exactly how a child sustained a particular injury, but it is possible to conclude whether the child sustained the injury in the context of a particular scenario of events. For example, it is possible to refute a story of a fall from an 18-inch high coffee table to a carpeted floor offered as the explanation for a massive head injury, although it may not be possible to determine exactly how the injury was sustained.

## INTERPRETATION OF INJURIES

Injury interpretation begins with identifying and categorizing each injury (e.g., abrasion, contusion, laceration, cut, stab). Each one is then thoroughly examined and documented, whether major or trivial. Medically trivial injuries, such as a small scrape, can be more forensically informative than injuries of more serious physiologic consequence. For example, the physiologically inconsequential shoe print abrasion on the skin overlying the lacerated liver reveals the identity of the striking object and the point of impact. Similarly, a mark associated with the fatal blow may be nondescript, whereas the instrument may leave a distinctive mark in another area. This type of information not only helps determine the nature of physiologically important injuries but can shed much light on other issues such as the nature of the instrument(s), the potential number of instruments, the site(s) of impact, and the minimum number of impacts.

The body of an allegedly abused child may be reexamined 24 hours after the original autopsy to allow further delineation of the external injuries and to allow for the appearance of other injuries that were not previously discernible. The phenomenon of "clearing" noninjured areas is caused by the autopsy-enhanced passive drainage of blood from the vasculature. Since extravascular blood in areas of injury does not drain, whereas blood in blood vessels does, the injured areas become more clearly delineated.

## AGING OF INJURIES

The characteristics of healing injuries aid in the assessment of how long before death they occurred. Since injury healing is progressive and predictable, the gross and microscopic appearance of the injury reflects its age. For example, contusions begin as clearly delineated red-blue marks, progress over days to become less defined yellow-green areas, and finally fade to indistinct brown marks within approximately a week to a month (Wilson, 1977). The chronology of the microscopic features of wound resolution has also been described (Raekallio, 1980). However, caution must be exercised when interpreting these timing features because a variety of factors can influence the appearance (and time course) of any particular injury (Wilson, 1977), including the victim's age and state of health; the injury site, depth, and size; the specific tissue injured; individual variations; the effects of therapy; and the development of complications such as infection. The chronology of fracture resolution has also been described (Zumwalt & Fanizza-Orphanus, 1990). The features of healing in visceral organ tissues are less well characterized than skin and bone but can be utilized within limits.

The interpretation of aging in an injury can provide absolute identification of when an injury occurred as specifically as a range of hours, days, or longer and the length of survival after the trauma was inflicted. The narrowness of the range is inversely proportional to the length of survival. This information is useful in determining who did and who did not have access to the child at the time the injury occurred, as well as evaluating the antemortem behavior of the child, for

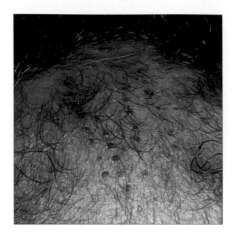

**Figure 25-3.** *Patterned injury. Rows of punctate abrasions caused by a hair brush.*

example, the onset of irritability, loss of appetite, or change in behavior. Injury aging can aid in determining when complications may have occurred after the initial injury, such as delayed rupture of the bowel following an initial non-transmural bowel wall laceration. Injury aging can also be used in a "relative" fashion to determine whether certain injuries occurred before or after others and if the injuries indicate one or more traumatic episodes occurred. The crucial information to make these determinations can be contained in a previous surgical specimen that was removed before the death occurred, for example, a bowel resection, followed by prolonged postsurgical survival. In these cases the medical examiner makes every effort to locate and examine the pertinent tissues.

## PATTERNED INJURIES AND INJURY PATTERNS

The interpretation of injuries involves the evaluation of each injury alone as well as in conjunction with coexistent wounds. This requires the recognition of patterned injuries and injury patterns. These factors must be considered in the light of historical data, findings at the scene of the injury, and the physical capabilities of the child.

### PATTERNED INJURIES

Although most injuries are relatively nonspecific, some contusions and abrasions have a configuration that reveals details about the instrument used to inflict the injury (**Figure 25-3**). Patterned injuries suggest and can be matched to a particular type of instrument or occasionally linked to a specific instrument (**Figures 25-4 to 25-7**). Parallel linear marks separated by a pale zone suggest a linear object such as a stick, rod, or belt (**see Figure 25-4a,b**). Curved marks are often caused by loops of cord (rope or electrical wire), clothes hangers, or other curved instruments (**Figure 25-5a,b**). Some instruments create a multiplicity of patterns, reflecting variations in the striking surface(s) of the instrument. In these cases, each pattern further defines the particular object (**Figure 25-6a to c**). Sometimes the appearance of the injuries indicates the use of multiple instruments to inflict the injuries (**Figure 25-7, a to e**).

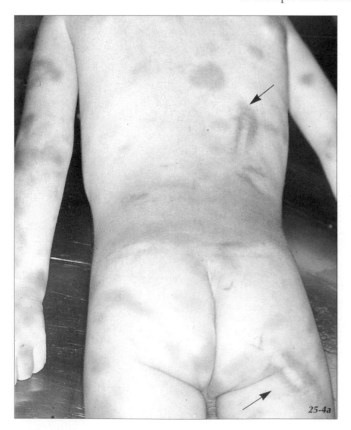

25-4a

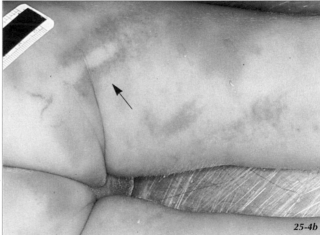

25-4b

**Figure 25-4a,b.** *Patterned injuries. Note linear marks (arrows) separated by a pale zone.*

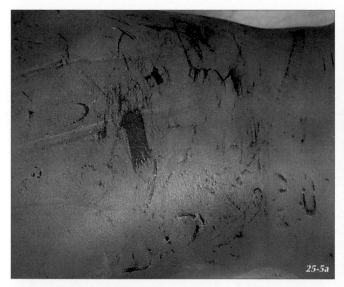

**Figure 25-5a,b.** *Patterned injuries.*

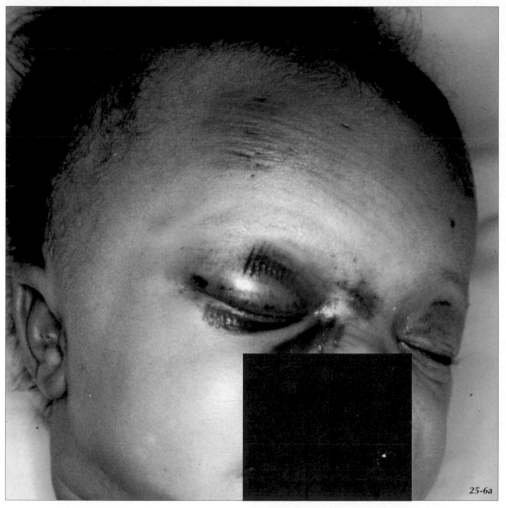

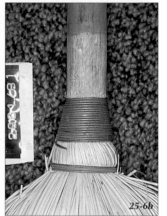

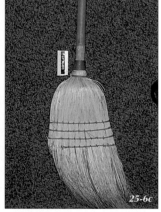

**Figure 25-6a to c.** *Patterned injury and object used. Forehead marks by the straw, orbital injuries by metal banding.*

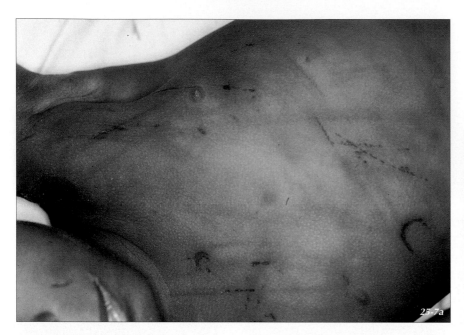

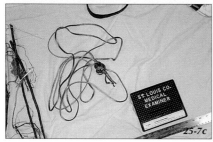
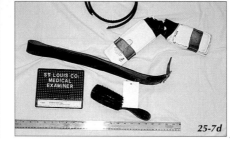
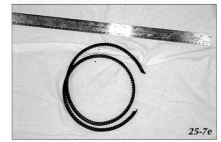

**Figure 25-7a to e.** *Injuries inflicted by multiple instruments.*

A particularly important patterned injury to recognize is the bite mark, which usually has little physiologic significance but has tremendous forensic value. Thorough examination and precise documentation of bite marks offer significant evidence. Swabbing of the bite can reveal serologic characteristics of the biter. Detailed analysis of the bite by an experienced forensic odontologist can indicate if the origin of the bite is human or animal, child or adult, self-inflicted or not; the injury can also be specifically matched to the bite of a particular individual. Comparison techniques may also eliminate a particular individual as having inflicted the bite.

The presence and characteristics of some injuries may not be readily apparent under sunlight or usual indoor lighting. Further delineation of some of these injuries may be accomplished by using alternative light source photography such as ultraviolet (West et al., 1992a, 1992b). Computer enhancement of photographs may also help discern previously unseen characteristics of injuries.

## BLUNT INJURY PATTERNS

Although most blunt injuries are nonspecific when considered in isolation, the overall number, location(s), and age(s) often form patterns that reveal their true nature. The sheer number of injuries can indicate abuse in the absence of a responsible contributory natural disease or other satisfactory explanation such as a motor vehicle crash.

The appearance of the wounds helps differentiate a single episode of injury from the classic pattern of repeated child battering. Injuries sustained in a single episode of violence will be at similar stages of healing, whereas those sustained during chronic battering are clearly of different ages. As mentioned previously, caution must be exercised when assessing the relative age of an injury to allow for the normal variation in healing that occurs in an individual. Influencing variations were listed previously.

The distribution of the injuries is also useful in distinguishing accidental versus intentional injuries. Unintentional injuries are sparse, tend to be superficial, and are often located on the forehead, zygoma, hands, shins, and knees—well-recognized points of impact (Norman et al., 1984). Intentional injuries tend to be multiple, often of various ages, bilateral (Laing, 1977), more extensive, of diverse types (O'Doherty, 1982), and in other locations (Hull, 1974; Pascoe et al., 1979) (**Figure 25-8a to c**). Specific patterns indicating the mechanics of injury production can also emerge, such as blunt head injury associated with "grip" bruises on the extremities and chest or the patterns of scalding by immersion.

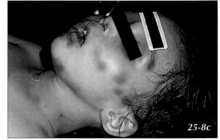

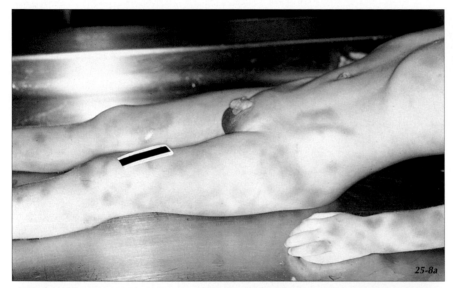

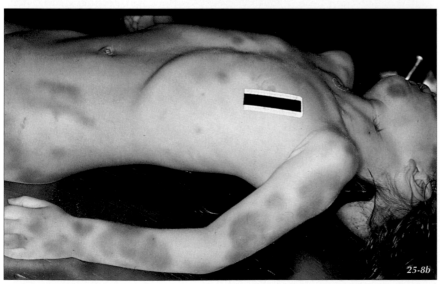

**Figure 25-8a to c.** *Locations of intentional injuries.*

## ◆LETHAL INJURIES

### HEAD INJURIES

The understanding of lethal head injuries in infants and children requires consideration of various differences between adults and children. The immature head is characterized by a flexible skull, patent sutures, incomplete myelinization, increased vasoreactivity, higher metabolic rates, larger cerebrospinal fluid space, and delicate blood vessels (Merten & Osborne, 1983). The type of head injuries resulting from accidental mechanisms in children through 24 months of age and those injuries resulting from nonaccidental infliction have been described and a differentiating algorithm devised for injury categorization (Duhaime et al., 1992).

### BLUNT HEAD TRAUMA

In addition to patterns of how injuries are sustained, certain lethal patterns are also evident among abused children. In 70% to 80% of fatal child abuse, death results from or involves blunt head injury (DiMaio & DiMaio, 1989). Children less than 2 years of age are at greatest risk to sustain this type of injury (Merten & Osborne, 1983). In fatally head-injured abused children under 2 years of age the median age is 8.7 months (Duhaime et al., 1992). In these children the external examination of the head usually reveals the presence of blunt injuries to the face, scalp, lips, buccal mucosa, or frenulum. Facial injuries, excluding superficial bruising over a zygoma or on the forehead or a superficial split lip in a mobile child, suggest abuse (Norman et al., 1984). Tears of the labial frenulum are common in children learning to walk but suggest abuse in children under the age of 6 months who are not ambulatory (Kenney, 1991). Cutaneous bruising in fatal head injuries is characteristically disproportionately less than the hemorrhage seen on the undersurface of the scalp or than the degree of craniocerebral injury. The nature of the scalp and the circumstances of the injury contribute to this phenomenon. The undersurface of the scalp must be examined to identify and localize any impact site(s) and not mistakenly exclude the presence of these injuries on the basis of the lack of visible or palpable areas on the external surface (**Figure 25-9a,b**). Subgaleal hemorrhage can also be related to hair pulling (Kempe, 1975).

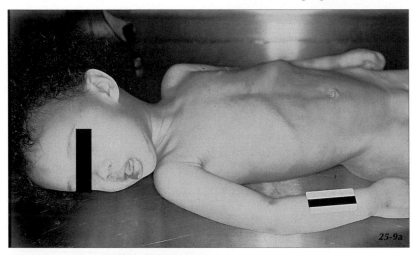

**Figure 25-9a,b.** *Blunt head trauma. The extent of the injury was not realized until the undersurface of the scalp was examined.*

### SKULL FRACTURE

A skull fracture in a fatally injured child is a very strong indicator of abuse unless the circumstances of the injury would be expected to generate a considerable amount of force, for example, a motor vehicle crash or a fall from a great height. Eighty percent of skull fractures related to abuse are found in children under the age of 1 year; these injuries are uncommon in children older than 2 years (Merten & Osborne, 1983). Although thin linear calvarial fractures, usually parietal in location, and ping-pong fractures can occasionally result from low-level falls (3 feet), such fractures are not associated with serious neurologic dysfunction except in the presence of a compression epidural hematoma (Helfer et al., 1977; Duhaime et al., 1992). More extensive and complex fractures reflecting greater translational force can be seen with falls from heights greater than 4 feet. Unless translational force is extreme, these fractures are associated with predominately focal damage and recovery of global neurologic function is usually rapid (Duhaime et al., 1992). The mildest recognizable consequence of angular deceleration to the brain—concussion—can be seen in low level falls (Duhaime et al., 1992). Concussion, skull fracture, and subdural hematoma have been described in falls from bunk beds (Selbst et al., 1990).

## INTRACRANIAL HEMORRHAGE

Various intracranial injuries are found in fatally abused children. Epidural, subdural, and subarachnoid hemorrhage can be present alone or in concert. Intracranial, extraparenchymal hemorrhage can act as a space-occupying lesion; however, it is not unusual for it to be clinically insignificant but forensically important as a marker indicating that significant force has been transmitted to the intracranial contents. Epidural and localized subarachnoid hemorrhages represent impact injuries. In contrast, diffuse subarachnoid hemorrhage and subdural hematomas are features of angular deceleration and are infrequent in non–motor vehicle accidents but are common in inflicted injury (Duhaime et al., 1992).

Brain findings depend on the mechanism of injury, the length of survival, and the age of the child, reflecting the state of the brain's myelination. Before the age of 5 months, blunt force injury to the brain results in shearing separation along the junction of the gray and white matter. These slit-like tears are characteristically found in the parasagittal frontal lobes and in the temporal lobes. They are usually associated with minimal hemorrhage (Lindenberg & Freytag, 1969). Old hemorrhage is differentiated from fresh hemorrhage by the presence of hemosiderin and/or gliosis. As myelination proceeds, the brain exhibits more typical adult contusions. However, the extent and magnitude of visible contusion rarely approach what is seen in adults. Localized cortical contusions can be seen in falls greater than 4 feet. Prominent cerebral edema is common (Zimmerman et al., 1978). Microscopic examination of infant brains sustaining lethal injuries often discloses the presence of axonal varicosities reflecting diffuse axonal injury. Diffuse axonal injury, a lesion commonly leading to death, reflects the application of severe angular deceleration to the brain, resulting in global cerebral dysfunction.

## SHAKING

The shaken infant syndrome typically involves children under the age of 15 months, with the median age being 3 months. In its pure form the fatal shaken infant syndrome is characterized by retinal hemorrhage, subdural/subarachnoid hemorrhage, and lethal damage to the central nervous system in conjunction with a lack of direct impact involving the head (**Figure 25-14**).

Since its characterization by Caffey (1972), the existence of this entity has been controversial. The controversy centers on whether shaking alone is sufficient to cause serious injury or death or if an impact involving the head must accompany the shaking. Using an experimental model, Duhaime and associates maintain that sufficient acceleration-deceleration forces cannot be attained via shaking alone to cause axonal tearing but require the addition of impact to account for the head injuries associated with the shaken infant syndrome (Duhaime et al., 1987). Others maintain that pure shaking can result in serious injury and death (Hadley et al., 1989; Alexander et al., 1990).

The separation of pure shaking from shaking with impact can be exceedingly difficult on clinical grounds. Significant impacts to the head, especially those involving broad and soft surfaces, may be associated with minimal or no external signs of injury. At autopsy the majority of cases involving impact will reveal hemorrhage in the undersurface of the scalp. This hemorrhage is often much more extensive than the external surface of the scalp would suggest (**see Figure 25-9a,b**). Some individuals note the presence of impact injuries to the head in clinically diagnosed cases of shaken infant syndrome and report never seeing a case without such an impact site identifiable at autopsy (DiMaio & DiMaio, 1989). However, I and others (Alexander et al., 1990) have seen cases where no impact site was identifiable during the autopsy. The lack of an impact site injury does not preclude an impact, since striking a broad soft surface may not create an identifiable injury

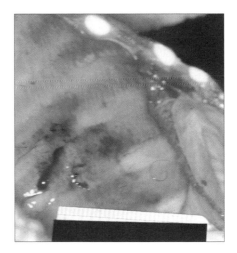

**Figure 25-10.** *Rib fractures.*

at the point of contact. I am aware of a shaking death committed by a paramour and reportedly witnessed by two teenage siblings of the deceased. The siblings described violent to-and-fro shaking with loss of consciousness by the deceased and specifically relate the lack of any impact to or by the head. I believe that a significant impact site in the scalp or the presence of a skull fracture precludes a definitive diagnosis of a pure shaken infant syndrome. These cases may best be referred to as the "shaken impact syndrome" (Bruce & Zimmerman, 1989). The incidence of impact trauma in cases clinically diagnosed as the shaken infant syndrome suggests that at least half of the deaths involving shaking are associated with impact (Alexander et al., 1990). (For a more in-depth discussion of the mechanisms of shaken infant syndrome, *see Chapter 1*.)

Although no single feature allows a definitive diagnosis of fatal shaking (with or without impact), it is convenient to reduce the syndrome to its component parts for the purposes of discussion.

The lethal component of this syndrome is injury to the brain and/or cervical spinal cord. Brain injury characteristically takes the form of brain swelling and diffuse axonal injury, which is manifest by the presence of axonal bulbs and varicosities **(see Figure 25-14a).** The development of the morphologically recognizable markers of axonal injury is time dependent, and their presence and appearance reflect the post-injury survival interval (Vowles, 1987). The lethal injury can also be a contusion of the cervicomedullary or proximal cervical spinal cord, as described by Hadley et al. (1989).

The second component of this syndrome is the presence of subdural and/or subarachnoid hemorrhage. The subdural hemorrhage is characteristically located over the cerebral convexities and is generally of small volume **(see Figure 25-14c).** Similarly, subarachnoid hemorrhage tends to be mild and patchy. The hemorrhages characteristically do not act as clinically significant space-occupying lesions but primarily serve as markers of intracranial angular energy transmission or movement.

Retinal hemorrhage, sometimes accompanied by detachment, is also characteristic of the shaken infant syndrome **(see Figure 25-14b).** Retinal hemorrhages reportedly occur in 66% to 100% of clinically diagnosed shaken infants (Ludwig, 1984; Hadley et al., 1989). This injury is not specific for shaking and can also occur with impact injuries, birth (approximately 10% to 40% of vaginally delivered babies—Sezen, 1970; Egge et al., 1980, 1981), sudden thoracic compression during cardiopulmonary resuscitation (rare), sudden elevation of head and/or neck intravascular pressure, and other causes of increased intracranial pressure (Tomaski & Rosman, 1975; Bacon et al., 1978). Retinal hemorrhages have also been related to endocarditis and hemorrhagic diatheses (McLellan et al., 1986). Old retinal hemorrhage is marked by the presence of hemosiderin deposition. In addition to retinal hemorrhage, retinal detachment and optic nerve sheath hemorrhage can also be seen.

In some cases of shaking, sentinel injuries may be present. These include contusions on the chest and/or arms created while gripping and shaking the child. Hemorrhage in the soft tissue of the upper neck as well as long bone metaphyseal fractures can also be associated with this entity (Caffey, 1946).

## Intrathoracic Injuries

Injuries to the trunk account for 10% to 25% of abuse deaths; the relative incidence of death increases with the age of the child (DiMaio & DiMaio, 1989). Blunt force injuries to the surface of the trunk are seldom unintentional if multiple and nontrivial.

Significant intrathoracic injuries reflect the application of severe force. Lethal intrathoracic injuries may include internal or external cardiac rupture, pneumothorax, and, rarely, flail chest. Hydrostatic right atrial tears can be caused by thoracic impacts or by compressive abdominal forces (Cumberland et al., 1991). Rib fractures resulting from abuse are common and, when present, are nearly always (90%) found in children under the age of 2 years (Leonidas, 1983) (**Figures 25-10 and 25-11**). Posterior rib fractures have been considered characteristic of abuse. Rib fractures rarely, if ever, occur in children as a result of cardiopulmonary resuscitation (Feldman & Brewer, 1984).

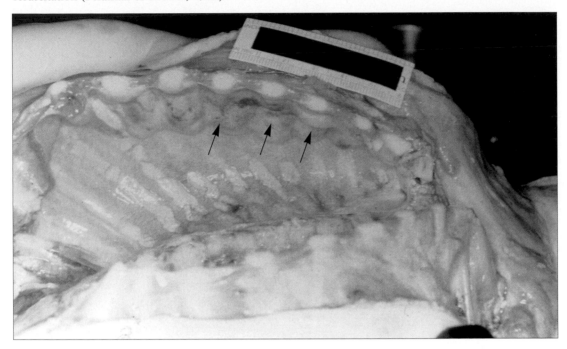

**Figure 25-11.** *Rib fractures (healing) (arrows).*

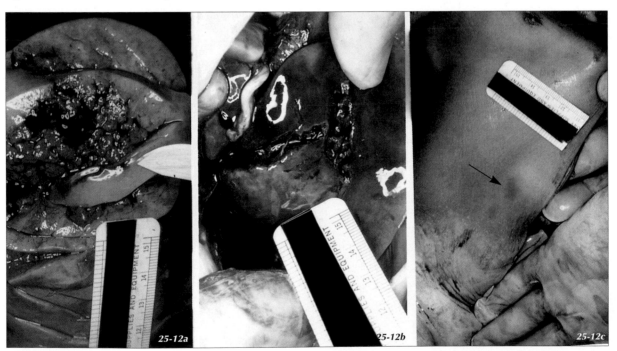

**Figure 25-12a,b.** *Liver laceration.* **c.** *Mild contusion (arrow) of external abdominal wall accompanying massive liver injury.*

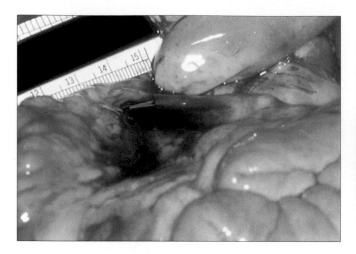

**Figure 25-13.** *Mesentery contusion.*

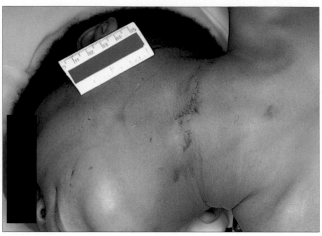

**Figure 25-15.** *Marks on neck in strangulation.*

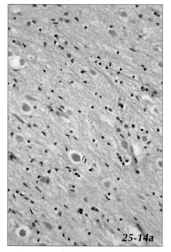

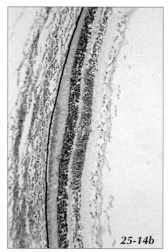

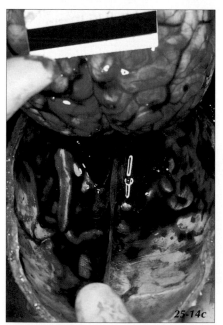

**Figure 25-14a.** *Diffuse axonal injury.*
**b.** *Retinal hemorrhage.* **c.** *Bilateral subdural hematomas.*

## INTRA-ABDOMINAL INJURIES

The most common lethal intra-abdominal injury is a ruptured liver (**Figure 25-12, a to c**). Half of the children with this injury display no externally visible injury to the abdominal wall (DiMaio & DiMaio, 1989). Common accompanying lesions include bowel serosal contusions, contusions and lacerations of the root of the small bowel mesentery (**Figure 25-13**), and perirenal soft tissue hemorrhage. Duodenal hematomas and lacerations occasionally occur and may not become apparent for an extended time after the injury. Death, often caused by peritonitis, sepsis, or some other complication, may not occur for days or weeks.

In intra-abdominal injury cases with prolonged survival, the medical examiner must evaluate previously resected tissue to determine the age of the initial injury. Gastric laceration is rare but can occur as a result of abdominal blows, especially if the stomach is distended at the time of impact (Case & Nanduri, 1983). Pancreatic injuries and secondary pancreatitis occasionally occur as a result of blows to the abdomen or back. Splenic and renal parenchymal injuries are uncommon in child abuse. Renal injuries are more likely to result from posterior or flank blows. As noted earlier, right atrial endocardial tears can result from abdominal compressive forces.

## MECHANICAL ASPHYXIA

Mechanical asphyxiation deaths of children can be particularly vexing because there can be minimal or no demonstrable injuries either externally or internally. The absence or paucity of findings is related to the size/strength disparity between assailant and victim and to the victim's inability to mount significant resistance or defense against the assault and to the ease with which mechanical asphyxia can be accomplished in this age group.

## STRANGULATION

Marks on the skin or in the soft tissues of the neck are usually present in strangulation, but can be absent (**Figure 25-15**). In contrast to adults, conjunctival and orbital petechiae are rarely seen in infants and are uncommon in children. The pliable cartilaginous nature of the larynx and hyoid bone in infants and children makes fractures of these structures unusual.

## SMOTHERING

Smothering is the most commonly employed method of mechanical asphyxiation used to kill infants and children. Findings, when present, can be restricted to mild facial bruising or abrasion or subtle intraoral injuries. Examination of the oral cavity, including the inner aspects of the lips, gums, buccal mucosa, and tongue, is critical when evaluating this type of death. In some cases, no injuries are present, and the autopsy findings are indistinguishable from those of children dying of SIDS. In these cases the cause of death determination relies heavily on other aspects of the medicolegal investigation. Rarely, evidence such as respiratory epithelium has been recovered from the suffocating agent, for example, a pillow (Luke, 1969). A few smothering incidents occurring in hospitals have been videotaped. Using smothering, it takes 70 to 90 seconds to induce a flat EEG and apnea. Unconsciousness follows a period of violent movement (Rosen et al., 1983; Southall et al., 1987; DiMaio & DiMaio, 1989).

## OVERLYING
Covert mechanical asphyxia can also take the form of overlying, in which the adult's body supposedly covers the child's body. Often the adult is obese and/or under the influence of alcohol or other intoxicants. Death results from chest compression with or without associated suffocation. Fatal overlying can be associated with a lack of identifiable external or internal injuries.

## CHOKING
Choking results from mechanical obstruction of the internal airway. The site of obstruction can be at the opening to the larynx or more distally in the airway. The obstruction can be caused by impacted material, tissue swelling (inflammatory or neoplastic), or both. In the case of impacted material the diagnosis rests on physically demonstrating the obstruction or documenting it by history in those cases where the material was expelled or removed during therapeutic activity.

Death caused by choking is usually accidental and is rarely homicidal. Homicide cases are often related to disciplinary activities. Force feeding can result in choking from a bolus of food in a manner similar to what has been termed a "cafe coronary." In other cases the aspiration of black pepper, usually administered as a punitive measure, has resulted in death (Adelson, 1964; Cohle et al., 1988) (**Figure 25-16a,b**). Pepper in the airway clogs the breathing tube with its bulk and irritates the tissues chemically.

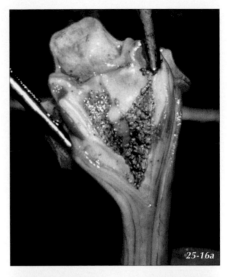
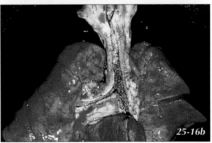

***Figure 25-16a,b.*** *Death caused by aspiration of black pepper.*

## OTHER MECHANISMS
Other modes of death associated with few, if any, physical findings include drowning (Nixon & Pearn, 1977; Pearn & Nixon, 1977; Griest & Zumwalt, 1989), electrocution, hypothermia (Zumwalt & Hirsch, 1980), hyperthermia (Zumwalt & Hirsch, 1980), and poisoning.

## POISONING
Another form of childhood homicide often characterized by few anatomic findings is the intentional introduction of toxic substances. This can take several forms; in classical poisoning, typical poisons are used (e.g., arsenic, fluoride, ethylene glycol); pharmaceuticals prescribed to family members or acquaintances may be administered; over-the-counter preparations, such as acetylsalicylic acid, may be given; or illicit substances such as cocaine or heroin (Rogers et al., 1976; Shnaps et al., 1981) may be provided to the child. Complete toxicologic screening coupled with specific indicated assays and a high index of suspicion are necessary to identify these agents (Rogers et al., 1976; Dine & McGroven, 1982; Case et al., 1983).

Death also can result from the administration of "nontoxic" substances in a toxic manner. Any substance can have deleterious effects if given in sufficient quantity or by an inappropriate route. For example, the administration of an excessive amount of table salt will induce hypernatremia (sodium excess with its attendant chemical imbalances), and the administration of excess water causes hyponatremia (a lack of sufficient sodium). Appropriate postmortem chemical studies of blood, vitreous fluid, and urine are necessary to evaluate these deaths. Since the substance is not always meaningfully measurable, its presence is only indicated by the physiologic aberration it induces. Excess administration of potassium is virtually undetectable at the time of autopsy, since a rapid rise in potassium occurs as a natural consequence of death. For further specific information about poisoning, *refer to Chapter 16, Poisoning.*

## ♦ INJURIES TO THE EXTREMITIES AND GENITALIA

Blunt force injuries to the extremities and genitalia are rarely lethal but are commonly found in fatally abused children. Nonlethal cutaneous injuries can serve as a marker for the mechanism of the lethal injury. For example, bruises on the extremities can be "grip" or "handle" markers. Injuries to the bones of the extremities are common, and their nature may be diagnostic of abuse. The recognition of nonlethal injuries can lead to the correct interpretation of how the lethal injury was sustained. Genital or rectal injuries can indicate sexual abuse or represent injuries inflicted as a disciplinary measure, perhaps related to toilet training.

## ♦ BURNS

Intentionally inflicted burns account for 10% to 25% of pediatric burns and have a disproportionate mortality, 30%, when compared to accidental burns, 2%. The mean age of the abused child sustaining a burn is 1 1/2 to 2 years, with the range being 1 month to 10 years (Purdue et al., 1988). A number of criteria have been proposed to help differentiate accidental burns from nonaccidental burns. These include evidence (physical or historical) of previous or concurrent injuries, the number of injuries, evidence of delay in seeking care, historical-physical-developmental discrepancies, pattern of burns, and location of burns (Stone et al., 1970). Intentionally inflicted burns occasionally are immediately lethal, but more commonly the child comes to medical attention and survives for a period of time before dying of complications such as sepsis or pneumonia. In these cases it is important to causally relate the death to the initial insult. In one third of cases of deliberately inflicted burns of obvious medical significance the caretaker seeks medical care only after an inordinate delay (Purdue et al., 1988), stating that "I didn't realize the burn was serious" or "We thought it would get better by itself." Some contact burns can be patterned, such as those caused by heating elements, or are of characteristic appearance, such as a burn from a cigarette. This pattern usually identifies the causative source of heat.

### SCALDING

Most burns in children are scalds, which account for 50% to 80% of burns up to the age of 4 or 5 years (Klasen, 1979; Thomas et al., 1984). Similarly, scalding is the most frequent form of burn abuse (Hight et al., 1979; Watkins et al., 1985). Scalding can occur at any age but typically occurs in the birth to 2-year age group (Rossignol et al., 1990). The age and motor abilities of the child must be considered when evaluating the nature of the injuries. For example, a 2 1/2- to 3-year-old unattended child could pull a pan of hot water off the stove or get into a tub of hot water but should be able to attempt to extricate himself from the water. A 6-month-old infant would not normally be expected to accomplish these tasks.

Burns caused by hot water immersion have a characteristic distribution that differentiates accidental scalds from intentional scalds. Body diagrams are useful in injury pattern interpretation. The differentiation of accidental (faucet burns, dousing from an overturned pan) from intentional (immersion) scalds requires knowledge of the distribution and depth of the burn, the temperature and nature of the scalding liquid, the duration of contact, the age of the child, the abilities of the child, the normal reaction to the alleged method of scalding, and the physical environment (floor, tub, etc.). Immersion burns tend to be of uniform depth with well-defined margins, whereas splash burns tend to be less well-defined, show a "run-down" pattern, and exhibit variable intensity. The distribution of immersion burns reflects the position the child assumed on being placed in the hot liquid. Protected areas are spared.

The temperature of the liquid and the length of immersion are critical in the production of scalding burns. Full-thickness scald burns of adult skin will occur in 1 to 3 seconds in 150°F water, 7 seconds if the water temperature is 140°F, 30 seconds at 130°F, and 2 minutes at 125°F (Moritz & Henriques, 1947). A child's skin is more sensitive than an adult's, and these times should be shorter in children. The average home water heater often delivers water hotter than 130°F. As part of the medicolegal death investigation or the police investigation, measurement of the water temperature from the tap and after the water sits in a receptacle for a specified period of time can help in verifying or refuting the alleged scalding mechanism, such as "The child was in the tub for less than 5 seconds before I pulled him out."

Intentional chemical burns and microwave injuries do occur but are uncommon. In the latter, tissue damage is proportional to tissue water content (Alexander et al., 1987).

## ◆ NEGLECT

Our society requires that caretakers provide the necessities of life, including food, hydration, clothing, shelter, and medical care. Intentional failure to fulfill these responsibilities constitutes neglect. Neglect can be either active or passive. Active neglect entails the deliberate withholding of life's necessities from the child. In passive neglect the child's welfare is overlooked because the caretaker's focus is elsewhere, such as may occur in prolonged bingeing or with psychotic episodes.

Lethal neglect usually results from malnutrition and dehydration (**Figure 25-17**), often accompanying a superimposed terminal process such as bronchopneumonia. Fatally starved children are typically less than 1 year old (Adelson, 1974). In these cases the nutritional history is out of line with the physical findings. "He hasn't been eating very well for the past 3 or 4 days" is offered as an explanation for marasmus, which is progressive, long-term wasting and emaciation.

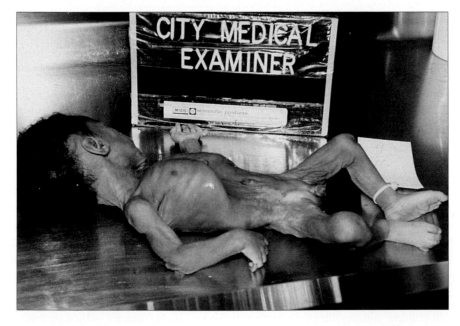

*Figure 25-17.* Lethal neglect resulting from malnutrition and dehydration.

## PHYSICAL FINDINGS

The deceased child's weight and height must be compared to birth sizes and plotted on standard growth curves. It is also useful to compare the postmortem size with any previous growth information about the child. The presence of some chronic disease or condition that could cause or contribute to the malnourishment or dehydration must be excluded (Adelson, 1974).

Other physical findings can suggest neglect. Digestive tract contents tend to be sparse, and any fecal material present tends to be dry. Dehydration is indicated by sunken orbits, skin tenting (delayed surface restoration when skin is stretched or elevated and released), "sticky" serosal surfaces, and electrolyte abnormalities in the vitreous (Coe, 1993). Thymic involution is common. Macrovesicular steatosis may reflect protein deficiency. The overall appearance of the child will point to chronic lack of care. Poor skin condition and chronic diaper rash from soiling are common.

The neglected child's environment generally reflects poor hygienic habits, marginal food supply, and substandard care of other children in the home. Prior health care is often lacking or delinquent.

Failure to provide safe environmental conditions for the child can result in death caused by extreme increases or decreases in body heat (hyperthermia or hypothermia) (Zumwalt et al., 1976; Zumwalt & Hirsch, 1980). Special care must be taken in evaluating the circumstances of these cases. Death can result from various manifestations of these conditions, such as myoglobinuria or pancreatitis. Perimortem failure of the body's thermoregulatory system and postmortem temperature alterations must not be confused with any antemortem temperature abnormalities.

## ALTERNATIVE CARE

Individuals have the right, in most cases, to refuse medical care or turn to nontraditional therapies. However, it is equally true that caretakers have a duty to provide adequate medical care to their charges. Death resulting from the intentional withholding of necessary care can be a form of neglect by omission.

A very controversial area involves the right of the parents to deny care on the basis of legitimate as opposed to convenient religious beliefs proscribing such activities or mandating nontraditional therapy such as prayer alone. This approach does not imply that the parents of these children do not care for or love their children. However, the freedom to practice their beliefs must be tempered with society's mandates regarding the welfare of their children and recognition of the consequences of spurning society's requirements.

When alternative care is involved in the death of a child, the medical examiner must obtain data to identify the cause of death, contributory conditions, and the presence and extent of any specific disease process. The nature and extent of the underlying disease process must be determined in evaluating whether the child could have been helped by current therapeutic regimens. Careful determination of the extent of the disease process can also allow an evaluation of caretaker explanations such as, "I didn't think the child was that sick."

*For further information refer to Chapter 18, Neglect and Abandonment.*

## ◆MUNCHAUSEN SYNDROME BY PROXY

A rare variant of chronic abuse is the Munchausen Syndrome by Proxy (Meadow, 1977). In this syndrome the child is brought to medical attention with an intentionally induced "disease" accompanied by a fictitious history. The caretaker most often responsible for inducing the illness is the mother, although other caretakers, including health care personnel, are occasionally responsible. Most instances of this syndrome are nonlethal, but some children do die. In a series of 19 cases, Meadow recorded 10% mortality (Meadow, 1982). Serious illness and death associated with this syndrome have been reportedly the result of hypoglycemia caused by the surreptitious injection of insulin, apnea due to the administration of succinylcholine, and smothering. It is important to recognize that the assault on the child can continue during and after hospitalization.

*For further information refer to Chapter 17, Munchausen Syndrome by Proxy.*

## ◆ SEXUAL ABUSE

The forensic postmortem examination of a child includes the evaluation for possible sexual abuse. Genital and anal injuries, the presence of sexually transmitted diseases, or circumstantial evidence pointing to possible sexual abuse should prompt a full sexual abuse evaluation. The lack of genital injuries does not exclude sexual abuse. A postmortem distended anus in the absence of other injuries must be interpreted with extreme caution because it could reflect only postmortem laxity.

*For further information refer to Chapters 8 and 9.*

## ◆ CONDITIONS THAT ARE NOT ABUSE

As evidenced by the preceding discussion, fatal child abuse can take on a stunning array of appearances. However, not all injuries are abusive in nature. An abused child can die of an unrelated accident or a natural condition. Various natural diseases and therapeutic measures can simulate to some degree the appearance of physical abuse and neglect. Trivial, innocently acquired scrapes and bruises must be recognized for what they are. Birth injuries need to be correctly identified.

### SUDDEN INFANT DEATH SYNDROME (SIDS)

SIDS is still generally recognized as the most common cause of death among children younger than 1 year of age. It is the "sudden death of an infant under 1 year of age which remains unexplained after the performance of a complete postmortem investigation including autopsy, examination of the death scene, and a review of the case history" (Willenger, 1989). The major abuse/neglect category that is likely to be confused with SIDS is mechanical asphyxia, notably suffocation. A thorough death investigation usually allows this distinction to be made. However, in some instances, to properly ascribe death to one or the other of these conditions is impossible. Deaths in which reasonable suspicion exists that the death is not innocuous should not be certified as SIDS but should be classified as undetermined (cause and manner of death).

### MONGOLIAN SPOT

Areas of hyperpigmentation such as the Mongolian spot should not be confused with injuries (Smialek, 1980) **(see Figure 25-2).** The lack of hemorrhage in the skin and soft tissues of the Mongolian spot differentiates this lesion from an antemortem injury.

### METABOLIC AND OTHER DISORDERS

Various conditions exist that may predispose a child to skeletal, cutaneous, visceral, or soft tissue damage or can manifest themselves as "pseudoinjuries," which must be differentiated from actual physical assaults. These conditions include osteogenesis imperfecti, some neoplasms, Caffey disease, congenital syphilis, kinky hair syndrome, coagulopathies, metabolic disorders, and some connective tissue diseases (Kirschner & Stein, 1985; Kaplan, 1986). Inborn errors of metabolism and poisoning share a variety of features, which can make differentiation difficult (Shoemaker et al., 1992; Woolf et al., 1992).

## INJURIES RELATED TO THERAPEUTIC INTERVENTION

A potential source of difficulty in evaluating the death of a child is the presence of injuries related to or allegedly explained by therapeutic or resuscitative intervention. Several types of contusions and ecchymoses can result from therapeutic endeavors (**Figure 25-18a,b**). Coagulation defects can intensify these lesions. Careful examination of areas of hemorrhage can reveal the true nature of the lesion, for example, needle or lancet punctures. The location of some contusions is also characteristic; examples include presternal contusion acquired during CPR, anterior arm and axillary fold hemorrhage caused by level of consciousness testing, and punctures on the soles of the feet related to neurologic evaluation. However, CPR-related facial bruises are distinctly uncommon (DiMaio & DiMaio, 1989).

***Figure 25-18a,b.*** *Contusions of the neck sustained during CPR.*

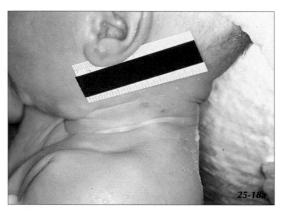 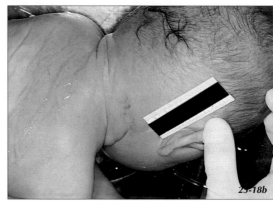

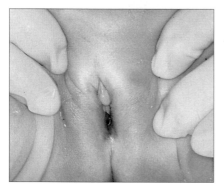

***Figure 25-19.*** *Catheterization injury.*

## IATROGENIC INJURIES

In some cases, intentionally inflicted injuries will be alleged as iatrogenic. Most notable in this group are rib fractures. In contrast to adults, rib fractures caused by CPR are very rare in children without a predisposing bone disease (Feldman & Brewer, 1984). Visceral injuries such as hepatic laceration can occur during resuscitation (Thaler & Krause, 1962; Moe, 1967). Retinal hemorrhage has also been reported to occur as a result of CPR but is rare in this setting (Carter, 1983; Kanter, 1986; Weedn et al., 1990). Injuries associated with medical intervention should be noted in the clinical record and, if they are unusual, communicated to the medical examiner (**Figure 25-19**).

## FOLK MEDICINE

Not only must the effects of traditional medical care be considered in evaluating an apparently injured child, but injuries related to nontraditional or "home" remedies must also be recognized. Such nontraditional practices include the application of hot coins to the skin (*Cao Gio*), dermal abrasion, cupping, plumbism, moxibustion, and *Caida de Mollera* (Guarnaschelli et al., 1972; Golden & Duster, 1977; Lock, 1978; Asnes & Wisotsky, 1981; Kempe, 1982; Feldman, 1984) *(see also Chapter 1, Identifying, Interpreting, and Reporting Injuries).*

## POSTMORTEM CHANGES

In addition to antemortem and perimortem artifacts, various postmortem alterations of the body can be confused with injuries that occurred before death. Included in this group are the irregular mottling of livor mortis, which can be confused with bruising, and postmortem insect bites (**Figure 25-20**) or other animal activity, which can be confused with abrasions. Careful examination of these "injuries" usually readily allows their separation from actual antemortem injuries.

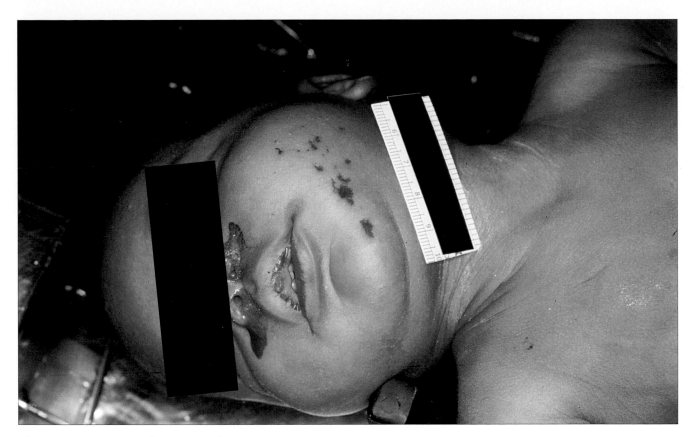

**Figure 25-20.** *Postmortem changes. Insect bites.*

## ♦ Organ and Tissue Transplantation Issues

An expanding role for the medical examiner in deaths related to abuse is in the area of postmortem retrieval of tissue and organs for transplantation. The current major limiting factor in many types of transplant surgery is the insufficient supply of suitable donor organs and tissues. Deaths coming under the jurisdiction of the medical examiner constitute a major potential source of such material. Within this large pool of potential donors is the numerically small population of lethally abused children. These children constitute an important group, since suitable pediatric organ and tissue donors are few. Legitimate concerns about the effects on pending legal proceedings frequently deter obtaining organs and tissues from allegedly abused children, curtailing access to this portion of the donor pool. To successfully fulfill society's need for these organs and tissues while at the same time meeting the requirements for potential legal actions necessitates close cooperation between all involved parties—medical, medicolegal, and legal personnel, as well as the family.

In general, no procedure can be carried out on the body of an individual whose death falls under medicolegal jurisdiction without the permission of the medical examiner. Unless otherwise specified by local statute or regulation, permission for organ and tissue retrieval must be obtained from the next of kin or legal guardian. The medical examiner cannot authorize donor harvesting, but such retrieval cannot proceed without his or her consent. The ability and willingness of the medical examiner to allow organ or tissue retrieval depend on applicable statutes and regulations, local custom, available resources, the particular organs and tissue requested, and the details of the particular death. As a general rule, the organ or tissue retrieval cannot interfere with the fulfillment of the medical examiner's statutory and professional responsibilities. However, cooperative planning among all concerned groups can lead to maximum organ and tissue utilization *and* maintain proper medicolegal evaluation of the death (National Association of Medical Examiners, 1991).

Several modifications to the usual medicolegal processing of the death can be used to facilitate satisfactory organ or tissue retrieval. Since the details of a particular death strongly influence which, if any, organs or tissues will be available for retrieval, it is advantageous when death appears likely or inevitable for the attending physician to report the impending death to the medical examiner. Such reporting facilitates harvesting of tissues and minimizes restrictions on organ and tissue retrieval. This also allows the medical examiner enough time to collect the necessary investigational information from other agencies. The intent is to allow the medical examiner to make an informed evaluation about which organs/tissues can be potentially retrieved and what further studies may be needed before any retrieval procedure. Following this, the family can be approached for their permission to retrieve the organs or tissues already pre-authorized by the medical examiner. In our experience this system works effectively and efficiently, and restriction of organ/tissue retrieval is minimized. Other procedures that can be indicated include examination before retrieval and photography of the victim at the hospital, preretrieval radiographic studies for medicolegal purposes, sample collection for toxicologic and other studies, medical examiner attendance at the retrieval procedure, intraoperative photographic and detailed descriptive documentation of organs or tissues before their removal, and indicated intraoperative biopsies. If the medical examiner does not attend the retrieval procedure and the operating surgeon detects an occult injury, the procedure should be halted pending further consultation with the medical examiner.

## ◆ BIBLIOGRAPHY

Adelson, L: Homicide by pepper, *J Forensic Sci* 9:391, 1964.

Adelson, L: *The Pathology of Homicide*, Charles C Thomas, Publisher, Springfield, IL, 1974.

Adelson, L: Pedicide revisited, *Am J Forensic Med Pathol* 12(1):16-26, 1991.

Alexander, R, et al: Incidence of impact trauma with cranial injuries ascribed to shaking, *Am J Dis Child* 144:724-726, 1990.

Alexander, RC, Surrell, JA, and Lohle, SP: Microwave oven burns to children: An unusual manifestation of child abuse, *Pediatrics* 79:255, 1987.

Asnes, RS, and Wisotsky, DT: Cupping lesions simulating child abuse, *J Pediatr* 99:267, 1981.

Bacon, CJ, Sayer, GC, and Howe, JW: Extensive retinal hemorrhage in infancy: An innocent cause, *Br Med J* 1:281, 1978.

Bite mark analysis. In D Averill, ed: *Manual of Forensic Odontology*, American Society of Forensic Odontology, 1991.

Brown, RH: The battered child syndrome, *J Forensic Sci* 21:65, 1976.

Bruce, D, and Zimmerman, R: Shaken impact syndrome, *Pediatr Ann* 18:482-494, 1989.

Caffey, J: Multiple fractures of long bones of children suffering from subdural hematoma, *Am J Radiol* 56:163-173, 1946.

Caffey, J: On the theory and practice of shaking infants: Its potential residual effects of permanent brain damage and mental retardation, *Am J Dis Child* 124:161-169, 1972.

Carter, JE: Whiplash shaking syndrome: Retinal hemorrhage and computerized axial tomography of the brain, *Child Abuse Negl* 7:279, 1983.

Case, M, and Nanduri, R: Laceration of the stomach by blunt trauma in a child: A case of child abuse, *J Forensic Sci* 28:496-501, 1983.

Case, MES, Short, CD, and Poklis, A: Intoxication by aspirin and alcohol in a child, *Am J Forensic Med Pathol* 4(2):149, 1983.

Coe, JI: Postmortem chemistry update, *Am J Forensic Med Pathol* 14:91-117, 1993.

Cohle, SD, Trestrail, JD, Graham, MA, et al: Fatal pepper aspiration, *Am J Dis Child* 142(6):633-636, 1988.

Cumberland, G, Riddick, L, and McConnell, C: Intimal tears of the right atrium of the heart due to blunt force injuries to the abdomen, *Am J Forensic Med Pathol* 12(2):102-104, 1991.

Davis, JH: Can sudden death be murder, *J Forensic Sci* 23:384, 1978.

DiMaio, DJ, and DiMaio, VJM: *Forensic Pathology*, Elsevier, New York, 1989.

Dine, MS, and McGroven, ME: Intentional poisoning of children: An overlooked category of child abuse: Report of 7 cases and review of literature, *Pediatrics* 70:32, 1982.

Duhaime, AC, Gennarelli, TA, Thibault, CE, Bruce, DA, Margulies, SS, and Wiser, R: The shaken baby syndrome: A clinical, pathological, and biomechanical study, *J Neurosurg* 66:409-415, 1987.

Duhaime, AC, et al: Head injury in very young children: Mechanisms, injury types, and ophthalmologic findings in 100 hospitalized patients younger than 2 years of age, *Pediatrics* 90:179-185, 1992.

Egge, K, Lyng, G, and Maltau, MJ: Retinal hemorrhages in the newborn, *Acta Ophthalmol* 58:231-236, 1980.

Egge, K, Lyng, G, and Maltau, MJ: Effect of instrumental delivery on the frequency and severity of retinal hemorrhages in the newborn, *Acta Obstet Gynecol Scand* 60:153-155, 1981.

Feldman, K: Pseudoabusive burns in Asian refugees, *Am J Dis Child* 138:768-769, 1984.

Feldman, KW, and Brewer, DK: Child abuse, cardiopulmonary resuscitation and rib fractures, *Pediatrics* 73:339-342, 1984.

Golden, S, and Duster, M: Hazards of misdiagnosis due to Vietnamese folk medicine, *Clin Pediatr* 10:949-950, 1977.

Griest, K, and Zumwalt, R: Child abuse by drowning, *Pediatrics* 83:41-46, 1989.

Guarnaschelli, J, Lee, J, and Pitts, FW: "Fallen fontanelle" (Caida de Mollera): A variant of the battered child, *JAMA* 222:1545, 1972.

Hadley, M, et al: The infant whiplash–shaken injury syndrome: A clinical and pathological study, *Neurosurgery* 24:536-540, 1989.

Helfer, RE, Slovis, TL, and Black, M: Injuries resulting when small children fall out of bed, *Pediatrics* 60:533-535, 1977.

Hight, D, Bakalar, N, and Hoyd, J: Inflicted burns in children, *JAMA* 242:517-520, 1979.

Hull, D: Medical diagnosis in the maltreated child. In J Carter, ed, Priory Press Ltd, London, 1974, Chapter 6.

Kanter, R: Retinal hemorrhage after cardiopulmonary resuscitation or child abuse, *J Pediatr* 108:430-432, 1986.

Kaplan, JM: Pseudoabuse: The misdiagnosis of child abuse, *J Forensic Sci* 31(4):1420-1428, 1986.

Kempe, CH: Uncommon manifestations of the battered child syndrome, *Am J Dis Child* 129(11):1265, 1975.

Kempe, CH: Cross cultural perspectives in child abuse, *Pediatrics* 69:497-498, 1982.

Kenney, J: Child abuse and neglect. In D Averill, ed: *Manual of Forensic Odontology*, American Society of Forensic Odontology, 1991.

Kirschner, R, and Stein, RJ: Mistaken diagnosis of child abuse: A form of medical abuse? *Am J Dis Child* 139:873, 1985.

Kleinman, PK, et al: Radiologic contributions to the investigation and prosecution of cases of fatal infant abuse, *New Engl J Med* 320:507-511, 1989.

Laing, SA: Bilateral injuries in childhood: An alerting sign, *Br Med J* 2:1355, 1977.

Leonidas, JC: Skeletal trauma in the child abuse syndrome, *Pediatr Ann* 12(12):875-881, 1983.

Lindenberg, R, and Freytag, E: Morphology of brain lesions from blunt trauma in early infancy, *Arch Pathol* 87:298, 1969.

Lock, M: Sears of experience: The art of moxibustion in Japanese medicine and society, *Cult Med Psychiatry* 2:151-175, 1978.

Ludwig, S: Shaken baby syndrome: A review of 20 cases, *Ann Emerg Med* 13:104-107, 1984.

Luke, JL: Recovery of intact respiratory epithelium from a cloth pillowcase four days following its utilization as a smothering instrument, *J Forensic Sci* 14(3):398-401, 1969.

McClain, P, et al: Estimates of fatal child abuse and neglect, United States, 1979 through 1988, *Pediatrics* 91:338-343, 1993.

McLellan, NJ, Prasad, R, and Punt, J: Spontaneous subhyaloid and retinal hemorrhages in an infant, *Arch Dis Child* 61:1130-1132, 1986.

Meadow, R: Munchausen Syndrome by Proxy: The hinterland of child abuse, *Lancet* 2:343, 1977.

Meadow, R: Munchausen Syndrome by Proxy, *Arch Dis Child* 57:92, 1982.

Merten, DF, and Osborne, DRS: Craniocerebral trauma in the child abuse syndrome, *Pediatr Ann* 12:12, 1983.

Moe, N: Complications following resuscitation, *Acta Med Scand* 182:773, 1967.

Moritz, AR, and Henriques, FC: Studies of thermal injury. II: The relative importance of time and surface temperature in the causation of cutaneous burns, *Am J Pathol* 23:695, 1947.

National Association of Medical Examiners: *Policy and Guidelines on Human Organ and Tissue Procurement*, The Association, St. Louis, 1991.

Nixon, J, and Pearn, J: Non-accidental immersion in bathwater: Another aspect of child abuse, *Br Med J* 1:271-272, 1977.

Norman, MG, Smialek, JE, Newman, DE, and Horembala, EJ: Postmortem examination on the abused child: Pathological, radiographic and legal aspects, *Perspect Pediatr Pathol* 8:313, 1984.

O'Doherty, N: *The Battered Child: Recognition in Primary Care*, Bailliere Tindall, London, 1982.

Pascoe, JM, Hildebrandt, HM, Terrier, A, et al: Patterns of skin injury in non-accidental and accidental injury, *Pediatrics* 64:245, 1979.

Pearn, J, and Nixon, J: Attempted drowning as a form of non-accidental injury, *Aust Paediatr J* 13:110, 1977.

Purdue, GF, Hunt, JL, and Prescott, PR: Child abuse by burning: An index of suspicion, *J Trauma* 28(2):221-224, 1988.

Raekallio, J: Histological estimation of the age of injuries. In J Perper and C Wecht, eds: *Microscopic Diagnosis in Forensic Pathology*, Charles C Thomas, Publisher, Springfield, IL, 1980.

Retinal hemorrhages in newborn infants, *Br J Ophthalmol* 55:248-253, 1970.

Rogers, D, Tripp, J, et al: Non-accidental poisoning: An extended syndrome of child abuse, *Br Med J* 1:793, 1976.

Rosen, CL, Frost, JD, et al: Two siblings with recurrent cardiorespiratory arrest: Munchausen Syndrome by Proxy or child abuse? *Pediatrics* 71:715, 1983.

Rossignol, AM, Locke, JA, and Burke, JF: Pediatric burn injuries in New England, *Burns* 16:41-48, 1990.

Schmitt, BD: Child abuse and neglect: Types, epidemiology and characteristics. In RG Sanger and DC Bross, eds: *Clinical Management of Child Abuse and Neglect: A Guide*, 1984.

Selbst, M, et al: Bunk bed injuries, *Am J Dis Child* 144:721-723, 1990.

Sezen, F: Retinal hemorrhages in newborn infants, *Br J Ophthalmol* 55:248-253, 1970.

Shnaps, Y, Frand, M, Rotem, Y, and Tirosh, M: The chemically abused child, *Pediatrics* 68:119, 1981.

Shoemaker, J, Lynch, R, Hoffmann, J, and Sly, W: Misidentification of propionic acid as ethylene glycol in a patient with methylmalonic acidemia, *J Pediatr* 120:417-421, 1992.

Smialek, J: Signatures of mongolian spots, *J Pediatr* 97:504, 1980.

Southall, DP, et al: Apneic episodes induced by smothering: Two cases identified by covert video surveillance, *Br Med J* 294:1637-1641, 1987.

Stone, N, Rinaldo, L, Humphrey, C, et al: Child abuse by burning, *Surg Clin North Am* 50:1419-1424, 1970.

Thaler, MM, and Krause, VW: Serious trauma in children after external cardiac massage, *N Engl J Med* 267:500, 1962.

Tomaski, LG, and Rosman, P: Purtscher retinopathy in the battered child syndrome, *Am J Dis Child* 1229:1335, 1975.

Vowles, G, et al: Diffuse axonal injury in early infancy, *J Clin Pathol* 40:185-189, 1987.

Watkins, A, Gagan, R, and Cupoli, JM: Child abuse by burning, *J Fla Med Assoc* 72:497-502, 1985.

Weedn, V, Mansour, A, and Nichols, M: Retinal hemorrhage in an infant after cardiopulmonary resuscitation, *Am J Forensic Med Pathol* 11(1):79-82, 1990.

West, M, et al: The detection and documentation of trace wound patterns by use of an alternative light source, *J Forensic Sci* 37:1480-1488, 1992a.

West, M, et al: Ultraviolet radiation and its role in wound pattern documentation, *J Forensic Sci* 37:1466-1479, 1992b.

Willenger, M: SIDS: A challenge, *J Natl Inst Health Res* 1:73, 1989.

Wilson, EF: Estimation of the age of cutaneous contusions in child abuse, *Pediatrics* 60:750, 1977.

Woolf, A, Wynshaw-Boris, A, Rinaldo, P, and Levy, H: Intentional infantile ethylene glycol poisoning presenting as an inherited metabolic disorder, *J Pediatr* 120:421-424, 1992.

Zimmerman, RA, Bilaniuk, LT, Bruce, D, et al: Computed tomography of pediatric head trauma: Acute general cerebral swelling, *Radiology* 126:403-408, 1978.

Zumwalt, RE, and Fanizza-Orphanus, AM: Dating of healing rib fractures in fatal child abuse, *Adv Pathol* 3:193-205, 1990.

Zumwalt, RE, and Hirsch, CS: Subtle fatal child abuse, *Hum Pathol* 11:167, 1980.

Zumwalt, RE, Petty, CS, and Holman, W: Temperatures in closed automobiles in hot weather, *Forensic Sci Gaz* 7:7, 1976.

# Legal Issues

Jesse A. Goldner, M.A., J.D.
Cassandra K. Dolgin, B.A., J.D.
Sandra H. Manske, R.N., M.A., J.D.

The identification and investigation of alleged child abuse and neglect for purposes of medical treatment, social service intervention, or criminal prosecution are likely to involve some aspect of the legal system as follows:

1.  Various state statutory provisions provide definitions of "child abuse" and "child neglect," although they may differ both from state to state and within a given state, depending on the objective in making the identification: for reporting to child protection agencies, for establishing a standard for juvenile court intervention, or for denominating behavior deemed unlawful and meriting punishment through the criminal justice system.

2.  State laws and regulations, as well as other legal rules, prescribe the manner in which child abuse and neglect cases are handled. They address both the method of reporting the incident to the appropriate state agency and how that agency is to respond to the report.

3.  The legal system not only controls what may transpire in a juvenile, criminal, or divorce court setting, but also dictates some of what should occur in the physician's office or hospital.

## ♦ An Historical Perspective

The United States initially adopted the legal view that children were a form of property of their parents from English common law (Horowitz & Davidson, 1984). Although the law did recognize the parental obligation to maintain, educate, and protect one's own child, the widely accepted maxims, "a man's home is his castle" and "spare the rod and spoil the child," reflected the reality that parental duties were relatively free from legal restrictions. Consequently, only cases of severe child abuse, involving cruel and merciless punishment or permanent physical injury, resulted in intervention and criminal prosecution (*State v. Jones*, 1886).

During the Industrial Revolution there was a greater willingness to recognize the need for child protection. This was manifested by legislation that limited child labor and provided for other forms of child protection. The early 19th century witnessed the limited adoption of state statutes authorizing the removal of children from neglectful environments. It was not until 1874, however, with the founding of the Society for the Prevention of Cruelty to Children, an outgrowth of the Society for the Prevention of Cruelty to Animals, that a significant push for legislative reform in the area of child maltreatment came into its own (Radbill, 1987).

State juvenile court systems, modeled after the Illinois Juvenile Court Act of 1899, emerged in the early 1900s. The development of these courts represented a direct exercise of the state's *parens patriae* authority, which justifies state intervention over parental objection in order to protect children (Bross, 1988). The exercise of such state power over a child is generally controlled by three principles:

*First, the power is based, primarily, on the presumption that children lack the mental competence and maturity possessed by adults. Second, before intervening the state must show that the child's parents or guardians are unfit, unable, or unwilling to care for the child. Finally, the state should exercise the parens patriae power solely to further the best interests of the child (Rosenberg & Hunt, 1984).*

The development of juvenile courts corresponded with the movement toward professionalism in social work and increased social services directed at child protection. Today the juvenile court exercises jurisdiction over minors brought within the system as a result of alleged abuse, neglect and abandonment, or incorrigibility and delinquency. These courts, as opposed to those that are part of the criminal justice system, afford the judge broad discretion in addressing the problems encountered by invoking state coercion to effectuate the social welfare system's goal of rehabilitation and treatment of abusive parents and other caretakers. The court's determination that a child is in need of supervision or assistance may result in court-ordered family services, placement of the child in foster care or a state youth facility, or, in extraordinary circumstances, termination of parental rights.

Differentiating between physical abuse and symptoms or injuries resulting from disease processes or accidents often proved difficult. The work of two physicians provided guidance. Radiologist Dr. John Caffey, in the early and mid-20th century, related previously unexplained X-ray findings to trauma that may have resulted from parental action. In the 1950s and early 1960s, Dr. C. Henry Kempe and his colleagues at the University of Colorado Medical School defined the "battered child syndrome" as an observable clinical condition capable of medical diagnosis. Together these discoveries had legal as well as medical significance (Kempe et al., 1962; Radbill, 1987).

Medical identification of certain nonaccidental physical injuries contributed not only to increased criminal prosecutions but also to legislative efforts to require the reporting of suspected cases of child abuse. In 1963 the U.S. Department of Health, Education, and Welfare's (now Health and Human Services) Children's Bureau developed a model child abuse reporting statute. By 1967 each state had enacted such a law. These first reporting statutes were narrow in purpose and scope. Their aim was simply to identify suspected child abuse, and only physicians were designated as mandatory reporters. As knowledge regarding child abuse increased, however, states refined these laws, expanding their purpose beyond mere identification to investigation and intervention, and broadening the group of mandated reporters (Fraser, 1978).

Recently the rehabilitative approach to dealing with child abuse and neglect cases, which has been favored in the treatment of physical and sexual abuse, has been subjected to extensive attack. Some critics have cited frustrations with the courts' ability to effectively intervene in many cases where such intervention seems necessary. Other critics point to the inability of professionals working in the area of mental health and child protection to change deviant behavior, particularly in a cost-effective way.

Consequently, at least to some extent, attention is shifting in two other directions. On the one hand, over the last decade, in an effort to increase the success of reliance on the judicial system to aid in the handling of these cases, many jurisdictions have passed statutes or issued judicial rulings designed to make testimony by a child easier and less traumatic in some or all of the different types of proceedings involving child abuse. These generally involve efforts to minimize the need for the child to be in the presence of the alleged abuser, while at the same time protecting the rights of defendants and others involved in these cases. These include, for example, the possible use of closed circuit cameras, videotaped testimony and courtroom screens, and the increased admissibility of hearsay evidence (Myers, 1986). Some limitations on the use of such techniques are reviewed later in this chapter. At the same time, increased efforts are being made to focus on prevention as perhaps the most cost-effective way of dealing with child abuse and neglect in the long run (Daro, 1988).

Generally, it is the state that responds to child maltreatment, but during the past quarter century, federal legislation has greatly influenced the states' legal response to child maltreatment. Beginning in 1974, the National Center on Child Abuse and Neglect was established by congressional mandate (Child Abuse Prevention and Treatment Act, 1974). The law imposed various requirements on the states as a condition for receiving federal funds for "developing, strengthening, and carrying out child abuse and neglect prevention and treatment programs." Presently, eligibility for funding under the legislation requires the establishment of state reporting laws, statutory immunity provisions for those who report suspected cases of abuse and neglect under state law, a state agency responsible for carrying out investigatory and treatment procedures, a state-wide central child abuse registry, provisions for confidentiality of registry records, and the appointment of a *guardian ad litem* for the child in cases involving judicial proceedings (Child Abuse Prevention and Treatment Act, 1974; Rosenberg & Hunt, 1984).

In 1980 the passage of additional federal legislation (Adoption Assistance and Child Welfare Act, 1980) required states to make reasonable efforts to avoid removing maltreated children from parental custody and mandated court or administrative review of state-supervised foster care placement at least every 6 months. This review determines the continuing necessity for and appropriateness of the placement, the compliance with an established case plan, and the extent of progress made toward alleviating or mitigating the cause of the placement. The review must also include a projected date for the child's return home, or, when return to the biological parent's home is unlikely, recommend placement for adoption or legal guardianship (Cunningham & Horowitz, 1989). The enactment of federal statutes concerning Native Americans (Indian Child Welfare Act, 1978) requires state agencies to make "active efforts" to provide services "designed to prevent the breakup of the Indian family."

Finally, federal legislation has enhanced intervention in child sexual abuse cases. Recent statutory measures impose criminal sanctions on any person who uses, or assists another in using, a minor to engage in sexually explicit behavior for the purpose of producing physical depictions of this behavior with the intent to distribute the material in interstate commerce (Federal Protection of Children Against Sexual Exploitation Act, 1986).

## ♦ REPORTING STATUTES AND CHILD PROTECTIVE SERVICES

The identification of abuse and neglect, the assessment of family social service needs, and the implementation of treatment programs and other intervention strategies for abused children and their families are carried out predominantly by state and county child protective service (CPS) agencies. Authorization for such action typically is found in state laws that establish and provide funding for these agencies and define the criteria for, and mode of, intervention. The primary purposes of CPS agencies are "(1) to protect and insure the safety of children who have been or are at risk of maltreatment, and (2) to provide services to alter the conditions which create risk of maltreatment in the future" (Cunningham & Horowitz, 1989).

A report to the state's child abuse and neglect hotline, made either by a professional involved with the child or by a neighbor or other nonmandated reporter, generally results in a referral to a CPS agency. Often such a referral results from a report to the local police. Occasionally the report is initiated by one parent with respect to the other in the context of a child custody dispute.

Child abuse and neglect reporting laws dictate the manner in which referrals are made to the CPS agency and also how the agency is to respond. Additionally, the statutes mandate other duties and rights of health care personnel and other reporters. These laws govern the central registries that maintain information regarding cases that have previously been investigated by the CPS agency. Finally, the laws often define the relationship between the CPS agency, the juvenile court, and various law enforcement agencies.

## REPORTING STATUTES

Each state, as well as the District of Columbia, Puerto Rico, and the Virgin Islands, has enacted its own child abuse and neglect reporting legislation. As a result, there is a lack of uniformity in statutory language and in the effect of the various laws. In particular, the statutes vary as to the precise definition of child abuse and the standards and procedures used for reporting suspected cases (Fraser, 1978). All of the statutes, however, share a common purpose and tend to follow a similar format based on the federally mandated requirements (Meriwether, 1986).

The purpose of every child abuse and neglect reporting statute is to protect the child from additional injury. Accordingly, statutes are written to encourage and facilitate reporting of suspected abuse or neglect. They are designed to promote early identification of the child in peril so that adequate investigation and treatment of the child, as well as of the family, when appropriate, can begin.

Every state reporting statute contains essentially the same elements, including (1) what must be reported (reportable conditions/definition of child abuse); (2) who must or may report; (3) when a report must be made (including the degree of certainty a reporter must have); (4) reporting procedures; (5) the existence and operation of a central registry; (6) rules regarding protective custody; (7) immunity for good faith reporters; (8) the abrogation of certain privileged communication rights that might otherwise apply; and (9) sanctions for failure to report. In addition, many child abuse reporting statutes provide for the taking of photographs or X-rays of the child when physical abuse is suspected, even in the absence of parental consent *(see Tables 26-1 to 26-4)*.

## WHAT MUST BE REPORTED

Every state reporting statute requires that mandated reporters report suspected child abuse and neglect (**Table 26-1**). Each state, however, defines child abuse and neglect differently; therefore reportable conditions vary among the states (Table 26-1). In general, reportable conditions include nonaccidental physical injury, neglect, sexual abuse, and emotional abuse.

## WHO MUST REPORT

Each state reporting statute designates who is required to report suspected child abuse and neglect (**Table 26-2**). Typically, these individuals include physicians, health care professionals, educators, and law enforcement personnel. Many states, however, have an even broader base of mandated reporters, including such professionals as coroners, dentists, probation officers, social workers, or other persons responsible for the care of children. Over 20 states require "any person" to report (Blue, 1988). In addition, the majority of state reporting statutes also provide for permissive reporting by nonmandated reporters.

| STATE | Mandatory Reporting Required | Permissive Reporting Allowed | Immunities | Civil Penalty | Criminal Penalty | Definition of Neglect | Definition of Emotional Injury | Definition of Medical Neglect | Definition of Physical Abuse | Definition of Sexual Abuse | Temporary Protective Custody | X-Ray/Photo | Emergency Treatment | Interagency Reporting |
|---|---|---|---|---|---|---|---|---|---|---|---|---|---|---|
| Alabama | X | X | X | | X | X | X | X | X | X | X | | X | X |
| Alaska | X | X | X | | X | X | X | X | X | X | X | X | | X |
| Arizona | X | | X | | X | | | | X | | | X | X | X |
| Arkansas | X | X | X | X | X | X | X | X | X | X | X | X | X | X |
| California | X | X | X | | X | X | X | X | X | X | | X | | X |
| Colorado | X | X | X | X | X | X | | X | | X | X | X | | X |
| Connecticut | X | | X | | X | X | X | X | X | X | X | X | X | X |
| Delaware | X | | X | | X | X | X | X | X | X | X | X | | X |
| District of Columbia | X | | X | | X | X | X | X | X | X | X | X | | X |
| Florida | X | | X | | X | X | X | X | X | X | X | X | X | X |
| Georgia | X | X | X | | X | X | | | | | | X | | X |
| Hawaii | X | X | X | | X | X | X | | | X | X | | | X |
| Idaho | X | | X | | X | X | X | X | X | X | X | | | X |
| Illinois | X | X | X | | | X | X | X | X | X | X | X | X | X |
| Indiana | X | X | X | | X | X | X | X | X | X | X | X | X | X |
| Iowa | X | X | X | X | X | X | | | X | X | X | X | | X |
| Kansas | X | X | X | | X | X | X | X | X | X | X | X | X | X |
| Kentucky | X | X | X | | | X | X | X | X | X | X | X | X | X |
| Louisiana | X | X | X | | X | X | X | X | X | X | X | | X | X |
| Maine | X | X | X | | | X | X | X | X | X | X | X | | |
| Maryland | X | | X | | | | | | X | X | X | | X | X |
| Massachusetts | X | X | X | X | X | | | | | X | X | X | | |
| Michigan | X | X | X | X | X | X | X | X | X | X | X | X | X | X |
| Minnesota | X | X | X | X | X | X | X | X | X | X | X | X | X | X |
| Mississippi | X | | X | X | | X | X | X | X | X | X | X | X | X |
| Missouri | X | X | X | | X | X | X | X | X | X | X | X | X | X |
| Montana | X | X | X | X | X | X | X | X | X | X | X | X | X | X |
| Nebraska | X | | X | | X | X | X | X | X | X | X | X | X | X |
| Nevada | X | X | X | | X | X | X | X | X | X | X | | X | X |
| New Hampshire | X | | X | | X | X | X | X | X | X | X | | X | X |
| New Jersey | X | | X | | X | X | X | X | X | X | X | | X | X |
| New Mexico | X | | X | | X | X | X | X | X | X | X | | X | X |
| New York | X | X | X | X | X | X | X | X | X | X | X | X | | |
| North Carolina | X | | X | | | X | X | X | X | X | X | | X | X |
| North Dakota | X | X | X | | X | X | X | X | X | X | X | X | X | X |
| Ohio | X | X | X | | X | X | X | X | X | X | X | X | X | X |
| Oklahoma | X | | X | | X | X | X | X | X | X | X | X | X | X |
| Oregon | X | | X | | X | X | X | X | X | X | X | X | X | X |
| Pennsylvania | X | X | X | | X | X | X | X | X | X | X | X | X | X |
| Rhode Island | X | | X | X | X | X | X | X | X | X | X | X | X | X |
| South Carolina | X | X | X | | X | X | X | X | X | X | X | X | X | X |
| South Dakota | X | X | X | | X | X | X | X | X | X | X | X | X | X |
| Tennessee | X | | X | | X | | | X | | X | X | X | X | X |
| Texas | X | | X | | X | | | X | | X | X | X | X | X |
| Utah | X | | X | | X | X | X | | X | X | X | X | X | X |
| Vermont | X | X | X | | X | X | X | X | X | X | X | X | | X |
| Virginia | X | X | X | | X | X | X | X | X | X | X | X | X | X |
| Washington | X | X | X | | X | X | | | X | X | X | X | X | X |
| West Virginia | X | X | X | | X | X | X | X | X | X | X | X | X | X |
| Wisconsin | X | X | X | | X | X | X | X | X | X | X | X | X | X |
| Wyoming | X | | X | | | X | X | X | X | X | X | X | X | |

**Table 26-1 General Provisions of Reporting Statutes.** *Derived from tables in Myers, JEB, and Peters, WD: Child Abuse Reporting Legislation in the 1980's, Denver, CO: American Humane Association, 1987. Used with permission.*

Table 26-2 (continued on following structure)

| STATE | Alcohol/Drug Abuse Counselor | Neighbor, Relative, Friend | Firefighter/Inspector | Physician/Surgeon | Osteopath | Dentist | Resident/Intern | Commercial Film & Photo Processor | Hospital/Institution Personnel | Health Practitioner or Professional | Chiropractor | Pharmacist | Nurses | Teachers/School Counselors | Other School Personnel/Administrator | Social Worker or Social Wk. Technician | Law Enforcement/Judge | Coroner/Medical Examiner | Psychologist/Mental Health Profes. | Optometrists | Podiatrist | Christian Science Pract. Religous Healers | Lic. Day Care Providers/Workers | Clergymen | Attorneys | Any Person Lic. to Practice Healing Arts | Emergency Medical Technician | Parole/Probation Officer | Foster Care/Child-Care Personnel | Homemaker | Any Public or Private Official | Any other person/Any Person |
|---|---|---|---|---|---|---|---|---|---|---|---|---|---|---|---|---|---|---|---|---|---|---|---|---|---|---|---|---|---|---|---|---|
| Alabama | | | | X | X | X | | | X | | | | X | X | X | X | X | X | X | X | X | | | X | | | X | | | | | |
| Alaska | | | | X | X | X | | | X | | | | X | X | X | X | X | | X | X | | | | X | X | | X | X | X | X | | |
| Arizona | | | | X | X | X | X | X | | | | | X | X | X | X | X | X | X | | X | | | X | X | | | | X | | | |
| Arkansas | | | | X | X | X | X | | X | | | | X | X | X | X | X | X | X | | | | | X | | | | | X | | | |
| California | | | | X | | X | X | X | | X | X | | X | X | X | | | | X | | | | X | X | X | | | | X | | | |
| Colorado | | | | X | X | X | X | | X | | | | X | X | X | | | X | X | X | X | | | X | | | | | X | | | |
| Connecticut | | | | X | X | X | X | | X | | | | X | X | X | X | X | X | X | X | X | | | X | X | | | | X | | | X |
| Delaware | | | | X | X | X | X | | | | | | X | X | X | X | X | X | X | | | | | | | | X | | | | | X |
| District of Columbia | | | | X | | | | | | | | X | X | X | X | X | X | | | X | | | | | | | | | | | | |
| Florida | | | | X | X | | | | X | X | X | | X | X | X | X | X | X | X | | | | X | X | | | | | X | | | X |
| Georgia | | | | X | X | X | X | | X | | | | X | X | X | X | X | | | | X | | | X | | | | | X | | | |
| Hawaii | | | | X | | X | | | | X | X | X | X | X | X | | X | | | | | | | X | | | X | | X | X | | |
| Idaho | | | | X | | X | | | | | | | X | X | | X | | X | | | | | | X | | | | | | | | X |
| Illinois | | | | X | X | X | | | X | | X | | X | | X | X | X | X | X | | X | X | | X | | | | | X | X | | |
| Indiana | | | | X | X | X | X | | X | | X | | X | X | X | X | X | | X | | | X | | | | | | | | | | X |
| Iowa | | | | X | X | X | X | | X | X | X | | X | X | X | X | X | | X | | | | | X | | | | | | | | |
| Kansas | | | X | | | X | X | | X | | | | X | X | X | X | X | | X | X | | X | X | | | X | X | | X | | | X |
| Kentucky | | | | X | X | X | X | | | X | X | | X | X | X | X | X | X | X | X | | | | | | | | | X | | | X |
| Louisiana | | | | X | | X | | | X | | | | X | X | | X | | | | | | | | | | | | | X | | | |
| Maine | | X | | X | X | X | X | | | X | | | X | X | X | X | X | | | X | X | | | | | | | | X | | X | X |
| Maryland | | | | | | | | | | X | | | X | | X | X | X | | | | | | | | | | | | | | | X |
| Massachusetts | | X | | X | X | X | X | | X | | | | X | X | X | X | X | | X | | X | | | X | | | X | X | X | | | |
| Michigan | | | | X | | X | | | | | | | X | X | X | X | X | | | X | | | | | | | | X | | | | |
| Minnesota | | | | | | | | | X | | | | X | X | X | X | | | | | | | | | X | | | | X | | | |
| Mississippi | | | | X | | X | X | | | | | | X | X | X | X | X | | X | | | X | X | | | | | | X | | | X |
| Missouri | | | | X | | X | X | | X | X | | | X | X | X | X | X | X | X | X | X | | | X | | | | X | X | | | |
| Montana | | | | X | X | X | X | | X | X | X | | X | X | X | X | X | X | | X | X | X | X | X | | | | | X | | | |
| Nebraska | | | | X | | | | | X | | | | X | X | X | X | | | | | | | | | | | | | | | | X |
| Nevada | X | | | X | | X | X | | X | | X | | X | X | X | X | X | X | X | X | X | | X | X | X | | X | X | X | | | |
| New Hampshire | | | | X | X | X | X | | X | | X | | X | X | X | X | X | X | X | | | | | X | X | | | | X | | | X |
| New Jersey | | | | | | | | | | | | | | | | | | | | | | | | | | | | | | | | X |
| New Mexico | | | | X | | X | | | | | | | X | X | | X | X | | | | | | | | | | | | | | | X |
| New York | | | | X | X | X | X | | X | | X | | X | | X | X | X | X | X | X | X | | | X | | | | | X | | | X |
| North Carolina | | | | | | | | | | | | | | | | | | | | | | | | | | | | | | | | X |
| North Dakota | | | | X | | X | | | X | | | | X | X | X | X | X | X | X | | | | | X | | | | | X | | | |
| Ohio | | | | X | | X | X | | X | | | | X | X | X | X | | X | X | | X | X | X | | X | | | | X | | | |
| Oklahoma | | | | X | X | X | X | | | | | | X | X | | | | | | | | | | | | | | | | | | X |
| Oregon | | | | | | | | | | | | | | | | | | | | | | | | | | | | | | | | X |
| Pennsylvania | | | | X | X | X | X | | X | | X | | X | X | X | X | X | X | X | X | X | | | X | X | | | | X | | | X |
| Rhode Island | | | | | | | | | | | | | | | | | | | | | | | | | | | | | | | | X |
| South Carolina | | | | X | | X | | | X | | | | X | X | | X | X | X | X | | | | X | X | | | | | X | | | |
| South Dakota | | | | X | X | X | X | | X | | | | X | X | X | X | X | X | X | X | X | | | | | | | X | | | | |
| Tennessee | | X | | X | X | | | | X | | X | | X | X | X | X | X | X | X | | | | | X | X | | | | X | | | X |
| Texas | | | | | | | | | | | | | | | | | | | | | | | | | | | | | | | | X |
| Utah | | | | | | | | | | | | | | | | | | | | | | | | | | | | | | | | X |
| Vermont | | | | X | X | X | X | | X | | X | | X | X | X | X | X | X | X | | | | | X | | | | | | X | | |
| Virginia | | | | | | X | | | X | | | | X | X | X | X | X | | X | | | | X | X | | X | | | X | X | | |
| Washington | | | | | | | | | | X | | X | X | X | X | X | | | | | | | | | | | | | X | | | |
| West Virginia | | | | | | | | | | | | | X | X | X | X | X | | X | | | | X | X | | | X | X | X | | | |
| Wisconsin | X | | | X | X | X | | | | X | X | | X | X | X | X | X | X | X | | X | | | X | | | | | X | | X | |
| Wyoming | | | | | | | | | | | | | | | | | | | | | | | | | | | | | | | | X |

**Table 26-2 Who Must Report Child Abuse and Neglect.** *Derived from tables in Myers, JEB, and Peters, WD: Child Abuse Reporting Legislation in the 1980's, Denver, CO: American Humane Association, 1987. Used with permission.*

## WHEN MUST A REPORT BE MADE

Child abuse reporting statutes dictate when a report must be made. Most statutes require reporters to make an immediate oral report by telephone, followed shortly thereafter by a written report to the appropriate state agency. This procedure facilitates an immediate investigatory response by the CPS agency, ensuring that the child is protected. It also establishes a permanent record of the alleged incident.

The degree of suspicion a reporter must reach before making a report is set out in the reporting statute and likewise varies from state to state. The original child abuse reporting statutes provided for a report to be made when there was "reason to believe" that a child had been abused (Fraser, 1978). Many states have expanded the requirement and now use language such as "cause to believe" or "reasonable cause to suspect" that a "child has been or may be subjected to abuse or neglect or observes a child being subjected to conditions or circumstances which would reasonably result in abuse or neglect." Practically, "cause to believe" and "reasonable cause to suspect" mean essentially the same thing for reporting purposes. As noted below, however, there may be a distinction in cases where civil liability for failure to report is at issue.

## REPORTING PROCEDURES

Each state statute specifies at least one agency to receive reports of suspected child abuse and neglect (**Table 26-3**). Traditionally, four different agencies have served as potential recipients for child abuse reports: social service agencies, police departments, health departments, and juvenile courts.

Most states have designated the department of social services, or a division within that department, as the appropriate agency to ultimately receive these reports. Some states designate only the department of social services, while other states designate two or more agencies such as the police and the department of social services to receive reports. These states generally require that all reports ultimately flow into the department of social services. A few states, however, permit the reporting to two or more agencies without requiring the coordination of information by any agency.

In many states the reporting statute specifies what information is to be included in the report. In other states the receiving agency determines, on a case-by-case basis, what information is required. Required information typically includes name, age, address, present location of the child, type and extent of the injuries, name and address of the parent(s) and/or caretaker(s) if known, and any other information that the reporter believes might be relevant. Most states require a mandated reporter to divulge his or her name and position, but permit a permissive reporter to remain anonymous.

Reporting statutes generally prescribe the time within which the CPS agency must initiate its investigation. In most instances this is within 24 hours of the receipt of a report.

## CENTRAL REGISTRIES

Reports received by a state's child abuse hotline are recorded in a central registry. Central registry records usually contain additional case information such as prior reports of child abuse and neglect and CPS case outcomes, treatment plans, and final dispositions at the CPS level. Nearly every state has established a central registry of child protection cases. Current exceptions include Minnesota, New Mexico, and Utah.

State law generally deems central registry records confidential and regulates their disclosure because they contain highly private data about individuals and families. Three general statutory approaches govern record accessibility: (1) Only individuals

| STATE | Department of Social Services | Law Enforcement | Central Registry |
|---|---|---|---|
| Alabama | X | X | |
| Alaska | X | X | |
| Arizona | X | X | |
| Arkansas | X | | |
| California | X | | |
| Colorado | X | X | |
| Connecticut | X | X | |
| Delaware | X | | |
| District of Columbia | X | X | |
| Florida | X | | |
| Georgia | X | | |
| Hawaii | X | X | |
| Idaho | X | X | |
| Illinois | X | | |
| Indiana | X | X | |
| Iowa | X | X | |
| Kansas | X | X | |
| Kentucky | X | | |
| Louisiana | X | X | |
| Maine | X | | |
| Maryland | X | X | |
| Massachusetts | X | | |
| Michigan | X | X | |
| Minnesota | X | X | |
| Mississippi | X | | |
| Missouri | X | | |
| Montana | X | X | |
| Nebraska | X | | |
| Nevada | X | | |
| New Hampshire | X | | |
| New Jersey | X | | |
| New Mexico | X | | |
| New York | | | X |
| North Carolina | X | | |
| North Dakota | X | | |
| Ohio | X | X | |
| Oklahoma | X | X | |
| Oregon | X | X | |
| Pennsylvania | X | | |
| Rhode Island | X | X | |
| South Carolina | X | X | |
| South Dakota | X | X | |
| Tennessee | X | X | |
| Texas | X | | |
| Utah | X | X | |
| Vermont | X | | |
| Virginia | X | | |
| Washington | X | X | |
| West Virginia | X | | |
| Wisconsin | X | X | |
| Wyoming | X | X | |

**Table 26-3 Mandated Recipients of Child Abuse and Neglect Reports.** *Derived from tables in Myers, JEB, and Peters, WD: Child Abuse Reporting Legislation in the 1980's, Denver, CO: American Humane Association, 1987. Used with permission.*

within a CPS agency may have access; (2) the CPS agency may issue regulations authorizing access by certain persons outside of the agency; or (3) state law may enumerate precisely which persons may have access. This third approach is most prevalent today. Those typically having access are law enforcement personnel investigating a report of child maltreatment, the treating physician, the CPS agency, the court, and persons conducting bona fide research (Besharov, 1978). In addition, the child's attorney or guardian ad litem generally is permitted to review registry records in instances when the CPS agency or law enforcement personnel refers the case to juvenile court and court involvement ensues. Registry information often is available for purposes of screening applicants for licenses to establish child care facilities, agencies/services/applicants for employment or volunteer work with such operations or with schools. Almost all states provide that prohibited disclosure is punishable as a misdemeanor (Horowitz & Davidson, 1984).

## PROTECTIVE CUSTODY

Nearly every state authorizes certain categories of individuals to take a child into protective custody if the individual concludes that the child would be seriously endangered if he or she remained with or was released to the parent or other caretaker. The child abuse reporting statutes designate who may take the child into custody, when, and under what circumstances. Depending on the particular statute, such individuals may include one or more of the following: police officers, physicians, juvenile or probation officers, and CPS professionals.

Some states require a court order, at least over the telephone if not in writing, before taking the child into custody against the parent's wishes. Other states directly authorize protective custody, provided that written notice or another document is filed with the juvenile court within 24 to 48 hours after the action is taken. In either case a custody hearing will typically be held at the juvenile court within a short period of time thereafter to review the initial decision to hold the child. Some states provide for protective custody when an authorized individual deems that there "is an imminent danger to the child's life or health." Other states allow protective custody when returning the child to his parent "would endanger his health or welfare" (Meriwether, 1986).

## IMMUNITY FOR GOOD FAITH REPORTERS

Individuals may be reluctant to report suspected child abuse. Potential reporters may fear that the suspected perpetrator will bring a lawsuit against them if the abuse is unconfirmed. To encourage reporting and alleviate this fear, every state's reporting statute extends some type of immunity from civil and criminal liability to persons making reports. Although such immunity provisions may not completely insulate the reporter from a lawsuit (that is, they cannot prevent the filing of an action against a reporter), they can make the successful litigation of such suits nearly impossible.

Some jurisdictions grant absolute immunity to mandated reporters (*Storch v. Silverman*, 1986). This means that the mandated reporter is protected even if the report was false and the reporter knew it to be false. Most jurisdictions, however, provide immunity only to an individual making a good faith report. In these states a reporter is liable only when the plaintiff can prove that the reporter made a false report and that the reporter knew that the report was false, or otherwise acted in bad faith or with a malicious purpose (*Gross v. Myers*, 1987).

## ABROGATION OF PRIVILEGED COMMUNICATIONS

Certain professionals owe their patients or clients a duty of confidentiality. This duty is incurred by virtue of the ethical obligations which the individual undertakes on becoming a professional and adopting the standards of that profession (Stromberg, 1988). Any breach of this obligation would ordinarily lead to a malpractice suit against the professional in which money might be awarded to the patient or client as compensation for damages sustained as a result of the breach of confidentiality. If the disclosure is mandated by a state statute, as in the instance of child abuse, however, no liability will result. Moreover, as discussed below, in such instances, the failure to make the disclosure, even in the face of an otherwise existing obligation of confidentiality, may, in fact, result in liability.

In addition to this obligation of confidentiality, certain professional communications are protected by a judicially or legislatively created testimonial privilege. Generally, a privilege operates to exclude information obtained in the course of a particular relationship from being presented as evidence at judicial proceedings.

The most common types of privileged communications are those between doctor-patient, husband-wife, attorney-client, social worker-client, and priest-penitent. States differ, however, as to which communications are protected by testimonial privilege. Most states abrogate all types of privileged communications in a child abuse case, except attorney-client (**Table 26-4**). Many states also refuse to intrude on the priest-penitent relationship.

Mandatory reporters must report suspected abuse or neglect, regardless of whether the abuse or neglect became apparent as a result of a confidential communication with the patient or client. Also, the professional must testify in juvenile court child protection cases when subpoenaed. In many jurisdictions this requirement to testify may also exist in criminal cases and in child custody cases in which allegations of child abuse are involved. Failure to testify when a judge orders that the testimony be given is likely to result in holding the witness in contempt and jailing the witness. In some states, however, if a claim of privilege is appropriately made, the testimony may be limited to information required to be reported under the reporting statute rather than to more extensive information about which the witness may have become aware (Stromberg, 1988).

## CRIMINAL SANCTIONS FOR FAILURE TO REPORT

Most states have provisions in their reporting statutes that make it a crime for a mandated reporter to knowingly fail to report suspected child abuse. Almost all of these statutes classify the offense as a misdemeanor and specify a maximum fine and/or jail sentence. Although criminal prosecutions for failure to report are rare, courts have ruled that physicians, including psychiatrists, may be subject to criminal penalty under the child abuse statute for failure to report suspected child abuse (*Groff v. State*, 1980; *Capaldi v. State*, 1988). The inclusion of a penalty provision serves a useful function for some reluctant professionals. They may find it more palatable to report suspected child abuse if they can explain to the child's family or caretaker that it is a crime for them not to make the report.

## SOCIAL SERVICE AND LAW ENFORCEMENT RESPONSE

A report of suspected child abuse or neglect to a state-maintained telephone "hotline" or to a local office in accordance with the state's child abuse reporting statute usually initiates the CPS process. At this early stage of the process, child abuse and neglect are often broadly defined. Individual local CPS offices and workers exercise wide discretion in how the agency will respond to individual reports of child maltreatment.

## VALIDATION OF REPORTS

As noted in the preceding discussion of reporting procedures, each state has enacted legislation prescribing criteria for case follow-up, which generally requires an investigation within a limited period of time. The primary aim of the investigation is to determine the validity of the report. If the case is "substantiated," "founded," or "indicated," a decision must be made regarding how to proceed.

| STATE | Physician/Patient | Professional/Patient | Elem./Second School Counselor/Student | Dentist/Patient | Husband-Wife Interspousal | Chiropractor/Patient | All Privileges except Atty/Client | Registered Nurse | Optometrist/Patient | Similar Privileges | Anyone Required to Report | Clergy/Penitent | Psychologist/Psychiatrist/Client | Social Worker/Client | Psychotherapist/Patient | Health Practitioner | Surgeon | Staff Members of Schools | Family Violence & Sexual Assault Advocate/Client |
|---|---|---|---|---|---|---|---|---|---|---|---|---|---|---|---|---|---|---|---|
| Alabama | | | | | | | X | | | | | | | | | | | | |
| Alaska | X | | | | X | | | | | | | | | | | | | | |
| Arizona | | | | | | | X | | | | | | | | | | | | |
| Arkansas | | | | | | | X | | | | | | | | | | | | |
| California | X | | | | | | | | | | | | | | X | | | | |
| Colorado | X | X | | | X | | | | | | | | | | | | | | |
| Connecticut | | | | | X | | | | | | | | | | | | | | |
| Delaware | | | | | X | | | | | | | | | | | | | | |
| District of Columbia | X | | | | X | | | | | | | | | | | | | | |
| Florida | | | | | X | | | | | | | | | | | | | | |
| Georgia | | | | | | | | | | | | | | | | | | | |
| Hawaii | X | | | | X | | | | | | | | | | | | | | |
| Idaho | | | | | X | | | | | | | | | | | | | | |
| Illinois | | | | | | | | | | | X | | | | | | | | |
| Indiana | X | | | | X | | | | | | | | | | | | | | |
| Iowa | | | | | X | | | | | | | | | | | | X | | |
| Kansas | X | | | | | | | | | | | | X | X | | | | | |
| Kentucky | X | X | | | | | | | | | | | | | | | | | |
| Louisiana | X | X | | | X | | | | | | | X | | | | | | | |
| Maine | X | | | | X | | | | | | | | | | X | | | | |
| Maryland | | | | | | | | | | | | | | | | | | | |
| Massachusetts | | | | | | | | | | | | | X | X | | | | | |
| Michigan | | | | | X | | | | | | | | | | | | | | |
| Minnesota | X | | X | X | X | | | X | | | | | | X | | | | X | |
| Mississippi | X | | | | | | | | | | | | | | | | | | |
| Missouri | | | | | X | | | | | | | | | | | | | | |
| Montana | X | | | | | | | | | X | | | | | | | | | |
| Nebraska | X | | | | X | | | | | | | | | | | | | | |
| Nevada | | | | | | | | | | X | | | | | | | | | |
| New Hampshire | | | | | X | | | | | | | | | | | | | | |
| New Jersey | | | | | | | | | | | | | | | | | | | |
| New Mexico | X | | | | | | | | | X | | | | | | | | | |
| New York | | | | | | | | | | | | | | | | | | | |
| North Carolina | X | | | | X | | | | | | | | | | | | | | |
| North Dakota | | | | | X | | | | | | | | | | | | | | |
| Ohio | X | | | | | | | | | | | | | | | | | | |
| Oklahoma | X | | | | | | | | | X | | | | | | | | | |
| Oregon | X | | | | X | | | X | | | | | | X | X | | | X | |
| Pennsylvania | | | | | | | | | | | X | | | | | | | | |
| Rhode Island | | | | | X | | | | | | | | | | | | | | |
| South Carolina | | X | | | X | | | | | | | | | | | | | | |
| South Dakota | X | | X | | X | | | | | | | | | | | | | | |
| Tennessee | | X | | | X | | | | | | | | | | X | | | | |
| Texas | | | | | X | | | | | | | | | | | | | | |
| Utah | X | | | | | | | | | | | | | | | | | | |
| Vermont | | | | | | | | | | | | | | | | | | | |
| Virginia | X | | | | X | | | | | | | | | | | | | | |
| Washington | X | | | | | | | | X | | | | X | X | | | | | |
| West Virginia | | | | | X | | | | | | | | | | | | | | |
| Wisconsin | X | | | | X | | | | | | | | | | | | | | |
| Wyoming | X | | | | X | | | | | | | | | X | | | | | |

**Table 26-4 Evidentiary Testimonial Abrogation of Privileges in Child Abuse Cases.** *Derived from tables in Myers, JEB, and Peters, WD: Child Abuse Reporting Legislation in the 1980's, Denver, CO: American Humane Association, 1987. Used with permission.*

If the child is not in the protective custody of a physician, the police, or the juvenile court at the time of the investigation, the CPS investigator must determine if there is imminent risk of harm to the child that would warrant the child's immediate removal from the home. If such action is needed, the police or the juvenile court may be contacted to facilitate this removal.

If the available evidence is insufficient to merit a finding of abuse or neglect, or if the investigation could not be completed, the case may be deemed "unsubstantiated" or "unfounded." The case may then be closed and all references to the report and case deleted from the central registry within a designated period of time, if no additional reports are made (Iverson & Segal, 1990). Central registries involve state collection of potentially inflammatory personal information. This gives rise to constitutional concerns regarding the rights to privacy and due process. Accordingly, many states have enacted procedures, by statute or state regulation, for the expungement of registry records. Expungement of records is based either on the child's attainment of a certain age, passage of a designated period of time since services were terminated, or a finding by the CPS agency that the report was unsubstantiated. In some states, individuals may formally challenge information contained in the registry through administrative or court procedures for the expungement or modification of records (*Roth v. Reagen*, 1988).

## INVESTIGATIVE PURPOSES AND PROCEDURES

Reporting statutes often detail the purpose of the investigation. Generally the goal is to evaluate the nature, extent, and cause of the abuse or neglect and to identify the person responsible. Efforts are also made to ascertain the names and conditions of other children in the home, the nature of the home environment, and the relationship of the child to the parents or other caretakers.

The investigative caseworker typically begins the process by contacting the individual who made the hot line report to confirm the information originally provided and to obtain additional information. The investigation consists of a series of interviews. Often the child is the next person interviewed. Preferably, this takes place in a neutral setting. The parents are also interviewed, often during a home visit. Thereafter, other persons named in the report who may have relevant information are questioned. These persons typically include teachers, physicians, neighbors, and other relatives (Levine, 1973; Hechler, 1988).

The CPS purpose when responding to a report of child maltreatment is distinct from the objectives of the criminal justice system. Yet, as noted, law enforcement personnel may be contacted by the CPS worker during the investigatory stage or they may already be otherwise involved. This is true in cases involving serious abuse, where there is a reason to believe that the parents are or may likely be resistant to CPS intervention, or if the CPS caseworker is concerned for his or her own safety.

State law provides the authority for CPS home visits, either expressly or through implication, but if individuals refuse to cooperate, a warrant or court order may be needed to gain access to a home. In addition, many state statutes, regulations, or case laws authorize CPS or law enforcement investigators to conduct examinations of the child or to refer the child for evaluation by medical personnel.

## CONSTITUTIONAL CONCERNS

Constitutional considerations are raised in the CPS investigative stage because the Constitution protects individuals against state action. CPS caseworkers act under "color of state law" (i.e., they carry out their investigative tasks pursuant to legislative authority). Protection under both federal and state constitutions may be implicated in such areas as home visits, child and parent interviews, and examinations of the child.

Search warrants are generally not required to conduct such visits or examinations. The burden of obtaining a warrant would seriously impair, if not frustrate, the state's effort to protect the child, particularly in emergency situations. There may, however, be constitutional limits on the nature and circumstances under which investigatory visits take place (*Daryl H. v. Coler*, 1986; Hardin, 1988). Usually the parent or guardian consents to the caseworker's or police officer's entry into the residence. Absent consent, or if the search exceeds the scope of the consent, any evidence found may be deemed inadmissible in any subsequent criminal proceeding. Similarly, statements made to investigators by a parent or other perpetrator may be inadmissible if a court finds that at the time of the questioning the individual was in custody or otherwise deprived of his freedom in some significant way (*People v. Hagar*, 1987; Hardin, 1988).

## TREATMENT AND REFERRAL OPTIONS

Following a determination of the validity of the allegation of abuse or neglect, a report is made to the agency's central registry. If the hotline referral is substantiated, a CPS caseworker, who may or may not have been involved in the initial investigation of the report, is usually assigned to the case. The caseworker develops a treatment plan and presents it to the family. CPS agencies offer various mental health and social services and seek voluntary acceptance of these recommended services. If the parent or guardian does not cooperate with the CPS agency, or if such voluntary treatment will not adequately protect the child, the investigative or treatment caseworker will request that a juvenile or probation officer file an abuse or neglect petition with the juvenile or family court or file such an action himself. Such an action will seek court intervention with the child and his or her family. Intervention may include temporary removal of the child from the home, court-ordered treatment, or, in some circumstances, termination of parental rights.

When the police have not been involved in the investigation, referral to a local law enforcement agency on completion of the CPS investigation may be mandated under state law, when the abuse is "substantiated" or meets the statutory requirements for criminal child or sexual abuse. In the absence of legislative direction, CPS regulations may require referral to prosecuting authorities or the police.

## CIVIL LIABILITY AND CHILD MALTREATMENT

Health care professionals and others engaged in protective services may be exposed to civil liability during the identification and investigation of alleged child abuse (Sprague & Horowitz, 1991).

## Failure to Report by Mandated Reporter

Violation of a statutory duty, such as the duty imposed on a mandated reporter to report suspected child abuse or neglect, is negligence *per se* (negligence in itself). Under this theory an injured child and his or her family could successfully sue a doctor or another mandated reporter for willingly or negligently failing to detect and report known or suspected child abuse. The suit could result in a judgment awarding monetary damages to compensate the patient for all injuries that occurred as a result of abuse or neglect after the time when a report should have been made. In the leading case on this issue the California Supreme Court held that a physician and his hospital employer may be liable for medical malpractice for failure to properly diagnose and treat the battered child syndrome when subsequent injuries occur (*Landeros v. Flood*, 1976).

In another case, which eventually settled out of court for $600,000, the child's mother and her boyfriend brought the child to the hospital with severe injuries twice within a 12-hour period. The hospital did not make a report of suspected child abuse at either time. The next day the mother and her boyfriend took the child to another hospital. The child was diagnosed with permanent brain damage.

The child's father sued the first hospital and others for negligence based on the first hospital's failure to report suspected child abuse (*Robinson v. Wical*, 1970).

It is in situations such as these that the precise language of the reporting statute may be of great legal significance. Seemingly minor differences in statutory language could have major implications for the outcome of a case. If the reporting statute's language mandates reporting when there is "cause to believe" that abuse has taken place, the statute is adopting a subjective standard. Under this standard, proof that the health care professional actually believed that abuse or neglect had occurred would be necessary. If "cause to suspect" was the applicable language, the standard would still be subjective, but a lesser degree of certainty would be required. Under either of these subjective standards, the plaintiff must establish that the reporter actually held the belief or suspicion and failed to report for liability to result.

Some jurisdictions require "reasonable cause to believe" or "reasonable cause to suspect." Here the jurisdiction is adopting an objective standard. Under the objective standard the test is what a reasonable person in the same situation as the professional would believe or suspect, regardless of the actual mindset of the professional (Fraser, 1978). Generally, the subjective standard is a more difficult one to meet.

## Other Bases of Liability of Reporters and Potential Defenses

In rare instances, civil actions may also be brought against health care professionals or others based on their conduct in connection with a child abuse or neglect case. Typically these lawsuits allege that the physician, social worker, or police officer, and their respective agencies negligently acted under the reporting statute, thereby causing harm to the parent or the child. A parent or child may bring an action seeking monetary damages for a wrongful report of child abuse, defamation and slander, negligent diagnosis or treatment, breach of confidentiality, overly-intrusive investigation, wrongful removal of a child from his or her home, wrongful institution or prosecution of an alleged offender, and wrongful examination of the child for signs of abuse (Besharov, 1984; Sprague, 1991). Willful conduct may also be alleged, including battery, false imprisonment, and/or malicious prosecution.

These claims are usually based on state tort (private or civil wrong or injury) law, which, through statute or common law (judicial precedent), recognizes that individuals in certain situations owe duties to one another. Violation of these duties can form the basis of an action for monetary damages. Similarly, an alleged violation of constitutional rights, either federal or state, may form the basis of a claim for damages (Sprague & Horowitz, 1991).

As previously noted, all jurisdictions provide absolute or limited immunity for the reporting of suspected child abuse. The same immunity provisions typically apply to other authorized actions taken by any individual in connection with the making of the report. Such actions include, for example, the taking of photographs and X-rays, the removal or retaining of the child, the disclosure of otherwise confidential or privileged information to CPS investigators, and the participation in any judicial proceedings that result from the reporting. Immunity provisions may preclude liability, but they cannot prevent the initiation of a civil action.

Initially, the court assumes that the plaintiff's allegations in the petition or complaint regarding the defendant's actions are true, without hearing any testimony. The court then determines if the immunity granted by the child abuse reporting statute was applicable. In jurisdictions that have adopted a rule of "absolute" immunity for statutorily prescribed activities of the defendants, the judge will dismiss the proceeding.

If, however, the jurisdiction has adopted a rule of "qualified" immunity (i.e., immunity only for actions undertaken in "good faith"), the court will allow the case to go to trial. The jury, or the judge acting as the finder of fact, will then hear testimony on behalf of each party from various witnesses regarding the allegations of the petition. If the alleged actions are proved to be true, but the trier of fact concludes that they were taken in good faith, the proceeding will be dismissed. Liability attaches only if the facts adduced at the trial prove both that the defendants engaged in the alleged behavior and that the defendants did not act in good faith.

## Additional Causes of Action Based on Failures to Protect the Child and Related Defenses

In situations involving state-employed child protection workers that resulted in the death or additional serious injury to the child, the child and an innocent parent or guardian may bring an action alleging that the public employees should have taken various steps to protect the child. The lawsuits may allege a failure to accept reports for investigation, a failure to adequately investigate reports, a failure to remove the child from the home, a failure to protect the child after return to the home, foster care, or a child care facility, or a failure to provide services leading to the return of the child (Sprague, 1991). These actions are also typically brought under state tort law.

Similar suits for damages have been brought charging violations of the federal Constitution. The typical allegation is that the officials' failure to act deprived them of their liberty in violation of the Due Process Clause of the Fourteenth Amendment to the United States Constitution. Specifically, the plaintiffs assert that substantive due process requires state agents to protect children referred as abused to child protection agencies. Nevertheless, in 1989 the United States Supreme Court limited the type of suit that could be brought in some of these cases (*DeShaney v. Winnebago County Dept. of Social Servs.*, 1989). The Court concluded that a state's failure to protect a child, not in the actual custody of the state, against violence generally will not constitute a violation of the Due Process Clause because the Clause imposes no duty on the states to provide members of the general public with adequate protective services. While the Clause forbids the state from depriving individuals of life, liberty, and property without due process of law, it only limits the state's power to act and does not impose an affirmative obligation to insure any minimal level of safety and security. Thus the constitutional issue is not whether the CPS agency, or another public actor, was aware of the danger to the child, but rather whether it limited or prevented the child from acting on his or her own behalf. Liability still could be found, however, under state rather than federal law, based on negligent conduct or in instances where a child is within the custody of a state agency.

In addition to any immunity provided under the reporting statute, civil liability may also be precluded by the "public duty" doctrine or rule (Prosser & Keeton, 1984). This rule generally applies only to health care professionals or other child care workers who are state employees. The rule provides that a public official is generally not liable to individuals for his or her negligence in discharging public duties. The rationale behind the rule is that the duty is owed to the public at large, rather than to any one individual. Liability will attach, however, where the duty is specifically owed an individual under state tort law. A special relationship between an individual and a public official or agency may be sufficient to give rise to liability for negligence in carrying out that duty (Prosser & Keeton, 1984). State reporting laws may be viewed as creating such a duty. Consequently, the public duty doctrine generally will not protect a physician or other health care professional employed by a public agency who undertakes to treat a child, but then fails to report child abuse or otherwise fails to comply with the specific requirements of the reporting statute.

Finally, in addition to legislating a statutory immunity for actions taken by reporters under the child abuse reporting laws, a number of states have enacted general immunity statutes that protect public employees from liability for injuries caused while acting within the scope of their employment (Prosser & Keeton, 1984). The underlying rationale is that the fear of being sued will infringe on the individual's discharge of his or her duty. In addition, even in the absence of a statutory provision, as a matter of common law, immunity may be affirmatively pled and judicially invoked by public employees.

As with the immunity provisions under the reporting statutes, "absolute immunity" applies to "public officials whose special functions or constitutional status requires complete protection from suit" (*Harlow v. Fitzgerald*, 1982), and extends to judges, legislators, and prosecutors, acting within their official capacity. Only "qualified" or "good faith immunity," on the other hand, is available to officials performing discretionary functions. But even such limited immunity may be sufficient to terminate a lawsuit based on insubstantial claims involving bare allegations of malice by government employees (*Harlow v. Fitzgerald*, 1982).

## ◆ THE LITIGATION OF CHILD ABUSE AND NEGLECT CASES

Court involvement in child abuse or neglect cases may occur in the form of a civil proceeding under specific child abuse or neglect statutes in a juvenile or family court; or in a criminal proceeding for homicide, assault or battery, or criminal child abuse or neglect. The issue may also be litigated in a child custody case related to a dissolution of marriage proceeding. A recent study examined more than 800 substantiated cases of intrafamilial child abuse and neglect reported in three counties across the country in the mid-1980s. Statistical analyses indicated that juvenile court proceedings were brought in just 21% of the cases and criminal prosecutions in only 4%, although treatment plans developed in some 75% of the cases and out-of-home placement occurred in 50% of the sample. Thus it is apparent that criminal prosecutions of the perpetrator remain relatively infrequent (Tjaden & Thoennes, 1992). Usually the state's goal of protecting the child in peril is met in a civil proceeding that takes place in a juvenile court or a family court.

This section reviews how child abuse cases generally proceed in juvenile, criminal, and divorce courts. It concludes with a discussion of the evidentiary rules that may arise in any trial dealing with child abuse.

### THE ROLE OF THE JUVENILE COURT AND ITS PROCEDURES

The role of the juvenile court or family court in child abuse cases is to (1) protect the child from further injury; (2) provide a fair and impartial hearing on the allegations in the petition; (3) consider recommendations of the child protection agency and other social service agencies; (4) implement a treatment plan for the child and/or the parent(s) when appropriate; and (5) protect the constitutional rights of both the child and the parents. The function of the court is not to punish but rather to work closely with the social service agencies to effect a treatment plan designed to protect the child. Generally the court attempts to improve the family situation so that the family is preserved (Johnson, 1975; Fox, 1984; Hertz et al., 1991), unless the child has suffered serious harm and would continue to be endangered if allowed to remain within that family.

Statutory provisions give these courts their specific powers. Typically, juvenile courts are authorized to adjudicate proceedings involving claims of abuse and neglect, dependency, and delinquency, as well as requests for the termination of parental rights (Johnson, 1975; Fox, 1984). There has been a long-standing debate, however, on whether the focus of juvenile court jurisdictional statutes, from a policy perspective, should be directed to intervention where there has been a showing of potentially harmful behavior of the parents or caretaker (Besharov, 1988) or only where there is a showing of harmful effects of such behavior on the child (Wald, 1975).

Some states have structured their juvenile justice system around family courts. Family courts generally have a broader jurisdiction than juvenile courts. This includes divorce and child custody, intrafamily assaults, and juvenile traffic offenses. Juvenile courts and family courts are courts of limited jurisdiction and thus are involved only in those types of cases which the state's statutes specifically authorize the court to hear. Moreover, these courts can issue orders only as specifically authorized by statute (Fox, 1984). Separate sets of state and local court rules may also govern the conduct of juvenile and family court procedures.

Child abuse and neglect proceedings usually involve bifurcated hearings. For the court to take any action with respect to the child, it first must determine that the child has, in fact, been abused or neglected and thus qualifies to be a "ward" of the court or "dependent" on the court for care and protection. This is often referred to as the "adjudicatory" stage or phase of the proceeding. If the court concludes that abuse or neglect has taken place, the child is considered to be under the "jurisdiction" of the juvenile court and the second phase or dispositional hearing is held. The dispositional hearing is designed to determine the appropriate intervention and to initiate a treatment plan.

The court may then order one or more of a variety of dispositions for the child. Additionally, the court may order dispositions for one or both of the parents. Generally, if the parent fails to comply with the juvenile court's order, the court cannot punish the parent by fines or imprisonment, but is restricted to conditioning the child's return to the home on the parent's obeying the court's order (Hertz et al., 1991). In very limited instances, in which the remedy of changing custody is not available or appropriate, the court may be authorized to hold the parent in contempt and jail the parent until the parent complies with the court's order.

Juvenile court proceedings generally are confidential and closed to the public and the press. In most instances, only those individuals directly involved are allowed access.

## PARTICIPANTS IN THE JUVENILE COURT PROCESS

Participants in a juvenile court child abuse proceeding may include the judge, the petitioner, the child, the parent or parents, an attorney for the petitioner, an attorney for the parent, a *guardian ad litem*, and sometimes an attorney for the child (Johnson, 1975; Fox, 1984).

## Judge

Child abuse cases in juvenile court are heard by a judge assigned to the juvenile court on a permanent or a rotating basis or by an attorney who is appointed to hear cases in juvenile court. These attorneys are called commissioners, masters, or referees.

The judge's initial responsibility in juvenile court child abuse cases is to protect the child's well-being and, in seeking to attain that goal, to see to it that proper procedures are observed. In addition, the judge is the trier of fact. Generally there are no juries. The judge rules on the admissibility of evidence and then decides, based on the evidence admitted, whether the child should be adjudicated and placed under the jurisdiction of the juvenile court. In the dispositional hearing the judge reviews the various recommendations and determines the appropriate disposition for the child.

## Petitioner

State statutes often restrict who may bring actions in juvenile court. Generally, a suit may be filed by probation officers, juvenile officers, officials of the state or local social service agency, or local county or prosecuting attorneys. In some states, "any interested person" can initiate a proceeding. The decision to initiate juvenile court proceedings is based on a variety of factors, including (1) the nature of injury involved; (2) the attitude of the family toward voluntary cooperation with social service agencies; and (3) prior history of abuse or neglect within the family.

## Child

The child is the subject of the juvenile court proceeding. The case is often named or "styled" "In the Interest of John Doe, a Child." The child may be called as a witness at the hearing by any of the parties and may be subject to cross-examination by other parties.

## Parents

Each parent of the child is entitled to notice of the hearing and in most jurisdictions is considered a party in the case. The parent, too, can be called as a witness and would then be subject to cross-examination. A parent can claim his or her constitutional right under the Fifth Amendment to refuse to respond to any question that might tend to be incriminating. Such a right may be limited if the state grants immunity to the parent whereby testimony given by the parent cannot then be used against him or her. In addition, the U.S. Supreme Court has held that, even without such a grant of immunity, a parent can be required to produce a child, in his or her custody, for a court hearing, at least in those instances where a parent has custody of a child pursuant to a court order resulting from child protection proceedings. Such action can be mandated even though it might tend to incriminate the parent and aid the state in criminally prosecuting the parent (*Baltimore City Dep't of Social Serv. v. Bouknight*, 1990).

## Attorney for the Petitioner

In most juvenile courts there will be a county, city, or corporation attorney who is employed full-time to represent the party instituting the court action. In some jurisdictions, CPS agencies have their own attorneys whose functions include bringing such juvenile court actions. In some localities the government contracts with private attorneys for representation. The petitioner's attorney drafts and files the petition and other necessary pleadings or motions. At the adjudicatory hearing the attorney for the petitioner attempts to establish, through the presentation of evidence, that the allegations in the petition are true. Then, at the dispositional hearing, the attorney attempts to convince the court to follow the recommendations of the petitioner regarding the child's future.

## Attorney for the Parent(s)

Because it is often the parent who is suspected of inflicting the harm or neglecting the child, the parent will typically want to be represented by an attorney in the juvenile court proceeding. In every state the parent has a right to be represented. In most jurisdictions the state will appoint an attorney if the parent is indigent, although this is not required by the U.S. Constitution. The right of a parent to appointed counsel may be granted by state statute. The U.S. Supreme Court has held that the Constitution does not require the appointment of counsel for parents in every parental termination proceeding (*Lassiter v. Department of Social Services*, 1981). The Court ruled that in the absence of an applicable state statute or rule regarding the appointment of an attorney for indigent parents, the decision to do so must be made by the trial judge on a case-by-case basis.

The attorney for the parent, of course, is required to protect the interests of the parent. In the adjudicatory hearing the parent's attorney usually tries to persuade the court that no abuse or neglect occurred, that any injury sustained was accidental, or alternatively that the perpetrator was someone other than the parent and the parent cannot be faulted for the perpetrator's conduct.

If the child is adjudicated to be within the jurisdiction of the juvenile court, the parent's attorney in a dispositional hearing will typically seek to have the child remain in the custody of his or her client or otherwise minimize the extent of official intervention in the family. The attorney must also protect the other interests of his or her client. The attorney must caution the client not to make statements that could be used against the parent in a later criminal prosecution. If there is a conflict of interest between the parents, it may be necessary for each parent to have his or her own attorney.

## Representation for the Child

Many states have enacted statutes that provide representation for the child in child protection proceedings. State laws vary, however, as to whether the child is to be represented by a *guardian ad litem* (guardian for this particular lawsuit), an attorney, or both. Frequently, one individual is appointed to both positions, although the responsibilities of the two differ.

Both the *guardian ad litem* and the attorney may present evidence and question witnesses at the adjudicatory hearing, and both may offer recommendations regarding the child's placement and treatment at the dispositional hearing.

The *guardian ad litem* represents the child's best interests in the child abuse or neglect proceeding. He or she must use independent judgment to determine the best interest of the child. The *guardian ad litem* is not the child's legal guardian and has no duties after the proceeding. An attorney must be an advocate for his client, in this case the child, and when the child is mature enough to express an opinion, counsel must generally advocate what the child determines to be in his or her own best interest.

## JUVENILE COURT PROCEDURES

### Petition

A juvenile court case involving abuse or neglect usually begins with the filing of a petition or complaint that alleges one or more specific instances of child abuse, neglect, or dependency. The petitioner is usually a juvenile probation officer or a representative of the state's department of social services charged with the investigation of allegations brought to the court by social service personnel, police, or other individuals. With the assistance of the attorney, the petitioner decides whether or not to file the action.

### Custody Hearing

The juvenile court will typically conduct a custody or detention hearing within a short time after a petition is filed. This allows the judge to review the initial decision to hold the child and to authorize continued placement outside the home. The hearing occurs only if the child has not been returned to his or her home pending further proceedings but rather remains in a hospital, other temporary shelter, or with relatives without the parents' consent. The temporary placement may have been authorized or arranged by the juvenile court, a probation officer, or a CPS worker. Before ordering the continuation of the protective custody, the judge generally must ascertain, pending a full hearing, that there is a substantial risk of immediate harm to the child and that there is no viable alternative for reducing that risk.

### Adjudicatory Hearing

In an adjudicatory hearing the state presents the evidence of abuse or neglect to the court. The only issue to be resolved is whether the child has been abused, neglected, abandoned, or otherwise comes within the jurisdiction of the court. In many instances the parent will admit the allegations or at least a sufficient part of them for the court to conclude that it is authorized to "take jurisdiction" or to "adjudicate" the child to be a ward of the court. In other situations, however, it is necessary for the attorney representing the petitioner to call witnesses to substantiate the facts alleged in the petition. Typical witnesses are doctors, police, teachers, child protection workers, relatives, parents, or other individuals who possess relevant information. Often a subpoena is issued to compel the witnesses' attendance at the proceedings.

The burden of proving child abuse or neglect in a juvenile court is on the party asserting the abuse or neglect, typically the state. The petitioner does not have to prove that a specific individual committed a certain abusive act, but only that the child's environment is injurious to his or her welfare or that those legally responsible for the child's care did not carry out their legal responsibility.

The standard of proof refers to the level of certainty by which the trier of fact must be convinced that the allegations in the petition are true. In a juvenile court child abuse case the standard is not that of "beyond a reasonable doubt," as in a criminal matter. State laws differ, however, as to whether the petitioner must prove child abuse or neglect by the standard of a "preponderance of the evidence" or by "clear and convincing evidence." Clear and convincing is higher than preponderance but lower than beyond a reasonable doubt. Proof by a "preponderance of the evidence" means that the petitioner must convince the judge that it is more likely than not that certain facts are true, by a 51% degree of certainty. A "clear and convincing evidence" standard requires proving that it is highly probable that the existence of those facts is true. The U.S. Supreme Court has concluded, however, that a burden of proof of at least "clear and convincing evidence" is constitutionally necessary when the petitioner seeks to terminate parental rights. Some states, however, do require the higher standard of proof of "beyond a reasonable doubt" for termination of parental rights (*Santosky v. Kramer*, 1982).

In most jurisdictions the judge has the authority to exclude individuals from the courtroom upon a finding that this is in the best interests of the child to do so. A judge may, for example, exclude a parent when the child is testifying to acts of abuse or neglect. Similarly, the judge may exclude a child, who might otherwise be entitled to be present, during medical or other testimony.

Rules of evidence do apply in juvenile court proceedings, but their application may be less strict and court procedures less formal than in criminal cases. Direct evidence (i.e., evidence by an eyewitness to the incident) is not necessary to prove child abuse or neglect. Rather, abuse or neglect can be proven by circumstantial evidence. The inference of abuse or neglect can be drawn from a combination of evidence, such as the nature and extent of the injuries, the lack of explanation for the injuries consistent with medical knowledge, the age of the child, and the fact that the parent was the custodian of the child at the time of the alleged abuse.

If the state fails to establish child abuse or neglect by the requisite standard of proof, the case is dismissed and no further action is taken. If, however, the child is adjudicated and the court takes jurisdiction over the child, the case proceeds to disposition.

## Dispositional Hearing

The appropriate placement for the child and the appropriate treatment, if any, for the child and the parent are determined at the dispositional hearing. The hearing may take place immediately after the adjudication or may be scheduled for a later date, pending the collection of additional information that might aid the judge in deciding the terms for the court order. Evidence submitted at the hearing usually focuses on the recommendations made to the judge by a court social worker, and in some situations by the *guardian ad litem*, regarding placement and treatment. Generally, state statutes give juvenile courts the authority to order a broad range of dispositions, but the specific powers granted to the court differ from state to state. Additionally, some states add a phrase such as "and such other orders as the court deems necessary." Common dispositional powers include (1) returning the child to the home with or without supervision; (2) giving physical custody to a relative; (3) placing the child in foster care; or (4), in severe cases, terminating the rights of the parent to the child.

Once a child has been adjudicated a ward of the juvenile court, the court retains "jurisdiction" or control over the child until the child either reaches the age of majority (as defined by state law, usually 18 years) or until the jurisdictional status is otherwise terminated by the court. Most juvenile courts hold periodic reviews to measure the progress of the case and to determine the need to modify previous orders. Review hearings are usually scheduled every 6 months to a year.

The most drastic measure a state may take to protect an abused or neglected child is the termination of parental rights. In essence, the court orders that the parent(s) no longer have any rights or duties with respect to the child (Wadlington et al., 1983). Termination of parental rights may be either voluntary or involuntary. State statutes specify the grounds and the specific circumstances under which parental rights may be terminated. Usually, involuntary termination is a disposition of last resort.

The most common grounds for termination of parental rights are abandonment, child abuse, or neglect. Statutes specify what conditions constitute abandonment for termination purposes. In some states, termination of parental rights is not an authorized disposition in the initial child abuse or neglect proceeding. Rather, it can only be ordered in situations where there is chronic failure to support the child or a consistent pattern of specific unacceptable parental behavior with respect to the child. Ordinarily the parent must be given sufficient time and opportunity to become a more adequate parent before termination. In some states a parent's severe chronic mental illness rendering him or her unable to adequately care for the child may also be grounds for termination of parental rights.

## CHILD ABUSE AND NEGLECT IN CRIMINAL COURT

The prosecution of individuals accused of crimes perpetrated against children, while not necessarily commonplace, has increased in recent decades, particularly in the area of child sexual abuse (Smith & Goretsky, 1992). This increase is due, in part, to advances made in identifying battered and sexually abused children and to the relaxation of evidentiary rules relating to victim competency, in-court testimony, and certain out-of-court statements (Kempe et al., 1962; Attorney General, 1984; Bulkley, 1985; MacMurray, 1989).

Although the juvenile court's involvement in these cases is based on the state's role as *parens patriae*, the criminal justice system's involvement is exercised under the state's police power, which authorizes official action to prevent identified harms to society. The use of this power serves to dissuade private retribution on the part of victims by placing responsibility for prosecuting alleged violations of the criminal law solely within the government's ambit. Criminal justice system activities include law enforcement investigations, criminal prosecutions, and sentencing proceedings. The substantive criminal law defines what conduct is criminal and provides the punishment to be imposed on an adjudication or finding of guilt.

### SUBSTANTIVE CRIMINAL LAW

State legislatures are responsible for declaring what conduct within their own jurisdictions is deemed criminal and subject to punishment. Similarly, the U.S. Congress provides for the punishment of activity determined to be harmful to society that occurs within certain territories under federal supervision.

In most jurisdictions, "child abuse" or "child neglect" is viewed as violating the prohibition of one or more of the following statutory crimes: murder, homicide, manslaughter, felonious restraint, false imprisonment, assault, battery, rape, statutory rape, deviant sexual assault, sexual assault, indecent exposure, child endangerment, reckless endangerment, and corruption of minors. A majority of jurisdictions do, however, have specific crimes of child abuse and child neglect. Depending on the alleged conduct and resulting harm to the victim, a criminal prosecution may be sought for one or more of these offenses. Conviction of more than one substantive crime arising from the same series of actions may be authorized, if the proof of each particular crime differs or overlaps (Perkins & Boyce, 1982; LaFave & Scott, 1986).

Crimes are further differentiated as felonies and misdemeanors. The boundary between which offenses constitute felonies and misdemeanors varies from state to state. In some jurisdictions the distinction between the two is based on whether ordered incarceration will take place in a local jail or in a state penitentiary, but more frequently the difference is in the prescribed minimum penalty in the event of a conviction. In general, a felony offense typically is punishable by 1 year or more of imprisonment. Sanctions imposed for a misdemeanor conviction usually involve incarceration for less than a year and/or a fine of $500 or less (LaFave & Scott, 1986). The distinction between misdemeanors and felonies is not only relevant to the potential punishment, but also to the resulting procedural consequences. Greater constitutional protection is offered to defendants in felony prosecutions, such as the right to a trial by jury (Perkins & Boyce, 1982). Defendants are entitled to appointed counsel for all felonies and in misdemeanors where the convicted defendant's punishment involves confinement (Whitebread & Slobogin, 1986).

## PROCEDURE IN CRIMINAL CASES

The precise procedure in criminal cases varies somewhat from state to state, but the sequence is basically the same (**Figure 26-1**) (Kamisar et al., 1986; Whitebread & Slobogin, 1986). Most frequently, the initial stage in the criminal justice system process is the police investigation. In cases of alleged child abuse, police involvement may (1) precede reporting to the CPS agency; (2) coincide with or accompany the CPS investigation; or (3) follow the CPS agency's substantiation of a reported allegation of maltreatment and referral to juvenile court and/or the law enforcement agency. Regardless of the time and manner in which law enforcement officers are notified of a suspected case, the police investigation is directed at goals separate from those of CPS investigations. The law enforcement agency's primary function is to determine whether a crime has occurred and, if so, whether there is sufficient evidence indicating the guilt of a particular person to justify arresting and charging the individual. CPS agencies are concerned with the identification of abuse for prevention and intervention purposes in the furtherance of child protection.

## Investigation

Police officers use a variety of investigative techniques, including pre-arrest questioning of possible suspects, interviewing witnesses or others with pertinent information, and collecting physical evidence. Care must be taken, however, to insure that a health care professional does not breach the obligation of confidentiality in an effort to cooperate with law enforcement personnel. Access to an individual's medical records or information should not be given to law enforcement personnel without a valid release of information, specific statutory authority, or a court order (Stromberg, 1988).

## Medical Records and Information

Health care professionals may wish to obtain a release of information authorizing the disclosure of information to police and prosecutors. Only half of the state statutes explicitly authorize and require the reporting of child abuse cases to the police. Such statutes may permit disclosure to certain law enforcement agencies or personnel of either specific facts or general medical or other reliable information known to health care personnel. In the absence of such specific authority, on occasion, police sometimes attempt to gain access to this information by threatening the health care professional with criminal charges based on other statutes. Such threats ought to be resisted.

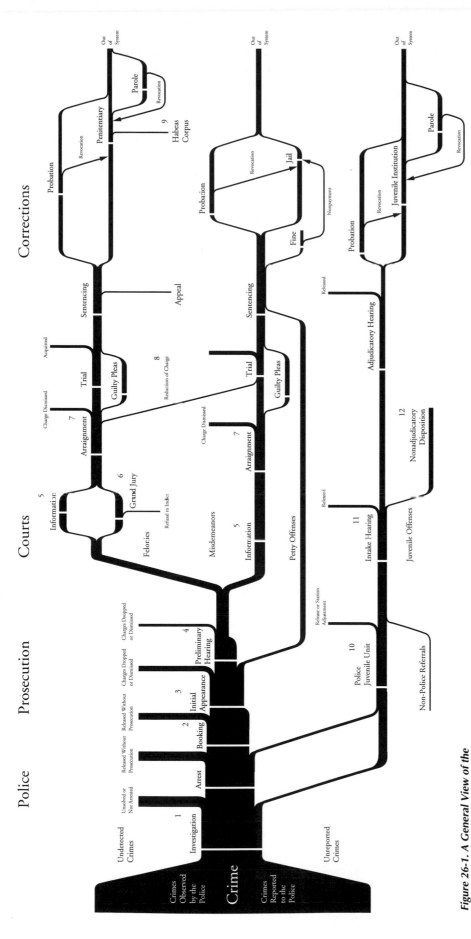

*Figure 26-1. A General View of the Criminal Justice System.* This chart seeks to present a simple yet comprehensive view of the movement of cases through the criminal justice system. Procedures in individual jurisdictions may vary from the pattern shown here. The differing weights of line indicate the relative volumes of cases disposed of at various points in the system, but this is only suggestive, since no nationwide data of this sort exist.

*Reprinted from: The Challenge of Crime in a Free Society, The President's Commission on Law Enforcement and the Administration of Justice, Washington, D.C., 1967.*

1. May continue until trial.

2. Administrative record of arrest. First step at which temporary release on bail may be available.

3. Before magistrate, commissioner, or justice of peace. Formal notice of charge, advice of rights. Bail set. Summary trials for petty offenses usually conducted here without further processing.

4. Preliminary testing of evidence against defendant. Charge may be reduced. No separate preliminary hearing for misdemeanors in some systems.

5. Charge filed by prosecutor on basis of information submitted by police or citizens. Alternative to grand jury indictment; often used in felonies, almost always in misdemeanors.

6. Reviews whether government evidence sufficient to justify trial. Some states have no grand jury system; others seldom use it.

7. Appearance for plea; defendant elects trial by judge or jury (if available); counsel for indigent usually appointed here in felonies. Often not at all in other cases.

8. Charge may be reduced at any time prior to trial in return for plea of guilty or for other reasons.

9. Challenge on constitutional grounds to legality of detention. May be sought at any point in process.

10. Police often hold informal hearings, dismiss or adjust many cases without further processing.

11. Probation officer decides desirability of further court action.

12. Welfare agency, social services, counseling, medical care, etc. for cases where adjudicatory handling not needed.

581

A few states still have misprision of felony statutes, which create an affirmative obligation to report a felony on the part of anyone with knowledge of its occurrence. Although some jurisdictions have statutes prohibiting the obstruction of justice or the hindering of prosecution, these, as well as misprision of felony laws, generally require an affirmative interference with an officer's lawful discharge of duties for the statute to apply (Perkins & Boyce, 1982; LaFave & Scott, 1986). Thus it would be permissible for the health care professional to refuse to disclose to the police otherwise confidential or privileged information.

On occasion, health care personnel may be presented with a *subpoena duces tecum* commanding the production of medical records (Stromberg, 1988). Subpoenas are generally issued in the name of a court clerk at the request of an attorney, but at this stage there has been no judicial determination that the record should, in fact, be disclosed without consent. In the absence of a release of information from an authorized individual such as a parent, a judge should be asked to rule on the question of whether the medical record should be released to avoid the possibility of liability for breach of confidentiality.

## Questioning of Suspects

As the police proceed with their investigation, possible suspects may be questioned. If an individual has been taken into custody or otherwise deprived of his freedom of action in any significant way, prior to questioning by law enforcement officials, the suspect must be given his "Miranda warnings" (*Miranda v. Arizona*, 1966; Whitebread & Slobogin, 1986). These warnings contain specific cautionary language informing the individual that he has a right to remain silent, that anything he says may be used against him in a court of law, that he has a right to an attorney, and that if he can't afford an attorney one will be appointed for him. If the warnings are not given, or if any statement or confession made was not voluntary, then the information may be excluded from evidence in any subsequent related criminal trial.

## Arrest and Booking

Before making an arrest (i.e., formally taking an individual into custody), law enforcement officers must have probable cause to believe that the arrestee is committing or has committed a felony, or that the arrestee committed a misdemeanor in the officer's presence (Whitebread & Slobogin, 1986). If, however, the crime is a misdemeanor not committed in the officer's presence, the policeman will have to obtain an arrest warrant from a magistrate or other judicial officer.

Once the police have probable cause to justify an arrest, they usually take the suspect into custody and process or "book" him or her. Fingerprints are made, and "mug shots" or booking photos are taken. How long the suspect can be held without judicial review is determined by state law. If an arrest warrant is not issued by a court before the termination of the prescribed time period, the police must release the suspect. In many jurisdictions an individual arrested has the right to have a bond commissioner or judge decide if he or she is to be released on personal recognizance or if a bail amount is to be set, pending prosecutorial review of the case and the possible issuance of formal charges.

## Prosecutorial Discretion

The investigating police officer presents the case to the prosecutor's office. The prosecutor possesses broad discretion regarding whether or not to file formal charges. This latitude finds support historically in American law. A number of factors generally influence the decision to file charges, including the strength of the available evidence, the harm caused by the offense, the victim's attitude toward pressing the case, the arrestee's prior criminal record, and the adequacy of alternative remedies apart from prosecution (LaFave & Israel, 1985).

Prosecutors sometimes are particularly reluctant to prosecute child abuse cases. They may believe that a criminal prosecution of a parent would impede the treatment and reunification of the family. More importantly, quite frequently a young child is the victim or otherwise is the primary or sole witness and concerns arise regarding both the child's credibility and the absence of other admissible evidence. Extensive cross-examination of a child witness may lead to confusion. Fears also exist that the child may be highly suggestible to influence by the perpetrator or other family members, causing an alteration of the content of the child's testimony at trial from the description of events provided earlier to the police and prosecutors. Sex abuse cases generate concerns that the jury will view the child as being prone to fantasy or being curious about sexuality and therefore apt to be confused. The extent to which these notions are valid is debatable. Many prosecutors, however, believe that the jury's possible concerns make it difficult to establish the elements of a criminal offense to the satisfaction of a jury "beyond a reasonable doubt" (Lloyd, 1981; Melton, 1981). Those relatively few cases in which prosecutions are brought generally involve sexual abuse, severe maltreatment, a nonparent perpetrator, an ethnic minority perpetrator, a female victim, or a victim who is 7 to 12 years of age (Tjaden & Thoennes, 1992).

Over the past decade, many prosecution offices have organized special units or assigned a limited number of prosecutors to pursue these cases. In such instances, expertise with these cases is developed and successful prosecutions may be more likely to occur.

If the prosecutor elects to bring criminal charges, a complaint is filed, and if an arrest warrant has not previously been obtained, the court generally will issue one upon the filing of the complaint. Further screening out of cases may occur as a result of a preliminary hearing or grand jury action, as described later.

## Initial Appearance

The arrestee, now referred to as the defendant, is presented before the court and advised of the formal charges contained within the complaint. This proceeding must occur within a specified period of time after arrest, as prescribed by law. At this hearing, bail and other possible conditions of release will be set or reviewed if initial determinations on these issues were made earlier. In felony cases a date will be set for a preliminary hearing on the charges, as described later, unless such a hearing is waived by the defendant or a grand jury issues an indictment in the interim. Defendants charged with misdemeanors are generally not entitled to preliminary hearings or grand jury indictments, and the case will be brought based solely on the prosecutor's charge (LaFave & Israel, 1985).

### Right to Counsel

At the initial appearance the court will generally inquire whether the defendant has retained counsel or wishes to do so. If the defendant is indigent, the court will appoint an attorney to represent the defendant. The attorney will either be a public defender or an attorney in private practice who has agreed to represent indigents. In either instance the attorney will be paid by the state (LaFave & Israel, 1985).

### Bail

Bail is usually viewed as a means of securing the defendant's presence at subsequent proceedings, and it also has come to be viewed as a way of helping to ensure the safety of the community. State and federal statutes may specify factors for the court to consider in determining whether bail should be set and in what amount. Typically, these factors include the seriousness of the offense, the strength of the case, the defendant's prior criminal record, and the defendant's background. The court may impose additional conditions of release. Appropriate conditions in child abuse cases may include a prohibition on contact with the victim, other members of the victim's family, or other witnesses.

Sometimes, particularly in homicide cases, the court will refuse to set bail or other conditions of release and instead will order that the defendant be held in jail pending the trial. Such preventive detention may be warranted upon a finding of future dangerousness or when there is a serious likelihood that the defendant will flee or otherwise attempt to obstruct justice (Whitebread & Slobogin, 1986). This measure may be appropriate in child abuse cases when there are concerns that the perpetrator will return to the child's home and either engage in further abuse or attempt to influence the child to recant accusatory statements.

## Preliminary Hearing

The preliminary hearing or grand jury is the next stage in the process. In many jurisdictions, individuals accused of crimes have a right to an adversarial preliminary hearing before a magistrate or judge. There, based on the evidence presented, the court determines whether probable cause exists to believe that a crime was committed and that the defendant was the perpetrator. Both the prosecution and the defense have the right to present evidence by subpoenaing witnesses and questioning them, as well as by the submission of documentary evidence such as medical and other reports.

The government carries the burden of proof. The defendant rarely presents affirmative evidence on his or her own behalf at this stage, although prosecution witnesses may be rigorously cross-examined. Probable cause will be found in practically all cases because the magistrate or judge generally does not have to weigh the credibility of the various witnesses unless the testimony is implausible or incredible. The only question is whether or not a jury, if it believed even some of the evidence presented, could find that a crime was committed and the defendant did it. If the judge concludes that a jury could so find, then the case is "bound over" for trial. The prosecutor will then issue a charge, usually called an information, based on what took place at the preliminary hearing. If no probable cause is found, the case must be dismissed and the defendant released (LaFave & Israel, 1985; Whitebread & Slobogin, 1986).

The preliminary hearing gives the defendant an opportunity to review the likely testimony to be presented against him. This may play a significant role in inducing him or her to enter a guilty plea. The defendant, of course, is entitled to attend the proceedings, although as described below, in some cases involving child abuse, limits may be placed on this right.

## Grand Jury

In federal felony prosecutions the Fifth Amendment to the U.S. Constitution requires that the case proceed only upon issuance of a grand jury indictment. A number of state constitutions contain comparable provisions. In some of those jurisdictions the preliminary hearing may be bypassed by the presentation of the case to a grand jury.

Grand jury review, whether or not subsequent to a preliminary hearing, also serves to provide a means of determining whether there is probable cause to proceed with prosecution against the defendant. But, unlike a preliminary hearing held before a judicial officer, the grand jury consists of a selected group of private citizens who review cases over a legislatively determined period of time.

The grand jury screening process differs fundamentally from the preliminary hearing in the manner in which it is conducted. The grand jury meets in closed session and only hears testimony from witnesses whom it or the prosecutor subpoenas. Members of the grand jury and the prosecutor may question the witnesses, but the defendant and his counsel are not permitted to attend the proceeding (LaFave & Israel, 1985; Whitebread & Slobogin, 1986). The grand jury mechanism may be preferable in cases involving child maltreatment because if the child is to be a witness, the grand jury procedure protects the child victim from the trauma of an additional confrontation with a perpetrator and an additional cross-examination by defense counsel. In some jurisdictions it may not even be necessary for the child victim to appear before the grand jury because a parent or law enforcement officer may be permitted to testify to what the child has stated or a videotape of the child's statement may be used in lieu of live testimony.

Upon a majority of the grand jurors finding sufficient evidence to justify prosecution, an indictment is signed by the members of the grand jury and designated a "true bill." The indictment, which sets forth a description of the offense, is then filed with the trial court. Return of a "no true bill" requires dismissal of the charges against the defendant.

## Arraignment

After the filing of either the prosecutor's information or the grand jury indictment with the court, the defendant is formally arraigned. The defendant appears before the court and is informed of the charges now pending against him or her. The defendant then enters a plea of not guilty or guilty. The question of the propriety of bail and other release procedures may again be explored.

## Pretrial Motions

Between entering a plea and the commencement of trial, the criminal defendant typically makes one or more pretrial motions, challenging such technical matters as the institution of the prosecution; the sufficiency of the indictment; the admissibility of expected physical evidence, statements, or confessions; the court's jurisdiction; and the physical location of the trial. In addition, the defendant will seek to "discover" certain materials from the prosecution and otherwise obtain information from witnesses who may testify against him. The extent to which this occurs is dependent on applicable law.

## Plea Bargaining, Guilty Pleas, and Dismissals

Before arraignment, plea bargaining between the prosecutor and defendant frequently occurs. Agreements derived from plea negotiations may take various forms. Such agreements can involve a plea of guilty to a less serious offense, a plea of guilty to the charged offense with a promise by the prosecutor to recommend a reduced sentence, or a plea of guilty to one or more charges in exchange for dismissal of other charges or a promise not to file additional charges. Justification for plea bargaining is found in the notion that it provides a quick disposition of cases necessitated by a system of justice that is already heavily overburdened. Plea bargaining is an important tool for the prosecutor when the child witness is reluctant to testify or the physical evidence of the crime is less than compelling.

The vast majority of criminal cases are disposed of by a guilty plea or by the dismissal of charges. In one study that examined a set of criminal filings in three counties across the country during the mid-1980s, 68% of the defendants entered guilty pleas to some or all of the charges and another 20% were dismissed before trial (Tjaden & Thoennes, 1992). These figures are consistent with national trends for all felony cases, where only 10% to 15% of the cases that reach the trial court actually go to trial (LaFave & Israel, 1985).

## Diversion

Diversion programs have emerged as a possible alternative to adjudication within the criminal justice system. Diversion involves halting or suspending formal criminal proceedings against a defendant without a formal conviction and requiring his or her participation in a therapeutic program. Diversion programs are a response to the difficulties in successfully prosecuting child maltreatment cases, particularly those involving sexual abuse.

Diversion generally is used only for misdemeanors or less serious or first felony complaints, and typically when the victim and the accused are family members. It may begin before the arrest or at any other stage before the commencement of the trial. Individuals selected for diversion are generally viewed as likely to participate in treatment and likely to benefit from it. Typically they are offered counseling directed at the abusive behavior, as well as career development, education, and supportive treatment services. If the participant responds favorably for a specified period of time, the court or the prosecutor or both will dismiss the case. If the defendant fails to meet the program's obligations, prosecution is resumed on the original criminal charge.

Jurisdictions vary in their use, if any, of diversion programs. Some states, by statute, specifically authorize diversion for particular crimes if certain criteria are met, while other jurisdictions provide for some degree of prosecutorial discretion or specific court involvement (LaFave & Israel, 1985; Kamisar et al., 1986). Similar schemes may be used as part of a condition of probation after a guilty plea or conviction at trial (Giarretto, 1976).

## Constitutional and Related Issues at Trial

The trial of any criminal case raises a broad array of constitutional and related issues, practically all of which are designed to protect the defendant and ensure a fair and impartial trial.

### Presumption of Innocence and Burden of Proof

The defendant is entitled to a presumption of innocence. This means that the prosecution has the burden of producing evidence of guilt and must persuade the trier of fact (the jury or the judge alone in a "bench trial") of the truth of each of the elements or legally significant facts of the offense with which the defendant is charged. Moreover, each of the elements must be proven by a high degree of evidence "beyond a reasonable doubt." Although it is difficult to define this standard, it is usually said that there must be "an abiding conviction, to a moral certainty, of the truth of the charge" (*Commonwealth v. Webster*, 1850).

### Privileges

The Fifth Amendment to the U.S. Constitution protects the defendant against compelled self-incrimination. This protection includes the right of the defendant not to take the witness stand and be forced to testify against himself.

In addition, statements admitting responsibility for abuse that are made to spouses, physicians, and other health care professionals may be excluded as a result of a claim of privilege (McCormick, 1984). The privilege may apply in criminal cases with respect to at least some of the information provided to health care professionals, even in the face of an abrogation of the privilege for civil child protection proceedings under a state's reporting statute (Stromberg, 1988).

### Searches, Seizures, and Confessions

As briefly noted in the discussion of social service and police response to reports of child abuse and neglect, an investigation of alleged child maltreatment may implicate a variety of constitutional issues that affect the admissibility of evidence at trial. These concerns are commonly based on activities such as the examination of the child, a search of a perpetrator's home, and statements obtained from the child's parent(s), guardian(s), or other possible perpetrators. The constitutional issues come into play not only in the context of potential civil liability of health care and child protection professionals, but also in criminal cases involving charges brought against perpetrators of child abuse and neglect.

Generally, constitutional provisions protect against intrusions by state authorities. Such authorities may include the police, child care workers, and even medical personnel employed by or acting on the direction of law enforcement or other state agencies. If such constitutional violations do occur, evidence that is obtained as a result of the violation may not be admitted in criminal prosecutions. Thus physical evidence that implicates a defendant may be excluded if it was seized in violation of the defendant's rights to be free from unreasonable searches and seizures under the Fourth Amendment to the U.S. Constitution. Similarly, confessions made in the absence of required Miranda warnings or as a result of police coercion may not be admissible at a criminal trial.

## Confrontation Clause

The Confrontation Clause of the Sixth Amendment to the U.S. Constitution is an area of constitutional law that has recently attracted attention from the U.S. Supreme Court. The clause often impacts the trial of criminal cases involving allegations of child abuse. The clause provides, in part, that "[i]n all criminal prosecutions, the accused shall enjoy the right ... to be confronted with the witnesses against him." The clause confers on a criminal defendant a right to confront witnesses at trial, both face-to-face and through cross-examination, and is designed to increase the defendant's ability to challenge the charges against him and to ensure an adversarial proceeding at trial (Whitebread & Slobogin, 1986). Confrontation Clause rights are also buttressed by rights under the Fourteenth Amendment's Due Process Clause, which prohibits a state from depriving an individual of liberty without due process of law.

The tension between the right to confrontation and attempts both by legislatures and individual judges to protect child victims from the potential trauma of confronting the abuser at trial or in pretrial proceedings is evident. Unlike the situation that may occur in both juvenile court and divorce-related hearings, where the court may be authorized in some circumstances to allow a child to testify "on camera" or in chambers and outside the presence of the alleged perpetrator, such testimony in a criminal case may violate the defendant's right to a public trial under the Sixth Amendment to the Constitution. It may also violate his or her right to confront witnesses and be present at trial under the Confrontation Clause. Finally, the First Amendment rights of the press and related rights of public access to trials may likewise be implicated (Whitebread & Slobogin, 1986).

A number of states have passed legislation providing for closed circuit and videotaped testimony in an effort to balance the competing interests of the child victims and the rights of criminal defendants. In addition, as discussed in the evidentiary section below, the Confrontation Clause may play a role in connection with the creation of various exceptions to the hearsay rule.

A violation of the Confrontation Clause may occur when the defendant is denied face-to-face confrontation with the witness. Although the defendant's right to be present extends to every stage of the trial, some exceptions do exist. The Supreme Court failed to find a violation of the Confrontation Clause when the defendant (but not his lawyer) was denied access to a pretrial hearing to determine the competency of two children who were victims of an alleged sex offense (*Kentucky v. Stincer*, 1985). The court noted, however, that the questions asked did not relate to the crime itself, and therefore the lack of the defendant's participation did not bear a substantial relationship to the defendant's opportunity to defend himself at trial. Moreover, the same questions were asked at trial where the defendant was present and there was full and complete cross-examination (LaFave & Israel, 1985).

The problem surrounding face-to-face confrontation is more likely when a child victim gives live testimony at trial, out of the presence of a defendant. In another case the U.S. Supreme Court reversed the conviction when a state law permitted a trial judge to order the placement of a large screen between the defendant and two

13-year-old girls who testified that he had sexually assaulted them. The court noted that the screen improperly prevented the witnesses from seeing the defendant and only allowed him to dimly perceive them. Justice O'Connor, who agreed with the reversal but filed a separate opinion, pointed out that the statute presumed that trauma would occur any time a young victim testified. She suggested that had there been an individualized finding by the trial judge that the child witnesses needed special protection, a different result might have ensued (Whitebread & Slobogin, 1986; *Coy v. Iowa*, 1988).

Soon thereafter the Supreme Court upheld a conviction under somewhat similar circumstances. In a 1990 case a state statute provided for a one-way television procedure if the trial judge decided that face-to-face testimony "will result in the child suffering serious emotional distress such that the child cannot reasonably communicate" (*Maryland v. Craig*, 1990). The statute provided that once this finding was made, the witness, prosecutor, and defense counsel would withdraw to a separate room, while the judge, jury, and defendant remained in the courtroom. The defendant could watch direct and cross-examination of the child over a video hookup and remain in electronic communication with his counsel. The court concluded that the central concerns regarding the Confrontation Clause were addressed under such a procedure. The court acknowledged the "growing body of academic literature documenting the psychological trauma suffered by child abuse victims who must testify in court." It concluded that as long as the trial judge decided, on a case-by-case basis, that such trauma would result if the child was faced with the defendant, and procedures such as those provided were followed to ensure the defendant's rights were respected, there was no constitutional violation (Whitebread & Slobogin, 1986).

## Trials

Defendants charged with felonies or misdemeanors punishable by more than 6 months in jail are entitled to jury trials. Juries generally comprise 12 persons, but in some jurisdictions, in certain cases, a jury of six is permissible. A defendant can waive his right to a jury trial and be tried by a judge alone. In felony trials a jury verdict either of guilt or acquittal must be unanimous. If the jury cannot come to a unanimous agreement, a mistrial results and the prosecution is terminated without a decision on the merits of the case. The state may not retry the defendant after an acquittal, but a subsequent prosecution may follow a mistrial.

## Sentencing

If there is a guilty verdict, a sentencing hearing is scheduled. Before the hearing a presentence report is completed, usually by the state's probation and parole department, to guide the judge in the sentencing decision. The report includes information about the defendant based on interviews with various individuals who have had contact with the defendant. The report may include the results of psychological testing or interviewing.

Both state and federal law define the range of permissible sanctions that may be imposed for the offense committed, including whether probation is available. In some jurisdictions, in some circumstances, the jury will recommend a punishment, which the judge can follow or choose to ignore in favor of a less severe penalty (Campbell, 1978).

In some situations the defendant may receive a prison sentence, but the sentence may be suspended with the defendant being placed on probation (with or without some limited period of incarceration) under the supervision of the probation department. A typical condition of probation in child abuse cases is a requirement of treatment for the defendant. The defendant's failure to attend or to participate in the treatment program can be viewed as a violation of probation, and the court might then reinstate the prison term originally decreed. Other conditions of probation may include an order to stay away from the victim and required payment to the victim for his or her treatment costs.

## Appeals and Post-conviction Actions

After a criminal conviction, direct appellate review is limited to a statutorily defined period of time and allows challenges to any alleged errors committed by the judge that occurred at trial. These include the judge's rulings on various motions that the defendant's attorney made before or at trial, on objections made to the admissibility of evidence, and on instructions the judge gave to the jury regarding the applicable law in the case. If the defendant's appeal is unsuccessful, he may make a "collateral attack" on the conviction. A collateral attack is usually based on constitutional challenges, such as a claim of ineffective assistance of counsel at trial or on appeal. The state, however, may not appeal from an acquittal.

## CHILD CUSTODY DISPUTES AND ALLEGATIONS OF ABUSE

### ARENAS OF LITIGATION

Sometimes allegations of child abuse arise in child custody disputes. Often they include claims of sexual abuse (Nicholson, 1988; Fahn, 1991). The parents may have been residing together as a family unit at the time, or the alleged behavior may have occurred subsequent to the break-up but pending judicial resolution of custody and visitation rights. Alternatively, the alleged incident might have taken place after a temporary or final custody decree, while the child was in the custody of a custodial parent, or during the course of visitation by the child with the noncustodial parent.

If no dissolution of marriage action has been filed, but there is a dispute concerning child custody, its resolution is likely to take place in the context of a juvenile court child protection proceeding as described earlier. In addition, most states have enacted legislation that provides for "civil orders of protection" for victims of domestic violence. Many of these statutes provide for judicial determination of custody rights with respect to the children of the parties involved in the context of such litigation (Finn, 1989).

Finally, the issue of child abuse may appear in any one of a number of stages of a court action related to the dissolution of a marriage of the child's parents. For example, together with or shortly after the filing of a petition for divorce, a motion may be filed requesting the court to issue an order providing for temporary custody and visitation pending the final hearing on the petition for a decree of divorce. At the final hearing, in which the court must determine provisions for joint or sole custody and visitation rights, the issue of child abuse may also be contested. Subsequent to the court issuing a final custody order, one or both of the parents may file motions to modify that order, alleging a change in the circumstances of the child or custodial parent. There, too, the question of child abuse may be litigated. State law or state or local court rules will determine whether it will be a juvenile or family court or a court of general civil jurisdiction that will rule on the custody issue in each of these contexts (Edwards, 1987).

Litigation of child custody disputes in each of these situations differs from that in the juvenile court/child protection context or the criminal context. The court here is engaging in a private dispute settlement function where it must choose between two or more individuals, each of whom claims an associational interest with the child. In the other situations described previously the court is enforcing standards of behavior believed necessary to protect the child or the greater society at large and, perhaps, to punish a wrongdoer (Mnookin, 1975).

## PROCEDURAL AND EVIDENTIARY RULES

The state's power to adjudicate private custody disputes, like its power in child protection cases, derives from the common law concept of the state as *parens patriae* (Cunningham & Horowitz, 1989). Each state, through legislation and judicial precedent, has prescribed both procedural and evidentiary rules that regulate how the issue is to be litigated as well as substantive rules to guide the court in determining what its orders regarding custody should be (Goldner, 1987; Clark, 1988).

Depending on the particular state, rules exist that permit or require the appointment of a guardian ad litem in child custody disputes. Similarly, under more or less restrictive circumstances, the trial judge may order that an investigation and report regarding custodial arrangements for the child be made by employees of public or private social service agencies or by other competent individuals. The child may be referred to professionals for diagnosis by the court or by the individual conducting the custody investigation. The investigator may consult with and obtain information from medical, psychiatric, or other experts who have previously dealt with the child. The judge may conduct in-chambers interviews with the child to ascertain custodial preferences or seek the advice of professional personnel in an effort to elicit such information most effectively. Some jurisdictions require the consent of all parties, in some circumstances, for the application of one or more of these unique procedural devices in a given child custody case. The manner in which a given state approaches these issues affects the court's ability to ascertain whether or not abuse or neglect has taken place. This, in turn, controls the extent to which the abuse or neglect then plays a role in the court's ultimate determination of contested custody questions.

Evidentiary rules control the extent to which professional privileges such as that between physician and patient, psychologist and client, and husband and wife limit the amount of information available to a court in making a child custody determination. Although most state reporting statutes seem to abrogate these privileges in child custody situations involving known or suspected child abuse or neglect (Stromberg, 1988), the precise language of the statutory provision that abrogates the privilege in a given state and possible judicial interpretations of that language could still affect whether or not related evidence is deemed admissible.

## SUBSTANTIVE STANDARDS

A majority of states currently provide that custody decisions turn on "the best interests of the child" or comparable language, as the substantive standard for making custody determinations (Clark, 1988). Likewise, visitation rights may be subject to a similar analysis. "The best interests of the child," however, can be an ambiguous standard. This standard essentially requires that a prediction be made in relation to the child's needs and each parent's ability to meet them.

The analysis of the phrase, when specified by the legislature, may provide guidelines that take into account a lengthy list of factors. These include matters such as (1) the wishes of the child's parents as to custody; (2) the wishes of the child; (3) the interaction and interrelationship of the child with his or her parents, siblings, and any other person who may significantly affect the child's best interests; (4) the child's adjustment to home, school, and community; (5) the mental and physical health of all individuals involved, including any history of abuse of any individuals involved; (6) the needs of the child for a continuing relationship with both parents and the ability and willingness of parents to actively perform their functions as mother and father for the needs of the child; (7) the intention of either parent to relocate his or her residence outside the state; (8) which parent is more likely to allow the child frequent and meaningful contact with the other parent; and (9) other considerations of environment, physical and emotional needs, intellectual stimulation, financial resources, moral development, and family makeup (Goldner, 1987; Clark, 1988).

When custody is contested, the judge must choose among various alternative arrangements, allocating between the two parents the rights and obligations relating to the child that were formerly shared by them. Although most jurisdictions now authorize awards of "joint custody" under which the parents continue to share rights and responsibilities with respect to the child after divorce, such an award is not required (Clark, 1988). In cases where child maltreatment is alleged, the court necessarily seeks to determine the truth of the accusations. When the allegations are substantiated, the judge should, of course, choose a custody arrangement that will maximize the child's safety.

## REVIEW AND MODIFICATION

Custody decisions are generally viewed as matters best left to the sound discretion of the trial court because of the fact-sensitive nature of the determinations, combined with the general lack of firm guidelines controlling "the best interests of the child" analysis (Oster, 1965; Pace, 1973). The wide latitude traditionally afforded to a trial court allows for a necessarily individualized case-by-case decision (Pearson & Ring, 1982). It does, however, limit the scope of review of an appellate court to that of reversal only for an "abuse of discretion." Thus, on appeal, a higher court generally will not re-evaluate the facts to determine whether, in its own view, a finding of child abuse perpetrated by the accused should have been made.

Legislation providing for modification of a child custody or visitation order commonly requires a showing of a "substantial or material change of circumstances" and that a modification will be in "the best interests of the child" (Atkinson, 1986). Allegations of abuse, formerly raised when custody was initially decided, will generally not constitute a change of circumstances without new evidence of abuse.

## Evidentiary Issues

The law of evidence is the system of rules and standards that regulates the admission of proof at the trial of any lawsuit (McCormick, 1984). In response to efforts to introduce various types of evidence, in the nature of both testimony and physical exhibits (sometimes called "real" evidence), objections may be made by opposing counsel. The trial judge must then rule on these objections and determine what actual evidence the finder of fact (which may be the jury, as in criminal cases, or the judge in juvenile court child protection cases or divorce cases) will be allowed to consider. The judge relies on established rules that are part of the law of evidence in making these determinations.

General rules of evidence may affect virtually any question that is asked of a witness during the trial. Particularly unique and difficult evidentiary issues do arise, however, in cases involving child abuse and neglect, and these warrant specific attention here. These issues include the possible use of circumstantial evidence, the competency of child witnesses, the use of hearsay testimony, limits regarding the scope of admissible expert testimony, and the use of various types of demonstrative evidence such as photographs and anatomically correct dolls.

Generally, the applicable rules of evidence in criminal child abuse prosecutions, civil juvenile court child protection proceedings, and child custody cases are the same. The rules may be somewhat "relaxed" in noncriminal proceedings in juvenile court or in divorce cases because a judge rather than a jury is the fact finder and, at least theoretically, has been trained to ignore inadmissible evidence in making his or her determination.

## DIRECT AND CIRCUMSTANTIAL EVIDENCE

Child abuse often does not yield a great deal of evidence that, under American rules of evidence, would be admissible in any of the trials or hearings related to child abuse. Most cases of child abuse occur in the child's home, and often the only people present are the child and the perpetrator. Even when others are present at the time of the incident, in many instances it is a member of the immediate family, such as a spouse who may be unwilling to testify or to testify truthfully, or a young child who is too immature to take the witness stand. Frequently the victim is too young or too immature to testify. Even if the child is mature enough to testify, he or she may be reluctant to do so or will change or recant his or her story. The alleged adult perpetrator typically contends that the child's injuries were accidental. Therefore direct evidence is usually sparse or nonexistent. Direct evidence is evidence which, if believed, resolves the matter in issue (McCormick, 1984).

Most of the available evidence in child abuse cases is circumstantial. Circumstantial evidence is evidence that is not based on actual personal knowledge or observation of the facts or events in controversy. Rather, it is based on facts from which deductions may be drawn, showing indirectly that certain events did take place or that certain other facts sought to be proved are true. Circumstantial evidence, even if believed, does not resolve the matter at issue. Additional reasoning must be applied to reach the proposition to which it is directed (McCormick, 1984).

For example, a witness' testimony that he saw X beat a child with a belt is direct evidence of whether X did, indeed, beat the child. Testimony that the child had belt marks on his back and legs, that the child was in X's custody, and that no one else had access to the child during the time when the marks were acquired would be strong circumstantial evidence that X beat the child. A case of child abuse may be proven entirely by circumstantial evidence, but there still must be sufficient evidence to convince the trier of fact.

In juvenile court proceedings, some courts have applied the doctrine of *res ipsa loquitur* to support an inference of child abuse. *Res ipsa loquitur* means "the thing speaks for itself." For example, child abuse may be inferred from the mere fact that the child sustained a particular injury, given the character of the injury and the surrounding circumstances (*S., In re*, 1965).

## COMPETENCY

An individual must be competent to testify as a witness at any trial or hearing (Melton et al., 1981). Competence to testify involves four factors: (1) a present understanding of the difference between truth and falsity and an appreciation of the obligation to speak the truth; (2) the mental capacity, at the time of the occurrence in question, to observe or receive accurate impressions of the event; (3) memory sufficient to retain an independent recollection of the observations; and (4) the capacity to communicate into words that memory and to understand questions about the event (Melton, 1981).

Historically, courts and legislatures created presumptions, depending on age, regarding the competency of children to testify. More recently, however, the trend has been to presume that all witnesses are competent to testify and to resolve doubts as to the credibility of the witness in favor of allowing the testimony and having the trier of fact decide what weight to give that testimony. A party can still challenge a witness, however, and the trial judge may prohibit the testimony if the judge finds that the witness did not meet one of the criteria just listed. Because judges would otherwise have the discretion to exclude testimony on the basis of competence, a number of jurisdictions have recently passed legislation that makes admissible *all* testimony by a child regarding evidence of child sexual abuse (Morey, 1985).

*HEARSAY*

In general, a witness can only testify to those facts about which he or she has personal knowledge. The witness may not testify to what others have said in an out-of-court or extra-judicial statement to prove the truth of the matter stated. Such secondhand information is called hearsay (McCormick, 1984). Hearsay evidence is usually inadmissible in a judicial proceeding. Hearsay is excluded to prevent the introduction of statements made by out-of-court declarants whose statements were not made under oath and whose credibility cannot be evaluated by the jury.

There are, however, certain recognized exceptions to the hearsay rule (McCormick, 1984). Each of these exceptions has been recognized in some or all jurisdictions. The exceptions typically have been created when the situation and the circumstances surrounding the declarant's statement increase the reliability of the out-of-court statement and thereby make the statement more trustworthy. For such statements to be admissible, however, they must meet the jurisdiction's requirements for that particular hearsay exception and, in criminal cases, not violate the Confrontation Clause of the U.S. Constitution. A number of the recognized exceptions to the hearsay rule are important in child abuse and neglect cases (Myers, 1987; Graham, 1988).

## Excited Utterances and Statements of Physical and Mental Conditions

One recognized hearsay exception is that for excited utterances. This exception allows for the admission of nonreflective statements regarding a startling event made while the declarant is still in a state of excitement. For example, a statement made by a child to a neighbor or the police that her mother beat her with a belt may be admissible if the court finds that the statement was made while the child was still excited and that the statement was impulsive and spontaneous rather than a product of reflective thought.

A related exception, recognized in most jurisdictions, is that for statements made to anyone regarding then existing physical conditions, including pain or other physical sensations. These are admissible to prove the truth of the statement, that is, they are admissible to prove that the physical condition or pain existed at the time the statement was made. Thus a statement made by a child to his or her mother, while pointing to a genital area, that "it hurts," could be admissible under this exception.

Similarly, most jurisdictions admit statements of the declarant's then existing state of mind or emotion. Thus, for example, in child custody litigation incident to a divorce, a child's statement to another individual regarding affection for or dislike of a parent will be admissible. Similarly, statements indicating fear of an abusive parent may also be admitted.

## Statements for Medical Diagnosis

In most jurisdictions there is a separate recognized exception authorizing the admission of statements made for purposes of medical diagnosis and treatment. Statements admissible under this exception may pertain to present or past conditions if they are made to a physician or the physician's agent, such as a nurse, technician, or receptionist. Such statements are admissible on the assumption that one generally does not fabricate statements to health care providers because the success of the patient's treatment depends on the accuracy of the information provided. Thus an affirmative response by a child to a question asked by a physician of whether anyone "touched you there" would be admissible as evidence to prove that the molestation had taken place.

Some courts also will admit statements that refer to the cause of the condition for which the declarant is seeking treatment, if the statements are reasonably pertinent to the diagnosis and are made in connection with the treatment. In the child abuse situation, a number of courts have reasoned that because the treatment of child abuse includes removing the child from the abusive setting, the doctor should attempt to ascertain the identity of the abuser. Therefore a child's statement to a physician to the effect that "Daddy hurt me" would be admitted.

## Present Sense Impressions

A few jurisdictions recognize an exception for "present sense impressions." These are statements describing or explaining an event or condition that are made while the declarant was perceiving the event or condition or immediately thereafter. For example, if a child was rescued while the abuse was taking place and immediately began to describe to the rescuer what had occurred, his or her statement may be admitted.

## Admissions by Parties

Another recognized exception to the hearsay rule is when the out-of-court statement is that of a party to the litigation and is relevant to the party's defense. For example, a parent-perpetrator may tell a neighbor, "I beat my child because he wet his pants." In a criminal case against the parent the neighbor could testify to this statement. Its admission in a juvenile court proceeding may depend on whether the parent is considered a party under the state's juvenile court rules.

## Business and Medical Records

Another exception to the hearsay rule allows the introduction of business records. This generally includes medical records. When business records are used to prove the truth of their contents, this constitutes hearsay. Such records, however, often are admitted under a recognized exception to the hearsay rule for records that are kept by a business in the regular course of its operation. The theory is that, if the "business" itself will rely on the accuracy of such records in carrying out its operations, a court should do likewise. For the record to be admitted there must be "foundational testimony" to the effect that the entry to the records was made accurately and promptly, that it was done in the course of usual business activity, and that the person recording the information had firsthand knowledge of the matter.

In most instances, medical records may be admissible as substantive evidence of the child's diagnosis, condition, medical history, and laboratory and X-ray findings under the business records exception to the hearsay rule. Medical records may also be used to refresh the physician's memory regarding the specific case when the physician is testifying at trial or giving evidence in a deposition. This use is appropriate whether or not the record is otherwise admissible as a business record.

Many courts are reluctant, however, to admit prognostic statements or statements concerning the cause of a condition that are contained in the medical record unless the doctor who wrote the statement is available for cross-examination or the statement was based on objective data rather than on data requiring speculation. For example, it would probably not be necessary to have a radiologist testify in court that the child has a spiral fracture of the femur. In this situation the record would be admissible to show that the child had the spiral fracture. Conversely, a doctor's statement that the spiral fracture of the femur was caused by child abuse, rather than by an accidental fall, would probably not be admitted into evidence unless the doctor was available for cross-examination.

Some jurisdictions have recognized a so-called "residual" exception to the hearsay rule. This permits the receipt of "reliable" hearsay evidence, which does not fit into an established exception, under limited situations, as long as the statement has "equivalent circumstantial guarantees of trustworthiness" to the recognized exceptions. Courts have sometimes relied on this exception in litigation involving children.

## Sexual Abuse Hearsay Exception

A number of jurisdictions, legislatively or by judicial decision, have created a new hearsay exception that authorizes the admission of out-of-court statements by children about sexual abuse (McCormick, 1984; Note, 1985; Myers, 1987). Often the sexual abuse hearsay exception's applicability is limited to criminal and/or juvenile court proceedings. This exception is similar to the residual exception, but only applies to children's statements about sexual abuse. The time, content, and circumstances of the statement must provide sufficient guarantees of trustworthiness. In addition, the child must either testify at the hearing or be unavailable. When unavailable, there must be additional corroborative evidence of the act which is the subject of the child's statement. These statutes allow a parent, doctor, or other individual to whom a child has made a statement regarding sexual abuse to testify to the child's description of what occurred, irrespective of whether or not the statement otherwise meets the requirements of another hearsay exception.

## Videotaping Statutes

Some state legislatures have passed statutes permitting a child's testimony to be preserved on videotape for presentation to a jury, thus enabling the child to avoid repeated appearances in court (McCormick, 1984; MacFarlane, 1985; Note, 1985). The statutes exempt from the ban on hearsay an audiovisually recorded statement of a child victim or witness that describes an act of sexual abuse or physical violence if certain requirements are met. The court must find that (1) the minor will suffer emotional or psychological stress if required to testify in open court; (2) the time, content, and circumstances of the statement provide sufficient guarantees of trustworthiness; and (3) certain other procedural requirements were met. Generally, the presence of the judge, the accused, or counsel is not required at the taping, and any person can conduct the interview. Before the statement is admitted, however, on the defendant's request, the court must provide for further questioning of the minor. The admission of the statement, however, does not preclude the court from allowing a party to call the minor as a witness, if justice requires.

In addition, these statutes authorize presenting the evidence of the statement of the child as the equivalent of testimony in the case, either by audiovisually recorded deposition or by closed circuit television. Such statutes specify who is to be present at the recording and authorize the exclusion of a party on a finding that his or her presence may cause severe emotional or psychological distress to the child. The use of such a recording is permitted provided the defendant can observe and hear the testimony and can consult with his or her lawyer.

## Confrontation Clause Issues

Although the rules regarding hearsay and its exceptions are generally applicable in juvenile, criminal, and divorce cases, particular note should be made of the interplay between these hearsay rules and a criminal defendant's rights under the Confrontation Clause of the Sixth Amendment to the U.S. Constitution. As noted in the discussion of criminal trials as well as in the discussion of hearsay, state legislatures and trial courts have endeavored to reduce the trauma a child might sustain from testifying in a criminal trial. Such protective measures may, however, violate the Confrontation Clause.

The Confrontation Clause and the hearsay rules are not one and the same. Nevertheless, they advance a number of similar values. As a matter of constitutional law, the right to confrontation (1) ensures that the witness will give his statements under oath, thus impressing him with the seriousness of the matter and guarding against a lie by the possibility of a penalty for perjury; (2) forces the witness to submit to cross-examination, which aids in the discovery of truth; and (3) permits the jury to observe the demeanor of the witness in making his or her statement, allowing it to assess credibility (*California v. Green*, 1970).

When the state seeks to admit hearsay evidence in a criminal case, the proper inquiry under the Confrontation Clause is said to be two-fold. First, where the declarant was available as a witness at trial, it must be asked whether the defendant was permitted an adequate opportunity for cross-examination. Second, and more important for present purposes, if the declarant was not present as a witness at trial, it must be asked whether the absence of the witness was necessary and whether there was sufficient "indicia of reliability" surrounding the out-of-court statement (McCormick, 1984; Whitebread & Slobogin, 1986). When the declarant is a child victim, the prosecutor must produce evidence of a good faith effort to obtain the presence of the witness, or establish that the witness is "not capable of testifying" as defined by state law. This may involve a showing that the witness is incompetent or that the child should be excused from testifying because the experience will cause additional trauma.

In a 1990 U.S. Supreme Court decision, a female defendant and her companion were convicted of lewd conduct against the companion's 2 1/2-year-old daughter (*Idaho v. Wright*, 1990). The conviction was successfully challenged by the female defendant on the ground that the trial court should not have admitted the pediatrician's testimony that the victim suggested to him that her father had abused her. The critical statements were made in response to the doctor asking whether her daddy touched her with his "pee-pee." The girl responded that "daddy does this with me. . .". The trial judge determined that the daughter was incompetent to testify and refused to allow her testimony, but he concluded that her statements to the pediatrician were reliable and admitted them under the state's "residual exception" to the hearsay rule. On appeal, the Supreme Court held that incriminating statements such as these, although otherwise admissible under an exception to the hearsay rule, may be prohibited under the Confrontation Clause. To be admitted, the prosecution must produce the declarant for cross-examination or establish the declarant's unavailability, as well as demonstrate that the statement bears adequate indicia of reliability. The court assumed that, given the incompetency finding, the child had in fact been "unavailable" for testimony. The question then became one of the reliability or trustworthiness of the statements. The court refused to adopt any hard and fast rules for professional interviews, such as a requirement that the statements be videotaped or that leading questions could not be used. It ruled that in determining reliability, factors relating to whether the child was likely to be telling the truth when the statements were made were to be considered and that these included the declarant's mental state, spontaneity, and consistent repetition; motive or lack of motive to make up a story; and the use of terminology unexpected of a child of that age. In this particular case, the court pointed out that the doctor had conducted the interview in a suggestive manner. Given the presumptive unreliability of the statements, the court concluded that there was no special reason for supposing that the statements were particularly trustworthy.

## EXPERT TESTIMONY

Generally, a witness is only permitted to testify to factual matters and may not offer an opinion or conclusion regarding the meaning of those facts. An expert witness, however, is allowed to give opinions in areas related to his or her expertise when the judge determines that such testimony is beyond the common knowledge of the trier of fact and will aid the trier of fact in deciding the issues in the case (McCormick, 1984). An expert witness is someone with specialized knowledge obtained through training and/or experience. To qualify as an expert, the witness will be required to state facts about his or her education and experience. The opposing attorney or the judge may ask additional questions regarding the witness' expertise. The trial judge is given great discretion in deciding whether the witness qualifies as an expert on the particular matter at issue.

Generally, physicians and other licensed or certified health care professionals have sufficient training and experience to express a medical opinion to help the judge or jury understand the medical aspects of the case. Therefore, in most situations, an individual with a medical degree will qualify as an expert witness. There is no requirement for subspecialization. The weight the fact finder, be it a judge or a jury, gives the physician's testimony may, however, be affected by such factors as board certification in the particular area involved, experience, publications, and the clarity of the witness' presentation concerning the pertinent condition.

## Battered Child and Failure-to-Thrive Syndromes

When physical abuse is alleged, expert medical testimony is often essential to establish that the injury was not accidental. In child abuse cases a physician usually qualifies as an expert who can give his or her opinion as to the nature of the child's injuries. Medical testimony that the child's injuries are consistent with the "battered child syndrome" is often allowed on the grounds that it is an accepted medical diagnosis (*State v. Best*, 1975; Boresi, 1989; *Estelle v. McGuire*, 1991). For example, patterned abrasions (belt, cord, stick) and certain fractures in young children (posterior rib fractures in different stages of healing) are powerful evidence of nonaccidental injury and child abuse.

"Failure-to-thrive" syndrome is another diagnosis generally recognized by the medical community and the courts. The syndrome describes a condition in which a very young child's height and weight consistently fall below the third percentile on the standard growth chart (Cunningham & Horowitz, 1989). Although similar growth patterns may be indicative of certain organic disease processes, they may be caused by parental neglect or deprivation, such as inadequate feeding and poor nutrition. Courts generally have accepted an expert's conclusion that the problem results from neglect when, subsequent to the child's hospitalization and receipt of proper nutrition, the child has gained substantial weight in a relatively short period of time (Goldner, 1979).

## Other Abuse-related Syndromes

Psychologists, social workers, and other mental health professionals may be called as expert witnesses in child abuse cases to testify to matters within their competence. Such areas include testimony regarding the emotional status of the child, conditions of the child's home, and parenting techniques. "Child abuse family profile," "child sexual abuse accommodation syndrome," and the "battering parent syndrome" are terms used to denote specific behavior patterns and characteristics common to children and families where child abuse has occurred. In a very few jurisdictions, testimony regarding the presence of these characteristics and syndromes common in abused children or in families in which abuse occurs may be offered into evidence by an expert to indicate the probability that the child has been abused. Courts in many jurisdictions are reluctant, however, to admit expert testimony regarding these syndromes because such syndromes are based on psychological factors that are speculative as compared to physical factors that are either concrete or qualitative (Boresi, 1989; Cunningham & Horowitz, 1989).

### DEMONSTRATIVE EVIDENCE

Demonstrative evidence consists of things rather than assertions of witnesses about things. Demonstrative evidence, such as photographs, medical illustrations or diagrams of the child's injuries, and X-rays, is frequently helpful in assisting the trier of fact in child abuse cases to understand a particular issue.

## Photographs, Drawings, and X-rays

Generally, demonstrative evidence will be admitted if a proper foundation is laid. Specifically, it must be shown that the demonstrative object is a fair and accurate representation of the thing it purports to represent or illustrate. For example, if a physician testifies about a child's bruises and cuts observed in the hospital and then is shown a picture of the child taken at approximately the same time the doctor examined the child, the doctor will be allowed to testify that the photo is a "true and accurate representation" of what he or she saw. Consequently, the photograph can then be admitted into evidence and shown to the trier of fact. Similarly, drawings that indicate the location of injuries may be admitted when the proper foundation is laid.

In a criminal prosecution for child abuse, admission of photographs of the child's injuries is left to the discretion of the judge because such photographs may inflame and prejudice a jury. The judge must balance the probative value of the pictures against their prejudicial effect in ruling on admissibility.

Generally, the child's X-rays will be admitted into evidence if accompanied by testimony explaining their relevance. X-rays may reveal certain types of fractures that, when found in a young child, are indicative of child abuse rather than accidental injury. For example, posterior rib fractures in different stages of healing in a young child are highly suggestive of physical abuse. Conversely, an X-ray may indicate an accident rather than child abuse. A fractured clavicle accompanied by bruises on the arms is indicative of an accidental fall.

## Anatomically Correct Dolls

The use of anatomically correct dolls is designed to reduce the trauma to child witnesses in sexual abuse cases. The dolls may ease the child's experience of testifying and assist the child who has difficulty relating events to the trier of fact using appropriate sexual or physiological terms (Cunningham & Horowitz, 1989). Some states have enacted legislation expressly permitting the use of such dolls during children's testimony. In addition, expert witnesses are sometimes permitted to describe or comment on a child victim's interactions with the dolls. Because the use of such dolls has sometimes been viewed as controversial, some jurisdictions bar their use in the courtroom (Ringland, 1986; *Amber, In re*, 1987; Dulka, 1988).

## ♦ BIBLIOGRAPHY

Adoption Assistance and Child Welfare Act, 1980. 42 U.S.C. *S* 670, et seq. (Supp. 1990).

*Amber, In re*, 191 Cal.App.3d 682 (1987).

Atkinson, J: *Modern Child Custody Practice*, Kluwer Law Book Publishers, New York, 1986.

Attorney General's Task Force on Family Violence, Final Report, Sept 1984.

*Baltimore City Dep't of Social Serv. v. Bouknight*, 493 U.S. 549 (1990).

Besharov, D: The legal aspects of reporting known and suspected child abuse and neglect, *Villanova L Rev* 23:458, 1978.

Besharov, D: Child welfare malpractice, *Trial* 20:56, March 1984.

Besharov, D: The need to narrow the grounds for state intervention. In D Besharov, ed: *Protecting Children from Abuse and Neglect: Policy and Practice*, Charles C Thomas, Publisher, Springfield, IL, 1988.

Blue, W: *State v. Williquette:* Protecting children from abuse through the imposition of a legal duty, *Am J Trial Ad* 12:171, 1988.

Boresi, K: Syndrome testimony in child abuse prosecutions: The wave of the future? *St Louis U Pub L Rev* 8:207, 1989.

Bross, D: Medical diagnosis as a gateway to the child welfare system: a legal review for physicians, lawyers and social workers, *Den U L Rev* 65:213, 1988.

Bulkley, J: Introduction: Background and review of child sexual abuse: Law reforms in the mid-1980's, *U Miami L Rev* 40:5, 1985.

*California v. Green*, 399 U.S. 149 (1970).

Campbell, AW: *The Law of Sentencing*, Lawyers Cooperative Publishing Co, Rochester, NY, 1978.

*Capaldi v. State*, 763 P.2d 117 (Okl. Cr. 1988).

Child Abuse Prevention and Treatment Act, 1974. 42 U.S.C. δ 5101 et seq. (Supp. 1990).

Clark, H: *Hornbook on the Law of Domestic Relations in the United States*, ed 2, West Publishing Co, St. Paul, MN, 1988.

*Commonwealth v. Webster*, 5 Cush. 295 (Mass. 1850).

*Coy v. Iowa*, 487 U.S. 1012 (1988).

Cunningham, C, and Horowitz, R: *Child Abuse and Neglect: Cases, Text and Problems*, American Bar Association, National Legal Resource Center for Child Advocacy and Protection, Washington, DC, 1989.

Daro, D: *Confronting Child Abuse: Research for Effective Program Design*, Free Press, New York, 1988.

*Daryl H. v. Coler* 801 F.2d 893 (7th Cir. 1986).

*DeShaney v. Winnebago County Dept. of Social Servs.*, 489 U.S. 189 (1989).

Dulka, M: Raising the standard for expert testimony: An unwanted obstacle in proving claims of child sexual abuse in dependency hearings, *Golden Gate L Rev* 18:443, 1988.

Edwards, L: The relationship of family and juvenile courts in child abuse cases, *Santa Clara L Rev* 27:201, 1987.

*Estelle v. McGuire*, 510 U.S., 112 S.Ct. 475 (1991).

Fahn, M: Allegations of child sexual abuse in custody disputes: getting to the truth of the matter, *Fam L Q* 25:193, 1991.

Federal Protection of Children Against Sexual Exploitation Act, 1986. 18 U.S.C. 2251, et seq. (Supp 1991).

Finn, P: Statutory authority in the use and enforcement of civil protection orders against domestic violence, *Fam L Q* 23:43, 1989.

Fox, SJ: *The Law of Juvenile Courts in a Nutshell*, ed 2, West Publishing Co, St. Paul, MN, 1984.

Fraser, B: A glance at the past, a gaze at the present, a glimpse at the future: A critical analysis of the development of child abuse reporting statutes, *Chi Kent L Rev* 54:641, 1978.

Giarretto, H: Humanistic treatment of father-daughter incest. In R Helfer and G Kempe, eds: *Child Abuse and Neglect: The Family and the Community*, Ballinger Publishing Co, Cambridge, MA, 1976.

Goldner, J: *Child Abuse and Neglect and the Law: Cases and Materials for Attorneys and Law Students*, Region VII Child Abuse and Neglect Resource Center, Institute of Child Behavior and Development, University of Iowa, Iowa City, 1979.

Goldner, J: *Missouri Dissolution of Marriage, Support and Child Custody*, Harrison Co, Norcross, GA, 1987.

Graham, M: The confrontation clause, the hearsay rule, and child sexual abuse prosecutions: The state of the relationship, *Minn L Rev* 72:523, 1988.

*Groff v. State*, 390 So.2d 361 (Fla. App. 1980).

*Gross v. Myers*, 748 P.2d 459 (Mont. 1987).

Hardin, M: Legal barriers in child abuse investigations: State powers and individual rights, *Wash L Rev* 63:493, 1988.

*Harlow v. Fitzgerald*, 457 U.S. 800 (1982).

Hechler, D: *The Battle and the Backlash: The Child Sexual Abuse War*, Lexington Books, Lexington, MA, 1988.

Hertz, R, Guggenheim, M, and Amsterdam, A: *Trial Manual for Defense Attorneys in Juvenile Court*, American Law Institute–American Bar Association, Philadelphia, 1991.

Horowitz, R, and Davidson, H: Protecting children from family maltreatment. In R Horowitz and H Davidson, eds: *Legal Rights of Children*, Shepard's/McGraw-Hill, Colorado Springs, CO, 1984.

*Idaho v. Wright*, U.S., 110 S.Ct. 3139 (1990).

Indian Child Welfare Act, 1978. 25 U.S.C. 1901, et seq. (Supp. 1990).

Iverson, T, and Segal, M: *Child Abuse and Neglect: An Information and Reference Guide*, Garland Publishing, Inc, New York, 1990.

Johnson, TA: *Introduction to the Juvenile Justice System*, West Publishing Co, St. Paul, MN, 1975.

Kamisar, Y, Lafave, N, and Israel, J: *Modern Criminal Procedure*, ed 6, West Publishing Co, St. Paul, MN, 1986.

Kempe, C, et al: The battered-child syndrome, *JAMA* 181:17, 1962.

*Kentucky v. Stincer*, 474 U.S. 15 (1985).

LaFave, W, and Israel, J: *Hornbook on Criminal Procedure* (with 1989 Supp), West Publishing Co, St. Paul, MN, 1985.

LaFave, W, and Scott, A: *Hornbook on Criminal Law*, ed 2, West Publishing Co, St. Paul, MN, 1986.

*Landeros v. Flood*, 551 P.2d 389 (Cal. banc 1976).

*Lassiter v. Department of Social Servs.*, 452 U.S. 18 (1981).

Levine, R: Caveat parens: A demystification of the child protection system, *U Pitt L Rev* 35:1, 1973.

Lloyd, D: The corroboration of sexual victimization of children. In J Bulkley, ed: *Child Sexual Abuse and the Law*, American Bar Association, National Legal Resource Center for Child Advocacy and Protection, Washington, DC, 1981.

MacFarlane, K: Diagnostic evaluations and the uses of videotapes in child sexual abuse cases. In *Papers From a National Policy Conference on Legal Reforms in Child Sexual Abuse Cases*, American Bar Association, National Legal Resource Center for Child Advocacy and Protection, Washington, DC, 1985.

MacMurray, B: Criminal determination for child sexual abuse prosecutor case-screening judgments, *J Interpersonal Violence* 4:233, 1989.

*Maryland v. Craig*, U.S., 110 S.Ct. 3157 (1990).

McCormick, C: *Hornbook on the Law of Evidence*, ed 3 (with 1987 Supp), West Publishing Co, St. Paul, MN, 1984.

Melton, G: Procedural reforms to protect child victim/witnesses in sex offense proceedings. In J Bulkley, ed: *Child Sexual Abuse and the Law*, American Bar Association, National Legal Resource Center for Child Advocacy and Protection, Washington, DC, 1981.

Melton, G, Bulkley, J, and Wulkan, D: Competency of children as witnesses. In J Bulkley, ed: *Child Sexual Abuse and the Law*, American Bar Association, National Legal Resource Center for Child Advocacy and Protection, Washington, DC, 1981.

Meriwether, M: Child abuse reporting laws: Time for a change, *Fam L Q* 20:141, 1986.

*Miranda v. Arizona*, 384 U.S. 436 (1966).

Mnookin, R: Child custody adjudication: Judicial functions in the face of indeterminacy, *Law Contemp Prob* 39:226, 1975.

Morey, R: The competency requirement for the child victim of sexual abuse: Must we abandon it? *U Miami L Rev* 40:245, 1985.

Myers, J: Hearsay statements by the child abuse victim, *Baylor L Rev* 38:775, 1986.

Myers, J: *Child Witness Law and Practice*, Wiley Law Publications, New York, 1987.

Nicholson, E, ed: *Sexual Abuse Allegations in Custody and Visitation Cases*, American Bar Association, National Legal Resource Center for Child Advocacy and Protection, Washington, DC, 1988.

Note: The testimony of child victims in sex abuse prosecutions: Two legislative innovations, *Harv L Rev* 98:806, 1985.

Oster: Custody proceeding: A study of vague and indefinite standards, *J Fam L* 5:21, 1965.

Pace, P: Custody and appellate courts, *Fam L* 3:27, 1973.

Pearson, J, and Ring, M: Judicial decision-making in contested custody cases, *J Fam L* 21:703, 1982.

*People v. Hagar*, 513 N.E.2d 628 (Ill. App. 1987).

Perkins, R, and Boyce, R: *Criminal Law*, ed 3, Foundation Press, New York, 1982.

Prosser, W, and Keeton, WP: *Hornbook on the Law of Torts*, ed 5 (with 1988 Supp), West Publishing Co, St. Paul, MN, 1984.

Radbill, S: Children in a world of violence: A history of child abuse. In R Helfer and R Kempe, eds: *The Battered Child*, The University of Chicago Press, Chicago, 1987.

Ringland, R: Child abuse evidence problems, *U Dayton L Rev* 12:27, 1986.

*Robinson v. Wical*, Civil No. 37607, Super. Ct. of Cal., San Luis Obispo, filed Sept 4, 1970.

Rosenberg, M, and Hunt, R: Child maltreatment. In N Reppucci et al, eds: *Children, Mental Health, and the Law*, Sage Publications, Beverly Hills, CA, 1984.

*Roth v. Reagen*, 422 N.W.2d 464 (Iowa 1988).

*S., In re*, 259 N.Y.S.2d 164 (Fam. Ct. 1965).

*Santosky v. Kramer*, 454 U.S. 745 (1982).

Smith, B, and Goretsky, S: The prosecution of child sexual abuse cases, *ABA Juv & Child Welf L Rptr* 11:78, 1992.

Sprague, M: Defining the risks after DeShaney. In M Sprague and R Horowitz, eds: *Liability in Child Welfare and Protection Work: Risk Management Strategies*, American Bar Association Center on Children and the Law, Washington, DC, 1991.

Sprague, M, and Horowitz, R, eds: *Liability in Child Welfare and Protection Work: Risk Management Strategies*, American Bar Association Center on Children and the Law, Washington, DC, 1991.

*State v. Best*, 232 N.W.2d 447 (S.D. 1975).

*State v. Jones*, 95 N.C. 588 (1886).

*Storch v. Silverman*, 231 Cal. Rptr. 27 (Cal. App. 1986).

Stromberg, C: *The Psychologist's Legal Handbook*, The Council for the National Register of Health Service Providers in Psychology, 1988.

Tjaden, P, and Thoennes, N: Legal intervention in child maltreatment cases, *Child Abuse Negl* 16:807, 1992.

Wadlington, W, Whitebread, C, and Davis, S: *Cases and Materials on Children in the Legal System*, Foundation Press, Mineola, NY, 1983.

Wald, M: State intervention on behalf of "neglected" children: A search for realistic standards, *Stan L Rev* 27:985, 1975.

Whitebread, L, and Slobogin, C: *Criminal Procedure*, ed 2 (with 1991 Supp), Foundation Press, New York, 1986.

# TESTIFYING

JAMES A. MONTELEONE, M.D.

Appearing in court to offer expert testimony is part of the process of working in child protection. The experience can be both unpleasant and confusing unless the physician is prepared for the environment of the courtroom and has researched his or her role in the situation. This chapter offers an overview of the legal environment, specific information concerning how to prepare for a courtroom experience, and the major elements of offering testimony.

## ◆ THE LEGAL ENVIRONMENT

Those working in medicine are accustomed to a team approach to achieve the well-being of the patient. The legal system presents an adversarial situation, where each lawyer attempts to prove the merits of his or her case and discredit the opposite view. The judge is most concerned with procedure and with ensuring that the case will be upheld under the scrutiny of courts of appeal. Finally, if there is a jury, it is largely peopled by individuals who are unschooled in technical medical matters and must see the case through the interpretative efforts of the witnesses and lawyers. It is into this arena that the physician is thrust and justice is sought.

Most child protection cases are heard in juvenile court. There is no jury, and decisions are made by the judge. Judges serving in these areas are generally sensitive to children's issues and base their decisions on achieving the best possible result for the child, yet protecting the rights of family and parents. However, it should be remembered that the trial consists of two sides presenting admissible evidence and that the better prepared, better qualified, most articulate lawyer frequently wins, whether justice is served or not.

The physician's role in this environment is quite different from the medical role normally assumed. Clinical judgments are questioned and dissected, frequently by nonphysicians, and time is just another tool, so delays and protracted proceedings are common, unlike the quick decisions needed in medicine. These aspects can make giving testimony a painful experience, although the vast majority of court appearances, even outside the juvenile court, are straightforward and professional.

It should be noted that only rarely is justice speedy. Delays and rescheduling of trial dates are normal, and it is advisable to be flexible in availability. Physicians are advised to work out an arrangement with the lawyer for whom they are testifying so that they can be on call and available and not sit and wait for hours to testify. If a long trip is required to appear in court, the physician should be certain that he or she is needed before undertaking the journey.

# ◆ PREPARATION FOR COURT APPEARANCE

Because lawyers are motivated to do the best for their clients and obtain a favorable result, the physician will be required to adhere to their instructions regarding appearance, demeanor, and delivery of information. This section will review these areas and offer guidance based on the typical courtroom experience.

## APPEARANCE

Because the physician is being called as an expert witness, it is best to appear professional and conservative. A coat and tie or conservative suit is preferred.

## DEMEANOR

The physician must keep his or her tone, attitude, and reactions consistent throughout testimony, whether direct questioning or cross-examination. It is best to be controlled, polite, slow to anger, humble, serious, and patient. A poor impression is left by those who are defensive, overbearing, tentative, smug, clever, amusing, or entertaining.

## DELIVERY OF INFORMATION

As in all public appearances, the physician must speak slowly and clearly, not mumbling words or sounding tentative. Credentials should be stated to establish the physician's qualifications as an expert witness. All questions should be answered honestly; if the physician does not know the answer, he or she should so state. Reluctance to answer any question may cast doubt on the physician's testimony in the minds of the judge and/or jury.

Witnesses tend to be at ease during direct questioning and then become tense on cross-examination. This change is manifest by shifts in posture and alterations in voice quality. The voice should be kept at an even tempo, and emphasis should be used in moderation to avoid giving the impression of being uncertain or anxious. Sitting quietly and in a relaxed manner is advised. This does not imply that the witness will not be nervous, but that the nervousness should be accepted and not allowed to hinder testimony.

Answers should be objective and impartial, avoiding a judgmental tone. The court will make judgments based on the testimony and presentation of material; however, if the physician feels strongly about a point, he or she should express this opinion. The role of the expert witness is to teach, and this attitude should be maintained during all questioning.

It is important to make eye contact with both the questioner and the judge or jury. The physician is there to provide information to them and should speak directly in doing this. During cross-examination, the lawyer may position himself or herself in such a way that eye contact with the jury is difficult. The physician may need to turn from the questioner to face the jury and reestablish eye contact.

The physician must listen carefully to the questions and be certain that all is understood before attempting to answer. Questions directed from the attorney for whose case the physician is testifying should be answered immediately; a delay in answering those from the opposing lawyer gives the attorney an opportunity to object if necessary. In all but one case, objections are to questions, not answers, and a witness should not be afraid of objections raised during questioning. The one exception is the objection that the witness's answer is unresponsive to the question, wherein the physician may be directed to respond more appropriately.

The terms used in testimony should be understandable to everyone present. Using highly technical or obscure terms to impress the judge or jury is inappropriate. If a technical term must be used, it should be explained without talking down to the audience, which could imply that they are unable to comprehend what is being said.

As stated earlier, the physician must not hesitate to state that he or she does not know the answer if that is the case. As an expert witness, the doctor must not go beyond the area of expertise; he or she may decline to answer or, if the physician feels able to present a reasonable answer, offer a qualified response, such as "My feeling on this is . . . . , but you should check with an expert in that field to be certain." If the physician is uncomfortable with answering any question, he or she should insist on the point of being not qualified to respond.

If a question is unclear or not understood, it is acceptable to ask that it be repeated. If the questioner points out something that should have been done and was not, it is best to admit that it was not done and avoid becoming defensive or apologize. Anger at being advised on a medical practice or procedure by someone outside of the medical field is unwise.

If the physician disagrees with authorities in the field, honestly stating this position is appropriate. However, he or she must be prepared to defend this position.

As a rule, only the information being asked for should be given; additional information should not be volunteered. Long, involved answers should be avoided, including narratives unless they are specifically required. The court and the lawyer will direct the physician when these detailed narratives are appropriate.

When the testimony is completed, the physician should wait to be excused by the court and should leave the courtroom unless requested to stay. No emotion, either positive or negative, should be shown. In addition, both before and after testimony, the physician should conduct himself or herself with circumspection because jurors, other witnesses, or investigators may be present and observing these actions.

## ◆ ELEMENTS OF GIVING TESTIMONY

It is essential that the physician read the case history and other materials carefully and thoroughly before the court appearance. Some lawyers expect that an expert witness will have total recall and be familiar with all elements of a case without looking at the record. Asking to see the chart during testimony to refresh memories and be certain of the facts in the case is acceptable and will enhance the chances for accurate presentation. However, the judge can forbid the witness to review the chart in court and the physician must be prepared to deal with this contingency.

The physician should review testimony with the lawyer for whom he or she is testifying before the actual court appearance. This is an opportunity to plan which questions will be asked by both sides and the physician can inquire as to why certain questions will be asked and why some will not be asked. In addition, the physician can suggest additional questions to strengthen the lawyer's case. However, in any case, the answers must be truly the physician's and not the lawyer's.

Whether or not this meeting took place can be the subject of questions by the cross-examiner. Frequently the witness is asked if he or she met with the lawyer before giving testimony, if the testimony was rehearsed, and if the answers were dictated by the lawyer. The most appropriate answer is, "Yes, we met. He [she] told me the questions that may be asked and instructed that I answer them honestly and in my own words."

The physician should review textbooks and key references to prepare to give testimony. More obscure references are generally not required; if asked to discuss an unfamiliar reference, it is appropriate to ask to see the reference being cited. It may be necessary to read the article while on the stand. The most critical points to be noted are the publication date and journal source. The material may be outdated, from a nonrefereed journal, or taken out of context and therefore not applicable. In choosing key references, the physician should be sure to choose those which are current and cite textbooks that are commonly accepted as reflecting contemporary practice.

If a deposition was taken previously, it should be reviewed in preparation for giving testimony. This will avoid the embarrassment of contradicting previous testimony without being able to offer a valid explanation of the difference. If views on a subject have changed over time, it is best to state this fact directly and not wait to have it presented in a negative light. A careful attorney will review all cases in which the physician may have testified and point out areas of seeming contradiction. The physician must be prepared to justify or clarify what has been stated previously.

In general an attorney does not ask questions to which he or she does not know the answer; the process is meant to bring information to light for the benefit of the jury or judge. Therefore it is best to avoid embellishing accomplishments or enhancing what appears in a deposition.

## PLOYS USED IN QUESTIONING AND HOW TO RESPOND

When a lawyer tries to put the witness at ease and induce a smile or laugh, the physician must be aware that smiling or laughing too long may give the impression that the situation is being taken too lightly. Maintaining a professional attitude is generally the best choice for a court appearance.

If the lawyer uses the title "Mr." rather than "Dr.," the physician should ignore the mistake. It may be a purposeful attempt to precipitate a negative reaction from the witness. Any mispronunciation of a technical term should also be ignored unless the witness is specifically asked to provide an accurate rendering. Correcting the lawyer may give the impression that the physician is pompous. If a correct pronunciation is given and the lawyer continues to mispronounce the term, this again should be overlooked rather than allowed to color the testimony. As stated previously, the physician should avoid technical terms if a more recognized and understood word is appropriate.

Conversations outside the courtroom should not involve the testimony being given. It is inappropriate to offer information beyond that given on the stand in any other situation.

Lawyers may try to rephrase testimony being given by the doctor, to enhance its presentation to the jury and/or judge. The physician must listen carefully to the edited version and make certain that it is an accurate rephrasing. Another ploy is to apply the answer to a different question. The physician must again evaluate each answer and make sure that it is what he or she really means.

In discussing a case involving multiple victims, the physician should be careful to focus on one victim at a time. If the lawyer switches back and forth from victim to victim, confusion may result in everyone's mind. If this ploy is attempted, it is best to ask to begin again and talk about each victim separately.

The lawyer may also ask several simple questions requiring a "yes" response and then insert one requiring a "no" response, hoping to catch the witness off-guard. This is called a "shotgun" approach. Each question should be listened to attentively and answered individually.

*An example of this technique is as follows:*

*While testifying in a child pornography case in which the expert testified to the ages of children in videos, these questions were asked:*

**Question:** Doctor, I am sure you have seen pictures of better quality than were present in that video. Is that correct?

**Answer:** Yes.

**Question:** Do different races and ethnic groups vary in the onset of puberty?

**Answer:** Yes.

**Question:** Are there differences between the sexes?

**Answer:** Yes.

**Question:** Is it true that pubertal changes will show as early as 8 years of age?

**Answer:** Yes.

**Question:** And as late as 16 years?

**Answer:** Yes.

**Question:** Even as late as 18 years?

**Answer:** Yes, but that is out of the range of normal.

**Question:** But possible?

**Answer:** Yes.

**Question:** It's possible that the children in the video could be 18 years old?

**Answer:** No. Though the videos were not of the best quality, there were a number of times where I could easily ascertain the development and age of the children. I feel confident the children were prepubertal and about 9 to 12 years of age.

Another multiple question ploy to beware of is the two-in-one question in which the response to the first part of the question differs from that to the second part. The witness tends to answer the second part of the question and leave the impression that it is appropriate for the entire question.

*This is an example:*

**Question:** Doctor, can gonorrhea be transmitted from objects, such as toilet seats and towels—you are aware of research which demonstrated that potential?

**Answer:** There are two parts to your question. Let me answer the second part first. Yes, there have been controlled studies in which a specimen carrying gonorrhea was placed on objects such as toilet seats and researchers were able to successfully transfer the organism to an agar plate over a number of hours. However, answering the first part of that question, no one has ever been able to demonstrate that gonorrhea is spread to humans in that manner. The literature clearly states that gonorrhea is sexually transmitted.

Regarding questions about references, if the physician is asked if he or she considers a particular reference or journal to be authoritative, or is asked to supply references considered authoritative, a correct response would be, "No reference is absolutely authoritative. No single source is the final word. Although previous reports play a role in making decisions, other important factors also play a part." If the physician declares that a particular reference is authoritative, he or she may be asked to agree with everything in that reference and even expected to justify all actions against that standard.

The questioner may try to imply or state that the physician's opinion is based on speculation or guesswork. The physician should not agree. Particular words to be wary of are *conjecture, supposition, theory,* and *assumption.* A recommended response is "No, my opinion is based on reasonable medical certainty."

The questioner may also try to minimize the findings being presented.

*For example, after testifying in a sexual abuse case and describing anal findings, the following cross-examination of one physician took place:*

**Question:** In your testimony you stated that you found a 2- to 3-millimeter tear of the anus. Is that correct?

**Answer:** Yes.

**Question:** How big is a millimeter?

**Answer:** One-tenth of a centimeter.

**Question:** And how big is a centimeter? Give it in terms we can relate to.

**Answer:** A centimeter is not quite a half an inch. The width of my little fingernail is 1 centimeter. (He held up his little finger to demonstrate.)

**Question:** Then we're talking about one-tenth of that, is that correct?

**Answer:** Yes.

**Question:** Here is a pen, Doctor. Would you show the jury on that piece of paper at the easel what 2 to 3 millimeters would be?

**Answer:** (The witness went to the board and drew two lines.) The space between those lines would be about 2 to 3 centimeters. The dimensions are relative . . .

**Question:** Never mind, Doctor, just answer the questions asked. The area you are speaking about is not much wider than the tip of the pen. I have had chapped lips with breaks larger than that.

At this point, the opposing attorney should have picked up on the witness' attempt to expand on the answer and, during reexamination, asked questions whose answers would put the injury in perspective.

In sexual abuse cases the legal proceedings frequently concentrate on physical findings. Yet the most important component in determining whether a child has been sexually abused is a credible disclosure. The physical findings should be put into perspective with statements during testimony such as, "The most important component in determining whether a child has been sexually abused is the disclosure. It must be remembered that the majority of children who have been sexually abused show no physical findings and many have no behavioral indicators. The physical findings and behavioral indicators can only support what the child says. If there are no witnesses, only two persons know what took place—the perpetrator and the victim. It comes down to whether or not you believe the child."

The opposing lawyer may try to set up a hypothetical situation and attempt to persuade the witness that it represents the case at hand when it, in fact, does not. The witness must be wary of questions starting with "What if . . ." and trying to make the witness believe that the lawyer knows something about the case that the witness does not. It is acceptable to ask if this is a hypothetical situation and answer within that context. The following is an exchange involving a hypothetical situation that was postulated during a case involving sexual abuse.

*The alleged perpetrator was the babysitter, and the individual who had interviewed the child was cross-examined as follows:*

**Question:** You stated that after you interviewed the child you felt that the child gave a credible statement and that, based on what the child said, you believed that she had been sexually abused by her babysitter. Is that correct?

**Answer:** Yes.

**Question:** What if I told you that the father and mother were in the process of a divorce? That the police had been called to the home by neighbors because of loud arguments between the mother and father. Would that change your conclusion?

**Answer:** I wasn't aware of that information. Is that true?

**Question:** Just answer the question. Would that change your conclusion?

**Answer:** No such information was in the chart when I interviewed her.

**Question:** Would that change your conclusion?

**Answer:** No. I still believe that the child was credible.

Although the witness stood by her original conclusion, that the child was credible, her reaction to the "what if" question left a different message.

*The situation would have been better handled, even if the hypothetical situation were true, by answering the question as follows:*

> "A divorce and custody situation could influence a child's disclosure. I was not aware of any such situation in this case, but had there been, I still feel the child gave a credible disclosure. I base that on the characteristics of a credible disclosure, which I discussed earlier."

Many questions cannot be properly answered with a *yes* or *no*, yet lawyers and the judge may demand they be answered that simply. A possible response might be the following:

> "I cannot answer that question with a yes or no. All things are not black and white; there are grays. May I expand on that answer?"

If the witness is not allowed to expand on the answer given, the lawyer for whom he or she is testifying should return to the question during redirect questioning and expose the entire answer.

In rebutting an answer from another expert, it is best to respond professionally and without rancor. An appropriate response might be, "Doctor _____ has a fine reputation. We do not agree on all issues."

Finally, the physician is trained to evaluate a patient and assess the merits of differential diagnoses as well as the primary diagnosis. In the witness chair the presentation of a differential diagnosis can imply doubt. If the physician is sure of the diagnosis offered and feels that there are no appropriate differential diagnoses, this should be stated clearly and defended upon cross-examination.

## QUESTIONS DESIGNED TO PUT THE WITNESS ON THE DEFENSIVE

Although there are difficult questions, as outlined above, not every question is a maneuver to entrap the witness. If the physician approaches testifying by regarding each question as a potential trap, the jury and judge may derive the impression that the witness is guarded and tentative, which can be detrimental to the case for which he is testifying.

There are sensitive issues that the physician may be called upon to discuss in testimony. Among them are the awarding of a fee for participation in the case, the charge of child advocacy, and the demand for documentation. These will be addressed with specific guidelines on how to handle them.

### FEE

The physician should not be embarrassed to admit when he or she is being paid for the time spent on the case. If the physician is asked if he or she is being paid to **testify** and how much, a proper response would be, "I am being paid **for the time I spend** on the case. Testifying is just one part of that time." In regard to the amount, giving the hourly fee that has been set is appropriate. Asking for compensation for the time spent on a case is perfectly acceptable.

### CHILD ADVOCACY

The physician, pediatrician, or family practitioner most often appears to protect the child, the victim in a case. Therefore usually the legal testimony offered will be to help the prosecution. However, the guiding principle should be to facilitate justice; this can be accomplished on the defendant's side in the case of misdiagnoses or conditions mistaken for abuse, as noted throughout this text. There should be no restriction put on working for the prosecution or defendant with regards to the work of testifying and offering expert review.

## DOCUMENTATION

In caring for any patient it is necessary to make the effort to document what has been done, clearly, in the patient's chart. While following a standard protocol is helpful, it is no guarantee that everything was accomplished in order or that all the elements of the protocol applied in the case under review. In testimony, if the physician states that he or she followed the standard protocol, the opposing attorney may attempt to present the physician as sloppy or careless by pointing out areas where there are deviations from that protocol. Another tactic is to give the jury or judge the impression that if something was not documented, it was not done. The jury, as less knowledgeable individuals, may not understand explanations offered by the physician and derive an unfavorable impression from this line of questioning. The lawyer may even attempt to portray an obscure incident or finding as a grave oversight, when the physician sees it as trivial and seemingly unworthy of mention.

It is important to remember to answer all questions calmly and with control. It is possible to explain that in standard procedure in medicine you document the positive and significant negative findings, but not necessarily the unimportant negative findings. If something is not documented, this does not necessarily mean that it was not done. An important observation to make to the jury is that if all thoughts, events, and negative findings were documented, the chart would be cumbersome and charting would require more time than would have been spent on caring for the patient.

## ◆ BIBLIOGRAPHY

Danner, D: Do's and don'ts for experts. In NT Shayne, Chairman: *Medical Evidence*, Practising Law Institute, 1980, pp. 347-351.

Horsley, JE, and Carlova, J: *Testifying in Court*, Medical Economics Books, Oradell, NJ, 1988.

# PREVENTION OF CHILD ABUSE

PEGGY S. PEARL, ED.D.

Child abuse prevention depends on neither a program nor a system of services, but must be founded on a society valuing its children. Within such a context the society will be willing to fund preventive services, programs, and policies rather than merely "attempting" to solve the crises caused by the lack of interest in children's welfare. **Table 28-1** lists some of the indicators that are apparent when a nation makes its children a high priority.

| Table 28-1. Indicators of a Nation with Children as a High Priority |
| --- |

Outraged citizens are motivated to action when they hear that children are being maltreated.

Adequate and affordable housing is available for all families.

Recreation and esteem-building activities are available to all children and families.

Mental health, medical, and dental care are accessible to all families.

Social service delivery systems are accessed by families in need of assistance before maltreatment occurs rather than systems that treat after abuse occurs or punish for maltreating.

Universal instruction in the care and guidance of children is found in the curriculum of all public and private schools (pre-kindergarten to grade 12 as well as adult continuing education).

Instruction in interpersonal communications, nonviolent conflict resolution, and resource management is provided for all students (pre-kindergarten to grade 12 as well as adult continuing education).

Job training and education programs provide all workers with access to jobs as an avenue out of poverty.

Workplace policies support families (i.e., parental leave; job sharing; flextime; employee assistance programs; dependent care assistance programs; mental health, medical, and dental insurance; career ladders; and employee wellness programs).

Nonviolent societal role models are highly visible.

All parents have access to self-help and support groups.

Adequate funding exists for research to build the database regarding environments that facilitate optimal development of individuals throughout the life span.

Legal systems, both criminal and civil, are properly funded, staffed, and trained to promptly and fairly resolve maltreatment cases.

Culturally and ethnically sensitive home-based parent education programs are available to all new parents.

Adequate salaries are provided for professionals who work in all child-related professions to attract and retain the best and the brightest in jobs caring for the nation's priority—children and their families.

Each individual is equally valued without regard for sex, race, ethnic background, ability, disability, or economic status.

## ◆PROGRAMS INVOLVING GOVERNMENT, THE JUDICIAL SYSTEM, AND THE PRIVATE SECTOR

The prevention of child abuse involves providing all parents with the necessary resources for successful parenting. The basic national commitment to children and the prevention of their maltreatment begins when the nation's leaders take the initiative to support families. However, society cannot assume that child abuse prevention is a function of government alone (Daro, 1988b; U. S. Advisory, 1990). The leaders must represent both the public and the private sectors (Kempe & Kempe, 1978; U. S. Advisory, 1990; Recommendations, 1991). The private sector must support families through interventions and prevention programs offered in the workplace as well as encourage and fund community-wide efforts on behalf of children. Workplace policies supportive of families include job sharing, flextime, mental health, medical, and dental insurance, parental leave, employee assistance programs, and dependent care assistance programs (Cohn, 1987). Recognizing the correlation between unemployment and child abuse and neglect, job training and full employment are important segments of a societal commitment to children (Daro, 1988b).

Comprehensive child abuse prevention includes action taken within the judicial system. The legal system—criminal, civil, and juvenile courts—must support laws and procedures both to ensure the protection of children and to support families. Judicial procedures should be sensitive to the needs of children and families. Additionally, there must be adequate numbers of well-trained judges, lawyers, and court support staff, as well as manageable caseloads, to address the complex and demanding nature of child abuse and neglect litigation. The legal system must be sensitive to the needs of abuse victims to prevent additional maltreatment of these vulnerable individuals within the system, as well as to protect children from continuing in abusive, dysfunctional families (U. S. Advisory, 1990; Recommendations, 1991). To continually monitor the effectiveness of the legal and protective service systems, each community should have active citizen advocacy groups (Martin, 1976; Donnelly, 1991; Recommendations, 1991). These groups continually work to ensure that the policies of the private and public sectors offer the most appropriate support for families and children.

## ◆PROGRAMS AND SERVICES NEEDED BY FAMILIES

Preventative services must be delivered by a holistic system of competent professionals who are highly trained in different aspects of child maltreatment (Oats & Cohn, 1997, Marshall, et al., 1997, Recommendations, 1991, and US Advisory Committee, 1993). Through systematic research of child maltreatment including primary, secondary and tertiary prevention, a multi-disciplinary knowledge base will be researched, field tested and communicated to all who work in the field. Adequate salaries must be provided for professionals who work in all child-related professions to attract and retain the best and brightest in jobs caring for the nation's priority–children and families. The current high turnover in human services professionals must be eliminated in a comprehensive, community based family support system staffed by individuals who can develop consistent, dependable long-term relationships with clients/patients (US Advisory Board on Child Abuse and Neglect, 1990).

To prevent child maltreatment, it is necessary that a wide range of training, services, resources, and policies be available to parents. These preventive strategies are commonly classified as *primary, secondary,* or *tertiary:*

*Primary prevention:* provides training, resources, and policies to _all_ parents to enhance their parenting and keep abuse from occurring. Examples include health care, adequate child care, supportive workplace policies, and life skills training for children.

*Secondary prevention:* provides training, resources, and policies to targeted high-risk populations to enhance their parenting skills, including training and services to victims to keep abuse from occurring in the next generation. Secondary prevention includes self-help groups for parents who consider themselves at risk for maltreating their children, home visitor programs for new parents, and parent education programs for adolescent parents.

*Tertiary prevention:* provides training, resources, and policies to enhance parenting to keep abuse from recurring once it has been identified. Among the programs included are respite day care for parents, treatment for abused and neglected children, crisis intervention services, counseling, and stress management training.

Within our society, basic prevention programs should be available to all parents before any maltreatment begins (Martin, 1976). All parents require access to parenting information, especially when they have their first children. Perinatal coaching, home visitor, Parents as Teachers, and parent aide programs have proven effective for parents with young children. Additionally, all parents must have access to health care both for themselves and for their children. All schoolchildren require life skills education, and all parents need stress management training and access to positive support services to help them cope with the stress of parenting. In our highly mobile society, many families lack the positive support of family and friends and, consequently, this support must be supplied by other sources, for example, the church, social organizations, or mental health agencies (Taylor & Beauchamp, 1988; Olds & Henderson, 1989; U. S. Advisory, 1990). Accessible and affordable child care must be available to all working parents, but especially to single parents and the "working poor" (Daro, 1988b). Treatment programs should be added within the penal systems for individuals of all ages—especially adolescent offenders—to prevent the abuse of children and women after incarceration. Additionally, all programs must be respectful of cultural issues in order to be effective.

In both private and public schools, children need instruction regarding positive ways to interact with others as much as they need instruction in math, English, and science. Life skills education should be integrated into the curriculum beginning with kindergarten and continuing into adult education. Life skills education includes nonviolent conflict resolution, stress management skills, resource management, effective decision making, and effective interpersonal communication, as well as information regarding child development and guidance (Martin, 1976; Kempe & Kempe, 1978; Daro, 1988a; Donnelly, 1991). Additionally, the basics of substance abuse prevention education currently advocated must be a component of education for parenting or life skills. Schools should provide the role model of positive discipline and not use corporal punishment.

Every community must make the accessibility of parent education classes part of a comprehensive adult education program. Effective classes will be respectful of cultural diversity. Topics suggested for these parent education classes include principles of child development, positive child guidance, and basics in child care, such as child nutrition and safety. One vital area that should be addressed with parents of children at any age is techniques to improve the parent-child interaction. Learning to play with and enjoy their children enhances both this interaction and the parents' pleasure in their parental role (Daro, 1988b & Pearl, In press).

Neighborhoods and communities should be "family friendly" contributing to the resilience of each individual—parent or child—in the community. This means opportunities for each citizen to be an integrated, active participant. Efforts should be made by each member in the community to engage or involve everyone else. The resilience in each individual is improved by the opportunity to both give and take in a caring atmosphere. That is to say, each individual needs the opportunity to help as well as seek help from others. Effective prevention programs must focus on community participation while strengthening community resources and responsibilities (Then, Thiessen, & Heinsohn-Krug, 1995).

Corporal punishment can easily become abuse when administered by parents who are angry and under stress. Therefore instruction in the positive methods of child guidance is required. Additionally, parents need to know constructive methods of coping with stress. Self-help groups such as Parents Anonymous (PA) give parents alternatives to abusing their children, emotionally or physically, and provide positive support networks when stress occurs. PA uses the Alcoholics Anonymous (AA) model of self-help, which has proven successful. Both primary and tertiary support groups should be developed to prevent and combat abuse.

To enhance parenting skills and competence as well as prevent child abuse, new parents benefit from various instruction and support services. The specific content and structure of these programs will vary, as well as the sponsoring agency or institution; however, *the goals of programs for new parents should include the following:*

1. Increasing the parent's knowledge of child development and the demands involved in parenting

2. Enhancing the parent's skill in coping with the stresses of infant and child care

3. Enhancing parent-child bonding, emotional ties, and communication skills

4. Increasing the parent's skill in coping with the stress of caring for children with special needs

5. Increasing the parent's knowledge about home and child management

6. Reducing the burden of child care

7. Increasing access to social and health services for all family members (Daro, 1988b)

Parent education offered as tertiary prevention for various types of maltreatment differs in informational need from primary or secondary programs and responds to separate service delivery systems. All programs should be culturally sensitive and targeted to the appropriate developmental level of the parents. Group parent education that emphasizes impulse control and alternative methods of discipline is particularly successful with physically abusive parents, whereas one-on-one, home-based services founded on individual counseling and problem-solving techniques are more effective with neglectful parents. Neglectful parents need instruction in practical child care tasks, for example, diapering and feeding an infant or distracting and communicating with a 2-year-old. Programs successful in preventing emotional abuse include group-based services that define nonphysical methods of discipline; emphasize the need for consistency in determining and implementing rules; and offer parents ways of demonstrating affection toward their children (Golub et al., 1987; Daro, 1988a).

## ◆ROLE OF THE MEDIA

The media must play a key role in the prevention of child abuse. As a major force in shaping public opinion, the media can offer responsible programming and reporting to de-emphasize the current societal acceptance of violence. Additionally, through judicial programming, the media can reverse the current trend toward a desensitization of individuals to the horrors of violence. As the acceptance and glamorization of violence are removed, a new message can be sent—that violence in all forms is inappropriate. The media can depict nonviolent methods of conflict resolution. The media has been involved in and should continue to play a role in educating the public as to the magnitude of the consequences of violence in the lives of families and possible alternatives. The media may also advocate policies beneficial to children and families. One important step involves portraying parenting as the important and valued job in our society it is and thereby increasing parental esteem and helping prevent child abuse.

# ◆PROGRAMS TO PREVENT NEGLECT AND SEXUAL ABUSE

Although different in form, child maltreatment practices share common causes and therefore the societal approaches to prevention impact most types of maltreatment. However, specific mention should be made about prevention programs for neglect and sexual abuse, since the causes of these types of maltreatment differ slightly from those of physical and emotional abuse.

## PREVENTION OF NEGLECT

To prevent child neglect, parents require the basic resources to provide proper care for their children. At some income levels parents cannot provide the necessary food, shelter, clothing, or mental health, medical, and dental care for their children (Helfer, 1987; U. S. Advisory, 1990; Recommendations, 1991). At this poverty level of existence, parents are also experiencing stress and are usually without adequate support systems. Currently in our society many individuals are employed full-time at jobs that do not pay enough to provide the basic needs for the family. Many more parents lack the job skills necessary for entry-level jobs; even if they had these skills, many entry-level jobs fail to provide medical and dental insurance. At the same time, national and state governments provide fewer mental health, medical, and dental services for citizens. The consequences of these two trends is that growing numbers of children are without adequate health care services (Daro, 1988b).

When society makes adequate child care a national priority, it ensures, through various public and private sector means, that all parents have access to the basic resources to care for their families. To care for our nation's children, all parents must have access to decent and affordable housing; adequate mental health, medical, and dental care; nutritious food; and developmentally appropriate child care services (Daro, 1988b; Olds & Henderson, 1989; Fink & McCloskey, 1990; U. S. Advisory, 1990; Recommendations, 1991). The cycle of poverty that results in the disintegration of families and an atmosphere of chronic violence must be interrupted with culturally sensitive programs that work, addressing housing, jobs, substance abuse treatment, family support, and so on (Donnelly, 1991).

To prevent neglect, parents must also function at optimal levels so they can focus on their children's needs. Many parents are impaired in their ability to parent because of substance abuse or psychopathologic disorders. To prevent child maltreatment these adults and adolescents must have access to culturally sensitive, developmentally appropriate substance abuse prevention and treatment programs and mental health services. These services must be available to all parents either free, at fees based on ability to pay, along sliding scales, or under provisions of employee insurance or employee assistance programs (Daro, 1988b; U. S. Advisory, 1990).

## PREVENTION OF SEXUAL ABUSE

In the last decade many programs to prevent sexual abuse were developed and widely implemented. Generally these sexual abuse prevention programs teach children how to protect themselves from abuse. Researchers and clinicians caution that the major responsibility for prevention of sexual abuse cannot be placed on the victims or potential victims because they are children. Sexual abuse prevention programs must focus on the perpetrator (Swift, 1979). The National Committee for the Prevention of Child Abuse developed a comprehensive strategy for preventing adults from becoming child sexual abusers.

*This prevention strategy includes the following:*

1. Education for adolescents and young children that provides all adolescents with quality sex education, including healthy sexuality, during the preteen and teenage years to enhance their knowledge of what is normal and abnormal.

2. Training for professionals and volunteers who work with children that teaches these individuals how to identify and help children who are being abused, how

to teach children to protect themselves from abuse, and how to detect those who may be potential molesters.

3. Education for parents that provides all new parents with quality education and support to enhance early attachment and bonding when their first babies are born. This should include information about appropriate and inappropriate touch and what to do about it. Parents need to know how to detect and handle in their own children symptoms that may indicate sexual abuse has occurred.

4. Institutional changes that ensure that all child-serving institutions and programs (e.g., schools, boys clubs, Girl Scouts, day care, etc.) train children in self-awareness and self-protection. Guidelines and regulations must be in place to screen, train, and monitor all volunteers and staff.

5. Media messages that create an environment in which the prevention programs and concepts just outlined will be effective by communicating two messages.

   *First, for adolescents and adults, messages that say:*
   Child sexual abuse is a crime.
   Help is available.
   Abuse is a chronic problem unless you get help.
   Children get hurt when you sexually abuse them.
   Children cannot consent to this kind of behavior.
   *Second, messages to children, including:*
   It's okay to say no.
   It's not your fault.
   Reach out for help if this begins to happen to you.
   Help is available for you (Cohn, 1986).

   The comprehensive child sexual abuse prevention strategy just outlined, like all prevention programs, strengthens individuals and families by enhancing parenting skills.

Since many sexual abuse perpetrators are former victims who commit their first offense during adolescence, it is essential that all victims receive treatment. In addition, all offenders must have treatment before being released to offend again. In the current era of increased criminalization of sexual maltreatment, all segments of the penal system must have mandatory treatment programs for individuals eligible for parole. Perpetrators who refuse to participate in a meaningful way in prison treatment programs should be denied their right to return to full community participation.

## ♦SUMMARY

All parents should have available to them the resources, education, and services needed to parent effectively. A comprehensive multidisciplinary approach to prevention is needed. No specific program or plan is most effective with all parents. A mix of family support programs is needed in both the private and public sectors to enhance parenting. Once abuse has occurred, various resources, educational programs, and services are needed to prevent additional abuse. Each family needs a culturally sensitive and developmentally appropriate individualized approach, with some requiring intense and ongoing services to prevent maltreatment (Daro & Gelles, 1992). Research has shown specific gains in the following areas after parental participation in secondary and tertiary prevention programs: improved mother-infant bonding and maternal capacity to respond to the child's emotional needs; demonstrated ability to care for the child's physical and developmental needs; fewer subsequent pregnancies; more consistent use of health care services and job training opportunities; and decreased reliance on the public welfare system, higher school completion rates, and higher employment rates (Daro, 1988b; Donnelly, 1991).

Prevention requires society's commitment to the care and total well-being of children. This commitment begins with individual attitudes that equally value all individuals. Additionally, the commitment must be backed by both the public and the private sectors and must extend beyond mere rhetoric to include allocating resources as well as changing existing attitudes, policies and statutes that do not conform to this commitment. Society must recognize the importance of parenting and then commit resources to assist all parents in performing this challenging and rewarding job.

## ◆ BIBLIOGRAPHY

Cohn, AH: Preventing adults from becoming sexual molesters, *Child Abuse Negl* 10(4):559-562, 1986.

Cohn, AH: Our national priorities for prevention. In RE Helfer and RS Kempe, eds: *The Battered Child*, University of Chicago Press, Chicago, 1987.

Conte, JR, Rosen, CR, and Saperstein, L: An analysis of programs to prevent the sexual victimization of children (paper presented at the Fifth International Congress on Child Abuse and Neglect), Montreal, 1984.

Daro, D: *Confronting Child Abuse: Research for Effective Program Design*, Free Press, New York, 1988a.

Daro, D: Intervening with new parents: An effective way to prevent child abuse (working paper 839), National Committee for the Prevention of Child Abuse, Chicago, 1988b.

Daro, D: Child sexual abuse prevention: Separating fact from fiction, *Child Abuse Negl* 15(1/2):1-4, 1991.

Daro, D, and Gelles, RJ: Public attitudes and behaviors with respect to child abuse prevention, *J Interpersonal Violence* 7(4):517-531, 1992.

Donnelly, AC: What we have learned about prevention: What we should do about it, *Child Abuse Negl* 15(1)99-106, 1991.

Dubowitz, H: Pediatrician's role in preventing child maltreatment, *Pediatric Clinics of North America* 37:989-1002, 1990.

Fink, A, and McCloskey, L: Moving child abuse and neglect prevention programs forward: Improving program evaluation, *Child Abuse Negl* 14(2):187-206, 1990.

Golub, JS, Espinosa, M, Damon, L, and Card, J: A videotape parent education program for abusive parents, *Child Abuse Negl* 11(1):255-265, 1987.

Helfer, RE: The developmental basis of child abuse and neglect: An epidemiological approach. In RE Helfer and RS Kempe, eds: *The Battered Child*, University of Chicago Press, Chicago, 1987.

Kempe, CH, and Kempe, RS: *Child Abuse*, Harvard Press, Cambridge, MA, 1978.

Marshall, WN, Jr. and Locke, C: Statewide survey of physician attitudes to controversies about child abuse, *Child Abuse Negl* 21(2):171-179, 1997.

Martin, HP: Summing up and moving on. In HP Martin, ed: *The Abused Child: A Multidisciplinary Approach to Developmental Issues and Treatment*, Ballinger Publishing Co, Cambridge, MA, 1976.

Mullen, PE, Martin, JC, Anderson, Romans, SE, and Herbison, GP: The long-term impact of physical, emotional, and sexual abuse of children: A community study, *Child Abuse Negl* 20(1):7-21, 1996.

Olds, DL, and Henderson, CR, Jr: The prevention of maltreatment. In D Cicchetti and V Carlson, eds: *Child Maltreatment: Theory and Research on the Causes and Consequences of Child Abuse and Neglect*, Cambridge University Press, Cambridge, England, 1989.

Pearl, PS: Why some parent education programs for parents of gifted children succeed and others do not? *Early Child Development and Care,* vol 130:41-48, 1997.

Recommendations for the 21st century, *Child Abuse Negl* 15(1):39-50, 1991.

Runtz, MG, and Schallow, JR: Social support and coping strategies as mediators of adult adjustment following childhood maltreatment, *Child Abuse Negl* 21(2):211-226, 1997.

Swift, C: The prevention of sexual abuse: Focus on the perpetrator, *J Clin Child Psychol* 133-136, 1979.

Taylor, DK, and Beauchamp, C: Hospital-based primary prevention strategy in child abuse: A multi-level needs assessment, *Child Abuse Negl* 12(3):343-354, 1988.

Thyen, U, Thiessen, R, & Heinsohn-Krug, M: Secondary prevention—serving families at risk, *Child Abuse Negl* 19(11):1337-1347, 1995.

Trundell, B, and Whatley, MH: School sexual abuse prevention: Unintended consequences and dilemmas, *Child Abuse Negl* 12(1):103-113, 1988.

US Advisory Board on Child Abuse and Neglect: *Child Abuse and Neglect: Critical First Steps in Response to a National Emergency,* Health and Human Services, Washington, DC, 1990.

Zellman, GL: The impact of case characteristics on child abuse reporting decisions, *Child Abuse Negl* 16:57-74, 1992.

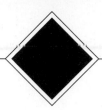

# INDEX

## A

AA; *see* Alcoholics Anonymous

Abandonment
    emotional, 344, 346
    neglect and, 339-356
    physical, 344
    temporary, 345
    termination of parental rights and, 579

Abandonment infanticide, 344

Abdomen, blunt trauma to, 69-70, 71

Abdominal injuries, 48-54

Abdominal radiographs, 74

Abnormal responses, psychological abuse and, 386-387

Abortion, therapeutic, 17

Abrasions, 538
    healing of, 169

Abrogation of privileged communication, reporting statutes
        and, 567-568, 569

Absolute immunity, legal issues and, 572, 574

Abstat, 443

Abuse
    allegations of, child custody disputes and, 193, 589-598
    child; *see* Child maltreatment
    Child Fatality Review Panel Data Report and, 498-499
    of discretion, legal issues and, 591
    elder, 398
    emotional; *see* Emotional abuse
    fetal; *see* Fetal abuse
    intrauterine; *see* Fetal abuse
    multiple personality disorder and, 278
    multiple-perpetrator, 378
    multiple-victim, 378
    neonatal, 36
    physical; *see* Physical abuse
    psychological; *see* Psychological abuse
    ritualistic, 138-140, 234-235, 378-379
    sexual; *see* Sexual abuse
    sibling, 3, 399, 401
    spouse, 17, 398, 410
    substance; *see* Substance abuse
    traumatizing, sexual abuse and, 406-407

Abused-to-abuser cycle, 409; *see also* Cycle of abuse

Abuse-related syndromes, child custody disputes and, 597

Abusive acts, sexual abuse and, 130

Abusive burns; *see* Burns, abusive

Acceleration-deceleration forces, shaken infant syndrome
        and, 13, 36, 43-44, 95, 99, 100, 493, 543

*Accident Facts*, 106

Accidental burns and conditions that are not abuse, 113-116

Accidental deaths, 87, 88

Accidental drownings, 16

Accidental injuries versus intentional injuries, 6-7, 494, 541

Accidents, 446, 533
    motor vehicle, 10, 436, 449

Acetylsalicylic acid, poisoning and, 547

Acid phosphatase, sexual abuse and, 168

Acidemia, methylmalonic, 5

Acquired immunodeficiency syndrome (AIDS), 303, 311

Acromial apophysis, 43

Actions, post-conviction, in criminal court, 589

Active inducer in Munchausen Syndrome by Proxy, 333

Active neglect, 549

Acute stress disorder, 286-287

Acyclovir in treatment of herpes simplex, 305, 309

ADA; *see* American Dental Association

ADA/Colgate Health Survey, 65

Addict
    doctor, in Munchausen Syndrome by Proxy, 333-334
    drug; *see* Substance abuse

ADHD; *see* Attention-deficit hyperactivity disorder

Adhesions, labial, in sexual abuse, 163

Adjudicatory hearing
    in juvenile court, 577-578
    legal issues and, 575, 577, 579

Admissions by parties, child custody disputes and, 594

Adolescent perpetrators, 405

Adolescent pregnancy, sexual abuse and, 132-133

Adolescents
    behavioral indicators of sexual abuse in, 189-190
    developmental stages of children related to art and, 252
    lying and, 226
    physical development of brain and, 214
    stress-related behaviors in, 188, 189

anterior chamber injury, 83

birth process causing, 80

cardiopulmonary resuscitation causing, 80

injury to cortical pathways, 83

lens dislocation, 83

lens subluxation, 83

neglect and, 83-84

nonabusive, 80-81

periorbital edema, 80-81

presenting signs of, 79

retinal hemorrhage, 80

ruptured vascular malformations causing, 80

sexual abuse and, 79, 83

shaken baby syndrome and, 81-82

subconjunctival hemorrhage, 80-81

team approach to, 84

vitreous hemorrhage, 82

Ophthalmologist in assessment of child maltreatment, 84

Opiates

endogenous, 293

poisoning and, 318

Oppositional disorder, 225, 409

Optic atrophy, 83

Optic nerve sheath hemorrhage, 544

Oral injuries, 59-66

burns and, 62

dental implications of child neglect, 63-64

dentistry in prevention of child maltreatment, 64-65

to gingiva, 61

to hard and soft palate, 62

in infants, 59-60

to labial frenula, 61-62

to lingual frenula, 61-62

to lips, 62

to oral soft tissues, 61-62

to teeth, 60-61

to tongue, 62

Organ transplantation issues, 553-554

Orthodontic appliances, damage to lips from, during trauma, 62

Osmolar gap in assessment of poisoning, 320

Osteogenesis imperfecta, 5, 54, 551

Osteogenic cells, dating skeletal injury and, 34

Osteomyelitis, 55

Osteopenia, 55

Osteopetrosis, 55

Out-of-body phenomenon, multiple personality disorder and, 272

Out-of-Home Investigations (OHI) Unit, 453, 461

Ovens, microwave, burns from liquids heated in, 123

Overlying, 422, 547

Overpressuring child, 372, 381-382

Overreporting of neglect, 341

Oxazepam in treatment of post-traumatic stress disorder, 294

# P

PA; *see* Parents Anonymous

PA x-ray film; *see* Posteroanterior x-ray film

Pain

congenital insensitivity to, 5, 54-55

post-traumatic, 399

Palatal contusions, 62

Palm of hand, burns of, 6, 113, 121

Pancreas, injuries to, 50-51

Pancreatic pseudocyst, 50

Pancreatitis, 50, 51, 74, 546, 550

P.A.N.D.A. Coalition; *see* Prevent Abuse and Neglect through Dental Awareness Coalition

Papanicolaou stain, herpes simplex and, 309

Papilledema, acute, 83

Parallel linear marks, 538

Parallel play, 227

Paramours, child abuse and, 187, 206, 423, 435, 439, 440, 443, 544

Paregoric, poisoning and, 317

*Parens patriae*, legal issues and, 559-560, 579, 590

Parent

abusive, responses of, to infant, 388

assessment of, 396

attorney for, in juvenile court, 576-577

characteristics of, in Munchausen Syndrome by Proxy, 331

in juvenile court, 576

maltreated as children, 387-388

maltreating, psychiatric characteristics of, 290-291

potentially abusive, red flag characteristics of, 515

Parent advocacy groups, 20

Parent Bonding Instrument, 285-286

Parental behaviors

corrupting, 372, 379-380

ignoring, 372, 373-375

indicating potential for psychological abuse, 389

isolating, 372, 376-377

overpressuring, 372, 381-382

rejecting, 372, 375-376

ritualistic abuse, 378-379

terrorizing, 372, 377-378

verbally assaulting, 372, 380-381

Parental custody refusal, neglect and, 345

Parental indicators, psychological abuse and, 387-389

Parental neglect, 236

Parental reasoning, cognitive-developmental stages of, 383-384

Parental rights, termination of, legal issues and, 579

Parent/caregiver interview outline, in sexual abuse, 193-196

Parent-child interaction

assessment of, 230, 387

failure to thrive and, 348

psychological abuse and, 388-389, 396

Parents Anonymous (PA), 614

Partial thromboplastin time (PTT), 74

Parties, admissions by, child custody disputes and, 594

Parulis, 63

Passive neglect, 549

Passive voice, questions in, legal issues and, 224

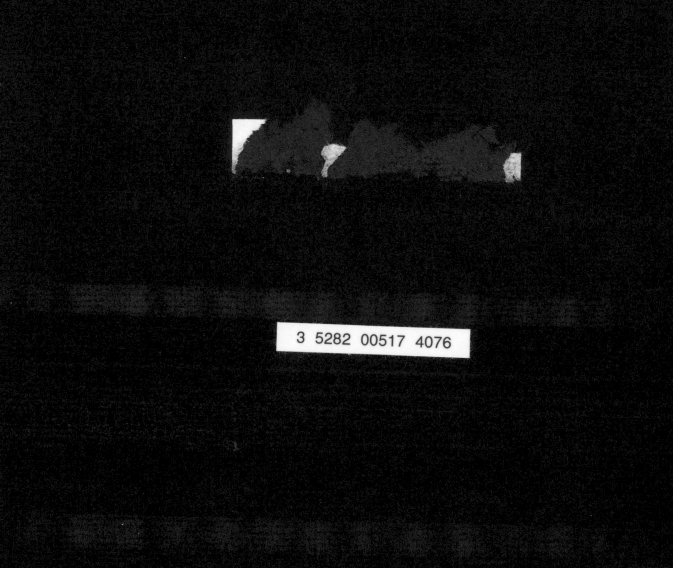